T0344440

Drug Allergy Testing

Drug Allergy Testing

DAVID A. KHAN, MD
Professor of Internal Medicine
University of Texas Southwestern Medical Center
Dallas, Texas

ALEENA BANERJI, MD
Associate Professor
Massachusetts General Hospital
Boston, Massachusetts

ELSEVIER

ELSEVIER

3251 Riverport Lane
St. Louis, Missouri 63043

Content Strategist: Kayla Wolfe
Content Development Manager: Taylor Ball
Content Development Specialist: Casey Potter
Publishing Services Manager: Deepthi Unni
Project Manager: Janish Ashwin Paul
Designer: Renee Deunow

Printed in United States of America

Last digit is the print number: 9 8 7 6 5 4 3 2 1

Working together
to grow libraries in
developing countries

www.elsevier.com • www.bookaid.org

List of Contributors

Aleena Banerji, MD
Associate Professor
Massachusetts General Hospital
Boston, MA, United States

Esther Barrionuevo, MD, PhD
Allergy Unit, IBIMA-Regional University Hospital of
  Malaga-UMA
Malaga, Spain

Jonathan A. Bernstein, MD
Professor of Clinical Medicine
Department of Internal Medicine
Division of Immunology/Allergy Section
Editor-in-Chief Journal of Asthma
University of Cincinnati College of Medicine
Cincinnati, OH, United States

Miguel Blanca, MD, PhD
Scientific Consultant
Allergy Service, Hospital Infanta Leonor,
Madrid, Spain

Natalia Blanca-Lopez, MD, PhD
Staff Member, Allergy Service, Hospital
Infanta Leonor, Madrid, Spain

Karen H. Blatman, MD
Division of Rheumatology, Immunology and Allergy
Department of Medicine
Brigham and Women's Hospital
Harvard Medical School
Boston, MA, United States

Kimberly G. Blumenthal, MD
Division of Rheumatology, Allergy, and Immunology,
  Department of Medicine, Massachusetts General
  Hospital, Boston, Massachusetts
Medical Practice Evaluation Center, Department of
  Medicine, Massachusetts General Hospital, Boston,
  Massachusetts Harvard Medical School, Boston,
  Massachusetts
Edward P. Lawrence Center for Quality and Safety,
  Massachusetts General Hospital, Boston,
  Massachusetts

Knut Brockow, MD
Department of Dermatology and Allergy Biederstein,
  Technische Universität München
Munich, Germany

Maria G. Canto, MD, PhD
Head of the Service, Allergy Service,
Hospital Infanta Leonor, Madrid, Spain

Mariana Castells, MD, PhD
Director, Drug hypersensitivity and Desensitization
  Center
Director Mastocytosis Center
Brigham and Women's Hospital
Professor in Medicine
Harvard Medical School
Boston, MA, United States

Melanie C. Dispenza, MD, PhD
Associate Professor of Medicine
Division of Allergy-Immunology
Northwestern University
Feinberg School of Medicine
Chicago, IL, United States

Anne M. Ditto, MD
Department of Allergy and Immunology
Northwestern University
Chicago, IL, United States

Inmaculada Doña, MD, PhD
Allergy Unit, IBIMA-Regional University Hospital of
  Malaga-UMA
Malaga, Spain

Joshua M. Dorn, MD
Division of Allergic Diseases, Department of Internal
  Medicine
Mayo Clinic
Rochester, MN, United States

Tahia D. Fernández, PhD
Research Laboratory, IBIMA-Regional University
  Hospital of Malaga-UMA
Malaga, Spain

Francesco Gaeta, MD, PhD
Allergy Unit, Presidio Columbus
Rome, Italy

Marlene Garcia-Neuer, MS
Division of Rheumatology, Immunology and Allergy
Department of Medicine, Brigham and Women's
    Hospital
Boston, MA, United States

Lene H. Garvey, MD, PhD
Associate Professor
Danish Anaesthesia Allergy Centre
Allergy Clinic, Department of Dermatology and
    Allergy
Gentofte Hospital, University of
    CopenhagenKildegårdsvej
28Hellerup, Denmark

Justin Greiwe, MD
Bernstein Allergy Group
Volunteer Faculty University of Cincinnati
Cincinnati, OH, United States

Jason H. Karnes, PharmD, PhD, BCPS
Assistant Professor
Department of Pharmacy Practice and Science,
    University of Arizona College of Pharmacy,
    Tucson, AZ
Division of Pharmacogenomics, Center for Applied
    Genetics and Genomic Medicine (TCAG2M),
    Tucson, AZ
Sarver Heart Center, University of Arizona College of
    Medicine, Tucson, AZ

David A. Khan, MD
Professor of Internal Medicine
University of Texas Southwestern Medical Center
Dallas, TX, United States

Merin Kuruvilla, MD
Assistant Professor of Medicine
Emory University School of Medicine
Atlanta, GA, United States

Tanya M. Laidlaw, MD
Assistant Professor of Medicine, Harvard Medical
    School
Director of Translational Research in Allergy
Brigham and Women's Hospital
Boston, MA, United States

David M. Lang, MD
Professor of Medicine and Chair,
Department of Allergy and Clinical Immunology,
    Co-Director, Asthma Center, Director, Allergy/
    Immunology Fellowship, Respiratory Institute
Cleveland Clinic, Cleveland, OH 44195

Yu Li, MS
Division of Rheumatology, Allergy, and Immunology,
    Department of Medicine
Massachusetts General Hospital
Boston, MA, United States
Medical Practice Evaluation Center, Department of
    Medicine, Massachusetts General Hospital, Boston,
    Massachusetts

Anne Y. Liu, MD
Division of Allergy and Immunology
Stanford University School of Medicine
Stanford, CA, United States

Stephen J. Lockwood, MD, MPH
Fellow, Clinical Unit for Research Trials in Skin
Department of Dermatology
Massachusetts General Hospital
Harvard Medical School
Boston, MA, United States

Donna Lynch, MSN, FNP-BC
Division of Rheumatology, Immunology and Allergy
Department of Medicine, Brigham and Women's
    Hospital
Boston, MA, United States

Eric Macy, MD, MS, FAAAAI
Allergy and Clinical Immunology
San Diego Kaiser Permanente Medical Center
Partner
Southern California Permanente Medical Group
Voluntary Health Sciences Assistant Clinical Professor
Division of Rheumatology, Allergy, and Immunology
Department of Medicine
UCSD School of Medicine

Kathleen Marquis, PharmD, PhD
Pharmacy Services
Brigham and Women's Hospital
Harvard Medical School
Boston, MA, United States

Sara M. May, MD
Assistant Professor
Division of Pulmonary, Critical Care, Sleep and
    Allergy
University of Nebraska Medical Center
Omaha, NE, United States

Jasmit S. Minhas, MD
Department of Internal Medicine, Lahey Hospital and
    Medical Center, Burlington, Massachusetts
Tufts University School of Medicine, Boston,
MA, United States

María I. Montañez, PhD
Research Laboratory, IBIMA-Regional University
    Hospital of Malaga-UMA
Malaga, Spain

Iris M. Otani, MD
Department of Medicine, Division of Pulmonary,
    Critical Care, Allergy and Sleep Medicine
University of California San Francisco
San Francisco, CA, United States

Miguel A. Park, MD
Assistant Professor
Division of Allergic Diseases
Mayo Clinic
Rochester, MN, United States

Rebecca Pavlos, PhD
Institute for Immunology and Infectious Diseases,
    Murdoch University
Murdoch, WA, Australia

Jonny Peter, MB ChB, MMed, FCP (SA), PhD
Allergology and Clinical Immunology, Department of
    Medicine
University of Cape Town
Cape Town, South Africa

Elizabeth Phillips, MD
Professor of Medicine
Physician Scientist
Director of Personalized Immunology, Oates Institute
    for Experimental Therapeutics
Nashville, TN, United States

Antonino Romano, MD
Allergy Unit, Presidio Columbus, Rome, Italy, IRCCS
    Oasi Maria S.S., Troina, Italy

Arturo P. Saavedra, MD, PhD
Associate Professor of Dermatology
Harvard Medical School
Vice-Chairman for Clinical Affairs and Medical
    Director
Massachusetts General Hospital
Boston, MA, United States

Rebecca Saff, MD, PhD
Massachusetts General Hospital
Instructor in Medicine, Harvard University
MA, United States

María J. Torres, MD, PhD
Allergy Unit, IBIMA-Regional University Hospital of
    Malaga-UMA
Malaga, Spain

Jason A. Trubiano, BBiomedSci MBBS (Hons)
Department of Infectious Diseases, Alfred Health &
    Monash University
Microbiology Unit, Alfred Pathology Service
Melbourne, VIC, Australia

Rocco L. Valluzzi, MD
Allergy Unit, Presidio Columbus, Rome, Italy,
    Department of Pediatrics, Division of Allergy,
    Pediatric Hospital Bambino Gesù, Rome, Vatican
    City, Italy

Gerald W. Volcheck, MD
Division of Allergic Diseases, Department of Internal
    Medicine,
Mayo Clinic
Rochester, MN, United States

Preface: Drug Allergy Testing

Drug allergies are a common problem worldwide with up to 10%–20% of hospitalized patients reporting drug allergies. Drug hypersensitivity reactions can range from benign rashes to potentially fatal multisystem reactions. In addition, many patients are inappropriately labeled as being allergic to a medication. However, even when incorrect, a label of drug allergy can be associated with higher morbidity. Despite all these factors, the approach to management of drug allergies is not uniform, with approaches that vary both locally and internationally.

This book will help address some of the unmet needs faced by practitioners who diagnose and manage patients with drug allergies. Although the primary focus of this book is on diagnostic testing in drug allergy, other aspects of drug hypersensitivity are addressed, including the epidemiology, immunopathology, clinical presentations, phenotypes, and drug desensitization. An international list of experts has been assembled to review the published literature and make evidence-based recommendations on specific aspects of drug allergy. We hope that this book will not only enhance your knowledge but also serve as a very practical resource for the diagnosis and management of a wide array of drug allergic reactions.

David A. Khan
Aleena Banerji

Contents

CHAPTER 1

Epidemiology of Drug Allergy

REBECCA SAFF, MD, PHD

KEY POINTS

- Adverse drug reactions (ADRs) represent an important health concern, particularly with unpredictable hypersensitivity reactions, but accurate data on the prevalence of DHRs have been difficult to obtain, because of the difficulty in classifying the type of reaction and the underlying mechanism.
- Cutaneous reactions are common, occurring in 2–10 per 1000 patients, and are frequently caused by antibiotics.
- Severe cutaneous adverse reactions (SCARs) are uncommon but can result in significant morbidity and mortality. Anaphylaxis due to medications, particularly antibiotics, is more common in adults than in children and is associated with more severe reactions, including fatal anaphylaxis.

Adverse drug reactions (ADRs) are defined by the World Health Organization as any noxious, unintended, and undesired effect of a drug that occurs at doses used for prevention, diagnosis, and treatment.[1] These are estimated to account for 3%–6% of all hospital admissions and to occur in 10%–15% of hospitalized patients.[2] In a national ambulatory care survey, 0.31% of visits were because of adverse effects of medications, representing an estimated 2.73 million visits annually.[3] Cutaneous reactions to drugs are among the most common clinical manifestations of adverse drug events and had an annual incidence of 2.26 per 1000 persons, with increasing incidence in older adults.[4] The actual incidence is likely even greater, as physicians often either do not recognize ADRs or attribute the symptoms to an underlying disease state. Although some ADRs present as minor symptoms, many are serious and can lead to death in about 0.2%–0.4% of hospitalized patients.[5] In addition, the cost of managing ADRs can be high, whether they occur in the inpatient or outpatient setting.

ADRs were originally classified into two types. Type A ADRs are predictable and dose dependent, and they comprise approximately 80% of reactions. Type A ADRs include drug-induced toxicity, pharmacologic side effects, and drug interactions, such as orthostatic hypotension with antihypertensive medications or bleeding with warfarin. Type B ADRs are unpredictable, dose independent, and unrelated to the drug's known pharmacology. Type B ADRs make up 10%–15% of reactions and include drug intolerance (an undesired drug effect produced by the drug at therapeutic or subtherapeutic doses), idiosyncratic reactions (uncharacteristic reactions that are not explainable in terms of the known pharmacologic effects of the

drug), and hypersensitivity reactions, which include both immunologically and nonimmunologically mediated events.[6,7] Other types have now been added, including chronic reactions related to both dose and time (Type C), delayed reactions (Type D), effects due to withdrawal of medication (Type E), and, most recently, the unexpected failure of therapy (Type F).

The World Allergy Organization defines the term *hypersensitivity* as objectively reproducible signs or symptoms initiated by exposure to a defined stimulus at a dose tolerated by normal persons and *drug allergy* as a drug hypersensitivity reaction (DHR) with a demonstrated immunologic mechanism.[8] Therefore, DHRs would include immune-mediated or allergic reactions as well as nonimmune-mediated reactions, although these terms are often used interchangeably in the literature (Table 1.1). The 2010 Drug Allergy Practice Parameters defines drug allergy as "an immunologically mediated response to a pharmaceutical and/or formulation (excipient) agent in a sensitized person." Drug allergy may be further classified by the Gell-Coombs classification as follows: IgE mediated (type I), cytotoxic (type II), immune complex (type III), and cellular mediated (type IV).[9] Although Gell-Coombs classification is helpful, it does not account for many common clinical manifestations. The classification of drug allergies is limited by our understanding of the underlying mechanisms.

Immune-mediated reactions include IgE-mediated events, such as anaphylaxis, and T cell–mediated events, including severe cutaneous adverse reactions (SCARs). DHRs can also include reactions that have an immunologic basis but do not require sensitization, such as direct mast cell activation by

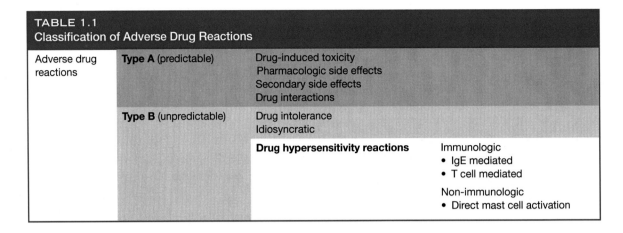

TABLE 1.1
Classification of Adverse Drug Reactions

Adverse drug reactions	**Type A** (predictable)	Drug-induced toxicity Pharmacologic side effects Secondary side effects Drug interactions	
	Type B (unpredictable)	Drug intolerance Idiosyncratic	
		Drug hypersensitivity reactions	Immunologic • IgE mediated • T cell mediated Non-immunologic • Direct mast cell activation

intravenous contrast or vancomycin. Distinguishing immune-mediated from nonimmune-mediated reactions can be difficult, as the clinical findings (such as urticaria from a nonsteroidal antiinflammatory drug [NSAID]) can be similar and have multiple possible underlying mechanisms.

Given the difficulty of defining the type of reaction and the underlying mechanism, it has been hard to determine the prevalence of DHR. Most studies are performed retrospectively, and the reactions are based primarily on clinical characteristics such as the symptoms and temporal relationship between drug use and disease onset. There are very few studies that confirm diagnosis of DHRs with in vivo or in vitro tests, and these are often done in small referral populations.

DRUG HYPERSENSITIVITY REACTIONS

There are a number of studies that have attempted to determine the rate of overall drug hypersensitivity events in specific clinical settings using skin manifestations as a marker of reaction. One of the first major studies that attempted to evaluate the prevalence of drug allergy in a prospective population was the Boston Collaborative Drug Surveillance Program. This was a prospective inpatient study initially reported in JAMA in 1976 which included 565 drug-attributed skin reactions that occurred among 22,227 monitored patients.[10] Allergic skin reactions occurred in slightly over 2% of hospitalized medical patients, and the primary cause was β-lactam antibiotics (52 of 1000 patients receiving ampicillin and 16 of 1000 patients receiving penicillin G). Because the average patient received about eight drugs, the rate of reactions per course of drug therapy was approximately 3 in 1000 courses. A follow-up study of the same population reported in 1986 confirmed the

reaction rate of 2.2% of patients, with the primary cause being β-lactam antibiotics.[11] Other prospective studies found rates of approximately 3 reactions per 1000 hospitalizations in inpatients, although these were limited to cutaneous reactions.[12–18] The most common cause of a cutaneous reaction in these studies was antibiotics, particularly β-lactam antibiotics, which were the implicated drug in 20% of reactions.

A 2003 study, in France, of patients with cutaneous allergic reactions verified by a dermatologist determined a prevalence of 3.6 per 1000 hospitalized patients.[18] Although the reactions were primarily exanthematous, they were responsible for hospitalization in 18% of the reacting patients and increased the duration of hospitalization in 14%. A 2006 prospective study in Mexico showed a prevalence of 7 per 1000 hospitalized patients, most frequently morbilliform rash, although 13% of the patients with reactions were identified as having a severe drug reaction.[19] An incidence of 2.2 per 1000 was found in a prospective study of Chinese patients, with morbilliform exanthema seen in 40% of patients.[20] In all these studies, antibiotics were the most common cause. Overall, the literature seems to suggest the incidence of cutaneous ADR ranges from 2 to 10 per 1000 patients, although only a small percentage of these are severe.

DHRs in the ambulatory setting are not as well studied as reactions that occur in the inpatient setting. In a review of ambulatory-based studies of adverse drug events, the overall rate of ADRs in the ambulatory setting was 15 per 1000 person-months, and skin symptoms, such as rash, itching, or edema, which can be associated with hypersensitivity reactions, were seen in 6.8% of the ADRs.[21] Using the National Ambulatory Care Survey (1995–2000) and National Hospital Ambulatory Care Survey (1995–2000), a rate of more than 100,000 outpatient visits annually for severe cutaneous reactions and about 2 million visits for likely drug-related immediate hypersensitivity reactions was found.[22] From these data, it was estimated that there are more than 500,000 outpatient visits for drug eruptions and drug allergies annually.

Given the difficulty of identifying true cases of DHRs in a population, a number of methods have been used to try to determine the true incidence. An electronic inpatient drug allergy reporting system was used to identify reactions in a general hospital in Singapore, which were then verified by an allergist.[17] Using this method, the incidence of drug allergy was 4.2 per 1000 hospitalizations. The rate of new DHRs during the course of inpatient treatment was 2.07 per 1000 hospitalizations with a mortality of 0.09 per 1000. Antimicrobials and antiepileptic drugs comprised 75% of the drug allergies reported. Cutaneous eruptions were the most common clinical presentation (95.7%), with maculopapular rash being the most common, and systemic manifestations occurred in 30%. However, underreporting was a problem and this likely underestimates the true incidence of DHRs. In Korea, a mandatory reporting system was used to identify DHRs, which were verified by allergists.[23] The incidence of DHRs was 1.8 per 1000 hospitalizations, with 70% cutaneous symptoms and 30% with systemic symptoms.

Billing codes have also been used to try to determine the rate of DHRs in large populations. Billing codes rely on heterogeneous coding of physicians and staff and can therefore miss potential reactions but could provide population data, allowing for a better understanding of the true burden of disease. Using billing codes validated by a chart review to identify allergic drug reactions, the estimated frequency of allergic drug reactions was found to increase from 0.49% of emergency department (ED) visits in 2001 to 0.94% in 2012.[24] Most reactions were attributed to antibiotics (42%), intravenous contrast (7%), and NSAIDs (6%). Validated codes could allow for better determination of incidence of DHRs using large datasets.

SEVERE CUTANEOUS ADVERSE REACTIONS

Severe cutaneous adverse reactions (SCARs) are delayed in onset and are mediated by CD4+ and CD8+ T lymphocytes. These include Stevens-Johnson syndrome (SJS), toxic epidermal necrolysis (TEN), drug-induced hypersensitivity syndrome or drug rash with eosinophilia and systemic symptoms (DIHS/DRESS), and acute generalized exanthematous pustulosis (AGEP). These reactions are rare but have severe morbidity and high mortality rates. The estimated morality rate is 10% for SJS, 30% for SJS/TEN, and almost 50% for TEN, and drugs are known to be the most common

cause of reactions.[25,26] As these reactions are primarily diagnosed clinically, true estimates are difficult to obtain. Because of the rarity of these reactions, with an incidence of 1.4–6 per million person-years, most data come from large retrospective studies.[2]

Both SJS and TEN are characterized by large areas of necrotic epidermal detachment and mucosal erosions and differ only in the amount of body surface areas involved; they are considered a spectrum of the same disorder. Large registries have found that the time to onset is typically within 4 weeks, although this varies depending on the culprit drug.[27,28] Antibiotics and antiepileptic medications are the most common culprits. In a large retrospective study of a European registry (EuroSCAR), the use of antibacterial sulfonamides, anticonvulsant agents, oxicam NSAIDs, allopurinol, chlormezanone, and corticosteroids were associated with increased risk of SJS/TEN.[29] In 2008, a follow-up study in this cohort not only confirmed increased risk of SJS/TEN with antiinfective sulfonamides, allopurinol, carbamazapine, phenobarbital, phenytoin, and oxicam-NSAIDs but also reported increased risk associated with nevirapine and lamotrigine.[28] In Japan, drugs were associated with 69% of cases of SJS and all cases of TEN, and the most common culprits were anticonvulsants, antibiotics, and NSAIDs.[30]

A recent report of the prevalence of SJS/TEN caused by medications in a large academic medical center in the United States found a rate of 375 patients per million, and antibiotics, particularly penicillins, cephalosporins, and sulfonamides, as well as macrolides and quinolones, were the most common culprits, followed by antiepileptics (particularly lamotrigine, phenytoin, carbamazepine, and phenobarbital) and NSAIDs.[31]

DIHS/DRESS is a rare, severe, and potentially fatal cutaneous ADR characterized by generalized maculopapular eruptions or erythroderma, high fever, lymphadenopathy, eosinophilia, atypical lymphocytes, and organ involvement. It is reported to occur in 1 in 1000 to 10,000 exposures, and its mortality is approximately 10%.[32,33] Aromatic antiepileptic drugs were the first described culprit medications, but many other drugs have been reported to be associated, including allopurinol, sulfonamides, dapsone, and minocycline.[34] The estimated risk at first or second prescription of an aromatic antiepileptic drug is 1–4.5 in 10,000.[35] In an Indian cohort, the most common culprits were aromatic anticonvulsants, lamotrigine, minocycline, salazopyrine, and dapsone.[36] In a large European case series, antiepileptic drugs were involved in 35%, allopurinol in 18%, antimicrobial sulfonamides and dapsone in 12%, and other antibiotics in 11%.[37] Glycopeptides have been shown to be a common culprit in some cohorts, particularly vancomycin.[38,39]

AGEP is an acute drug reaction characterized by the development of numerous small, nonfollicular, sterile pustules accompanied by leukocytosis and fever. It has been associated with aminopenicillins, pristinamycin, quinolones, hydroxychloroquine, sulfonamide antibiotics, terbinafine, and diltiazem.[40] AGEP is rare, with an incidence of one to five patients per million per year.[41] The EuroSCAR study found a mean age of 56 years and a male:female ratio of 0.8:1.[40] The predominance in women was also seen in case series from Asia.[42]

ANAPHYLAXIS

Anaphylaxis is a rapid, life-threatening hypersensitivity reaction, typically representing an IgE-mediated reaction. The incidence of anaphylaxis has been increasing over time, and is estimated to be 50–100 cases per 100,000 person-years.[43] Anaphylaxis is most commonly caused by foods in pediatric populations, but drugs are a significant trigger in older populations. In retrospective reviews of patients treated in the emergency room for anaphylaxis, drugs were the cause of anaphylaxis in 36% of cases in Italy, 28% in Australia, and 46% in Belgium.[44–46] In contrast, drugs were found as a cause in 5% of pediatric cases of anaphylaxis seen in the emergency room in studies in Australia.[47,48] The European Anaphylaxis Registry also found that only 5% of reactions were caused by medications in children, and these were predominantly in adolescents, with antibiotics and analgesics being the most common culprits.[49] A study using data from ED visits in Florida used a combination of billing codes to identify patients with drug-related anaphylaxis, finding that adults had twice as much relative risk as children.[50] A study in children seen in the ED for drug-related anaphylaxis, using a combination of drug-specific billing codes and billing codes for anaphylaxis, symptoms of anaphylaxis, or shock, found a medication-induced anaphylaxis rate of 1.6 per 100,000 among children.[51]

In a retrospective review of acute anaphylaxis in adults resulting in admission, drugs, particularly antibiotics and NSAIDs, were the most common cause.[52] Patients with drug-induced anaphylaxis were older and more often had cardiovascular symptoms. Drugs were identified as the cause of anaphylaxis in 50% of cases in a retrospective review in Thailand, with 37% of cases occurring during hospitalization.[53] In a study of anaphylaxis occurring during admission in China, 89.8% of cases were triggered by medications, specifically antibiotics in 29.6%, radiocontrast media in 16.7%, and chemotherapy in 11.1%.[54]

Antibiotics are most commonly implicated in anaphylaxis, particularly β-lactam antibiotics. IgE-mediated reactions occur in 0.04%–0.015% of penicillin-treated subjects, and anaphylaxis occurs in approximately 0.001%.[55] NSAIDs and radiocontrast media are also important causes of anaphylaxis, although these are predominantly non-IgE mediated. NSAIDs (25.5%) and antibiotics (23.5%) were the most common cause of drug-induced anaphylaxis in a study in an emergency room in Hong Kong.[56]

Drugs are an important cause of anaphylaxis in the perioperative period, and the incidence of hypersensitivity reactions during anesthesia is approximately 1 in 5000, although this varies by country.[2] The most common culprits identified are antibiotics and neuromuscular blocking agents, with striking differences between countries.[57–59] In France, the most common causes of anaphylaxis have consistently been neuromuscular blocking agents, latex, and antibiotics.[60,61] In the United States, antibiotics are the more common culprit, particularly cefazolin.[57,62]

Death from anaphylaxis is a rare event and occurs in only 0.12 to 1.06 deaths per million person-years, although medications have been associated with more severe reactions and have been found as one of the most common causes of fatal anaphylaxis.[63,64] In a study of anaphylaxis-related deaths in the US National Mortality Database using billing codes to identify patients, 58.8% of the 2458 anaphylaxis-related deaths were due to medications, and there was a significant increase over the 12 year study period, with antibiotics accounting for 40% of the cases in which a drug was specified.[65]

PEDIATRIC DRUG ALLERGY

Although the reported incidence of ADRs is lower in the pediatric populations as compared with adults, they remain an important consideration. The overall incidence of ADRs was 10.9% in hospitalized children and 1.0% in outpatient children with a rate of hospital admission due to ADRs of 1.8%.[66] A review of ADRs in a children's hospital found that 0.4%–10.3% of all pediatric hospital admissions were ADR-related (2.9% overall incidence) and that 0.6%–16.8% of all children exposed to a drug during hospital stay experienced an ADR.[67] Antibiotics and antiepileptics were the most frequently reported therapeutic class associated with ADRs in the inpatient setting, and antibiotics and NSAIDS were frequently reported as associated with ADRs in the outpatient setting.[67] These studies did not further characterize ADRs into allergic and nonallergic. A 10-year retrospective review of ADRs at a pediatric hospital categorized ADRs into pharmacologic or allergic/idiosyncratic.[68] The overall incidence was 1.6%, and 51% were allergic/idiosyncratic. Similar to adults, antibiotics (33%) were the most common drug class associated with ADRs, followed by narcotic analgesics (12%) and anticonvulsants (11%).

Patients who experienced ADRs before hospital admission, or who reacted to medications during surgery, were more likely to experience severe reactions. Of these severe reactions, 40% were from chemotherapeutic agents and 24% were hypersensitivity reactions to anticonvulsants and resulted in serious or fatal ADRs.

LIMITATIONS IN DIAGNOSIS

Reported DHRs are common in the medical record and are often overdiagnosed because of false association of symptoms with medications, improper documentation, and incorrect classification. However, reactions may also be underreported and underdiagnosis can lead to serious adverse consequences. A predictive model for diagnosis of ADRs based on variables in the clinical history estimated true ADRs to occur in 20% of patients with reported allergies and ruled out possible allergic reactions in 52%, although mathematical modeling has limitations.[69] A study of over 1300 immediate DHRs in France in which the authors confirmed the reaction with skin testing and drug provocation tests found that only 17.6% of patients were positive for immediate hypersensitivity reactions.[70] The drugs responsible were β-lactams (30.3%), aspirin (14.5%), other NSAIDs (11.7%), paracetamol (8.9%), macrolides (7.4%), and quinolones (2.4%). A Spanish study of almost 5000 DHRs, were carefully reviewed and the mechanism determined using in vivo and in vitro testing, confirmed allergic cause in one-third of cases.[71] Before evaluation, based on clinical history, 37% of episodes were attributed to NSAIDS, 29.4% to β-lactams, 15% to non-β-lactam antibiotics, and 18.4% to other drugs. Following evaluation, over 37.4% were found to have an allergic cause with hypersensitivity to multiple NSAIDs and β-lactams predominating.

Antibiotics represent the most common cause of DHRs, with penicillin as the most common antibiotic causing allergy and reported in about 8% of individuals using healthcare in the United States.[72] However, after formal evaluation, greater than 90% of patients can tolerate penicillins.[73,74] There are many causes for this discrepancy, including misclassification of the original reaction as well as the known loss of sensitivity over time. Strategies to evaluate reported penicillin allergy are being evaluated, and there is evidence to show that penicillin allergy increases hospital stay, cost of care, and the use of broader-spectrum antibiotics, as well as increased *Clostridium difficile*, methicillin-resistant *Staphylococcus aureus*, and vancomycin-resistant enterococci prevalence.[75,76] Penicillin skin testing can decrease the use of broad-spectrum antibiotics and may potentially decrease the cost of care.[73,74] Guidelines to increase penicillin skin testing and the use of β-lactams in patients with reported allergy have shown that appropriate use is not associated with increased ADRs and correlates with a decrease in alternative antibiotic exposure.[73,77]

RISK FACTORS

Reactions to drugs are complex responses that are influenced by environmental factors, patient characteristics, and properties of the drug itself. Risk factors for cutaneous ADRs include viral infections, particularly human immunodeficiency virus (HIV), connective tissue disease including systemic lupus erythematosus, viral and autoimmune hepatitis, and non-Hodgkin's lymphoma.[18,19] Certain classes of drugs are associated with a higher frequency of reaction as they can act as haptens or prohaptens or bind covalently to immune receptors, increasing the risk of reaction.

Females have been shown to develop DHRs more frequently than males. Overall, females appear to be more affected than males.[71,78,79] In a study of allergy consults, there were twice as many female consults for drug allergy as male consults.[80] As previously discussed, DHRs are more common in adults than in children. Family history of drug allergy is a risk factor for reactions, and ethnicity and genetics appear to be increasingly important as we gain more insights into the mechanisms of the reactions.

GENETICS

Genetic factors that influence drug allergy are under intense investigation but are still largely unknown. The best understood mechanism is in SCAR, particularly SJS/TEN, as the mechanism is understood to involve the presentation of antigen in HLA to activate T cells. Given that the frequency of HLA types varies in ethnic populations, this has led to a better understanding of increased risk of SJS/TEN in certain populations with certain drugs. In 1982, the HLA-Bw44 antigen was found to be associated with ocular involvement in Stevens-Johnson in a white population.[81] Since that time, HLA associations have been described to a number of drugs.

HLA-B*5801 has been clearly associated with allopurinol in both SJS/TEN and DIHS in a number of populations, particularly SJS/TEN in Han Chinese from Taiwan.[82] This was subsequently seen in multiple populations, including Japanese and Europeans.[83,84] A meta-analysis found increased risk of allopurinol-induced

SJS/TEN in both Asian and non-Asian populations with HLA-B*5801, although the gene appears to be necessary but not sufficient, and research continues into other genetic factors that might be involved.[85]

HLA-B*15:02 was strongly associated with carbamazepine-induced SJS/TEN in Han Chinese population.[82] The association has been validated in many populations in Southeast Asia, including Thailand, Hong Kong, and India.[86–88] Genetic screening of HLA-B*1502 before the use of carbamazepine for patients with Asian ancestry is recommended by US Food and Drug Administration.

One of the best understood genetic predispositions to drug allergy is seen in abacavir hypersensitivity reactions. Abacavir causes a hypersensitivity reaction that occurs in 5%–8% of patients during the first 6 weeks of treatment resulting in fever, rash, and gastrointestinal and respiratory symptoms. Immediate discontinuation is required, and continued exposure or rechallenge can lead to more severe and potentially life-threatening reactions. In 2002, an association with a specific HLA allele was reported.[89,90] This was confirmed in multiple subsequent studies. In 2008, the utility of screening for HLA-B*5701 before starting abacavir was clearly demonstrated, and screening is now a standard clinical practice.[91,92]

In IgE-mediated reactions, studies reported in multiple populations have shown that genes that are involved in IgE production, particularly those of the IL-13 and IL-4 pathways, are important in β-lactam allergy.[93,94] Polymorphisms in the IL-4/IL-13 axis and related cytokines were reported to increase the risk of β-lactam-mediated reactions.[95] A strong association seen in β-lactam allergy is with a polymorphism in galectin-3, which binds IgE.[96] Variants in genomewide association studies in β-lactam allergy have shown the likely importance of HLA-DRA.[97]

CONCLUSIONS

ADRs represent an important health concern, particularly with unpredictable hypersensitivity reactions, but accurate data on the prevalence of DHRs have been difficult to obtain, because of the difficulty in classifying the type of reaction and the underlying mechanism. Cutaneous reactions are common, occurring in 2–10 per 1000 patients, and are frequently caused by antibiotics. SCARs are uncommon but can result in significant morbidity and mortality. Anaphylaxis due to medications, particularly antibiotics, is more common in adults than in children and is associated with more severe reactions including fatal anaphylaxis.

Risk factors include environmental factors, properties of the drug itself, and patient characteristics with pharmacogenetics increasingly recognized and providing an opportunity for screening. Moving forward, standardizing terminology, improving our understanding of the immune mechanism, and validating diagnosis with in vitro and in vivo testing will allow for a better of understanding of DHRs and their prevention and treatment.

REFERENCES

1. International drug monitoring: the role of national centres. Report of a WHO meeting. *World Health Organ Tech Rep Ser*. 1972;498:1–25.
2. Thong BY, Tan TC. Epidemiology and risk factors for drug allergy. *Br J Clin Pharmacol*. 2011;71(5):684–700.
3. Aparasu RR, Helgeland DL. Utilization of ambulatory care services caused by adverse effects of medications in the United States. *Manag Care Interface*. 2000;13(4):70–75.
4. Koelblinger P, et al. Skin manifestations of outpatient adverse drug events in the United States: a national analysis. *J Cutan Med Surg*. 2013;17(4):269–275.
5. Lazarou J, Pomeranz BH, Corey PN. Incidence of adverse drug reactions in hospitalized patients: a meta-analysis of prospective studies. *JAMA*. 1998;279(15):1200–1205.
6. Bousquet PJ, et al. Pharmacovigilance of drug allergy and hypersensitivity using the ENDA-DAHD database and the GALEN platform. The Galenda project. *Allergy*. 2009;64(2):194–203.
7. Doña I, et al. Trends in hypersensitivity drug reactions: more drugs, more response patterns, more heterogeneity. *J Investig Allergol Clin Immunol*. 2014;24(3):143–153. quiz 1 p. following 153.
8. Johansson SG, et al. Revised nomenclature for allergy for global use: report of the nomenclature review committee of the World Allergy Organization, October 2003. *J Allergy Clin Immunol*. 2004;113(5):832–836.
9. Parameters JTFOP, et al. Drug allergy: an updated practice parameter. *J Allergy Clin Immunol*. 2010;105(4):259–273.
10. Arndt KA, Jick H. Rates of cutaneous reactions to drugs. A report from the Boston Collaborative Drug Surveillance Program. *JAMA*. 1976;235(9):918–923.
11. Bigby M, et al. Drug-induced cutaneous reactions. A report from the Boston Collaborative Drug Surveillance Program on 15,438 consecutive inpatients, 1975 to 1982. *JAMA*. 1986;256(24):3358–3363.
12. Allain H, et al. Undesirable dermatologic results of drugs. Result of a drug monitoring survey. *Ann Med Interne (Paris)*. 1983;134(6):530–536.
13. Classen DC, et al. Computerized surveillance of adverse drug events in hospital patients. *JAMA*. 1991;266(20):2847–2851.
14. Rademaker M, Oakley A, Duffill MB. Cutaneous adverse drug reactions in a hospital setting. *N Z Med J*. 1995;108(999):165–166.

15. Hunziker T, et al. Comprehensive hospital drug monitoring (CHDM): adverse skin reactions, a 20-year survey. *Allergy*. 1997;52(4):388–393.

16. Sharma VK, Sethuraman G, Kumar B. Cutaneous adverse drug reactions: clinical pattern and causative agents–a 6 year series from Chandigarh, India. *J Postgrad Med*. 2001;47(2):95–99.

17. Thong BY, et al. Drug allergy in a general hospital: Results of a novel prospective inpatient reporting system. *Ann Allergy Asthma Immunol*. 2003;90(3):342–347.

18. Fiszenson-Albala F, et al. A 6-month prospective survey of cutaneous drug reactions in a hospital setting. *Br J Dermatol*. 2003;149(5):1018–1022.

19. Hernández-Salazar A, et al. Epidemiology of adverse cutaneous drug reactions. A prospective study in hospitalized patients. *Arch Med Res*. 2006;37(7):899–902.

20. Tian XY, et al. Incidence of adverse cutaneous drug reactions in 22,866 Chinese inpatients: a prospective study. *Arch Dermatol Res*. 2015;307(9):829–834.

21. Thomsen LA, et al. Systematic review of the incidence and characteristics of preventable adverse drug events in ambulatory care. *Ann Pharmacother*. 2007;41(9):1411–1426.

22. Stern RS. Utilization of hospital and outpatient care for adverse cutaneous reactions to medications. *Pharmacoepidemiol Drug Saf*. 2005;14(10):677–684.

23. Park CS, et al. The use of an electronic medical record system for mandatory reporting of drug hypersensitivity reactions has been shown to improve the management of patients in the university hospital in Korea. *Pharmacoepidemiol Drug Saf*. 2008;17(9):919–925.

24. Saff RR, et al. Utility of ICD-9-CM codes for identification of allergic drug reactions. *J Allergy Clin Immunol Pract*. 2016;4(1):114–119.e1.

25. Auquier-Dunant A, et al. Correlations between clinical patterns and causes of erythema multiforme majus, Stevens-Johnson syndrome, and toxic epidermal necrolysis: results of an international prospective study. *Arch Dermatol*. 2002;138(8):1019–1024.

26. Borchers AT, et al. Stevens-Johnson syndrome and toxic epidermal necrolysis. *Autoimmun Rev*. 2008;7(8):598–605.

27. Rzany B, et al. Epidemiology of erythema exsudativum multiforme majus, Stevens-Johnson syndrome, and toxic epidermal necrolysis in Germany (1990–1992): structure and results of a population-based registry. *J Clin Epidemiol*. 1996;49(7):769–773.

28. Mockenhaupt M, et al. Stevens-Johnson syndrome and toxic epidermal necrolysis: assessment of medication risks with emphasis on recently marketed drugs. The EuroSCAR-study. *J Investig Dermatol*. 2008;128(1):35–44.

29. Roujeau JC, et al. Medication use and the risk of Stevens-Johnson syndrome or toxic epidermal necrolysis. *N Engl J Med*. 1995;333(24):1600–1607.

30. Yamane Y, Aihara M, Ikezawa Z. Analysis of Stevens-Johnson syndrome and toxic epidermal necrolysis in Japan from 2000 to 2006. *Allergol Int*. 2007;56(4):419–425.

31. Blumenthal KG, et al. Stevens-Johnson syndrome and toxic epidermal necrolysis: a cross-sectional analysis of patients in an integrated allergy repository of a large health care system. *J Allergy Clin Immunol Pract*. 2015;3(2):277–280.e1.

32. Roujeau JC, Stern RS. Severe adverse cutaneous reactions to drugs. *N Engl J Med*. 1994;331(19):1272–1285.

33. Criado PR, et al. Drug reaction with eosinophilia and systemic symptoms (DRESS)/drug-induced hypersensitivity syndrome (DIHS): a review of current concepts. *An Bras Dermatol*. 2012;87(3):435–449.

34. Peyrière H, et al. Variability in the clinical pattern of cutaneous side-effects of drugs with systemic symptoms: does a DRESS syndrome really exist? *Br J Dermatol*. 2006;155(2):422–428.

35. Cho YT, et al. Co-existence of histopathological features is characteristic in drug reaction with eosinophilia and systemic symptoms and correlates with high grades of cutaneous abnormalities. *J Eur Acad Dermatol Venereol*. 2016;30.

36. Sasidharanpillai S, et al. Severe cutaneous adverse drug reactions: a clinicoepidemiological study. *Indian J Dermatol*. 2015;60(1):102.

37. Kardaun SH, et al. Drug reaction with eosinophilia and systemic symptoms (DRESS): an original multisystem adverse drug reaction. Results from the prospective RegiSCAR study. *Br J Dermatol*. 2013;169(5):1071–1080.

38. Lin YF, et al. Severe cutaneous adverse reactions related to systemic antibiotics. *Clin Infect Dis*. 2014;58(10):1377–1385.

39. Blumenthal KG, et al. Peripheral blood eosinophilia and hypersensitivity reactions among patients receiving outpatient parenteral antibiotics. *J Allergy Clin Immunol*. 2015;136(5):1288–1294.e1.

40. Sidoroff A, et al. Risk factors for acute generalized exanthematous pustulosis (AGEP)-results of a multinational case-control study (EuroSCAR). *Br J Dermatol*. 2007;157(5):989–996.

41. Sidoroff A, et al. Acute generalized exanthematous pustulosis (AGEP)–a clinical reaction pattern. *J Cutan Pathol*. 2001;28(3):113–119.

42. Chang SL, et al. Clinical manifestations and characteristics of patients with acute generalized exanthematous pustulosis in Asia. *Acta Dermato-venereol*. 2008;88(4):363–365.

43. Tejedor-Alonso MA, Moro-Moro M, Múgica-García MV. Epidemiology of anaphylaxis: contributions from the last 10 years. *J Investig Allergol Clin Immunol*. 2015;25(3):163–175. quiz follow 174–175.

44. Pastorello EA, et al. Incidence of anaphylaxis in the emergency department of a general hospital in Milan. *J Chromatogr B Biomed Sci Appl*. 2001;756(1–2):11–17.

45. Brown AF, McKinnon D, Chu K. Emergency department anaphylaxis: A review of 142 patients in a single year. *J Allergy Clin Immunol*. 2001;108(5):861–866.

46. Mostmans Y, et al. Anaphylaxis in an urban Belgian emergency department: epidemiology and aetiology. *Acta Clin Belg*. 2016;71(2):99–106.

47. Braganza SC, et al. Paediatric emergency department anaphylaxis: different patterns from adults. *Arch Dis Child.* 2006;91(2):159–163.

48. de Silva IL, et al. Paediatric anaphylaxis: a 5 year retrospective review. *Allergy.* 2008;63(8):1071–1076.

49. Grabenhenrich LB, et al. Anaphylaxis in children and adolescents: The European anaphylaxis registry. *J Allergy Clin Immunol.* 2016;137(4):1128–1137.e1.

50. Harduar-Morano L, et al. A population-based epidemiologic study of emergency department visits for anaphylaxis in Florida. *J Allergy Clin Immunol.* 2011;128(3):594–600.e1.

51. West SL, et al. Population-based drug-related anaphylaxis in children and adolescents captured by South Carolina Emergency Room Hospital Discharge Database (SCERHDD) (2000-2002). *Pharmacoepidemiol Drug Saf.* 2007;16(12):1255–1267.

52. Cianferoni A, et al. Clinical features of acute anaphylaxis in patients admitted to a university hospital: an 11-year retrospective review (1985-1996). *Ann Allergy Asthma Immunol.* 2001;87(1):27–32.

53. Jirapongsananuruk O, et al. Features of patients with anaphylaxis admitted to a university hospital. *Ann Allergy Asthma Immunol.* 2007;98(2):157–162.

54. Tang R, et al. Clinical characteristics of inpatients with anaphylaxis in China. *Biomed Res Int.* 2015;2015: 429534.

55. Parameters JTFoP, et al. The diagnosis and management of anaphylaxis: an updated practice parameter. *J Allergy Clin Immunol.* 2005;115(3 suppl 2):S483–S523.

56. Smit DV, Cameron PA, Rainer TH. Anaphylaxis presentations to an emergency department in Hong Kong: incidence and predictors of biphasic reactions. *J Emerg Med.* 2005;28(4):381–388.

57. Guyer AC, et al. Comprehensive allergy evaluation is useful in the subsequent care of patients with drug hypersensitivity reactions during anesthesia. *J Allergy Clin Immunol Pract.* 2015;3(1):94–100.

58. Kuhlen JL, et al. Antibiotics are the most commonly identified cause of perioperative hypersensitivity reactions. *J Allergy Clin Immunol Pract.* 2016;4(4):697–704.

59. Mertes PM, et al. Epidemiology of perioperative anaphylaxis. *Presse Med.* 2016;45(9):758–767.

60. Mertes PM, et al. Anaphylaxis during anesthesia in France: an 8-year national survey. *J Allergy Clin Immunol.* 2011;128(2):366–373.

61. Dong SW, et al. Hypersensitivity reactions during anesthesia. Results from the ninth French survey (2005–2007). *Minerva Anestesiol.* 2012;78(8):868–878.

62. Gurrieri C, et al. Allergic reactions during anesthesia at a large United States referral center. *Anesth Analg.* 2011;113(5):1202–1212.

63. Kuruvilla M, Khan DA. Anaphylaxis to drugs. *Immunol Allergy Clin North Am.* 2015;35(2):303–319.

64. Brown SG, et al. Anaphylaxis: clinical patterns, mediator release, and severity. *J Allergy Clin Immunol.* 2013;132(5):1141–1149.e5.

65. Jerschow E, et al. Fatal anaphylaxis in the United States, 1999–2010: temporal patterns and demographic associations. *J Allergy Clin Immunol.* 2014;134(6):1318–1328.e7.

66. Clavenna A, Bonati M. Adverse drug reactions in childhood: a review of prospective studies and safety alerts. *Arch Dis Child.* 2009;94(9):724–728.

67. Gallagher RM, et al. Adverse drug reactions causing admission to a paediatric hospital. *PLoS One.* 2012;7(12): e50127.

68. Le J, et al. Adverse drug reactions among children over a 10-year period. *Pediatrics.* 2006;118(2):555–562.

69. Hierro Santurino B, et al. A predictive model for the diagnosis of allergic drug reactions according to the medical history. *J Allergy Clin Immunol Pract.* 2016;4(2):292–300.e3.

70. Messaad D, et al. Drug provocation tests in patients with a history suggesting an immediate drug hypersensitivity reaction. *Ann Intern Med.* 2004;140(12):1001–1006.

71. Doña I, et al. Drug hypersensitivity reactions: response patterns, drug involved, and temporal variations in a large series of patients. *J Investig Allergol Clin Immunol.* 2012;22(5):363–371.

72. Macy E. Penicillin and beta-lactam allergy: epidemiology and diagnosis. *Curr Allergy Asthma Rep.* 2014;14(11):476.

73. Rimawi RH, et al. The impact of penicillin skin testing on clinical practice and antimicrobial stewardship. *J Hosp Med.* 2013;8(6):341–345.

74. del Real GA, et al. Penicillin skin testing in patients with a history of beta-lactam allergy. *Ann Allergy Asthma Immunol.* 2007;98(4):355–359.

75. Macy E, Contreras R. Health care use and serious infection prevalence associated with penicillin "allergy" in hospitalized patients: A cohort study. *J Allergy Clin Immunol.* 2014;133(3):790–796.

76. Picard M, et al. Treatment of patients with a history of penicillin allergy in a large tertiary-care academic hospital. *J Allergy Clin Immunol Pract.* 2013;1(3):252–257.

77. Blumenthal KG, et al. Impact of a clinical guideline for prescribing antibiotics to inpatients reporting penicillin or cephalosporin allergy. *Ann Allergy Asthma Immunol.* 2015;115(4):294–300.e2.

78. Barranco P, López-Serrano MC. General and epidemiological aspects of allergic drug reactions. *Clin Exp Allergy.* 1998;(28 suppl 4):61–62.

79. Haddi E, et al. Atopy and systemic reactions to drugs. *Allergy.* 1990;45(3):236–239.

80. Ibáñez MD, Garde JM. Allergy in patients under fourteen years of age in Alergológica 2005. *J Investig Allergol Clin Immunol.* 2009;(19 Suppl 2):61–68.

81. Mondino BJ, Brown SI, Biglan AW. HLA antigens in Stevens-Johnson syndrome with ocular involvement. *Arch Ophthalmol.* 1982;100(9):1453–1454.

82. Chung WH, et al. Medical genetics: a marker for Stevens-Johnson syndrome. *Nature.* 2004;428(6982):486.

83. Lonjou C, et al. A European study of HLA-B in Stevens-Johnson syndrome and toxic epidermal necrolysis related to five high-risk drugs. *Pharmacogenet Genomics.* 2008;18(2):99–107.

84. Kaniwa N, et al. HLA-B locus in Japanese patients with anti-epileptics and allopurinol-related Stevens-Johnson syndrome and toxic epidermal necrolysis. *Pharmacogenomics.* 2008;9(11):1617–1622.

85. Somkrua R, et al. Association of HLA-B*5801 allele and allopurinol-induced Stevens Johnson syndrome and toxic epidermal necrolysis: a systematic review and meta-analysis. *BMC Med Genet.* 2011;12:118.

86. Man CB, et al. Association between HLA-B*1502 allele and antiepileptic drug-induced cutaneous reactions in Han Chinese. *Epilepsia.* 2007;48(5):1015–1018.

87. Locharernkul C, et al. Carbamazepine and phenytoin induced Stevens-Johnson syndrome is associated with HLA-B*1502 allele in Thai population. *Epilepsia.* 2008;49(12):2087–2091.

88. Mehta TY, et al. Association of HLA-B*1502 allele and carbamazepine-induced Stevens-Johnson syndrome among Indians. *Indian J Dermatol Venereol Leprol.* 2009;75(6):579–582.

89. Hetherington S, et al. Genetic variations in HLA-B region and hypersensitivity reactions to abacavir. *Lancet.* 2002;359(9312):1121–1122.

90. Mallal S, et al. Association between presence of HLA-B*5701, HLA-DR7, and HLA-DQ3 and hypersensitivity to HIV-1 reverse-transcriptase inhibitor abacavir. *Lancet.* 2002;359(9308):727–732.

91. Mallal S, et al. HLA-B*5701 screening for hypersensitivity to abacavir. *N Engl J Med.* 2008;358(6):568–579.

92. Saag M, et al. High sensitivity of human leukocyte antigen-b*5701 as a marker for immunologically confirmed abacavir hypersensitivity in white and black patients. *Clin Infect Dis.* 2008;46(7):1111–1118.

93. Oussalah A, et al. Genetic variants associated with drugs-induced immediate hypersensitivity reactions: a PRISMA-compliant systematic review. *Allergy.* 2016;71(4):443–462.

94. Khan DA. Pharmacogenomics and adverse drug reactions: primetime and not ready for primetime tests. *J Allergy Clin Immunol.* 2016;138(4):943–955.

95. Yang J, Qiao HL, Dong ZM. Polymorphisms of IL-13 and IL-4-IL-13-SNPs in patients with penicillin allergies. *Eur J Clin Pharmacol.* 2005;61(11):803–809.

96. Cornejo-García JA, et al. A non-synonymous polymorphism in galectin-3 lectin domain is associated with allergic reactions to beta-lactam antibiotics. *Pharmacogenomics J.* 2016;16(1):79–82.

97. Guéant JL, et al. HLA-DRA variants predict penicillin allergy in genome-wide fine-mapping genotyping. *J Allergy Clin Immunol.* 2015;135(1):253–259.

CHAPTER 2

Economic Impact of Drug Allergy

YU LI, MS • JASMIT S. MINHAS, MD • KIMBERLY G. BLUMENTHAL, MD, MSC

KEY POINTS

- Adverse drug reactions and hypersensitivity reactions are clinically diverse and impose a range of economic impacts on the healthcare system.
- Mild cutaneous hypersensitivity reactions have a lower per case economic impact than more severe reactions such as the severe cutaneous adverse reactions, which pose a significant economic burden as a majority of patients require hospitalization in specialized units.
- Unverified drug allergies, especially unverified penicillin allergy, lead to more costly alternative drugs being used and other economic consequences, such as longer length of hospital and healthcare-associated infections.
- Cost-effectiveness analyses in drug hypersensitivity have demonstrated that genetic screening in specific populations for severe cutaneous adverse reactions is cost-effective.

INTRODUCTION

As the cost of healthcare is increasing in the United States, limiting unnecessary treatment and preventing adverse events that result from treatment have become increasingly important. Adverse and hypersensitivity reactions to drugs are clinically diverse and impose a range of economic impacts on the healthcare system. In this chapter, we summarize data on the cost of adverse and hypersensitivity reactions (HSRs). We include a summary of the cost of inaccurately reported allergies and identify areas where cost-effectiveness analyses have been performed. Throughout this chapter, all costs have been converted into inflation-adjusted 2016 US dollars.

COST OF ADVERSE DRUG REACTIONS, ADVERSE DRUG EVENTS, AND HYPERSENSITIVITY REACTIONS

Adverse drug events (ADEs) are patient injuries caused by a drug given as part of a medical intervention.[1] ADEs include physical harm, mental harm, and loss of function. ADEs can further be distinguished as either preventable ADEs, which result from medication errors, or nonpreventable ADEs, which are analogous to adverse drug reactions (ADRs, Fig. 2.1). About one in five ADRs is a result of an immune-mediated reaction to a drug or an HSR.[2]

Cost of Adverse Drug Events and Adverse Drug Reactions

US-based studies reported a cost of $3,023 to $3,897 for each ADE and $7,036 for each ADR (Table 2.1).[3,4]

Treatment for conditions as seemingly benign as drug-induced anemia can cost from $7023 to $10,182 per patient.[5] Outside the United States, the costs of ADRs ranged from $946 per patient in Taiwan to $3,813 per ADR-related admission in Singapore.[6,7] Studies in Canada, China, France, Germany, and Italy have also reported similar costs for ADEs and ADRs (Table 2.1).[8–13] In the United States, ADRs cost 4.2 billion dollars every year,[14] as they comprise 3%–6% of all hospital admissions and occur in 10%–15% of inpatients.[15] Estimated costs from abroad range from $13 million in Singapore[7] to $2.5 billion in Germany.[8]

Cost of Hypersensitivity Reactions

Drug HSRs, comprising 20% of ADRs,[16] range from mild (e.g., benign rashes) to severe, such as the reactions of anaphylaxis, angioedema, acute interstitial nephritis (AIN), Stevens-Johnson syndrome (SJS), toxic epidermal necrolysis (TEN), acute generalized exanthematous pustulosis (AGEP), erythema multiforme (EM), and drug rash eosinophilia and systemic symptoms (DRESS) syndrome.

Prior economic analyses of HSRs are limited. However, a few studies have defined the costs of mild cutaneous reactions, severe cutaneous reactions, drug-induced anaphylaxis, drug-induced angioedema, and SJS/TEN. To date, no studies have reported the costs of serum sickness–like reactions, AIN, or other Severe cutaneous adverse reactions (SCARs, including EM, DRESS syndrome, and AGEP).

The average cost of mild cutaneous hypersensitivities, such as rash, urticaria/hives, and itching, was

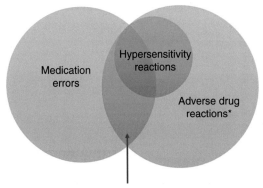

Preventable adverse drug events

FIG. 2.1 Relationship between medication errors, adverse drug events, adverse drug reactions, and hypersensitivity reactions.
*adverse drug reactions are nonpreventable adverse drug events.

estimated at $274 per episode.[17] However, urticaria that required hospitalization cost 23-fold more ($6,293).[18] Some drugs associated with cutaneous reactions can pose a higher economic burden without a hospital admission because of chronicity. For example, toxic dermatitis from molecularly targeted chemotherapeutics can cost up to $2,057 per patient.[10,19]

In a drug allergy epidemiology study in the United States, anaphylaxis was found to cost $1,708 per event if the patient was seen only in the emergency department, but $9,565 to $14,268 if the anaphylactic episode resulted in hospitalization.[18,20] A French study identified the direct medical cost of drug-induced anaphylaxis as $2,602 per patient, with total cost even higher (about $3,000) when the nonmedical cost of absenteeism was considered.[11] Although limited data exist, the cost of drug-induced angioedema for patients requiring hospitalization was found to be similar to that of drug-induced anaphylaxis ($9,564).[18]

TABLE 2.1
Cost of Adverse Drug Events (ADEs), Adverse Drug Reactions (ADRs), and Hypersensitivity Reactions

Author	Year	Country	Medical Setting	Adverse Reaction Type	Cost Per Patient
ADVERSE DRUG EVENTS					
Classen[4]	1997	United States	All	Attributable cost to ADEs	$3,023[a]
Bates[3]	1997	United States	All	Adjusted total cost per ADE Adjusted total cost per preventable ADE	$3,897[b] $7,036
Oderda[17]	2003	United States	Surgery	Increased cost in ADE patients Nausea/vomiting Rash/hives/itching	$935[c] $668 $274
Meier[8]	2015	Germany	All	Community-acquired ADEs Preventable ADEs	$3,097[d] $2,977
ADVERSE DRUG REACTIONS					
Schlienger[12]	1998	Canada	Epilepsy	Serious ADRs	$3,376[e]
Moore[9]	1998	France	All	All	$11,517[f]
Liao[6]	2013	Taiwan	All	Cutaneous ADRs	$946[g]
Qing-ping[13]	2014	China	All	All Serious ADRs	$32.35[h] $1,160
Ko[7]	2014	Singapore	Oncology	ADR-related admission	$3,813[i]
HYPERSENSITIVITY REACTIONS					
Flabbee[11]	2008	France	All	Anaphylaxis	$3,121[j]
Lin[18]	2010	United States	All	Angioedema Anaphylaxis Urticaria Allergy unspecified	$8,690[k] $9,565 $6,294 $5,507
Borovicka[19]	2011	United States	Oncology	Dermatologic toxicities	$2,057[l]

TABLE 2.1
Cost of Adverse Drug Events (ADEs), Adverse Drug Reactions (ADRs), and Hypersensitivity Reactions—cont'd

Author	Year	Country	Medical Setting	Adverse Reaction Type	Cost Per Patient
Giuliani[10]	2013	Italy	Non–small cell lung cancer	Mild rash Moderate rash Severe rash	$217 to $621[m] $603 to $1,423 $633 to $1,453
Banerji[20]	2014	United States	All	Anaphylaxis emergency department visit Anaphylaxis hospitalization	$1,708[n] $14,268
Le[5]	2015	United States	Hepatitis C	Rash	$7,001[o]
Dilokthorn-sakul[25]	2016	Thailand	All	Stevens-Johnson syndrome Toxic epidermal necrolysis	$1,019 $1,660

[a]Cumulative inflation rate from 1997 to 2016 was 50.2%.
[b]Cost per ADE event; cumulative inflation rate from 1997 to 2016 was 50.2%.
[c]Cumulative inflation rate from 2003 to 2016 was 31.0%.
[d]Currency rate for Euro to USD in 2015 was 1.110; cumulative inflation rate from 2015 to 2016 was 1.7%.
[e]Cumulative inflation rate from 1998 to 2016 was 47.9%.
[f]Cost per hospital bed per year; currency rate for British Pound to USD in 1998 was 1.657; cumulative inflation rate from 1998 to 2016 was 47.9%.
[g]Cumulative inflation rate from 2013 to 2016 was 3.3%.
[h]Currency rate for Chinese Yuan to USD in 2014 was 0.162; cumulative inflation rate from 2014 to 2016 was 1.8%.
[i]Cost per admission; currency rate for Singapore dollar to USD in 2014 was 0.789; cumulative inflation rate from 2014 to 2016 was 1.8%.
[j]Currency rate from Euro to USD in 2008 was 1.471; cumulative inflation rate from 2008 to 2016 was 12.0%. Direct cost for anaphylaxis was $2602 2016 USD; indirect cost was $518 USD.
[k]Cost per hospitalization; cumulative inflation rate from 2010 to 2016 was 10.5%.
[l]Cumulative inflation rate from 2011 to 2016 was 7.2%.
[m]Currency rate from Euro to USD in 2013 was 1.328; cumulative inflation rate from 2013 to 2016 was 3.5%.
[n]Cost per index event; cumulative inflation rate from 2014 to 2016 was 1.8%.
[o]Cumulative inflation rate from 2015 to 2016 was 1.7%.

Severe cutaneous adverse reactions (SCARs) are of lower incidence and prevalence but have a substantial morbidity and mortality that confer a large economic burden per case. Most patients with SJS or TEN require hospitalization, with over half (55%) admitted to a specialized unit,[21] such as an intensive care unit or burn unit. Prior studies found that the duration of hospital stay for SJS was 4–25 days, and for TEN, 17–26 days.[22,23] SJS carries a mortality rate of 1%–10% and TEN carries a mortality rate of 25%–40%.[21,24] Given these data, the estimated cost of SJS and TEN would sum to tens or even hundreds of thousands of dollars per case. However, only one prior study assessed the cost of SJS and TEN and identified a cost of $1019 and $1600, respectively, per patient.[25] This lower-cost assessment may be due to the underlying differences in healthcare costs or treatments in the country that conducted the study (Thailand).

COSTS OF OVERREPORTING ALLERGIES

Approximately 20%–35% of the US population reports at least one prior medication "allergy" (i.e., ADR).[26,27] Overreporting of inaccurate allergies to medications can adversely affect the quality of care patients receive and can also lead to unnecessary costs. The problem with overreported drug allergies is most clearly demonstrated by reviewing the impact of reporting an allergy to penicillin antibiotics.

Patients who self-report an allergy to penicillin receive broader-spectrum, and often less effective or more toxic, antimicrobial agents.[28–30] The use of alternative antibiotics to β-lactams is associated with increased treatment failures, increased ADEs, and higher rates of colonization/infection with resistant bacterial organisms, such as methicillin-resistant *Staphylococcus aureus* (MRSA).[30,31] Because as few as 1%–5% of patients who report a penicillin allergy are truly allergic,[32] the negative downstream consequences of overreported penicillin allergy may be avoidable. Although the total economic impact of reported penicillin allergy is unknown, prior studies have assessed many components of costs related to overreported penicillin allergy.[33-38]

Pharmacy costs have been compared in patients with and without a reported penicillin allergy.[33,34,38-40] The average wholesale price for penicillins and cephalosporins is generally less than that of β-lactam alternative antibiotics (Fig. 2.2).[41,42] However, pharmacy acquisition costs vary, hospitals have distinct cost-to-charge ratios, and drug costs change as generic options become available.[43] Although studies have used different pharmacy costs in their studies, all prior studies have found the costs of antibiotics for penicillin-"allergic" patients higher than the costs of those without reported penicillin allergy,[34,38-40] with a difference from $10.53 to $581.70 per patient.[34,35,38]

In a retrospective case-cohort study of Kaiser Permanente, patients with a reported penicillin allergy had longer length of hospital stay (0.68 more days for females and 0.35 days for males) and higher infection rate from *Clostridia difficile*, Methicillin-resistant *Staphylococcus aureus* (MRSA), and vancomycin-resistant *Enterococcus*.[33] The authors estimated that treating alleged penicillin-"allergic" patients costs about 10 times as much as the cost of penicillin allergy evaluation, which they estimated would cost $133 per nurse-performed skin test.[33] Although this skin test cost estimate did not include all costs associated with material, time, personnel, and the downstream consequences from testing (e.g., adverse events that result from the testing),[44-48] large cost savings

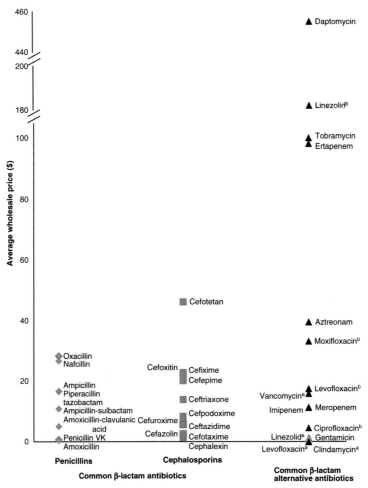

FIG. 2.2 Average wholesale price per day for a standard dose for common β-lactam and alternative antibiotics. *a*, parenteral; *b*, oral.

might be realized with a testing program, especially if penicillin allergy evaluation averts healthcare-associated infections, which cost up to $45,000 each.[36,37,49]

Because comprehensive penicillin allergy screening detects few positives, allergy evaluation methods beyond skin testing may be even more cost-effective.[32,50–52] Alternative approaches include using oral challenges (also called test doses or drug provocation testing)[53] or guidelines that use both penicillin skin testing and challenge procedures.[54] Prior studies found that oral challenge alone (i.e., without prior skin testing) leads to a cost saving, with the price of testing reduced by 35% ($69).[50] An oral challenge study for amoxicillin allergy in Canadian children demonstrated a high predictive value and saved $182,393 per year compared with full skin testing and oral challenge.[55] An inpatient guideline that used challenge doses for low-risk patients resulted in 164 fewer penicillin skin tests used and saved $60,694.[54] Simulation data similarly support that when test dose or full dose challenges can be performed safely, it is more cost-effective than a full evaluation with penicillin skin testing.[56]

COST-EFFECTIVENESS ANALYSES IN DRUG HYPERSENSITIVITY

Cost-effectiveness analyses (CEAs) are performed either using data from randomized controlled trials or using literature-based data that populate a computer simulation model.[57] The results of CEAs are generally reported as incremental cost-effective ratio (ICER), but other outcomes beyond life expectancy can also be used (e.g., cost per allergic reaction averted). The ICER is calculated from the difference in cost between two healthcare programs divided by the difference in their outcomes, presented in cost per quality-adjusted life-year (QALY).[58] In the United States, we conventionally use $50,000 per QALY as the threshold for determining interventions that are cost-effective.[59] To date, CEAs in drug hypersensitivity have been limited.

Genetic Screening in Drug Hypersensitivity

There are associations between severe HSRs and specific class I major histocompatibility complex molecules (i.e., MHC or HLA), including abacavir and HLA-B*57:01, carbamazepine and HLA-B*15:02, and allopurinol and HLA-B*58:01 as well as HLA-A*31:01. Because the prevalence of genetic traits, the cost of genetic testing, and the price of mainstream and alternative treatments vary widely across countries, regions, and ethnicities, genetic screening for severe HSRs have been studied in CEAs across different healthcare settings (Fig. 2.3). For example, HLA-B*57:01 testing before abacavir administration has been shown to be cost-effective in the United States (ICER = $41,087 per QALY), but not in Singapore ($211,764 per QALY to $942,664 per QALY), where the HLA-B*57:01 frequency varies among Chinese, Malay, and Indian populations.[60,61]

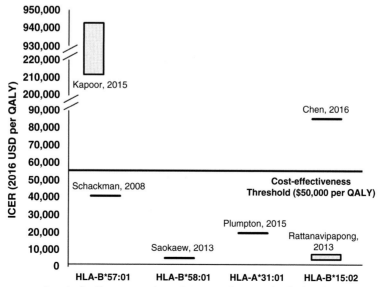

FIG. 2.3 Summary of cost-effectiveness analyses from genetic screening in drug hypersensitivity. Values or ranges of incremental cost-effectiveness ratios were represented in 2016 USD per QALY for corresponding HLA haplotype screening.[60,61,66–69] *HLA*, human leukocyte antigen; *ICER*, incremental cost-effectiveness ratio; *QALY*, quality-adjusted life-year; *USD*, United States dollar.

Aspirin Desensitization

In a CEA of aspirin desensitization for aspirin-exacerbated respiratory disease and cardiovascular protection,[62] ambulatory aspirin desensitization was cost-effective at $7,577 per QALY gained, compared with usual care. Additionally, for patients who required aspirin for cardioprotection, this analysis identified that aspirin desensitization was less expensive than usual care with $3,499 per QALY gained. This was compared with clopidogrel as alternative therapy, which was less favorable, but still cost-effective, at $11,426 per QALY gained.

SUMMARY

Adverse and hypersensitivity reactions have diverse clinical morbidity and mortality, reflected in their distinct but substantial economic burdens. For many adverse and hypersensitivity reactions, our understanding of healthcare resource utilization is still limited.

As US healthcare costs continue to increase despite no measurable improvement in health outcomes, healthcare spending must be targeted toward interventions that result in improved outcomes with fewer costs. With the passage of the Affordable Care Act and increasing formations of accountable care organizations, payment incentives will change toward adoption of the most cost-effective treatments.[63–65] Further economic analyses and CEAs related to drug allergy may help improve clinical outcomes and reduce healthcare costs.

REFERENCES

1. Bates DW, Cullen DJ, Laird N, et al. Incidence of adverse drug events and potential adverse drug events. Implications for prevention. ADE prevention study group. *JAMA.* 1995;274(1):29–34.
2. Kelly WN. Potential risks and prevention, Part 1: fatal adverse drug events. *Am J Health Syst Pharm.* 2001;58(14):1317–1324.
3. Bates DW, Spell N, Cullen DJ, et al. The costs of adverse drug events in hospitalized patients. Adverse drug events prevention study group. *JAMA.* 1997;277(4):307–311.
4. Classen DC, Pestotnik SL, Evans RS, Lloyd JF, Burke JP. Adverse drug events in hospitalized patients. Excess length of stay, extra costs, and attributable mortality. *JAMA.* 1997;277(4):301–306.
5. Le TK, Macaulay D, Kalsekar A, et al. Costs and resource utilization associated with anemia and rash in chronic hepatitis C patients treated with direct-acting antiviral agents in the United States. *Clin Ther.* 2015;37(8):1713–1725. e3.
6. Liao PJ, Shih CP, Mao CT, Deng ST, Hsieh MC, Hsu KH. The cutaneous adverse drug reactions: risk factors, prognosis and economic impacts. *Int J Clin Pract.* 2013;67(6):576–584.
7. Ko Y, Gwee YS, Huang YC, Chiang J, Chan A. Costs and length of stay of drug-related hospital admissions in cancer patients. *Clin Ther.* 2014;36(4):588–592.
8. Meier F, Maas R, Sonst A, et al. Adverse drug events in patients admitted to an emergency department: an analysis of direct costs. *Pharmacoepidemiol Drug Saf.* 2015;24(2):176–186.
9. Moore N, Lecointre D, Noblet C, Mabille M. Frequency and cost of serious adverse drug reactions in a department of general medicine. *Br J Clin Pharmacol.* 1998;45(3):301–308.
10. Giuliani J, Marzola M. The management of skin toxicity during erlotinib in advanced non-small cell lung cancer: how much does it cost? *Cutan Ocul Toxicol.* 2013;32(3):248–251.
11. Flabbee J, Petit N, Jay N, et al. The economic costs of severe anaphylaxis in France: an inquiry carried out by the allergy vigilance network. *Allergy.* 2008;63(3):360–365.
12. Schlienger RG, Oh PI, Knowles SR, Shear NH. Quantifying the costs of serious adverse drug reactions to antiepileptic drugs. *Epilepsia.* 1998;39(suppl 7):S27–S32.
13. Qing-ping S, Xiao-dong J, Feng D, et al. Consequences, measurement, and evaluation of the costs associated with adverse drug reactions among hospitalized patients in China. *BMC Health Serv Res.* 2014;14:73.
14. Aspden P, Wolcot J, Bootman JL, Cronenwett LR. *Preventing Medication Errors: Quality Chasm Series.* Washington, DC: National Academies Press; 2006. http://www.nationalacademies.org/hmd/Reports/2006/Preventing-Medication-Errors-Quality-Chasm-Series.aspx.
15. Thong BY, Tan TC. Epidemiology and risk factors for drug allergy. *Br J Clin Pharmacol.* 2011;71(5):684–700.
16. Uetrecht J, Naisbitt DJ. Idiosyncratic adverse drug reactions: current concepts. *Pharmacol Rev.* 2013;65(2):779–808.
17. Oderda GM, Evans RS, Lloyd J, et al. Cost of opioid-related adverse drug events in surgical patients. *J Pain Symptom Manage.* 2003;25(3):276–283.
18. Lin RY, Shah SN. Increasing hospitalizations due to angioedema in the United States. *Ann Allergy Asthma Immunol.* 2008;101(2):185–192.
19. Borovicka JH, Calahan C, Gandhi M, et al. Economic burden of dermatologic adverse events induced by molecularly targeted cancer agents. *Arch Dermatol.* 2011;147(12):1403–1409.
20. Banerji A, Rudders S, Clark S, Wei W, Long AA, Camargo Jr CA. Retrospective study of drug-induced anaphylaxis treated in the emergency department or hospital: patient characteristics, management, and 1-year follow-up. *J Allergy Clin Immunol Pract.* 2014;2(1):46–51.
21. Sekula P, Dunant A, Mockenhaupt M, et al. Comprehensive survival analysis of a cohort of patients with Stevens-Johnson syndrome and toxic epidermal necrolysis. *J Invest Dermatol.* 2013;133(5):1197–1204.
22. Chan HL, Stern RS, Arndt KA, et al. The incidence of erythema multiforme, Stevens-Johnson syndrome, and toxic epidermal necrolysis. A population-based study with particular reference to reactions caused by drugs among outpatients. *Arch Dermatol.* 1990;126(1):43–47.

23. Morici MV, Galen WK, Shetty AK, et al. Intravenous immunoglobulin therapy for children with Stevens-Johnson syndrome. *J Rheumatol*. 2000;27(10):2494–2497.

24. Harr T, French LE. Toxic epidermal necrolysis and Stevens-Johnson syndrome. *Orphanet J Rare Dis*. 2010;16(5):39.

25. Dilokthornsakul P, Sawangjit R, Inprasong C, et al. Healthcare utilization and cost of Stevens-Johnson syndrome and toxic epidermal necrolysis management in Thailand. *J Postgrad Med*. 2016;62(2):109–114.

26. Zhou L, Dhopeshwarkar N, Blumenthal KG, et al. Drug allergies documented in electronic health records of a large healthcare system. *Allergy*. 2016;71(9):1305–1313.

27. Macy E, Ho NJ. Multiple drug intolerance syndrome: prevalence, clinical characteristics, and management. *Ann Allergy Asthma Immunol*. 2012;108(2):88–93.

28. Picard M, Begin P, Bouchard H, et al. Treatment of patients with a history of penicillin allergy in a large tertiary-care academic hospital. *J Allergy Clin Immunol Pract*. 2013;1(3):252–257.

29. Lutomski DM, Lafollette JA, Biaglow MA, Haglund LA. Antibiotic allergies in the medical record: effect on drug selection and assessment of validity. *Pharmacotherapy*. 2008;28(11):1348–1353.

30. MacFadden DR, LaDelfa A, Leen J, et al. Impact of reported beta-lactam allergy on inpatient outcomes: a multicenter prospective cohort study. *Clin Infect Dis*. 2016. http://dx.doi.org/10.1093/cid/ciw462.

31. Baxter R, Ray GT, Fireman BH. Case-control study of antibiotic use and subsequent clostridium difficile-associated diarrhea in hospitalized patients. *Infect Control Hosp Epidemiol*. 2008;29(1):44–50.

32. Macy E, Ngor EW. Safely diagnosing clinically significant penicillin allergy using only penicilloyl-poly-lysine, penicillin, and oral amoxicillin. *J Allergy Clin Immunol Pract*. 2013;1(3):258–263.

33. Macy E, Contreras R. Health care use and serious infection prevalence associated with penicillin "allergy" in hospitalized patients: a cohort study. *J Allergy Clin Immunol*. 2014;133(3):790–796.

34. Li M, Krishna MT, Razaq S, Pillay D. A real-time prospective evaluation of clinical pharmaco-economic impact of diagnostic label of 'penicillin allergy' in a UK teaching hospital. *J Clin Pathol*. 2014;67(12):1088–1092.

35. King EA, Challa S, Curtin P, Bielory L. Penicillin skin testing in hospitalized patients with beta-lactam allergies: effect on antibiotic selection and cost. *Ann Allergy Asthma Immunol*. 2016;117(1):67–71.

36. Zimlichman E, Henderson D, Tamir O, et al. Health care-associated infections: a meta-analysis of costs and financial impact on the US health care system. *JAMA Intern Med*. 2013;173(22):2039–2046.

37. Stone PW, Glied SA, McNair PD, et al. CMS changes in reimbursement for HAIs: setting a research agenda. *Med Care*. 2010;48(5):433–439.

38. MacLaughlin EJ, Saseen JJ, Malone DC. Costs of beta-lactam allergies: selection and costs of antibiotics for patients with a reported beta-lactam allergy. *Arch Fam Med*. 2000;9(8):722–726.

39. Satta G, Hill V, Lanzman M, Balakrishnan I. beta-lactam allergy: clinical implications and costs. *Clin Mol Allergy*. 2013;11(1):2. http://dx.doi.org/10.1186/1476-7961-11-2.

40. Borch JE, Andersen KE, Bindslev-Jensen C. The prevalence of suspected and challenge-verified penicillin allergy in a university hospital population. *Basic Clin Pharmacol Toxicol*. 2006;98(4):357–362.

41. Kimberlin DW, Brady MT, Jackson MA, Long SS. *Red Book*American Academy of Pediatrics ; 2015. http://redbook.solutions.aap.org/book.aspx?bookid=1484.

42. Gencarelli DM. Average wholesale price for prescription drugs: is there a more appropriate pricing mechanism? *NHPF Issue Brief*. 2002;(775):1–19.

43. Riley GF. Administrative and claims records as sources of health care cost data. *Med Care*. 2009;47(7 suppl 1):S51–S55.

44. Demeere N, Stouthuysen K, Roodhooft F. Time-driven activity-based costing in an outpatient clinic environment: development, relevance and managerial impact. *Health Policy*. 2009;92(2–3):296–304.

45. Kaplan RS, Porter ME. How to solve the cost crisis in health care. *Harv Bus Rev*. 2011;89(9):46–52. 54, 56–61 passim.

46. Waago-Hansen C. How time-drive activity-based costing (TDABC) enable better use of existing resources in order to improve return on investment (ROI) in modern healthcare and hence facilitates a sustainable healthcare system. *theHealth*. 2014;5(1):3–8.

47. McLaughlin N, Burke MA, Setlur NP, et al. Time-driven activity-based costing: a driver for provider engagement in costing activities and redesign initiatives. *Neurosurg Focus*. 2014;37(5):E3.

48. Yun BJ, Prabhakar AM, Warsh J, et al. Time-driven activity-based costing in emergency medicine. *Ann Emerg Med*. 2016;67(6):765–772.

49. Council PHCCC. *The Impact of Healthcare-associated Infections in Pennsylvania 2010*; 2012. http://www.phc4.org/reports/hai/10/docs/hai2010report.pdf.

50. Ferre-Ybarz L, Salinas Argente R, Gomez Galan C, Duocastella Selvas P, Nevot Falco S. Analysis of profitability in the diagnosis of allergy to beta-lactam antibiotics. *Allergol Immunopathol (Madr)*. 2015;43(4):369–375.

51. Bourke J, Pavlos R, James I, Phillips E. Improving the effectiveness of penicillin allergy de-labeling. *J Allergy Clin Immunol Pract*. 2015;3(3). 365–334 e361.

52. Moral L, Garde J, Toral T, Fuentes MJ, Marco N. Short protocol for the study of paediatric patients with suspected betalactam antibiotic hypersensitivity and low risk criteria. *Allergol Immunopathol (Madr)*. 2011;39(6):337–341.

53. Iammatteo M, Blumenthal KG, Saff R, Long AA, Banerji A. Safety and outcomes of test doses for the evaluation of adverse drug reactions: a 5-year retrospective review. *J Allergy Clin Immunol Pract*. 2015;3(5):826–827.

54. Blumenthal KG, Shenoy ES, Varughese CA, Hurwitz S, Hooper DC, Banerji A. Impact of a clinical guideline for prescribing antibiotics to inpatients reporting penicillin

or cephalosporin allergy. *Ann Allergy Asthma Immunol.* 2015;115(4):294–300. e292.

55. Mill C, Primeau MN, Medoff E, et al. Assessing the diagnostic properties of a graded oral provocation challenge for the diagnosis of immediate and nonimmediate reactions to amoxicillin in children. *JAMA Pediatr.* 2016;170(6):e160033.

56. Phillips E, Louie M, Knowles SR, Simor AE, Oh PI. Cost-effectiveness analysis of six strategies for cardiovascular surgery prophylaxis in patients labeled penicillin allergic. *Am J Health Syst Pharm.* 2000;57(4):339–345.

57. Weinstein MC, Stason WB. Foundations of cost-effectiveness analysis for health and medical practices. *N Engl J Med.* 1977;296(13):716–721.

58. Gafni A, Birch S. Incremental cost-effectiveness ratios (ICERs): the silence of the lambda. *Soc Sci Med.* 2006;62(9):2091–2100.

59. Grosse SD. Assessing cost-effectiveness in healthcare: history of the $50,000 per QALY threshold. *Expert Rev Pharmacoecon Outcomes Res.* 2008;8(2):165–178.

60. Schackman BR, Scott CA, Walensky RP, Losina E, Freedberg KA, Sax PE. The cost-effectiveness of HLA-B*5701 genetic screening to guide initial antiretroviral therapy for HIV. *AIDS.* 2008;22(15):2025–2033.

61. Kapoor R, Martinez-Vega R, Dong D, et al. Reducing hypersensitivity reactions with HLA-B*5701 genotyping before abacavir prescription: clinically useful but is it cost-effective in Singapore? *Pharmacogenet Genomics.* 2015;25(2):60–72.

62. Shaker M, Lobb A, Jenkins P, et al. An economic analysis of aspirin desensitization in aspirin-exacerbated respiratory disease. *American Academy of Allergy.* 2008;121(1):81–87.

63. Berwick DM, Hackbarth AD. Eliminating waste in US health care. *JAMA.* 2012;307(14):1513–1516.

64. Koh HK, Sebelius KG. Promoting prevention through the affordable care act. *N Engl J Med.* 2010;363(14):1296–1299.

65. Orszag PR, Emanuel EJ. Health care reform and cost control. *N Engl J Med.* 2010;363(7):601–603.

66. Saokaew S, Tassaneeyakul W, Maenthaisong R, Chaiyakunapruk N. Cost-effectiveness analysis of HLA-B*5801 testing in preventing allopurinol-induced SJS/TEN in Thai population. *PLoS One.* 2014;9(4):e94294.

67. Plumpton CO, Yip VL, Alfirevic A, Marson AG, Pirmohamed M, Hughes DA. Cost-effectiveness of screening for HLA-A*31:01 prior to initiation of carbamazepine in epilepsy. *Epilepsia.* 2015;56(4):556–563.

68. Chen Z, Liew D, Kwan P. Real-world cost-effectiveness of pharmacogenetic screening for epilepsy treatment. *Neurology.* 2016;86(12):1086–1094.

69. Rattanavipapong W, Koopitakkajorn T, Praditsitthikorn N, Mahasirimongkol S, Teerawattananon Y. Economic evaluation of HLA-B*15:02 screening for carbamazepine-induced severe adverse drug reactions in Thailand. *Epilepsia.* 2013;54(9):1628 1638.

CHAPTER 3

Drug Allergy: Definitions and Phenotypes

KNUT BROCKOW, MD

DEFINITIONS

Adverse drug reactions (ADRs) are unwanted effects of drug administration, regardless of etiology and pathogenic mechanisms. The World Health Organization defines an ADR as a noxious, unintended, and undesired effect of a drug, which occurs at doses used in humans for diagnosis, prophylaxis, and therapy.[1,2] It should be noted that errors in drug administration or compliance, therapeutic failures, accidental poisoning, and drug abuse do not fall under this definition. ADRs occur in about 10%–20% of all hospitalized patients.[3] When a new drug is marketed, only a few patients are likely to have been exposed to it.[2] The most common pharmacologic/toxic drug-induced reactions are uncovered in the adverse event profile of a drug during this phase and during postmarketing surveillance. Typical uncovered reactions are called "predictable."

Thus, pharmacologists have proposed a classification of ADRs based on predictability into two major subtypes,[4] which is also occasionally used in the allergy literature:

1. Type A reactions, which are dose-dependent and predictable, and
2. Type B reactions, which are not dose-dependent and unpredictable.

Two other minor subtypes of chronic ADRs, which are associated with long-term therapy (e.g., dependency, carcinogenic effects), are of no relevance for drug allergy. Examples of predictable Type A reactions include (1) unwanted side effects of a drug, such as the sedating effects of an antihistamine; (2) secondary events, such as pseudomembranous colitis after antibiotic-induced alteration of the bacterial gut flora; or (3) drug interactions. Unpredictable Type B reactions do occur in only 15% of ADRs but are often severe and account for significant morbidity and mortality.[5,6] The allergy classification of ADRs into toxic reactions, which are related to the known toxic properties of the drug (corresponding mostly to pharmacologic Type B reactions) and drug hypersensitivity reactions

(DHRs) corresponding widely, but not completely, to Type B reactions, is more suitable for allergists and immunologists. DHRs are defined as objectively reproducible symptoms or signs initiated by exposure to a defined drug at a dose tolerated by normal persons.[7] This implies an unexpected occurrence depending on individual predisposition. The International Consensus on Drug Allergy (ICON) further specifies that DHRs clinically mostly resemble allergic reactions.[5] The pharmacologic and the allergy definitions are not fully congruent. DHRs may in a few cases be predictable. For example, very good predictability exists for drug reaction with eosinophilia and systemic symptoms (DRESS) syndrome to abacavir by HLA status.[8] In addition, DHRs are not really dose-independent, although they often have a very low threshold. Allergists should rather stick to the allergy classification, which is less dependent on predictability and dose-dependency.

The terms "drug allergy" and "drug hypersensitivity" are not considered interchangeable terms.[5] "From an allergist's perspective the term 'drug allergy' is typically used to describe DHRs that are immune mediated."[6] "Nonallergic drug hypersensitivity" refers to reactions in which other pathogenic mechanisms play a role.[9] These mechanisms have been described only partially, e.g., urticaria to acetylsalicylic acid because of alterations in the arachidonic acid pathway. For general communication, when an allergic drug reaction is suspected, DHR is the preferred term because true drug allergy and nonallergic DHR cannot be differentiated by the clinical picture, chronology, or the drug concerned.[5] Drug intolerance (pharmacologic toxicity of a drug given at therapeutic dosages), idiosyncratic reactions (nonimmunologic hypersensitivity that is not explicable by the pharmacologic properties of a drug), and pseudoallergy, which has been used as an alternative term to describe drug idiosyncrasy showing the typical picture of an immediate-type (IgE-mediated) allergic reaction, are included in the category of nonallergic DHR (Table 3.1; Fig. 3.1).[6,7]

TABLE 3.1
Definitions

- *Adverse drug reaction*: A harmful and unintended reaction that occurs alongside the intended principal effect of a drug, for which a causal relationship between the use of the drug and the adverse reaction is suspected except therapeutic failures, intentional overdosage, abuse of the drug, or errors in administration.

- *Drug hypersensitivity reactions*: They are objectively reproducible symptoms or signs initiated by exposure to a defined drug at a dose tolerated by a normal person. They cannot be explained by the normal toxic properties of a drug and need a special predisposition of a patient to develop a reaction. They are further subdivided into drug allergy and nonallergic drug hypersensitivity.

- *Drug allergy*: Immunologically mediated response to a drug (pharmaceutical agent and/or excipient) in a sensitized person.

- *Nonallergic drug hypersensitivity*: Drug hypersensitivity not associated with immunologic humoral or cellular sensitization, i.e., not explainable by one of the four immunologic mechanisms described by Coombs and Gell. Nonallergic drug hypersensitivity can be further subdivided into drug intolerance, drug idiosyncrasy, pseudoallergy, and PI reactions (see below).

- *Drug intolerance*: Undesirable and unexpected pharmacologic toxic effect that occurs at unusually low doses of a drug. It may be caused by underlying abnormalities of metabolism, excretion, or bioavailability of the drug.

- *Drug idiosyncrasy*: Abnormal and unexpected effect unrelated to the intended pharmacologic action of a drug. The mechanism is often unknown but the reaction is reproducible on readministration.

- *Pseudoallergy*: Drug idiosyncrasy with immediate systemic symptoms that mimic anaphylaxis but are caused by non-IgE-mediated release of mediators from mast cells and basophils.

- *Pharmacologic interaction with the drug (PI reaction)*: Nonallergic idiosyncratic reaction caused by noncovalent, HLA-dependent direct activation of a T cell receptor as an off-target effect.

Adapted from Drug allergy: an updated practice parameter. *Ann Allergy Asthma Immunol*. 2010;105:259–273 and Brockow K, Przybilla B, Aberer W, et al. Guideline for the diagnosis of drug hypersensitivity reactions: S2K-Guideline of the German Society for Allergology and Clinical Immunology (DGAKI) and the German Dermatological Society (DDG) in collaboration with the Association of German Allergologists (AeDA), the German Society for Pediatric Allergology and Environmental Medicine (GPA), the German Contact Dermatitis Research Group (DKG), the Swiss Society for Allergy and Immunology (SGAI), the Austrian Society for Allergology and Immunology (OGAI), the German Academy of Allergology and Environmental Medicine (DAAU), the German Center for Documentation of Severe Skin Reactions and the German Federal Institute for Drugs and Medical Products (BfArM). *Allergo J Int*. 2015;24:94–105.

For describing the mechanism of a DHR, the Coombs and Gell classification is still valid.[10] The majority of reactions are IgE mediated (Type I) and T cell mediated (Type IV), whereas cytotoxic (Type II) and immune complex (Type III) reactions to drugs are rare. T cell reactions have been subdivided into Type IVa to Type IVd reactions according to the regulatory mechanisms, composition of the T cell infiltrate, and mediators released.[11] An alternative nonallergic HLA-dependent noncovalent mechanism directly activating the T cell receptor as an off-target effect of the drug has been described for exanthems and named pharmacologic interaction (PI) mechanism.[11] The mechanisms of DHR are described in detail in Chapter 4.

PHENOTYPING OF DRUG HYPERSENSITIVITY REACTIONS BY CHRONOLOGY

A pretest assessment and classification of a given DHR is needed to determine the optimal evaluation and management plan. Clinical DHR can be classified according to (1) chronology, (2) clinical manifestation, and the (3) involved drug (Table 3.2), which all carry important information on probability assessment. According to the time interval between the drug intake and the onset of the clinical reaction, immediate (acute) reactions have been differentiated from nonimmediate (late) reactions.[5] Initially, immediate reactions have been defined to occur within 1 h.[12-14] In the ICON consensus, this time interval has been extended up to 6 h.[5]

Immediate reactions mostly manifest with urticaria, angioedema, or anaphylaxis and are either IgE mediated or nonallergic. Nonimmediate reactions are, in the majority of cases, different forms of exanthems and caused by an allergic type IV reaction or by the PI mechanism.[11] The typical time interval between the drug intake and the occurrence of clinical reactions is given in Table 3.3.[7] However, it is important to clearly separate the classification based on chronology from that on clinical manifestation into two different entities. As the history of the patient may be incorrect or as

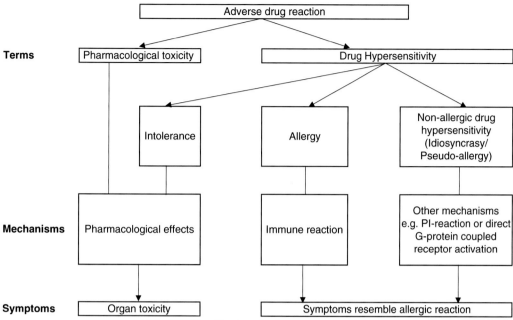

FIG. 3.1 Classification of adverse drug reactions.

TABLE 3.2
Phenotyping of Drug Hypersensitivity Reactions

Criterion	Clinical Information	Typical Time Interval Between the Start of Drug to the Onset of Reaction
1. Time interval to reaction (chronology)	a. In already sensitized patients:	
	a1. Immediate reaction (acute)	≤6 h (by definition)
	a2. Nonimmediate reaction (late)	>6 h (by definition)
	b. In de novo sensitization while on treatment: Typical sensitization latency	5–10 days
2. Clinical manifestations	a. Flushing, urticaria, angioedema, anaphylaxis	≤6 h
	b. Maculopapular exanthem, SDRIFE, fixed drug eruption, AGEP, SJS, TEN, DRESS, vasculitis	>6 h
	c. Specific symptoms: e.g., hepatitis, cytopenia, autoimmune diseases (e.g., lupus erythematosus)	>6 h
3. Mechanisms	a. Immediate: Immunologic immediate-type hypersensitivity (Type I, IgE-mediated drug allergy): typical manifestations are listed in 2.a Nonallergic immediate hypersensitivity: typical manifestation are listed in 2.a	≤6 h
	b. Nonimmediate: Immunologic delayed-type hypersensitivity: (Type IV, T cell-mediated drug allergy): typical manifestations are listed in 2.b Nonimmunologic PI reaction: typical manifestations are listed in 2.b	1–10 days (in rare cases and repeat reactions >6 h)
	c. Other immunologic hypersensitivity reactions (Type II, Type III according to Coombs and Gell, IgG-, IgA-, or IgM-mediated): cytopenias, serum sickness, allergic vasculitis	>24 h

AGEP, acute generalized exanthematous pustulosis; *DRESS*, drug reaction with eosinophilia and systemic symptoms; *PI*, pharmacologic interaction; *SDRIFE*, systemic drug-related intertriginous and flexural exanthema; *SJS*, Stevens-Johnson syndrome; *TEN*, toxic epidermal necrolysis.

TABLE 3.3
Overview of Common Clinical Phenotypes in Drug Hypersensitivity

	Primary Manifestations	Severity Sign	Time Delay[a]	Duration	Typical Elicitors
Urticaria	Single wheals or widespread urticaria, pruritus	Symptoms from other organ systems: part of anaphylaxis?	≤6 h, often <1 h	<24 h (single wheal)	NSAIDs, β-lactams, muscle relaxants, RCM, quinolones
Angioedema	Deep swelling usually on face (eyelids, lips), less often on extremities and genitals	Symptoms from other organ systems: part of anaphylaxis? Upper airway obstruction	≤6 h, often <1 h	Hours to 4 days	See above, ACE inhibitors
Anaphylaxis	Multiorgan involvement of the skin, gut, respiratory, and/or cardiovascular tract	Hypotension, tachycardia, unconsciousness, dyspnea, wheezing: respiratory or cardiovascular involvement	≤6 h, often <1 h	Typically <1–2 h	See above (urticaria)
Maculopapular exanthem	Macules, papules often on the trunk, pruritus	May be accompanied by mild fever and eosinophilia	4–14 days	1–2 weeks	β-lactams, other antibiotics, RCM, anticonvulsants
SDRIFE	Macules, papules in intertriginous areas, pruritus, later scaling	May be accompanied by mild fever and eosinophilia	4–14 days	1–2 weeks	Aminopenicillins
Fixed drug eruption	Erythematous plaque, violaceous/hyperpigmented, single or multiple lesions	Blister may be present. Generalized bullous fixed drug eruption	30 min to 2 days	Weeks	NSAIDs, sulfonamides, tetracyclines
Vasculitis	Purpuric papules primarily on lower extremities	Necrotizing lesions. Systemic involvement (especially kidney, GI)	7–21 days	Weeks	NSAIDs, antibiotics, diuretics
AGEP	Pustules on edematous erythema often in intertriginous areas, later scaling	Fever, neutrophilia, leukocytosis	1–2 days (antibiotics) 4–14 days (others)	Weeks	β-lactams, pristinamycin, quinolones, chloroquine
DRESS	Widespread macules, papules, often on the trunk, edematous face, fever, eosinophilia, lymphadenopathy, hepatitis, other organ involvement	Severe hepatitis, myocarditis, interstitial pneumonitis, nephritis, thyroiditis, arthritis	2–8 weeks	Weeks to months	Anticonvulsants, allopurinol, sulfonamides, minocycline, nevirapine, dapsone
SJS	Dusky red lesions, atypical confluent target lesions, blisters, <10% of skin detached, fever, mucosae involved	Progression to TEN, severe systemic symptoms, visceral organ involvement, high fever	4–42 days	Weeks to months	Anticonvulsants, sulfonamides, allopurinol, NSAIDs
TEN	See SJS, >30% of skin detached	Severe systemic symptoms, visceral organ involvement, renal insufficiency, high fever	4–42 days	Weeks to months	Allopurinol, sulfonamides, anticonvulsants, oxicam NSAIDs

TABLE 3.3
Overview of Common Clinical Phenotypes in Drug Hypersensitivity—cont'd

	Primary Manifestations	Severity Sign	Time Delay[a]	Duration	Typical Elicitors
Others	Anemia, or leukopenia, or thrombocytopenia, or drug fever, or drug hepatitis or drug-induced lupus	Dyspnea, infection, bleeding, visceral organ involvement	Variable	Variable	β-lactams, others

AGEP, acute generalized exanthematous pustulosis; *DRESS*, drug reaction with eosinophilia and systemic symptoms; *NSAIDs*, nonsteroidal antiinflammatory drugs; *RCM*, radiocontrast media; *SDRIFE*, systemic drug-related intertriginous and flexural exanthema; *SJS*, Stevens-Johnson syndrome; *TEN*, toxic epidermal necrolysis.
[a]From the start of drug use to the onset of reaction.

rare exceptions may occur, anaphylaxis 7 h after the last drug intake would be classified as nonimmediate, even though an immediate-type (IgE-mediated) mechanism might be involved. Drugs typically inducing immediate, nonimmediate, or both reactions are known. The most common immune elicitors are given in the following section on clinical phenotypes and in Table 3.3.

PHENOTYPING OF DRUG HYPERSENSITIVITY REACTIONS BY CLINICAL MANIFESTATIONS

Clinical Phenotypes Often Associated With Immediate (Acute) Drug Hypersensitivity Reactions and typical elicitors

The following phenotypes are seen in the majority of cases associated with immediate acute DHRs (Table 3.3).

Urticaria and angioedema

Urticaria is a common skin eruption characterized by wheals usually associated with pruritus.[15,16] A wheal is a transient flat or elevated, pale-red macula caused by edema and vasodilatation in the upper part of the dermis. It measures from millimeters up to several centimeters. Lesions typically appear within few minutes to hours after drug intake. The number, size, and shape of lesions vary widely. A single lesion usually resolves within 24 h at one location. However, an outbreak of urticaria with migrating and changing lesions may last several days to weeks.

Angioedema is a pale or erythematous swelling, affecting mainly the face, lips, tongue, oral mucosa, male genitalia, hands, and feet because of a deeper edema of the dermis. When the larynx or pharynx is involved, a life-threatening situation may develop. Angioedema causes less itching; patients rather report a feeling of pressure. The evolution is slower than urticaria and may last up

several days if bradykinin is involved days. Urticaria or angioedema is often elicited by acetylsalicylic acid and other nonsteroidal antiinflammatory drugs, β-lactam antibiotics, muscle relaxants, radiocontrast media, quinolones, and other antibiotics.[17,18] Those drugs are also the most common elicitors for anaphylaxis. Specifically for angioedema, ACE inhibitor-induced reactions are quite common and may develop even years after the start of intake, which is an exception from the rule that urticaria, angioedema, and anaphylaxis are mostly immediate (acute) reactions.

Anaphylaxis

Anaphylaxis involves more than one organ out of the skin, gastrointestinal tract, respiratory system, and cardiovascular system. The clinical presentation may be variable. Often, the reaction starts with the skin manifestations of pruritus, urticaria, and/or angioedema. Additionally, the gastrointestinal tract may be involved with nausea, abdominal pain, vomiting, and/or diarrhea. Typical respiratory tract involvement may be rhinoconjunctivitis, dyspnea, wheezing, and coughing. Cardiovascular events include a drop of blood pressure, tachycardia, fainting, and unconsciousness. Severe respiratory and cardiovascular manifestations may be the primary manifestations in perioperative anaphylaxis.

Clinical Phenotypes Often Associated With Nonimmediate (Late) Drug Hypersensitivity Reactions and typical elicitors

In nonimmediate (late) hypersensitivity reactions, exanthems are the most common presentations (Table 3.3). An exanthem is a rapidly erupting widespread rash. This has been first described by the ancient Greeks as a specific sign of an infectious disease, such as measles, chicken pox, or rubella, but nowadays, it is also a common manifestation of a DHR. Also, some skin diseases or autoimmune diseases can be exanthematic in their appearance. The majority of drug-induced exanthems are maculopapular. However, vesicular, pustular, bullous, lichenoid, and other lesions may develop in an exanthem. The following entities are recognized and associated with nonimmediate DHRs.

Maculopapular exanthem

The most frequent DHRs are benign maculopapular exanthems (MPEs) often reported as "drug rashes" or "drug eruptions."[18] They are the most common cutaneous DHRs and observed in 2% of hospitalized patients.[19] MPEs usually appear between 4 and 14 days after a new drug has been started; however, in a sensitized individual, initial symptoms already may appear as early as about 6 h and develop into a typical exanthem after 1 or 2 days. Occurrence of a MPE a few days after the drug intake has been stopped is also possible. Erythematous macules and infiltrated papules are the primary lesions. The trunk and the proximal extremities are most often involved in a symmetric distribution. However, widespread exanthems may generalize, become confluent, and develop into an erythroderma. Typically, there is no scaling in the early phase but in the later clearing phase, desquamation is common. Mucous membranes are normally not involved. Pruritus is typical, and low-grade fever may occur. Exanthems are caused by T cell-mediated (Type IV) drug hypersensitivity or by the PI mechanism.[11] Common elicitors of MPEs are β-lactam antibiotics, other antibiotics, sulfonamides, radiocontrast media, and antiepileptic drugs.

Symmetric drug-related intertriginous and flexural exanthem

A special pattern of a maculopapular exanthem with a characteristic distribution pattern, involving flexural and intertriginous areas, is called symmetric drug-related intertriginous and flexural exanthem (SDRIFE).[20] Typically, a sharply delineated erythema of the perigenital and perianal area, as well as the axillae and other intertriginous folds, is seen. Males are more often affected than females. Few pustules may be observed and there may be an overlap with acute generalized exanthematous pustulosis. The patients are generally well without systemic symptoms and signs. Postexanthematous desquamation is often seen. Main elicitors of SDRIFE are aminopenicillins.

Acute generalized exanthematous pustulosis

Disseminated nonfollicular small sterile pustules on a widespread confluating exanthem are the mainstay of acute generalized exanthematous pustulosis.[21,22] Intertriginous areas and the trunk are often involved. Several pustules may become confluent and form large, very superficial, bullous or pustular lesions. Clearing of these lesions is associated with extensive scaling. Patients do have fever and leukocytosis with neutrophilia and often eosinophilia. Typical elicitors are aminopenicillins and cephalosporins. A reaction develops after 1–2 days of systemic intake of aminopenicillins and needs longer time intervals for most other drugs, e.g., diltiazem.

Bullous exanthems

Small isolated vesicles and pustules may develop in any MPE. The more severe bullous entities are called Stevens-Johnson syndrome (SJS) and toxic epidermal necrolysis (TEN).[23] Both are differentiated from erythema exsudativum multiforme by the absence of typical target lesions: Erythema exsudativum multiforme is mainly caused by viral infections, whereas SJS and TEN are in the majority of cases caused by drugs. SJS and TEN start within the first 4–6 weeks of treatment with small blisters arising on purple (multiform) macules. Lesions are widespread and usually predominant on the trunk, causing painful skin. Bullous lesions develop fast, often within 12 h, on the skin and on mucous membranes (oral, genital, conjunctival, perianal). Atypical flat multiform target lesions are often present. Patients are severely ill and often develop fever. The area of confluated bullae leading to detachment of the skin is <10% (as calculated in burns) of the total body surface in SJS, 10%–30% in SJS/TEN overlap, and >30% in TEN. Nicolsky's sign is positive. Lethality is dependent on age, the extent of skin detachment, and how early the culprit drug was stopped. A prognostic score has been published assessing severity.[24] Typical drugs to induce SJS and TEN are allopurinol, bacterial sulfonamides, oxicam NSAIDs, nevirapine, and antiepileptics.[21]

Drug reaction with eosinophilia and systemic symptoms

DRESS is a severe skin reaction also involving internal organs.[25] Erythematous central facial swelling is typical and often an early sign. The presentation of the rash may vary from typical macules and papules to multiform, eczematous, or purpuriform lesions. Fever, malaise, and lymphadenopathy are mostly present. In the peripheral blood, eosinophilia, leukocytosis, and atypical lymphocytes are often found persisting for several days. Agranulocytosis and anemia may occur. Concerning further involvement of other internal organs, hepatitis and an elevation of liver enzymes or nephritis are most commonly found. Other visceral organ involvement, such as arthritis, myositis, or pneumonitis, is less often seen. A validation score has been published, which may aid in the diagnosis.[25] The exanthem typically starts relatively late, 2–12 weeks after the start of treatment. Lethality is about 2% and often related to liver failure. Even after the discontinuation of drug treatment, further flares are common. This has been linked to reactivation of herpesviruses (human herpesvirus 6, Epstein-Barr Virus, cytomegalovirus), which is commonly detected in DRESS. Common eliciting drugs for DRESS are not only antiepileptics, such as carbamazepine, lamotrigine, phenobarbital, and phenytoin, but also allopurinol, minocycline, sulfonamides and nevirapine.

Fixed drug eruption
Fixed drug eruption manifests with a characteristic erythematous to violatious, sometimes edematous, macule or plaque, which may become bullous in the center. This lesion always occurs at the same localization in less than 2 days on reexposure to the culprit drug. The lesion heals typically leaving a residual hyperpigmentation. Sometimes multilocular fixed drug eruptions do occur. If they are bullous, they are called generalized bullous fixed drug eruption (GBFDE). In contrast to patients with SJS/TEN, patients with GBFDE have no systemic symptoms, the lesions are well demarcated, and the mucous membranes are rarely or only minimally involved.[26] NSAIDs, tetracyclines, sulfonamides, antibiotics, and phenytoin are common elicitors for fixed drug eruptions.

Vasculitis
Hypersensitivity vasculitis is a quite typical manifestation in dermatology. Histologically, it is characterized by leukocytoclastic vasculitis and clinically by palpable purpuric macules and papules predominantly in the dependent areas, particularly on the legs. Hemorrhagia, blister formation, and ulcerations may develop. Vasculitis is only rarely elicited by drugs. However, nonsteroidal antiinflammatory drugs, sulfonamide antibiotics, and diuretics are among the drugs that have been reported to elicit drug-induced vasculitis. Discontinuation of the culprit drug is mandatory. Other forms of systemic vasculitis have to be differentiated.

Organ-specific and miscellaneous drug reactions
If fever is the only manifestation of a DHR, it is called drug fever.[27] Headaches and myalgias may be present. Several drugs have been described to elicit isolated drug fever, e.g., antibiotics, sulfonamides, and cytostatics.

General symptoms, such as fever, malaise, headaches, and fatigue, may be associated with other DHRs. Internal organ affections mostly involve circulating blood cells and the liver. Eosinophilia is common in DHRs. IgG-mediated cytopenia or cytotoxic immune cytopenia occur and may manifest as hemolytic anemia, leukocytopenia, or thrombocytopenia. Drug-induced hepatitis is a well-described entity.[28] More rarely, interstitial nephritis can be caused by drugs. Lymphadenopathy, pneumonitis, pancreatitis, myocarditis, thyroiditis, and gastrointestinal tract involvement has been observed in few patients. Fever, arthralgias, macular or urticarial exanthems and lymphadenopathy are typical for an entity named serum sickness syndrome. In the past, it has been commonly seen 1–3 weeks after the administration of heterologous serum. Currently, it is mainly reported after the use of penicillins and cephalosporins (particularly cephachlor) after a latency period of 6–8 h.

Drug-induced autoimmune disease
Drugs can induce autoimmune responses, such as those seen in patients with prolonged DRESS syndrome. It also may lead to drug-induced lupus erythematosus characterized by the sudden onset of fever, malaise, myalgia, arthralgia, and sometimes erythematous macules on light-exposed skin with or without atrophy and scaling.[29] Skin lesions may resemble typical lupus erythematosus lesions. Antinuclear antibodies are commonly positive and directed against nuclear histone H2B for drug-induced systemic lupus, whereas anti-Ro/SSA and anti-La/SSB are more common in cutaneous drug-induced lupus. Many elicitors of drug-induced lupus have been reported, such as TNF-blockers, interferons, and terbinafine.[30]

REFERENCES
1. International drug monitoring: the role of national centres. Report of a WHO meeting. *World Health Organ Tech Rep Ser*. 1972;498:1–25.
2. Bousquet PJ, Demoly P, Romano A, et al. Pharmacovigilance of drug allergy and hypersensitivity using the ENDA-DAHD database and the GALEN platform. The Galenda project. *Allergy*. 2009;64:194–203.
3. Gomes ER, Demoly P. Epidemiology of hypersensitivity drug reactions. *Curr Opin Allergy Clin Immunol*. 2005;5:309–316.
4. Rawlins MD, Thompson JW. Mechanisms of adverse drug reactions. In: Davies DM, ed. *Textbook of Adverse Drug Reactions*. Oxford: Oxford University Press; 1991:18–45.
5. Demoly P, Adkinson NF, Brockow K, et al. International Consensus on drug allergy. *Allergy*. 2014;69:420–437.

6. Drug allergy: an updated practice parameter. *Ann Allergy Asthma Immunol.* 2010;105:259–273.

7. Brockow K, Przybilla B, Aberer W, et al. Guideline for the diagnosis of drug hypersensitivity reactions: S2K-Guideline of the German Society for Allergology and Clinical Immunology (DGAKI) and the German Dermatological Society (DDG) in collaboration with the Association of German Allergologists (AeDA), the German Society for Pediatric Allergology and Environmental Medicine (GPA), the German Contact Dermatitis Research Group (DKG), the Swiss Society for Allergy and Immunology (SGAI), the Austrian Society for Allergology and Immunology (OGAI), the German Academy of Allergology and Environmental Medicine (DAAU), the German Center for Documentation of Severe Skin Reactions and the German Federal Institute for Drugs and Medical Products (BfArM). *Allergo J Int.* 2015;24:94–105.

8. Phillips EJ, Chung WH, Mockenhaupt M, Roujeau JC, Mallal SA. Drug hypersensitivity: pharmacogenetics and clinical syndromes. *J Allergy Clin Immunol.* 2011;127(suppl 3):S60–S66.

9. Johansson SG, Bieber T, Dahl R, et al. Revised nomenclature for allergy for global use: Report of the Nomenclature Review Committee of the World Allergy Organization. *J Allergy Clin Immunol.* October 2003;2004(113):832–836.

10. Gell P, Coombs R. The classification of allergic reactions underlying disease. In: Gell P, Coombs R, eds. *Clinical Aspects of Immunology.* Oxford: Blackwell Science; 1963.

11. Pichler WJ. Delayed drug hypersensitivity reactions. *Ann Intern Med.* 2003;139:683–693.

12. Brockow K, Romano A, Blanca M, Ring J, Pichler W, Demoly P. General considerations for skin test procedures in the diagnosis of drug hypersensitivity. *Allergy.* 2002;57:45–51.

13. Torres MJ, Blanca M, Fernandez J, et al. Diagnosis of immediate allergic reactions to beta-lactam antibiotics. *Allergy.* 2003;58:961–972.

14. Romano A, Blanca M, Torres MJ, et al. Diagnosis of non-immediate reactions to beta-lactam antibiotics. *Allergy.* 2004;59:1153–1160.

15. Goldsmith L, Katz S, Gilchrest B, Paller A, Leffell D, Wolff K. *Fitzpatrick's Dermatology in General Medicine.* 8th ed. Columbus, OH, USA: Mc Graw Hill Education; 2012.

16. Bircher AJ. Uncomplicated drug-induced disseminated exanthemas. *Chem Immunol Allergy.* 2012;97:79–97.

17. Schnyder B. Approach to the patient with drug allergy. *Med Clin North Am.* 2010;94:665–679.

18. Roujeau JC. Clinical heterogeneity of drug hypersensitivity. *Toxicology.* 2005;209:123–129.

19. Fiszenson-Albala F, Auzerie V, Mahe E, et al. A 6-month prospective survey of cutaneous drug reactions in a hospital setting. *Br J Dermatol.* 2003;149:1018–1022.

20. Hausermann P, Bircher AJ. SDRIFE - another acronym for a distinct cutaneous drug exanthema: do we really need it? *Dermatology.* 2007;214:1–2.

21. Paulmann M, Mockenhaupt M. Severe drug-induced skin reactions: clinical features, diagnosis, etiology, and therapy. *J Dtsch Dermatol Ges.* 2015;13:625–645.

22. Sidoroff A, Dunant A, Viboud C, et al. Risk factors for acute generalized exanthematous pustulosis (AGEP)-results of a multinational case-control study (EuroSCAR). *Br J Dermatol.* 2007;157:989–996.

23. Bastuji-Garin S, Rzany B, Stern RS, Shear NH, Naldi L, Roujeau JC. Clinical classification of cases of toxic epidermal necrolysis, Stevens-Johnson syndrome, and erythema multiforme. *Arch Dermatol.* 1993;129:92–96.

24. Bastuji-Garin S, Fouchard N, Bertocchi M, Roujeau JC, Revuz J, Wolkenstein P. SCORTEN: a severity-of-illness score for toxic epidermal necrolysis. *J Invest Dermatol.* 2000;115:149–153.

25. Kardaun SH, Sekula P, Valeyrie-Allanore L, et al. Drug reaction with eosinophilia and systemic symptoms (DRESS): an original multisystem adverse drug reaction. Results from the prospective RegiSCAR study. *Br J Dermatol.* 2013;169:1071–1080.

26. Lipowicz S, Sekula P, Ingen-Housz-Oro S, et al. Prognosis of generalized bullous fixed drug eruption: comparison with Stevens-Johnson syndrome and toxic epidermal necrolysis. *Br J Dermatol.* 2013;168:726–732.

27. Johnson DH, Cunha BA. Drug fever. *Infect Dis Clin North Am.* 1996;10:85–91.

28. Podevin P, Biour M. Drug-induced "allergic hepatitis". *Clin Rev Allergy Immunol.* 1995;13:223–244.

29. Rubin RL. Drug-induced lupus. *Expert Opin Drug Saf.* 2015;14:361–378.

30. Lowe GC, Henderson CL, Grau RH, Hansen CB, Sontheimer RD. A systematic review of drug-induced subacute cutaneous lupus erythematosus. *Br J Dermatol.* 2011;164:465–472.

CHAPTER 4

Immune Mechanisms of Drug Allergy

KATIE D. WHITE, MD, PHD • KATHERINE KONVINSE, MSC • RANNAKOE
LEHLOENYA, MD • ALEC REDWOOD, PHD • ELIZABETH J. PHILLIPS, MD

KEY POINTS

- Many adverse drug reactions (ADRs) are not predictable based solely on the pharmacologic action of the drug.
- We now know that these reactions stem from specific off-target drug activity that includes the interaction of drugs with immune receptors and pharmacologic drug effects such as those seen in non-IgE-mediated mast cell activation syndrome
- Some reactions that display a clinical phenotype consistent with an immunologically mediated reaction, such as anaphylaxis, angioedema, urticaria, maculopapular exanthema, fever, and internal organ involvement (e.g., hepatitis), are related to an adaptive immune response and are associated with immunologic memory.
- These reactions encompass a number of phenotypically distinct clinical diagnoses that comprise both B cell–mediated (antibody-mediated, Gell-Coombs Types I–III) and purely T cell–mediated reactions (Gell-Coombs Type IV).

INTRODUCTION

Adverse drug reactions (ADRs) are major causes of iatrogenic, and potentially preventable, patient morbidity and mortality. These reactions are the source of approximately 3%–6% of inpatient admissions, are estimated to be the fourth most common cause of death, and comprise 5%–10% of inpatient costs that total over $4 billion annually in the United States alone.[1-4] Many ADRs are not predictable based solely on the pharmacologic action of the drug, and we now know that these reactions stem from specific off-target drug activity that includes the interaction of drugs with immune receptors and pharmacologic drug effects such as those seen in non-IgE-mediated mast cell activation syndrome (Fig. 4.1). Some reactions that display a clinical phenotype consistent with an immunologically mediated reaction, such as anaphylaxis, angioedema, urticaria, maculopapular exanthema, fever, and internal organ involvement (e.g., hepatitis), are related to an adaptive immune response and are associated with immunologic memory. These encompass a number of phenotypically distinct clinical diagnoses that comprise both B cell–mediated (antibody-mediated, Gell-Coombs Types I–III) and purely T cell–mediated reactions (Gell-Coombs Type IV).

Gell-Coombs Classification of Immune-Mediated Adverse Drug Reactions

According to the Gell and Coombs schema, developed in 1963, drug hypersensitivity reactions are classified into four types based on the immune mediators of disease. This mechanism-based classification system is still widely used today.

Type I, also known as immediate, hypersensitivity reactions, typically occurs within 30–60 min, but can occur within seconds, of drug exposure, depending on the mode of drug administration. On the first exposure to the implicated drug, drug-specific IgE antibodies are formed and bind to Fcε receptors on the surface of mast cells and basophils. Later exposure to the same drug results in cross-linking of cell-bound antibodies on the mast cells and basophils, leading to cell degranulation and the release of histamine, leukotriene, prostaglandin, and a variety of other immune mediators (Fig. 4.2). The principal effects of these products are vasodilation, increased vessel permeability, smooth muscle contraction, and leukocyte extravasation into tissues, resulting in clinical features ranging from irritating (pruritus) to life-threatening (anaphylaxis). Urticarial rash, flushing, angioedema, and gastrointestinal symptoms are also typical of Type I hypersensitivity reactions. Drugs commonly associated with Type I hypersensitivity reactions include antimicrobials, neuromuscular blocking agents, some NSAIDS, proton pump inhibitors, insulin, and chimeric monoclonal antibodies. These reactions are associated with immunologic memory; however, immune responses are lost over time. For instance, for patients with a history of IgE-mediated hypersensitivity to

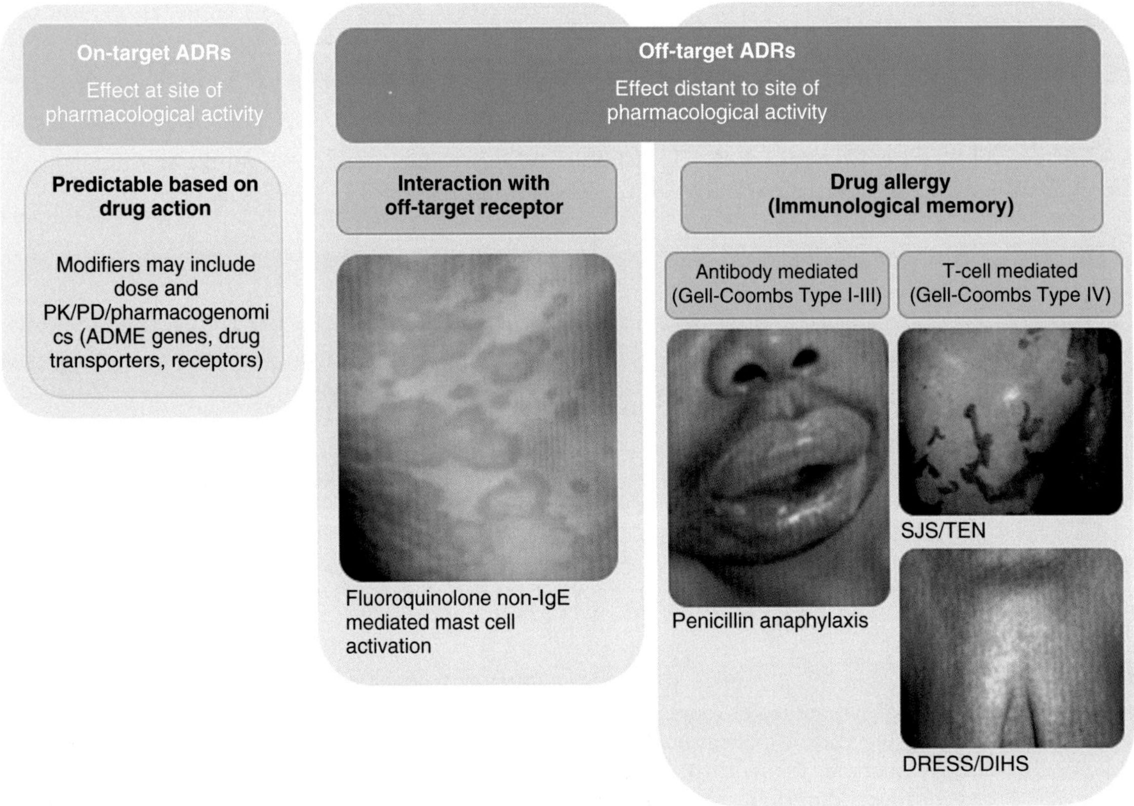

FIG. 4.1 **Classification of Adverse Drug Reactions (ADRs).** ADRs may result from either on-target or off-target interactions between the drug and cellular proteins. On-target adverse effects, traditionally referred to as Type A reactions, account for the majority of ADRs (≥80%) and are generally predictable based on the pharmacology of the drug. Variation in the cellular processes that modulate drug absorption, distribution, metabolism, and excretion (ADME); drug transporters; target receptor expression; and drug dosing or administration errors contribute to ADRs that are primarily mediated by pharmacologic mechanisms. Although off-target adverse effects account for a smaller proportion of total ADRs (≤20%), the cost, morbidity, and mortality associated with these reactions is significant. Off-target reactions may occur by both nonimmune-mediated and immune-mediated mechanisms. For example, the non-IgE-mediated mast cell activation syndrome, which phenotypically resembles anaphylaxis, has recently been shown in a murine model to result from off-target binding of drug to G protein–coupled receptors without the involvement of the adaptive immune system.[8] The immune-mediated ADRs include both B cell/antibody and T cell–mediated reactions (Type I–IV reactions according to the Gell-Coombs schema). It should be noted that all ADRs are dose-dependent although the degree to which drug concentration contributes to phenotype varies for individual reactions. (Adapted from Peter JG, Lehloenyz R, Dlamini S, Risma K, White KD, Konvinse KC, Phillips EJ. Severe delayed cutaneous and systemic reactions to drugs: a global perspective on the Science and Art of Current Practice. *J Allergy Clin Immunol Prac.* 2017;5(3):547–563.)

β-lactam antibiotics, as determined by clinical history and skin test reactivity, approximately 10% of patients per year will lose skin test reactivity to penicillins and other β-lactams.[5,6] Lack of reexposure to the implicated drug may explain some of this phenomenon, but it has also been observed that resensitization to the drug is uncommon even in the setting of repeat exposure.[7] The term "pseudoallergic" or "anaphylactoid" is used

to describe reactions that appear clinically similar to Type I hypersensitivity reactions but are not mediated by cross-linking of IgE antibodies. These reactions may be triggered by peptidergic drugs such as ciprofloxacin signaling through a specific mast cell–related G protein–coupled receptor.[8]

Type II hypersensitivities are IgG or IgM (non-IgE) antibody–mediated reactions, which typically occur

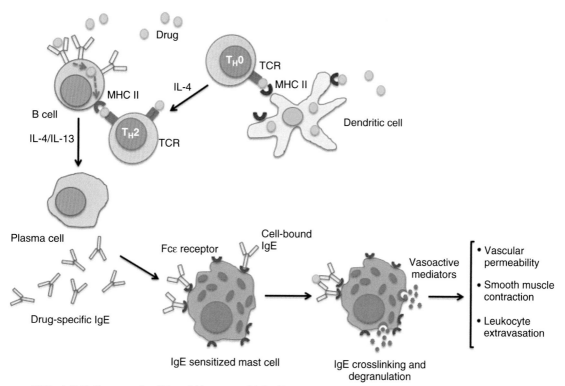

FIG. 4.2 **Pathogenesis of Type I Hypersensitivity Reactions.** In Type I hypersensitivity reactions, dendritic cells bind and internalize drug antigen for presentation to T_H0 (naïve) CD4+ T cells. In the presence of IL-4, the naïve T cell develops into a drug-specific T_H2 cell. Drug antigen is processed by the B cell and is presented to the drug-specific T_H2 cells. T_H2 cells produce cytokines (IL-4, IL-13) that induce B cell differentiation into a plasma cell that secretes drug-specific IgE. Soluble IgE then binds to $Fc\varepsilon$ receptors on the surface of mast cells and basophils. A second encounter with drug induces cross-linking of cell surface–bound IgE antibodies to induce mast cell degranulation with the release of soluble mediators that cause vascular permeability, smooth muscle contraction, and leukocyte extravasation into tissues.

minutes to several hours after drug exposure. These reactions occur when IgG or IgM antibodies bind cell surface–associated drug or drug metabolite. These antibody-coated cells are recognized and killed by innate immune cells, such as natural killer (NK) cells, monocytes, and macrophages, which bind to the target cells via the Fc region of the antibody. Clinically, Type II hypersensitivities may present as drug-induced hemolytic anemia (some β-lactam antibiotics, quinidine, α-methyldopa), thrombocytopenia (quinine, acetaminophen, vancomycin, and sulfonamide antibiotics), or granulocytopenia (some anticonvulsants, pyrazolone drugs, thiouracil, sulfonamides, and phenothiazines).

Type III, also known as immune complex, hypersensitivity reactions occur when an antibody (IgG > IgM) binds to a soluble antigen (often a drug or a drug metabolite), forming a circulating immune complex, which can deposit into small vessels, joints, and renal glomeruli, resulting in serum sickness reactions. These small immune complexes induce complement fixation and unlike larger immune complexes are not cleared from the circulation by macrophages. Clinically, these reactions are characterized by fever, lymphadenopathy, urticaria, joint pain, and proteinuria. Drugs known to cause Type III hypersensitivity reactions include penicillins, cephalosporins, sulfonamides, trimethoprim–sulfamethoxazole, ciprofloxacin, tetracycline, lincomycin, NSAIDS, and carbamazepine.

Type IV, also known as delayed, hypersensitivities are T cell–mediated reactions that occur days to weeks after drug initiation. The clinically relevant T cell–mediated drug reactions are collectively referred to as the drug hypersensitivity syndromes (DHSs) and have been classified into delayed exanthema without systemic symptoms (maculopapular eruption or MPE), contact dermatitis, drug-induced hypersensitivity syndrome (DIHS)/drug reaction with eosinophilia and systemic symptoms (DRESS), Stevens-Johnson syndrome/toxic epidermal necrolysis (SJS/TEN), acute generalized exanthematous pustulosis (AGEP), fixed drug eruption, and single organ involvement pathologies such as drug-induced liver disease (DILI) and pancreatitis.[9,10] In general, these reactions result from drug interaction with immune receptors involved in T cell immune activation, leading to aberrant CD4+ or CD8+ T cell immune responses. The rest of this chapter will focus on the immunopathogenesis of Type IV delayed hypersensitivity drug reactions with particular reference to SJS/TEN, DRESS/DIHS, and a unique, systemic T cell–mediated DHS termed the abacavir hypersensitivity syndrome (AHS).

THE IMMUNOPATHOGENESIS OF T CELL–MEDIATED DRUG HYPERSENSITIVITY SYNDROME: ESTABLISHED MODELS

The role of T cells as pathogenic mediators of many DHSs has been firmly established. As described in Chapter 5, many Type IV DHSs are strongly associated with variation in the class I and class II HLA genetic loci, which encode the restricting elements for CD8+ and CD4+ T cells, respectively. Three nonmutually exclusive models describe how a small-molecule pharmaceutical might interact with immune proteins to elicit T cell reactivity. These are the hapten/prohapten model, the pharmacologic interaction (p-i) model, and the altered peptide repertoire model (Fig. 4.3).

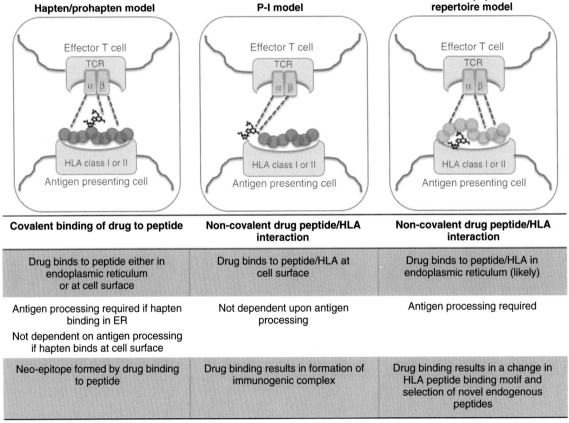

Hapten/prohapten model	P-I model	Altered peptide repertoire model
Covalent binding of drug to peptide	**Non-covalent drug peptide/HLA interaction**	**Non-covalent drug peptide/HLA interaction**
Drug binds to peptide either in endoplasmic reticulum or at cell surface	Drug binds to peptide/HLA at cell surface	Drug binds to peptide/HLA in endoplasmic reticulum (likely)
Antigen processing required if hapten binding in ER Not dependent on antigen processing if hapten binds at cell surface	Not dependent upon antigen processing	Antigen processing required
Neo-epitope formed by drug binding to peptide	Drug binding results in formation of immunogenic complex	Drug binding results in a change in HLA peptide binding motif and selection of novel endogenous peptides

FIG. 4.3 **Models of T Cell Activation by Small Molecules.** Three models have been proposed to explain T cell stimulation by small-molecule pharmaceuticals. The hapten/prohapten model postulates that the drug binds covalently to peptide (either in the intracellular environment before peptide processing and presentation or at the cell surface) to generate a neoantigen that stimulates a T cell response. The p-i model proposes that a small molecule may bind to HLA in a noncovalent manner to directly stimulate T cells. The altered peptide model postulates that a small molecule can bind noncovalently to the MHC binding cleft to alter the specificity of peptide binding. This results in the presentation of novel peptide ligands to elicit an immune response.

For DHSs that adhere to the hapten/prohapten model, the drug or drug metabolite binds covalently to an endogenous protein that then undergoes intracellular processing to generate a pool of chemically modified peptides. When presented in the context of HLA proteins, these modified peptides will be recognized as "foreign" by T cells and elicit an immune response.[11,12] Examples of DHS that are associated with hapten modification of endogenous proteins include the binding of penicillin derivatives to serum albumin[13] and protein modification by the nitroso-sulfamethoxazole.[14]

Under the p-i model, the offending drug is postulated to bind noncovalently to either the T cell receptor (TCR) or HLA protein in a peptide-independent manner to directly activate T cells. This model has been hypothesized to explain in vitro T cell reactivity that is labile (i.e., reactivity is abrogated by washing drug from the surface of antigen presenting cells [APCs]) and/or is observed within seconds of drug exposure, a time course too short to require intracellular antigen processing.[15,16]

In DHSs that adhere to the altered peptide repertoire model, the offending drug occupies a position in the peptide-binding groove of the HLA protein, thereby changing the chemistry of the binding cleft and the peptide specificity of HLA peptide presentation. It is proposed that peptides presented in this context are recognized as "foreign" by the immune system and therefore elicit a T cell response.[17,18]

Stevens-Johnson Syndrome and Toxic Epidermal Necrolysis

SJS and TEN are two of the most severe immune mediated ADRs (IM-ADRs) with an estimated patient mortality rate over 30% at 1 year following the disease onset.[19] Cardinal features of SJS/TEN include widespread epidermal necrosis, resembling a severe burn injury and manifesting clinically with skin, mucous membrane, and eye involvement (Fig. 4.1). SJS/TEN is considered to be a disease with a cohesive immunopathogenesis and is defined by the percentage of body surface area (BSA) involvement (SJS: 10% BSA affected; SJS/TEN overlap: 10%–30% BSA affected; TEN: >30% BSA affected). Internal organ failure and secondary complications such as infection, thrombosis, and deconditioning are frequently associated with SJS/TEN. Furthermore, the long-term sequelae of this disease, including scarring, blindness, and psychiatric illness, are a source of significant disability for survivors. Multiple studies have demonstrated strong associations between carriage of class I HLA alleles and risk of drug-induced SJS/(for full descriptions

see Chapter 5). The best characterized examples of these associations include carriage of HLA-B*15:02 and risk of carbamazepine-induced SJS/TEN in Southeast Asian populations and carriage of HLA-B*58:01 and risk of allopurinol-induced SJS/TEN in both European and Southeast Asian populations, among others.[20–25] Cytotoxic CD8+ T cells, NK cells, and CD3+CD56+ NK T cells (NKT cells) are enriched in blister fluid samples obtained from patients with acute SJS/TEN, and these cells are the primary mediators of pathogenesis (Fig. 4.4).[26–29] Granulysin, a cytotoxic peptide produced by CD8+ T cells, NK cells, and NKT cells, is an important mediator of epidermal cell death in SJS/TEN. Granulysin is present in high concentrations in blister fluid. Serum levels of granulysin associate with the severity of acute SJS/TEN and predict mortality.[30,31] Immunohistochemical analyses of skin biopsies taken during acute SJS/TEN show that early lesions are characterized by the infiltration of CD14+CD16+CD11c+HLA-DR+ monocytes into the epidermis and dermoepidermal junction before the onset of epidermal damage. These cells express CD137 and the costimulatory molecules CD80 and CD86 and are characteristic of monocytes poised to facilitate the proliferation of cytotoxic T cells recruited to the site of pathology.[32]

More recent studies applying next-generation sequencing technologies demonstrate that in some cases of HLA-B*15:02-associated carbamazepine-SJS/TEN, the repertoire of CD8+ T cells recruited to the blister fluid are enriched for T cells bearing a common CDR3 sequence and that this dominant clonotype is shared among multiple patients with carbamazepine-SJS/TEN (unpublished data). Another study, however, focusing on allopurinol-SJS/TEN using similar methods to evaluate the TCR repertoire, demonstrated some clonotypic restriction of TCR usage within individual patients but no public TCR common to multiple patients.[30]

Drug Reaction With Eosinophilia and Systemic Symptoms

Drug reaction with eosinophilia and systemic symptoms (DRESS) presents as a widespread rash of varying severity without skin separation or blistering and is often accompanied by fever, internal organ involvement (usually hepatitis), and hematologic abnormalities (often atypical lymphocytes and/or eosinophilia) (Fig. 4.1). Diffuse lymphadenopathy, pneumonitis, encephalitis, cardiac failure (myocarditis), and nephritis are variable features of this syndrome, which may mimic a viral illness. The onset of symptoms typically occurs 2–8 weeks following initiation of the inciting

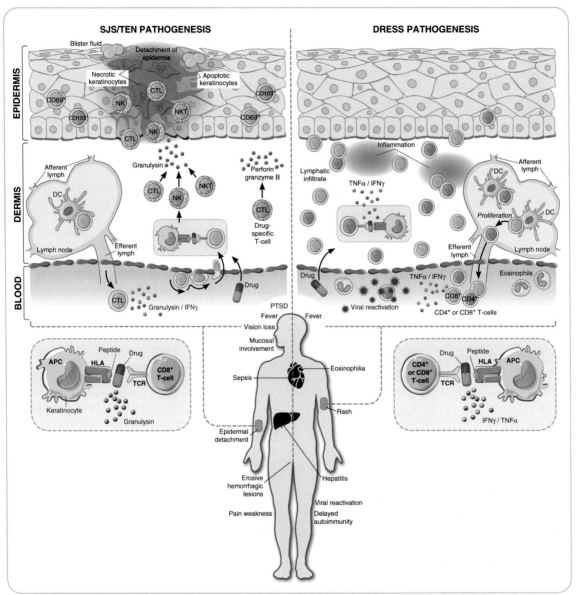

FIG. 4.4 **Current Models of Stevens-Johnson Syndrome/Toxic Epidermal Necrolysis (SJS/TEN) and Drug Reaction With Eosinophilia and Systemic Symptoms (DRESS) Pathogenesis.** Widespread epidermal necrosis is a hallmark of SJS/TEN. It is likely that this process is initiated by drug interaction with HLA present on the surface of epidermal keratinocytes in an allotype-specific manner. Drug-peptide–HLA interaction generates an immunogenic epitope that is recognized by CD8+ effector T cells, NK cells, and NKT cells to stimulate a cytotoxic response. Keratinocyte death is mediated by granulysin, a cytotoxic peptide release by drug-reactive effector cells, leading to epidermal detachment and the formation of fluid filled bullae and sloughing. The dermis is the primary skin compartment involved in DRESS pathogenesis. Both effector T cells (CD8+ and CD4+) and CD4+FoxP3+ regulatory T cells contribute to disease. DRESS is also associated with reactivation of human herpesviruses although the exact role of viral reactivation in DRESS pathogenesis is currently unclear. (Adapted from Peter JG, Lehloenyz R, Dlamini S, Risma K, White KD, Konvinse KC, Phillips EJ. Severe delayed cutaneous and systemic reactions to drugs: a global perspective on the Science and Art of Current Practice. *J Allergy Clin Immunol Prac.* 2017;5(3):547–563.)

drug, and symptoms can persist for weeks. Prolonged or recurrent symptoms, sometimes weeks following the cessation of the offending drug, as well as late-onset autoimmune diseases including thyroiditis, systemic lupus, and type I diabetes, are not uncommon following resolution of acute disease.[33] Numerous drugs are associated with the development of DRESS, including the antiretrovirals (abacavir, nevirapine, fosamprenavir), allopurinol, antiepileptic medications (carbamazepine, phenytoin, phenobarbital and lamotrigine), β-lactam antibiotics, NSAIDs, and sulfa antimicrobials.

DRESS is associated with expansion of circulating and dermal-infiltrating effector T cells as well as $CD4^+FoxP3^+$ regulatory T cells (Tregs).[34,35] Skin-homing $CD4^+FoxP3^+$ T cells are postulated to limit the severity of acute disease by suppressing effector T cell responses.[36] Reactivation of human herpesviruses (HHVs), in particular HHV-6, but also Epstein-Barr virus (EBV), HHV-7, and cytomegalovirus, is universally observed during acute and recovery phase disease (Fig. 4.4). HHV-6 and EBV reactivation has been observed as early as 2–3 weeks after the onset of rash, and antiviral $CD8^+$ effector T cells are expanded during this phase of disease. Whether viral replication contributes to the events inciting DRESS or is the result of general immune dysfunction, such as breakdown of Treg suppressor function or the upregulation of the HHV-6 receptor, CD134, on $CD4^+$ T cells, has not been defined.[35-38] Nevertheless, viral replication and a virus-specific T cell response likely contribute to the clinical features of DRESS, including prolonged duration, multiorgan involvement, and relapsing disease following withdrawal of glucocorticoid steroids.

Drug-Specific Models: The Aromatic Amine Anticonvulsants

Carbamazepine is an aromatic amine anticonvulsant used for the treatment of epilepsy, bipolar disorder, and trigeminal neuralgia. Multiple DHS are associated with carbamazepine, including SJS/TEN, MPE, and DRESS/DIHS. Carriage of the HLA-B*15:02 allele was first associated with carbamazepine-induced SJS/TEN in Han Chinese patients (negative predictive value [NPV] approaches 100%) and later to others of Southeast Asian ethnicity.[20,39] Mutagenesis studies demonstrate that carbamazepine binding to HLA-B*15:02 maps to the B pocket of the peptide-binding groove with a likely primary contact at the Arg62 residue, a conserved amino acid among HLA B75 serotypes. Additional contacts at the Asn63, Ile95, and Leu156 residues also likely participate in carbamazepine–B*15:02 interactions, as

alteration of these residues results in reduced affinity of carbamazepine binding.[40] The observation that neither drug nor antigen processing is required for T cell activation supports the p-i model of drug–immune receptor interaction.[40]

Recent experiments aimed at defining the $CD8^+$ T cell repertoire in carbamazepine-SJS/TEN have employed next-generation sequencing of circulating and blister fluid–derived T cells from multiple Taiwanese patients with HLA-B*15:02-associated carbamazepine-SJS/TEN. These studies have identified a shared $CD8^+$ T cell clonotype, bearing a common CDR3 sequence, that is present in blood and blister fluid among patients with carbamazepine-SJS/TEN but not in the peripheral blood of drug-tolerant controls or in blister fluid from patients with SJS/TEN secondary to another causative drug (Hung and Chung, unpublished data and Chung et al.[30]) This is significant as it suggests for the first time the concomitant involvement of both a specific HLA allotype and a specific TCR clonotype in the pathogenesis of a serious DHS and in this case SJS/TEN.

Drug-Specific Models: Allopurinol

Allopurinol is a xanthine oxidase inhibitor used to treat hyperuricemia/gout and is associated with DHS of primarily cutaneous phenotype in approximately 2% of patients who initiate therapy. The HLA-B*58:01 genotype is associated with allopurinol-induced SJS/TEN and DRESS/DIHS in persons of Han Chinese ancestry (100% NPV, 3% positive predictive value [PPV]), an association that has since been identified in other Asian populations.[24,41,42] Oxypurinol, the active metabolite of allopurinol, is the primary agent in the pathogenesis in allopurinol-DHS. In vivo, allopurinol is rapidly metabolized to oxypurinol ($T_{1/2} = 1-2\,h$ for allopurinol; oxypurinol is metabolized within 15 h in the setting of normal renal function). In keeping with the necessity of noncovalent and dose-dependent interactions between oxypurinol immune receptors (HLA and/or TCR) to activate T cells, in the setting of renal insufficiency, oxypurinol accumulates and serum concentrations of oxypurinol remain elevated for considerably longer periods. As such, impaired renal function and increased plasma concentrations of oxypurinol correlate with disease severity and mortality in allopurinol-SJS/TEN/DRESS.[31,43]

Cell culture experiments have shown that T cells isolated from patients with allopurinol-DHS expand and acquire effector functions following stimulation with allopurinol or oxypurinol but that high concentrations of oxypurinol (up to 100 μg/mL, 10× that expected with a therapeutic dose) are the primary drivers of T cell reactivity.[30,44] These findings are consistent with observations that allopurinol is rapidly converted to oxypurinol in vivo and that elevated serum concentrations of oxypurinol in the setting of delayed renal clearance contribute to risk of allopurinol-DHS. In vitro generation of allopurinol- and oxypurinol-reactive T cell lines was shown to be independent of intracellular metabolism or antigen processing, consistent with a p-i mechanism of drug-HLA-peptide–TCR interaction.[45,46] Mutagenesis studies suggest that oxypurinol binds in the HLA-B*58:01 peptide-binding groove and that binding is likely dependent on the presence of Arg97 because mutation of this residue to valine substantially decreases T cell proliferation in the presence of oxypurinol relative to wild-type HLA-B*58:01.[45] In silico modeling experiments predict that oxypurinol docks within the F-pocket of HLA-B*58:01 and that stable association requires the formation of a hydrogen bond with Arg97, consistent with site-directed mutagenesis data. These studies also suggest that allopurinol binding to HLA-B*58:01 occurs at reduced affinity than that predicted for oxypurinol, which supports the in vivo and in vitro data, showing that reactivity is mediated by oxypurinol in a dose-dependent manner.[46]

The mechanisms by which oxypurinol stimulates TCRs are currently under investigation. One study that examined the CD8+ T cell repertoire among blister fluid and peripheral blood cells obtained from multiple patients with allopurinol-associated SJS/TEN by bulk next-generation TCR sequencing demonstrated some degree of clonotypic restriction for some, but not all, patients and no evidence of a shared clonotype as seen for carbamazepine-associated SJS/TEN.[30] Which, if any, of these clonotypes mediates pathogenesis is not known. Granulysin is a key mediator of this disease and levels of granulysin correlate with disease severity and mortality in allopurinol-SJS/TEN and DRESS.[31]

Drug-Specific Models: Abacavir Hypersensitivity Syndrome

Abacavir is a guanosine analog that is used as part of combination antiretroviral therapy for the treatment of HIV-1 infection. In early studies, hypersensitivity type reactions were reported in approximately 5%–8% of patients within the first 6 weeks following the initiation of abacavir. These reactions were named the abacavir hypersensitivity syndrome and were characterized by fever, malaise, gastrointestinal and respiratory symptoms, and/or generalized rash. In 2002, a strong association between carriage of the HLA class I allele HLA-B*57:01 and AHS was reported.[47] Key clinical studies that confirmed the immunologic basis of this syndrome included the application of abacavir in varying concentrations in a patch test on the skin that demonstrated consistent and visibly positive results indicative of in vivo T cell responses to abacavir in HLA-B*57:01 positive AHS patients.[48] These observations were followed by the PREDICT-1 and SHAPE trials, which showed that screening for and exclusion of HLA-B*57:01 carriers from abacavir drug exposure could completely eliminate the incidence of immunologically confirmed (patch test positive) AHS with a 100% NPV and a 55% PPV.[49,50]

The functional basis for AHS was defined in 2012 with the simultaneous publication of two crystal structures of HLA-B*57:01 in complex with abacavir and peptide.[17,18] These studies supported an altered peptide repertoire model for abacavir-specific activation of T cells. According to this model abacavir binds to the HLA-B*57:01 peptide-binding groove underneath the C-terminus of the bound peptide, and this induces a change in the binding properties of HLA-B*57:01 such that peptides with a small aliphatic C-terminal residue (Ile, Leu, Val) are preferentially selected, a repertoire that is distinct from that presented by HLA-B*57:01 in the absence of drug binding. Approximately 20%–45% of the peptides eluted from abacavir-treated HLA-B*57:01 APCs were distinct from those recovered from untreated cells, illustrating the dramatic shift in the repertoire of HLA-B*57:01 bound peptide in the presence of abacavir. This work defined the altered peptide repertoire model of DHS and predicts that in the context of drug, self-peptides that are normally not "seen" by the immune system are presented to T cells and recognized as "foreign" to elicit an immune response.

Unexplained Features of T Cell–Mediated Adverse Drug Reactions

There remain many unanswered questions regarding the immunopathogenesis of T cell–mediated DHS. First, all of the T cell–mediated DHS described in this chapter are generally characterized by a high NPV for HLA association (approaching 100% in many cases) but a low PPV meaning that only a small proportion of those carrying an HLA risk allele will develop DHS. For instance, why is it that 55% of HLA-B*57:01 carriers will develop a hypersensitivity reaction in response to abacavir exposure but only 3% of HLA-B*15:02 carriers exposed to carbamazepine will develop SJS/TEN? What immunologic factors differ among those individuals who develop DHS and those who carry the risk HLA allele but tolerate the drug? Second, what might explain the variable clinical phenotypes of T cell–mediated

DHS? AHS is characterized predominantly by systemic symptoms and internal organ involvement and is less commonly associated with rash. In contrast, carbamazepine-associated DHS most commonly manifest as severe cutaneous and systemic reactions such as SJS/TEN and DRESS. Carbamazepine causes the full spectrum of DHS (SJS/TEN, DRESS, AGEP, FDE, MPE, DILI) and specific phenotypes have been associated with carriage of different HLA alleles. What explains the phenotypic variation seen among these HLA-restricted DHS? Third, there exists wide variability in the timing of clinical onset of many DHS. For instance, immunologically mediated abacavir hypersensitivity, defined as patch test positive HLA-B*57:01 positive abacavir reactivity, occurs in a narrow time window of <2 days to 3 weeks from the first exposure to drug. SJS/TEN has a shorter latency period than DRESS and typically occurs 4–28 days following the first drug exposure. Many carbamazepine-associated DHS have been observed to occur over a broad and longer timeframe with the onset of symptoms often occurring later, 2–8 weeks after drug therapy. Factors playing into the variable timing of these syndromes are currently unclear. Finally, in some cases, immunologically mediated drug-specific recall reactions have been demonstrated years after drug exposure and withdrawal. For example, abacavir-specific in vivo (skin patch test) and ex vivo (ELISpot) responses remain positive years after clinical abacavir hypersensitivity in the absence of subsequent reexposure to abacavir. Similarly, long-lived T cell responses have been observed in patients with history of carbamazepine-SJS/TEN years after clinical DHS. Factors that lead to the maintenance of this long-lasting memory T cell response and the specific antigen leading to the maintenance of this response are similarly unknown.

Ongoing work to define the pathogenesis of immune-mediated ADRs might shed light on these outstanding questions. One focus of current research seeks to evaluate the role of preexisting memory T cell responses in the pathogenesis of DHS. It has been shown that T cells isolated from abacavir-naïve, HLA-B*57:01 positive individuals proliferate and become activated in response to abacavir exposure in 14-day cell culture systems and that abacavir-reactive T cells derive from both memory and naïve T cell populations.[51] These findings raise the possibility that a proportion of drug-reactive T cells may stem from memory populations that were generated before drug exposure against an unrelated antigen, such as an infectious pathogen. If this hypothesis is correct, then the requirement for preexisting memory T cells may, at least in part,

explain the low PPV for HLA allele carriage as a sole predictor of DHS risk, the rapid onset of symptoms following drug exposure in some DHS, the variable phenotypes seen among different HLA- and drug-specific DHS, and the long-lasting immunologic memory after drug withdrawal. Other avenues of research that may define components of the immunopathogenesis of T cell–mediated DHS include investigations into how variation in genes encoding proteins that are involved in drug metabolism and/or intracellular peptide processing and presentation, such as the cytochrome P450 (CYP) enzymes and/or endoplasmic reticulum aminopeptidase variants, might contribute to DHS risk in the setting of HLA risk allele carriage.[52-54]

FUTURE RESEARCH AND IMPLICATIONS FOR CLINICAL PRACTICE

Identification of patients who are at risk for an ADR via pharmacogenomics screening before drug administration is desirable given the substantial cost, morbidity, and mortality associated with these reactions. Methods to incorporate such screening strategies into clinical practice have been successfully implemented for a small number of well-characterized T cell–mediated DHS. For example, it is now a standard-of-care practice to test patients for carriage of the HLA-B*57:01 gene before the initiation of abacavir and to exclude any patient who carries this allele from receiving abacavir. This practice has eliminated AHS in populations where screening is routinely performed. From a drug safety standpoint, the 100% NPV for lack of reaction in the absence of allele carriage in the target population, the low number needed to test to prevent one case, and the paucity of safe and efficacious therapeutic alternatives are critical for incorporation of these screening strategies into clinical care. However, given the low PPVs for the HLA-associated ADRs defined to date, screening strategies that focus solely on HLA genotyping will inevitably result in the denial of therapy to a large number of carriers of HLA risk alleles who would ultimately tolerate the drug in question without complication and benefit from its use. Further delineation of the factors that contribute to DHS risk, in addition to HLA genotype, will be critical to defining disease pathogenesis and potentially allow us to refine our screening protocols to more precisely identify those patients who are truly at risk for ADR. This will, in turn, improve drug safety, improve the efficiency of drug design, and reduce the cost of drug development.

ABBREVIATIONS

ADR   Adverse drug reaction
AGEP   Acute generalized exanthematous pustulosis
AHS   Abacavir hypersensitivity syndrome
APC   Antigen presenting cell
BSA   Body surface area
CDR   Complementarity-determining regions
DHS   Drug hypersensitivity syndrome
DIHS   Drug-induced hypersensitivity syndrome
DILI   Drug-induced liver injury
DRESS   Drug reaction with eosinophilia and systemic symptoms
EBV   Epstein-Barr virus
HLA   Human leukocyte antigen
HSV   Herpes simplex virus
MPE   Maculopapular eruption
NPV   Negative predictive value
PK/PD   Pharmacokinetic/pharmacodynamic
NSAID   Nonsteroidal anti-inflammatory drug
PPV   Positive predictive value
SJS   Stevens-Johnson syndrome
TCR   T cell receptor
TEN   Toxic epidermal necrolysis

ACKNOWLEDGMENTS

National Institute of Health:1P50GM115305-01 (EJP, KK, KDK), 1R01AI103348-01 (EJP), 1P30AI110527-01A1 (EJP), 5T32AI007474-20 (EJP), 1 R13AR71267-01(EJP), National Health & Medical Research Council of Australia (EJP,AR), Australian Centre for HIV and Hepatitis Virology Research (EJP).

REFERENCES

1. Lazarou J, Pomeranz BH, Corey PN. Incidence of adverse drug reactions in hospitalized patients: a meta-analysis of prospective studies. *JAMA*. 1998;279(15):1200–1205.
2. Hakkarainen KM, Hedna K, Petzold M, Hagg S. Percentage of patients with preventable adverse drug reactions and preventability of adverse drug reactions–a meta-analysis. *PLoS One*. 2012;7(3):e33236.
3. Kongkaew C, Noyce PR, Ashcroft DM. Hospital admissions associated with adverse drug reactions: a systematic review of prospective observational studies. *Ann Pharmacother*. 2008;42(7):1017–1025.
4. Pirmohamed M, James S, Meakin S, et al. Adverse drug reactions as cause of admission to hospital: prospective analysis of 18 820 patients. *Bmj*. 2004;329(7456):15–19.
5. Sullivan TJ, Wedner HJ, Shatz GS, Yecies LD, Parker CW. Skin testing to detect penicillin allergy. *J Allergy Clin Immunol*. 1981;68(3):171–180.
6. Blanca M, Torres MJ, Garcia JJ, et al. Natural evolution of skin test sensitivity in patients allergic to beta-lactam antibiotics. *J Allergy Clin Immunol*. 1999;103(5 Pt 1):918–924.
7. Hershkovich J, Broides A, Kirjner L, Smith H, Gorodischer R. Beta lactam allergy and resensitization in children with suspected beta lactam allergy. *Clin Exp Allergy*. 2009;39(5):726–730.
8. McNeil BD, Pundir P, Meeker S, et al. Identification of a mast-cell-specific receptor crucial for pseudo-allergic drug reactions. *Nature*. 2014;519.
9. Pavlos R, Mallal S, Ostrov D, et al. T cell-mediated hypersensitivity reactions to drugs. *Annu Rev Med*. 2014;66.
10. White KD, Gaudieri S, Phillips E. HLA and the pharmacogenomics of drug hypersensitivity. In: Padmanabhan S, ed. *Handbook of Pharmacogenomics and Stratefied Medicine*. Elsevier, Inc; 2014:437–465.
11. Pichler W, Yawalkar N, Schmid S, Helbling A. Pathogenesis of drug-induced exanthems. *Allergy*. 2002;57(10):884–893.
12. Pichler WJ. Delayed drug hypersensitivity reactions. *Ann Intern Med*. 2003;139(8):683–693.
13. Padovan E, Mauri-Hellweg D, Pichler WJ, Weltzien HU. T cell recognition of penicillin G: structural features determining antigenic specificity. *Eur J Immunol*. 1996;26(1):42–48.
14. Naisbitt DJ, Gordon SF, Pirmohamed M, et al. Antigenicity and immunogenicity of sulphamethoxazole: demonstration of metabolism-dependent haptenation and T-cell proliferation in vivo. *Br J Pharmacol*. 2001;133(2):295–305.
15. Pichler WJ, Beeler A, Keller M, et al. Pharmacological interaction of drugs with immune receptors: the p-i concept. *Allergol Int*. 2006;55(1):17–25.
16. Pichler WJWS. Interaction of small molecules with specific immune receptors: the p-i concept and its consequences. *Curr Immunol Rev*. 2014;10:7–18.
17. Ostrov DA, Grant BJ, Pompeu YA, et al. Drug hypersensitivity caused by alteration of the MHC-presented self-peptide repertoire. *Proc Natl Acad Sci USA*. 2012;109(25):9959–9964.
18. Illing PT, Vivian JP, Dudek NL, et al. Immune self-reactivity triggered by drug-modified HLA-peptide repertoire. *Nature*. 2012;486(7404):554–558.
19. Lee HY, Chung WH. Toxic epidermal necrolysis: the year in review. *Curr Opin Allergy Clin Immunol*. 2013;13(4):330–336.
20. Chung WH, Hung SI, Hong HS, et al. Medical genetics: a marker for Stevens-Johnson syndrome. *Nature*. 2004;428(6982):486.
21. Kulkantrakorn K, Tassaneeyakul W, Tiamkao S, et al. HLA-B*1502 strongly predicts carbamazepine-induced Stevens-Johnson syndrome and toxic epidermal necrolysis in Thai patients with neuropathic pain. *Pain Pract*. 2012;12(3):202–208.
22. Mehta TY, Prajapati LM, Mittal B, et al. Association of HLA-B*1502 allele and carbamazepine-induced Stevens-Johnson syndrome among Indians. *Indian J Dermatol Venereol Leprol*. 2009;75(6):579–582.

23. Then SM, Rani ZZ, Raymond AA, Ratnaningrum S, Jamal R. Frequency of the HLA-B*1502 allele contributing to carbamazepine-induced hypersensitivity reactions in a cohort of Malaysian epilepsy patients. *Asian Pac J Allergy Immunol.* 2011;29(3):290–293.

24. Hung SI, Chung WH, Liou LB, et al. HLA-B*5801 allele as a genetic marker for severe cutaneous adverse reactions caused by allopurinol. *Proc Natl Acad Sci USA.* 2005;102(11):4134–4139.

25. Lonjou C, Borot N, Sekula P, et al. A European study of HLA-B in Stevens-Johnson syndrome and toxic epidermal necrolysis related to five high-risk drugs. *Pharmacogenet Genom.* 2008;18(2):99–107.

26. Le Cleach L, Delaire S, Boumsell L, et al. Blister fluid T lymphocytes during toxic epidermal necrolysis are functional cytotoxic cells which express human natural killer (NK) inhibitory receptors. *Clin Exp Immunol.* 2000;119(1):225–230.

27. Leyva L, Torres MJ, Posadas S, et al. Anticonvulsant-induced toxic epidermal necrolysis: monitoring the immunologic response. *J Allergy Clin Immunol.* 2000;105 (1 Pt 1):157–165.

28. Nassif A, Bensussan A, Dorothee G, et al. Drug specific cytotoxic T-cells in the skin lesions of a patient with toxic epidermal necrolysis. *J Invest Dermatol.* 2002;118(4):728–733.

29. Nassif A, Bensussan A, Boumsell L, et al. Toxic epidermal necrolysis: effector cells are drug-specific cytotoxic T cells. *J Allergy Clin Immunol.* 2004;114(5):1209–1215.

30. Chung WH, Pan RY, Chu MT, et al. Oxypurinol-specific T cells possess preferential TCR clonotypes and express granulysin in allopurinol-induced severe cutaneous adverse reactions. *J Invest Dermatol.* 2015;135(9):2237–2248.

31. Chung WH, Chang WC, Stocker SL, et al. Insights into the poor prognosis of allopurinol-induced severe cutaneous adverse reactions: the impact of renal insufficiency, high plasma levels of oxypurinol and granulysin. *Ann Rheum Dis.* 2015;74(12):2157–2164.

32. Tohyama M, Watanabe H, Murakami S, et al. Possible involvement of CD14+ CD16+ monocyte lineage cells in the epidermal damage of Stevens-Johnson syndrome and toxic epidermal necrolysis. *Br J Dermatol.* 2012;166(2):322–330.

33. Shiohara T, Kano Y, Takahashi R, Ishida T, Mizukawa Y. Drug-induced hypersensitivity syndrome: recent advances in the diagnosis, pathogenesis and management. *Chem Immunol Allergy.* 2012;97:122–138.

34. Morito H, Ogawa K, Fukumoto T, et al. Increased ratio of FoxP3+ regulatory T cells/CD3+ T cells in skin lesions in drug-induced hypersensitivity syndrome/drug rash with eosinophilia and systemic symptoms. *Clin Exp Dermatol.* 2014;39(3):284–291.

35. Takahashi R, Kano Y, Yamazaki Y, Kimishima M, Mizukawa Y, Shiohara T. Defective regulatory T cells in patients with severe drug eruptions: timing of the dysfunction is associated with the pathological phenotype and outcome. *J Immunol.* 2009;182(12):8071–8079.

36. Shiohara T, Ushigome Y, Kano Y, Takahashi R. Crucial role of viral reactivation in the development of severe drug eruptions: a comprehensive review. *Clin Rev Allergy Immunol.* 2015;49(2):192–202.

37. Miyagawa F, Nakamura Y, Miyashita K, et al. Preferential expression of CD134, an HHV-6 cellular receptor, on CD4T cells in drug-induced hypersensitivity syndrome (DIHS)/drug reaction with eosinophilia and systemic symptoms (DRESS). *J Dermatol Sci.* 2016;83(2):151–154.

38. Picard D, Janela B, Descamps V, et al. Drug reaction with eosinophilia and systemic symptoms (DRESS): a multiorgan antiviral T cell response. *Sci Transl Med.* 2010;2(46):46ra62.

39. Tangamornsuksan W, Chaiyakunapruk N, Somkrua R, Lohitnavy M, Tassaneeyakul W. Relationship between the HLA-B*1502 allele and carbamazepine-induced Stevens-Johnson syndrome and toxic epidermal necrolysis: a systematic review and meta-analysis. *JAMA Dermatol.* 2013;149(9):1025–1032.

40. Wei CY, Chung WH, Huang HW, Chen YT, Hung SI. Direct interaction between HLA-B and carbamazepine activates T cells in patients with Stevens-Johnson syndrome. *J Allergy Clin Immunol.* 2012;129(6):1562–1569. e5.

41. Tassaneeyakul W, Jantararoungtong T, Chen P, et al. Strong association between HLA-B*5801 and allopurinol-induced Stevens-Johnson syndrome and toxic epidermal necrolysis in a Thai population. *Pharmacogen Genom.* 2009;19(9):704–709.

42. Kaniwa N, Saito Y, Aihara M, et al. HLA-B locus in Japanese patients with anti-epileptics and allopurinol-related Stevens-Johnson syndrome and toxic epidermal necrolysis. *Pharmacogenomics.* 2008;9(11):1617–1622.

43. Ng CY, Yeh YT, Wang CW, et al. Impact of the HLA-B(*)58:01 Allele and Renal Impairment on Allopurinol-Induced Cutaneous Adverse Reactions. *J Invest Dermatol.* 2016;136(7):1373–1381.

44. Yun J, Mattsson J, Schnyder K, et al. Allopurinol hypersensitivity is primarily mediated by dose-dependent oxypurinol-specific T cell response. *Clin Exp Allergy.* 2013;43(11):1246–1255.

45. Lin CHC, Chen JK, Ko TM, et al. Immunologic basis for allopurinol-induced severe cutaneous reactions: HLA-B*58:01-restricted activation of drug-specific T cells and molecular interaction. *J Allergy Clin Immunol.* 2015;135(4):1063–1065 .

46. Yun J, Marcaida MJ, Eriksson KK, et al. Oxypurinol directly and immediately activates the drug-specific T cells via the preferential use of HLA-B*58:01. *J Immunol.* 2014;192(7):2984–2993.

47. Mallal S, Nolan D, Witt C, et al. Association between presence of HLA-B*5701, HLA-DR7, and HLA-DQ3 and hypersensitivity to HIV-1 reverse-transcriptase inhibitor abacavir. *Lancet.* 2002;359(9308):727–732.

48. Phillips EJ, Sullivan JR, Knowles SR, Shear NH. Utility of patch testing in patients with hypersensitivity syndromes associated with abacavir. *Aids.* 2002;16(16):2223–2225.

49. Mallal S, Phillips E, Carosi G, et al. HLA-B*5701 screening for hypersensitivity to abacavir. *N Engl J Med.* 2008;358(6):568–579.

50. Saag M, Balu R, Phillips E, et al. High sensitivity of human leukocyte antigen-b*5701 as a marker for immunologically confirmed abacavir hypersensitivity in white and black patients. *Clin Infect Dis.* 2008;46(7):1111–1118.

51. Lucas A, Lucas M, Strhyn A, et al. Abacavir-reactive memory T cells are present in drug naive individuals. *PLoS One.* 2015;10(2):e0117160.

52. Chung WH, Chang WC, Lee YS, et al. Genetic variants associated with phenytoin-related severe cutaneous adverse reactions. *JAMA.* 2014;312(5):525–534.

53. Yuan J, Guo S, Hall D, et al. Toxicogenomics of nevirapine-associated cutaneous and hepatic adverse events among populations of African, Asian, and European descent. *Aids.* 2011;25(10):1271–1280.

54. Pavlos R, Strautins K, James I, Mallal S, Redwood AJ, Phillips E. Variation in EraP Influences Risk fr HLA-B*57:01 Positive Abacavir Hypersensitivity. 23rd Conference on Retroviruses and Opportunistic Infections (CROI); Boston, MA; 2016.

55. Peter JG, Lehloenyz R, Dlamini S, Risma K, White KD, Konvinse KC, Phillips EJ. Severe delayed cutaneous and systemic reactions to drugs: a global perspective on the Science and Art of Current Practice. *J Allergy Clin Immunol Prac.* 2017;5(3):547–563.

CHAPTER 5

Pharmacogenomics of Drug Allergy

REBECCA PAVLOS, PHD • JASON KARNES, PHARMD, PHD, BCPS •
JASON TRUBIANO, BBIOMEDSCI, MBBS (HONS) •
JONNY PETER, MB CHB, MMED, FCP (SA), PHD • ELIZABETH PHILLIPS, MD

KEY POINTS

- Adverse drug reactions (ADRs) are associated with high global morbidity and mortality, significantly impacting the health care system.
- There is need to understand both patient- and drug-related risk factors and mechanisms involved in these diverse reactions.
- Pharmacogenomics refers to the effect of multiple genes on drug responses and may include genes that affect pharmacokinetics, pharmacodynamics, and susceptibility to hypersensitivity responses.
- The majority (>80%) of ADRs are pharmacologically mediated on- or off-target reactions and develop in a concentration-dependent manner. Pharmacologically driven ADRs can be mild (headache, gastrointestinal effects) or life-threatening as with warfarin-induced severe bleeding.

INTRODUCTION

Adverse drug reactions (ADRs) are associated with high global morbidity and mortality, significantly impacting the health care system. There is need to understand both patient- and drug-related risk factors and mechanisms involved in these diverse reactions. Pharmacogenomics refers to the effect of multiple genes on drug responses and may include genes that affect pharmacokinetics, pharmacodynamics, and susceptibility to hypersensitivity responses. The majority (>80%) of ADRs are pharmacologically mediated on- or off-target reactions and develop in a concentration-dependent manner. Pharmacologically driven ADRs can be mild (headache, gastrointestinal effects) or life-threatening as with warfarin-induced severe bleeding. They are a result of a complex interplay of modifiable and unmodifiable factors such as weight, kidney and liver function, genetics, underlying disease and drug-drug interactions.

Immune-mediated adverse drug reactions (IM-ADRs), considered as off-target reactions, comprise <20% of all ADRs.[1] IM-ADRs encompass a number of phenotypically distinct clinical diagnoses that are associated with immunologic memory of varying duration and include both B cell–mediated (antibody-mediated, Gell-Coombs types I-III) and purely T cell–mediated (Gell-Coombs type IV) reactions (Fig. 5.1).[2,69] Type I reactions are typically immediate,

IgE-mediated reactions, usually occurring within 1 h after drug administration, and mainly cause urticaria, angioedema, bronchospasm, pruritus, and anaphylaxis. Penicillin allergy is an example of a Type I ADR commonly seen in clinical practice. Type IV reactions, in contrast, are delayed hypersensitivity reactions (HSRs) mediated by drug-reactive T lymphocytes. These reactions present as a variety of clinical phenotypes, including severe cutaneous syndromes (acute generalized exanthematous pustulosis and Stevens-Johnson syndrome [SJS]/toxic epidermal necrolysis [TEN]), systemic reactions (abacavir [ABC] hypersensitivity syndrome [HSS] and drug rash eosinophilia and systemic symptoms [DRESS]), or organ-specific manifestations (drug induced liver injury [DILI]) (see Chapter 4).[3] ABC HSS and carbamazepine-induced SJS/TEN are arguably the best characterized CD8+ T cell–mediated ADRs.

In addition to the ADRs that are primarily pharmacologically or immunologically mediated, some ADRs that seem to have an immunologic or allergic phenotype, (such as urticaria or angioedema), are not well correlated with markers of an adaptive immune response, Examples of such reactions, which are often called "pseudoallergic" or "anaphylactic," include various mechanisms of non-IgE-mediated mast-cell activation.

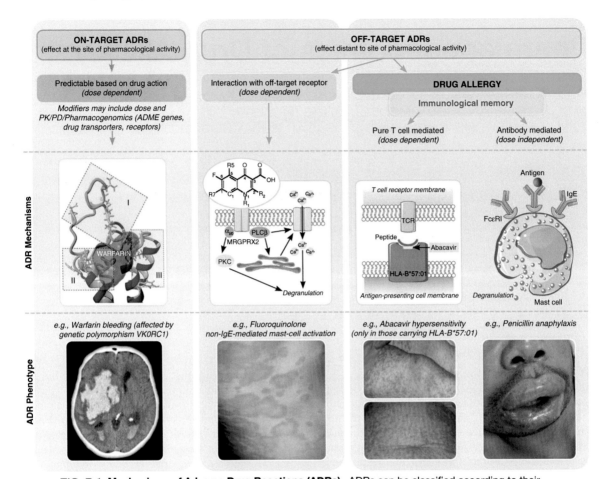

FIG. 5.1 **Mechanisms of Adverse Drug Reactions (ADRs).** ADRs can be classified according to their on-target versus off-target interactions between the drug and cellular components. Both on-target and off-target effects can demonstrate concentration-exposure relationships that may differ between individuals based on acquired or genetic host factors. The interaction between the drug and the target may relate to both the dose and/or duration of treatment. On-target or pharmacologic reactions generally relate to an augmentation of the known primary therapeutic and pharmacologic action of a drug (e.g., bleeding related to warfarin) and off-target effects can occur by mechanisms that are both directly immune mediated and associated with immunologic memory of varied duration (drug allergy), and mechanisms without immunologic memory that may have an "immunologic phenotype." These reactions are often mediated through a pharmacologic interaction (e.g., aspirin exacerbated respiratory disease or non-IgE-mediated mast-cell activation seen with fluoroquinolones and opioids). Off-target reactions that are nonimmunologically mediated are often dose dependent, whereas immunologically mediated off-target reactions associated with immunologic memory can be both dose dependent (T cell–mediated reactions) or dose independent (recognition and amplification of small amounts of antigen in the case of IgE-mediated reactions). Predisposition to both on-target and off-target reactions is driven by not only genetic variation but also ecologic factors that can vary over the course of an individual's lifetime. (Adapted from White KD, Chung WH, Hung SI, Mallal S, Phillips EJ. Evolving models of the immunopathogenesis of T cell-mediated drug allergy: The role of host, pathogens, and drug response. *J Allergy Clin Immunol.* 2015;136(2):219–234, quiz 35.[61])

REACTIONS LACKING IMMUNOLOGIC MEMORY

Reactions With a Pharmacologic Component

Drug pharmacokinetics is influenced by absorption (typically from the gastrointestinal tract), distribution throughout bodily tissues, metabolism, and excretion. Although complex modeling is necessary to predict drug concentrations accurately, multiple genetic variants have been shown to increase or decrease the risk of pharmacologic ADRs, with variants in drug metabolism (both phase I and phase II) or transport genes being the most extensively investigated. There are many examples where genetic variation influences the drug concentration and these pharmacogenomic drug-gene pairs have a large effect, have clinical relevance, and can be leveraged to predict the occurrence of pharmacologic ADRs (Table 5.1).

To predict which patients will develop pharmacologic ADRs, individuals are often classified into categories of enzyme activity: poor metabolizer, intermediate metabolizer, extensive metabolizer (EM), and ultrarapid metabolizer (UM).[4] The enzyme cytochrome P450 (CYP)2D6, responsible for metabolizing about 20% of commonly used drugs such as antidepressants, antipsychotics, and opioid analgesics, contains over 100 polymorphisms that allow classification of enzyme activity in this manner (Table 5.1).[5] For example, a patient taking codeine characterized as a *CYP2D6* UM has an increased risk of a morphine toxicity-related ADR when given the same dose as a *CYP2D6* EM patient. Testing for *CYP2D6* variants before codeine administration allows the drug dose to be tailored to metabolizer status to reduce the risk of ADRs. Many similar examples exist in which variability in drug-metabolizing enzymes confer an increased risk of an ADR (see the online US Food and Drug Administration [FDA] resource, "Table of Pharmacogenomic Biomarkers in Drug Labeling").[6]

Phase I enzymes, such as CYP enzymes, metabolize the parent drugs into their metabolites, whereas phase II enzymes conjugate these metabolites with endogenous chemicals to facilitate excretion. An example of variants in phase II enzymes that affect the risk of ADRs is thiopurine S-methyltransferase (TPMT) (Table 5.1), which is primarily responsible for the addition of a methyl group to the chemotherapeutic purine derivatives 6-mercaptopurine and azathioprine, which subsequently inactivates these agents. Patients treated for inflammatory bowel disease with thiopurine may suffer from toxicities such as neutropenia if they carry reduced function polymorphisms in *TPMT*.[7] A reduced dosage of these agents is recommended in patients who carry *TPMT* mutations.

In addition to drug-metabolizing enzymes, variants in drug transporters also affect pharmacologic ADR risk. For example, the organic anion transporter (OATP) 1B1, encoded by the *SLCO1B1* gene, is responsible for transporting some drugs from the blood into hepatocytes (Table 5.1) and particular variants show reduced function of the transporter, resulting in a reduced drug concentration in the liver and an increased blood concentration. For example, simvastatin is commonly used to reduce cholesterol and prevent cardiovascular events and patients with particular *SLCO1B1* mutations can experience a reduced efficacy of simvastatin and a drug-induced myopathy.[8] Such patients may benefit from receiving an alternate cholesterol-lowering drug that is not transported by SLCO1B1.

Reactions With an Off-Target Pharmacologic and/or Immunologic Component

Non-IgE-mediated mast-cell activation

Mast-cell degranulation by certain drugs, including antibiotics (i.e., fluoroquinolones), opioids, antiplatelet agents/nonsteroidal antiinflammatories (e.g., aspirin), and neuromuscular blocking agents, have been historically reported. These reactions have the clinical phenotype of anaphylaxis but lack evidence of IgE cross-linking/FcɛR signaling, leading to the nomenclature of anaphylactoid or "pseudoallergic." The mechanisms of non-IgE-mediated mast-cell degranulation ADRs have been poorly understood, but several new pharmacogenomic candidates have been identified, such as the human G protein–coupled receptor MAS Related GPR Family Member X2 (MRGPRx2). *MrgprX2* is orthologous to *MrgprB2* in the mouse and is uniquely expressed by connective tissue mast cells.[9,10] Mutant *MrgprB2* mice and human mast cell lines have been utilized to demonstrate mast-cell reactivity to several FDA-approved drugs in an *MrgprX2/B2*-dependent manner. These drugs include peptidergic drugs, such as icatibant, that are introduced subcutaneously or intramuscularly and induce injection-site reactions (local swelling or flare, pain, and pruritus), and intravenously applied drugs (associated with skin flushing or rash, changes in blood pressure or heart rate, and bronchospasms). A tetrahydroisoquinoline motif appears to be key in *MrgprB2*-dependent activation of mast cells and is shared by several drugs, including members of the nicotinic receptor antagonist nonsteroidal neuromuscular blocking drugs, and the fluoroquinolone family of antibiotics has a similar motif.[9,11] Furthermore, naturally occurring loss- or gain-of-function mutations are known to alter the activity of *MrgprX1*, the analogous G protein–coupled receptor expressed in dorsal root ganglia neurons, which mediates pain and histamine-independent itch.[12]

TABLE 5.1
Genetic Biomarkers for Selected Pharmacologic Adverse Drug Reactions (ADRs)

Gene	Major Alleles	Drug	ADR
PHASE 1 DRUG-METABOLIZING ENZYMES			
DPYD	*2A, *13, D949V	5-Fluorouracil, capecitabine	Myelosuppression, neurotoxicity, hand-and-foot syndrome
CYP2B6	*6, *16, *18	Efavirenz	CNS side effects
CYP2C19	*2, *3, *17	Clopidogrel TCAs SSRIs	Stent thrombosis, bleeding Anticholinergic, CNS, and cardiac effects CNS effects (e.g., insomnia, headache), gastrointestinal dysfunction, and sexual dysfunction
CYP2D6	*1 × N, *2, *3, *4, *5, *67, *10, *17, *41	Codeine, tramadol TCAs Antipsychotics Carvedilol, metoprolol, propranolol, timolol	Respiratory depression Anticholinergic, CNS, and cardiac effects Extrapyramidal symptoms Heart block
CYP2C9	*2, *3	Phenytoin Warfarin	Phenytoin toxicity Bleeding
PHASE II DRUG-METABOLIZING ENZYMES			
G6PD	Mediterranean, Canton, Kaiping, etc.	Rasburicase, dapsone, sulfonylureas	Hemolytic anemia, methemoglobinemia
GSTM1	*B, *0	Busulfan	Venoocclusive disease
UGT1A1	*28	Atazanavir Irinotecan	Jaundice Neutropenia, diarrhea
UGT1A8	*2	Mycophenolate	Diarrhea
UGT2B7	*2	Diclofenac	Hepatotoxicity
NAT2	*4, *5, *6, *7, *10, *14, *17, *18	Isoniazid Hydralazine Sulfasalazine	Neurotoxicity Lupus-like syndrome Hemolytic anemia
TPMT	*2, *3A, *3B, *3C	Azathioprine, mercaptopurine, thioguanine	Neutropenia
DRUG TRANSPORTERS			
SLCO1B1	*1B, *5, *15, *16, *17	Simvastatin	Myopathy

CNS, central nervous system; CYP, Cytochrome P450; DYPD, Dihydropyrimidine Dehydrogenase; G6PD, Glucose-6-Phosphate Dehydrogenase; GSTM1, Glutathione S-Transferase Mu 1; NAT2, N-Acetyltransferase 2; SSRI, selective serotonin reuptake inhibitor; TCA, tricyclic antidepressant; TPMT, Thiopurine S-Methyltransferase; UGT, UDP Glucuronosyltransferase.
* allele

Several other antimicrobials, including vancomycin, amphotericin B, rifampin, and teicoplanin, are capable of producing nonspecific mast-cell degranulation in "red man syndrome," which is characterized by flushing and/or an erythematous rash that affects the face, neck, and upper torso.[13] To date, the mechanism driving red man syndrome remains unknown, because drugs such as vancomycin do not appear to interact with mas-related G protein–coupled receptors (unpublished data).[14]

Aspirin exacerbated respiratory disease
Nonsteroidal anti-inflammatory drug (NSAID)-exacerbated respiratory disease (i.e., aspirin exacerbated respiratory disease [AERD]) is a disorder characterized by

the intolerance of aspirin and other nonselective cyclo-oxygenase (COX) inhibitors in 7%–14% of patients with asthma.[15,16] The syndrome is characterized by upper and lower airway symptoms in combination with other classical signs of immediate hypersensitivity, including urticaria, angioedema, or facial flushing after NSAID exposure. NSAID reactions that lack an adaptive immune response and immunologic memory are linked to the inhibition of the COX-1 enzyme, which results in decreased inflammatory prostanoids, especially prostaglandin E_2. Prostaglandin E_2 maintains a critical "check" against 5-lipoxygenase activity and mast-cell activation, and a dysregulated function subsequently reduces the inhibition of the 5-lipoxygenase–leukotriene C4 (LTC4) synthase pathway, which converts arachidonic acid to the cysteinyl leukotrienes, and also results in enhanced mast-cell activation (release of histamine, tryptase, and prostaglandin D2).[17]

Patients susceptible to these reactions typically present with cross-intolerance to multiple NSAIDs, rather than an isolated agent. Genetic predictors of these reactions to aspirin, and NSAIDs more broadly, have been examined and belong to the arachidonic acid pathway (Arachidonate 5-Lipoxygenase [*ALOX5*], Leukotriene C4 Synthase [*LTC4S*], Thromboxane A2 Receptor [*TBXA2R*], Prostaglandin E Receptor 4 [*PTGER4*]), the membrane-spanning 4A gene family, and the histamine production pathway and also include the proinflammatory cytokines (Tumor Necrosis Factor [*TNF*], Transforming Growth Factor Beta 1 [*TGFB1*], Interleukin 18 [*IL-18*]).[18] In addition, genome-wide association studies (GWAS) have identified Centrosomal Protein 68 (*CEP68*) and *HLA-DPB1* as the strongest candidates associated with AERD.[19,20]

Other NSAID reactions. Cutaneous hypersensitivities to aspirin and other NSAID drugs can be classified as per the European Academy of Allergy and Clinical Immunology definitions, including (1) NSAID-exacerbated cutaneous (chronic urticaria) disease and (2) NSAID-induced urticaria/angioedema (isolated or cross-reactive).[21] An association with human leukocyte antigen (HLA) genes (*HLA-DRB1*, *HLA-B44*, *HLA-Cw5*) and arachidonic acid pathway genes (*ALOX5*, *ALOX5AP*, *ALOX15*, *TBXAS1*, Prostaglandin D2 Receptor [*PTGDR*], Cysteinyl Leukotriene Receptor 1 [*CYSLTR1*]) has been identified as predictors of these immune-mediated cutaneous NSAID ADRs.[22–26] As yet, there has been a limited number of genomic studies examining immune-mediated immediate hypersensitivity outside of antibiotics and antiinflammatories, namely, for biological therapies.[27,28] There currently remains an absence of pharmacogenomics studies incorporating identified genes to diagnostics

and therapeutic approaches for patients with NSAID-related chronic or acute urticaria.

Drug-induced thrombocytopenia

Drug-induced thrombocytopenia presents as moderate to severe thrombocytopenia (a platelet count of $<50 \times 10^9$/L) and spontaneous bleeding varying from simple ecchymoses, petechiae, and mucosal bleeding to life-threatening spontaneous intracranial hemorrhage. Drug-induced thrombocytopenia disorders can be a consequence of two mechanisms, either decreased platelet production caused by bone marrow suppression or accelerated immune-mediated destruction of platelets, referred to as drug-induced immune thrombocytopenia (DITP). Nonimmune thrombocytopenia results from a loss of cellularity within the bone marrow and an impairment of megakaryocyte proliferation and maturation, thereby leading to decreased platelet production. Chemotherapeutic agents are most often implicated in non-immune-mediated thrombocytopenia.[29] Several theories have been proposed to explain the development of DITP[1]: classic drug-dependent platelet antibodies (quinine-type)[2]; hapten-induced antibodies (e.g., penicillin)[3]; fiban-dependent antibodies (e.g., tirofiban)[4]; Fab-binding monoclonal antibodies (e.g., abciximab)[5]; drug-induced autoantibody formation (e.g., gold); and[6] immune complex formation (e.g., heparin). Multiple medications may cause DITP, with quinine, quinidine, trimethoprim-sulfamethoxazole, and vancomycin most often implicated.[30] The detection of drug-dependent platelet antibodies in vitro can confirm the diagnosis of DITP.

Heparin-induced thrombocytopenia. Heparin and related anticoagulants are associated with the development of heparin-induced thrombocytopenia in up to 2.4% of treated patients with thromboembolic disorders. Heparin-induced thrombocytopenia (HIT) is an immune-mediated, off-target effect with a 30% mortality rate with a unique kinetics that does not resemble either a typical primary or a secondary immune response. An increased risk is seen with a higher heparin dose and longer duration of treatment, major invasive surgery or trauma, and other classic risk factors for thromboembolism.[31]

HIT is associated with the development of antibodies to complexes of heparin and platelet factor 4 (PF4), a protein normally found in the α granules of platelets.[32] The anti-PF4/H response shows a unique profile that cannot be explained by a secondary response, a memory response, or general nonspecific activation of memory B cells.[33] Patients exhibit several unique features, including an early peak in anti-PF4/H IgG antibodies even in heparin-naive patients, which are increased in the context of trauma or inflammation. Some anti-PF4H/H antibodies show characteristics of autoantibodies in binding to PF4 on platelets even in the absence of heparin. Conversely, anti-PF4H/H Ab titers typically decrease rapidly, unlike in a secondary immune response.[33]

Up to 50% of heparin-treated patients will develop PF4/heparin antibodies, but the vast majority do not progress to full-blown HIT. Clinicians test for PF4/heparin antibodies to aid in the diagnosis of HIT, but these tests have a high false-positive rate. Other diagnostic tests for HIT include functional assays such as the serotonin release assay, which tests platelet reactivity to heparin in vitro. Owing to assay limitations in clinical testing and the inability to predict HIT in heparin-treated patients, the identification of genetic risk factors for HIT is necessary. Identified genetic polymorphisms associated with HIT include the gene coding for the Fcγ receptor RIIIA (*FCGR3A*) expressed by monocytes/macrophages[34–37] and variants in the T cell death associated gene 8 (*TDAG8*).[38] However, none of these identified genetic risk factors to date reliably predict HIT and further research is required.

REACTIONS INVOLVING IMMUNOLOGIC MEMORY

Immediate/Accelerated Immune-Mediated Reactions

Immediate reactions (<1 h after drug administration) and early accelerated reactions (<6 h after drug administration) are commonly mediated via IgE-dependent pathways. Accelerated reactions that occur between 6 and 72 h after dosing are more likely to be mediated by T cells or by a non-IgE-mediated mechanism. Most genetic studies to date have focused on immediate drug hypersensitivity to β-lactams, aspirin, or NSAIDs,[18] and although a small number of GWAS have examined antibiotic-associated ADRs, a single implicated gene(s) has been elusive. However, for the β-lactams the greatest association appears in the HLA class 2 antigen-presenting genes, cytokines (*IL4, IL4R, IL13, IL18, IL10*), and production and release of preformed mediators (Galectin 3 [*LGALS3*] as the strongest predictor).[23,39–42]

Delayed Immune Reactions
Human leukocyte antigen
T cells recognize peptides that are displayed on the cell surface bound to an HLA molecule via the T cell receptor (TCR). Class I major histocompatibility complex (MHC) molecules (HLA-A, -B and -C) are expressed by all nucleated cells and interact with an appropriate TCR on the surface of CD8+ T cells, whereas the expression of class II MHC (HLA-DM, HLA-DO, HLA-DP, HLA-DQ, and HLA-DR) is restricted to professional antigen-presenting cells that present foreign antigens to TCRs of CD4+ T cells. In support of an adaptation of conventional presentation of peptides together with HLA molecules from antigen-presenting cells, there are many well-characterized examples of drug hypersensitivity with strong HLA associations (Table 5.2). The online resource, the HLA Adverse Drug Reaction Database, provides a comprehensive database of published risk and protective HLA associations for the majority of drugs linked to delayed HSSs.[43]

Several models have been proposed to explain how smaller synthetic compounds are recognized by T cells and how they are able to elicit an immune response. These include the hapten/prohapten hypothesis and the "pharmacological interaction of drugs with immune receptors" (P-I) model. These models are explained in detail in Chapter 4. The *P-I model* of drug hypersensitivity is based on the hypothesis that drugs can form noncovalent bonds with immune receptors. This broad concept can cover the direct interaction of drugs with antigen-presenting HLA molecules or stimulation of the TCR. The *Altered Peptide Model* is an expansion of the P-I concept and provides an explanation for the development of ABC HSS. The crystal structure of ABC bound to HLA-B*57:01 shows that ABC binds noncovalently to the floor of the peptide-binding groove of HLA-B*57:01, altering the chemistry and shape of the antigen-binding cleft[44,45] and the subsequent repertoire of peptides presented to T cells.

Other HSRs with well-characterized class I HLA associations include carbamazepine SJS/TEN with *HLA-B*15:02*, allopurinol SJS/TEN and DRESS with *HLA-B*58:01*, dapsone DRESS with *HLA-B*13:01*, and flucloxacillin-induced DILI in carriers of *HLA-B*57:01* (Table 5.2; Fig. 5.2).[48,49,56,57] These syndromes have much lower positive predictive values for the implicated HLA alleles when compared with *HLA-B*57:01* and ABC HSS[58] (Table 5.2). Determining the reason why some individuals with risk alleles do not develop drug HSR syndromes but others do is a remaining challenge in ADR research.

PHARMACOGENOMIC SCREENING
Although many candidate genes have been identified as significant in the development of both "on target" and "off target" driven ADRs, the implementation

TABLE 5.2
Adverse Drug Reactions With Well-Defined HLA Associations

Drug ADR	HLA Allele	HLA Carriage Rate	Disease Prevalence	OR	NPV	PPV	NNT to prevent "1"	HLA screening
Abacavir Hypersensitivity syndrome	B*57:01	5%–8% Caucasian <1% African/Asian 2.5% African American	8% (3% true HSR and 2%–7% false-positive diagnosis	960	100% for patch test confirmed	55%	13	Yes
Allopurinol SJS/TEN and DRESS/DIHS	B*58:01	9%–11% Han Chinese 1%–6% Caucasian	1/250–1/1000	>800	100% in Han Chinese	3%	250	Yes
Carbamazepine SJS/TEN	B*15:02	10%–15% Han Chinese <0.1% Caucasian	<1–6/1000 (Han Chinese)	>1000	100% in Han Chinese (with other B75 serotype)	3%	1000	Yes
Dapsone DRESS/DIHS	B*13:01	2%–20% Chinese 28% Papuans/Australian Aboriginals 0% European/African 1.5% Japanese	1%–4% Han Chinese	20	99.8%	7.8%	84	Yes?
Flucloxacillin DILI	B*57:01	As above	8.5/100 000	81	99.99%	0.12%	13,819	?

ADR, adverse drug reaction; *DIHS*, drug-induced hypersensitivity syndrome; *DILI*, drug induced liver injury; *DRESS*, drug rash eosinophilia and systemic symptoms; *HLA*, human leukocyte antigen; *HSR*, hypersensitivity reaction; *NNT*, number needed to treat; *NPV*, negative predictive value; *OR*, odds ratio; *PPV*, positive predictive value; *SJS*, Stevens-Johnson syndrome; *TEN*, toxic epidermal necrolysis.

of any pharmacogenomic test must be cost-effective in clinical practice. As such, the ADRs must have severe clinical or economic consequences, exhibit a well-established association between genotype and clinical phenotypes, and have a high positive predictive value of the associated gene variant for the ADR phenotype.[59,60] These factors determine the cost and number of patients required to be tested to avoid one ADR case and have implications for patients who may unnecessarily be denied optimal treatment, who carry risk alleles but would not have developed an adverse reaction. The presence of alternative drugs that have a wider safety margin and/or do not require genetic testing is another factor that may affect the likelihood of a successful translation of pharmacogenetics testing into routine clinical practice. Of the 27

factors that are necessary for translation of a pharmacogenetics test into clinical practice, it is estimated that 10 related to the characteristics of the test allele, the drug, and the drug toxicity may be nonmodifiable, whereas general factors relating to the research/clinical environment, the ability to generate high-level evidence, laboratory support, and design and implementation of clinical systems may be dynamic over time, determined largely by the burden of a particular ADR (Table 5.3).[62,70]

Screening for risk HLA genes in delayed ADRs is a successful example of pharmacogenomic screening. The first global screening program for *HLA-B*57:01* before starting ABC therapy has successfully eradicated reported cases of ABC HSS in areas where routine HLA-B*57:01 screening has been introduced.[63,64] The high

Year		Drug Reaction	HLA Association
2002	CHRONOLOGY OF THE GENETICS OF SEVERE T CELL–MEDIATED ADRS	ABACAVIR HSR	HLA-B*57:01
2004		Carbamazepine SJS/TEN	HLA-B*15:02
2005		Allopurinol DRESS/SJS/TEN Nevirapine rash/hepatitis	HLA-B*58:01 HLA-DRBA*01:01
2008		Other Aromatic amine anticonvulsants Nevirapine HSR	HLA-B*15:02 HLA-B*14:02/Cw8
2009		Nevirapine rash Flucoxacillin DILI	HLA-B*35:05 HLA-B*57:01
2011		Carbamazepine SJS/TEN/DRESS/MPE Methazolamide SJS/TEN Amox-clav DILI Lapatinib DILI Nevirapine HSR (cutaneous)	HLA-A*31:01 HLA-B*59:01 HLA-A*02:01/DRB1*15:01 HLA-DQA1*02:01 CYP2B6 516 G→T
2013		Carbamazepine SJS/TEN Nevirapine hepatitis Nevirapine SJS/TEN Nevirapine SJS/TEN	other B75 serotype HLA HLA-B*58:01 and HLA-DRB1*01:02 HLA-C*04:01 CYP2B6 516 G→T and 983 T→C
2014		Phenytoin SJS/TEN>DRESS>MPE Thiopurine pancreatitis	CYP2C9*3 HLA-DRB1*07:01/DQA1*02:01
2015		Carbimazole/methimazole aganulocytosis	HLA-B*38:02
2016		Antithyroid drug agranulocytosis	HLA-B*27:05

FIG. 5.2 **Chronology of Genetics of Severe T Cell–Mediated Adverse Drug Reactions.** The discovery of the association of abacavir hypersensitivity and *HLA-B*57:01* was the breakthrough observation that first linked drug hypersensitivity to class I–restricted, T cell–driven mechanisms.[46,47] Since then, associations between class I human leukocyte antigen (HLA) alleles and severe immunologically mediated drug reactions have dominated. The early examples of carbamazepine and *HLA-B*15:02* in Stevens-Johnson syndrome/toxic epidermal necrolysis (SJS/TEN) in Asians and allopurinol and *HLA-B*58:01* in severe cutaneous adverse reactions have also provided key insights into hypersensitivity reaction (HSR) pathogenesis.[48–50] In some examples, such as amoxicillin-clavulanate drug-induced liver disease in Northern Europeans, class I/II pairings appear important, whereas others, such as nevirapine hypersensitivity with hepatotoxicity phenotype, appear restricted primarily to class II HLA alleles.[51,52] Drug metabolism also confers independent risk for some adverse drug reactions such as phenytoin with *CYP2CP*3*[53] and cutaneous nevirapine hypersensitivity with *CYP2B6 516G>T*.[54,55] *DILI*, drug induced liver injury; *MPE*, maculopapular exanthema.

TABLE 5.3
Prerequisites for Widespread Incorporation of Pharmacogenetic Testing Into Routine Clinical Practice, Illustrated by Key Examples of ADRs With Strong HLA Associations

Prerequisites	DRUG/HLA ASSOCIATION		
	ABC	CBZ	ALL
TEST			
1. HLA allele is strongly associated with the toxicity, and the negative predictive value of the test is high across all populations*	+++	++	++
2. The number of patients needed for testing to prevent a case of toxicity is low*	+++	++	++
3. HLA allele is prevalent in a large, nondisenfranchised population*	++	++	++
DRUG			
4. Drug exhibits favorable attributes, such as good efficacy, convenience in dosing and administration, tolerability, and pill burden*	+++	++	+++
5. Alternative drug(s) that do not require pharmacogenetic testing are either absent or have negative attributes*	++	+	+++
DRUG TOXICITY			
6. Toxicity is severe and persistent* (i.e., not isolated mild rash)	++	++	++
7. Toxicity is readily and accurately phenotyped*	+	++	++

Prerequisites	DRUG/HLA ASSOCIATION		
	ABC	CBZ	ALL
8. An adjunctive diagnostic test, such as skin patch testing or ex vivo testing (e.g., ELISpot) can improve phenotypic precision	+++	++	+[a]
ENVIRONMENT			
9. Champions available (e.g., clinical academics, industry [if drug not off patent*], professional bodies, regulatory agencies, guideline committees, patient advocacy groups, laboratory providers, and the media), willing, and able to drive pharmacogenetic test development and implementation	+++	++	++
GENERATION OF HIGH-LEVEL EVIDENCE			
10. Case-control studies with estimated predictive values based on the assumed prevalence of the HLA allele	++	++	++
11. Population-based cohort studies with directly calculated predictive values of the test	++	++	++
12. Open screening studies	++	++	+
13. Supportive experimental data	+++	++	++
14. Blinded randomized controlled trials	+++	−	−
15. Evidence across ethnic groups and geographic areas to determine the clinical settings that the test may be applied to	+++	++	++
16. Cost-effectiveness data	++	++	++
DEVELOPMENT AND AVAILABILITY OF APPROPRIATE LABORATORY SUPPORT			
17. No patent restriction on use of the test*	++	++	++
18. Development of simple, inexpensive, robust, unambiguous laboratory tests	+++	++	+
19. Rapid and simple report and interpretation	+++	++	++
20. Development of reagents (e.g., mAbs, PCR-based kits)	+++	++	+
21. Global distribution and commercialization of allele-specific test	+++	+	+
22. Allele-specific quality assurance targeted to avoid false-negative results and consequent morbidity or mortality	+++	+	+
23. Reimbursement of test	+++	++[b]	+/−[c]
DESIGN AND IMPLEMENTATION OF APPROPRIATE CLINICAL SYSTEMS			
24. Education of clinicians, nurses, pharmacists, phlebotomists, and patients	+++	++	++
25. Systems to ensure appropriate and routine triggering of ordering of the test	+	+	+
26. Systems in the clinic to ensure the correct blood samples are sent to the correct laboratory for analysis	+	+	+
27. Systems to ensure test results and correct interpretation are rapidly transmitted to, retained by, and acted on by the health care team and patient	+	+	+

ABC, abacavir/HLA-B*57:01 association; *ADR*, adverse drug reaction; *ALL*, allopurinol/HLA-B*58:01 association; *CBZ*, carbamazepine/HLA-B*15:02 association; *HLA*, human leukocyte antigen; *mAb*, monoclonal antibody; *PCR*, polymerase chain reaction.

A number of prerequisites that must be in place for successful integration of pharmacogenetic testing into routine clinical care are listed. Typically, all of these prerequisites must be satisfactorily fulfilled for the incorporation of the testing to be successful. Many of the necessary attributes associated with the test, drug, toxicity, and environment are not modifiable (indicated by *), whereas other critical elements, such as the availability of a sufficient amount of evidence of the appropriate type and adequate laboratory and clinical systems, can be developed with sufficient time and resources. +++ prerequisite present and very strongly influential, ++ prerequisite present and strongly influential, + prerequisite present and moderately influential, − prerequisite absent.

Reproduced with permission from Clarivate Analytics (formerly the IP & Science Division of Thomson Reuters) and Phillips EJ, Mallal SA. HLA and drug-induced toxicity. *Curr Opin Mol Ther.* 2009;11(3):231–242 © Clarivate Analytics.

[a]Allopurinol and oxypurinol patch testing have no utility in the clinical setting; the oxypurinol lymphocyte transformation test has correlated with the phenotype of allopurinol drug rash eosinophilia and systemic symptoms and Stevens-Johnson syndrome/toxic epidermal necrolysis.

[b]HLA-B*15:02 is now reimbursed by governmental programs in many parts of Southeast Asia, the United Kingdom, and some third-party payers in the United States.

[c]HLA-B*58:01 is still not routinely covered in most areas.

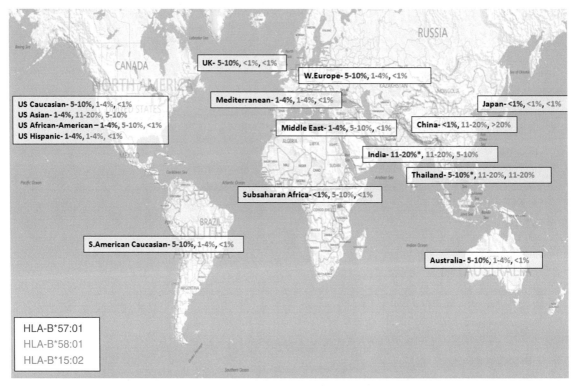

*High prevalence of HLA-B*57:01 refers to Northern Thailand and Northern India only with intermediate percentages or <1% prevalence reported in other regions*

FIG. 5.3 **Global Frequencies of Human Leukocyte Antigen (HLA) Risk Alleles for Delayed Adverse Drug Reactions.** Geographic distribution and frequency of the key drug hypersensitivity reaction (HSR) alleles associated with abacavir HSS, allopurinol drug rash eosinophilia and systemic symptoms (DRESS)/drug-induced hypersensitivity syndrome (DIHS)/hypersensitivity syndrome (HSS) and Stevens-Johnson syndrome/toxic epidermal necrolysis (SJS/TEN) and carbamazepine SJS/TEN. Red, HLA-B*57:01 frequency; blue, HLA-B*58:01 frequency; and green, HLA-B*15:02 frequency. (Adapted from Ref. 70.)

positive predictive value of *HLA-B*57:01* for ABC HSS (55%) has meant that this has been a cost-effective approach. For *HLA-B*15:02*-driven CBZ SJS/TEN, the prevalence of *HLA-B*15:02* is the highest among Asian populations (0.057 to 0.145 in Han Chinese, 0.085 to 0.275 in Thais, and 0.12 to 0.157 in Malays) compared with European (0.01 to 0.02), Japanese (0.002), and Korean populations (0.004) (Fig. 5.3). Studies based in Taiwan and Thailand have demonstrated the utility and cost-effectiveness of *HLA-B*15:02* screening in such populations where the risk allele is most common.[65,66] Other screening programs currently being implemented or evaluated include *HLA-B*58:01* testing before allopurinol initiation and *CYP2C9*3/HLA-B*15:02/HLA-B*13:01* screening before phenytoin prescription in Southeast Asians.[67-69]

Future research into the pharmacogenomics of ADRs will focus on additional risk factors that will influence the development of these syndromes. Ideally, some of these findings will be translated to personalized medicine whereby a range of risk factors can be explored within an individual before administration of risk medications. For many drug-gene pairs, the necessary prerequisites for successful translation into screening programs may be lacking. Regardless of whether genetic testing can be successfully translated into clinical practice it provides considerable insight and clues into the mechanisms and immunopathogenesis of associated drug HSSs. It is likely that this knowledge will be most useful in improving preclinical screening and drug development, to better the understanding of mechanisms by which drugs cause adverse reactions and the specific risk factors involved.

ACKNOWLEDGEMENT

National Institute of Health:1P50GM115305-01, 1R01 AI103348-01, 1P30AI110527-01A1, 5T32AI007474-20, 1 R13AR71267-01, National Health & Medical Research Council of Australia, Australian Centre for HIV and Hepatitis Virology Research.

REFERENCES

1. White KD, Chung WH, Hung SI, Mallal S, Phillips EJ. Evolving models of the immunopathogenesis of T cell-mediated drug allergy: The role of host, pathogens, and drug response. *J Allergy Clin Immunol*. 2015;136(2):219–234. quiz 35.
2. Gell PGH CR. The classification of allergic reactions underlying disease. In: Gell PGH CR, ed. *Clinical Aspects of Immunology*. 2nd ed. Oxford: Blackwell Scientific; 1963.
3. Pirmohamed M, Aithal GP, Behr E, Daly A, Roden D. The phenotype standardization project: improving pharmacogenetic studies of serious adverse drug reactions. *Clin Pharmacol Ther*. 2011;89(6):784–785.
4. Caudle KE, Dunnenberger HM. *Standardizing Terms for Clinical Pharmacogenetic Test Results: Consensus Terms from the CLINICAL Pharmacogenetics Implementation Consortium (CPIC)*; 2016.
5. Gaedigk A, Sangkuhl K, Whirl-Carrillo M, Klein T. Prediction of CYP2D6 phenotype from genotype across world populations. *Genet Med*. 2016;19.
6. FDA US. Table of pharmacogenomic biomarkers in drug labeling. Available from: http://www.fda.gov/drugs/sciencere search/researchareas/pharmacogenetics/ucm083378.htm.
7. Liu YP, Wu HY, Yang X, Xu HQ, Li YC, Shi DC, et al. Association between thiopurine S-methyltransferase polymorphisms and thiopurine-induced adverse drug reactions in patients with inflammatory bowel disease: a meta-analysis. *PLoS One*. 2015;10(3):e0121745.
8. Link E, Parish S, Armitage J, Bowman L, Heath S, Matsuda F, et al. SLCO1B1 variants and statin-induced myopathy–a genomewide study. *N Engl J Med*. 2008;359(8):789–799.
9. Subramanian H, Gupta K, Ali H. Roles of Mas-related G protein-coupled receptor X2 on mast cell-mediated host defense, pseudoallergic drug reactions, and chronic inflammatory diseases. *J Allergy Clin Immunol*. 2016;138(3):700–710.
10. Tatemoto K, Nozaki Y, Tsuda R, Konno S, Tomura K, Furuno M, et al. Immunoglobulin E-independent activation of mast cell is mediated by Mrg receptors. *Biochem Biophys Res Commun*. 2006;349(4):1322–1328.
11. McNeil BD, Pundir P, Meeker S, Han L, Undem BJ, Kulka M, et al. Identification of a mast-cell-specific receptor crucial for pseudo-allergic drug reactions. *Nature*. 2015;519(7542):237–241.
12. Heller D, Doyle JR, Raman VS, Beinborn M, Kumar K, Kopin AS. Novel Probes Establish Mas-Related G Protein-Coupled Receptor X1 Variants as Receptors with Loss or Gain of Function. *J Pharmacol Exp Ther*. 2016;356(2):276–283.
13. Wilson AP. Comparative safety of teicoplanin and vancomycin. *Int J Antimicrob Agents*. 1998;10(2):143–152.
14. Sivagnanam S, Deleu D. Red man syndrome. *Crit Care*. 2003;7(2):119–120.
15. Berges-Gimeno MP, Simon RA, Stevenson DD. The natural history and clinical characteristics of aspirin-exacerbated respiratory disease. *Ann Allergy Asthma Immunol*. 2002;89(5):474–478.
16. Rajan JP, Wineinger NE, Stevenson DD, White AA. Prevalence of aspirin-exacerbated respiratory disease among asthmatic patients: A meta-analysis of the literature. *J Allergy Clin Immunol*. 2015;135(3):676–681. e1.
17. Laidlaw TM, Boyce JA. Aspirin-Exacerbated Respiratory Disease–New Prime Suspects. *N Engl J Med*. 2016;374(5):484–488.
18. Oussalah A, Mayorga C, Blanca M, Barbaud A, Nakonechna A, Cernadas J, et al. Genetic variants associated with drugs-induced immediate hypersensitivity reactions: a PRISMA-compliant systematic review. *Allergy*. 2016;71(4):443–462.
19. Kim JH, Park BL, Cheong HS, Bae JS, Park JS, Jang AS, et al. Genome-wide and follow-up studies identify CEP68 gene variants associated with risk of aspirin-intolerant asthma. *PLoS One*. 2010;5(11):e13818.
20. Park BL, Kim TH, Kim JH, Bae JS, Pasaje CF, Cheong HS, et al. Genome-wide association study of aspirin-exacerbated respiratory disease in a Korean population. *Human Genet*. 2013;132(3):313–321.
21. Kowalski ML, Woessner K, Sanak M. Approaches to the diagnosis and management of patients with a history of nonsteroidal anti-inflammatory drug-related urticaria and angioedema. *J Allergy Clin Immunol*. 2015;136(2):245–251.
22. Ayuso P, Plaza-Seron Mdel C, Dona I, Blanca-Lopez N, Campo P, Cornejo-Garcia JA, et al. Association study of genetic variants in PLA2G4A, PLCG1, LAT, SYK, and TNFRS11A genes in NSAIDs-induced urticaria and/or angioedema patients. *Pharmacogenet Genom*. 2015;25(12):618–621.
23. Cornejo-Garcia JA, Gueant-Rodriguez RM, Torres MJ, Blanca-Lopez N, Tramoy D, Romano A, et al. Biological and genetic determinants of atopy are predictors of immediate-type allergy to beta-lactams, in Spain. *Allergy*. 2012;67(9):1181–1185.
24. Pacor ML, Di Lorenzo G, Mansueto P, Martinelli N, Esposito-Pellitteri M, Pradella P, et al. Relationship between human leucocyte antigen class I and class II and chronic idiopathic urticaria associated with aspirin and/or NSAIDs hypersensitivity. *Mediators Inflammation*. 2006;2006(5):62489.
25. Quiralte J, Sanchez-Garcia F, Torres MJ, Blanco C, Castillo R, Ortega N, et al. Association of HLA-DR11 with the anaphylactoid reaction caused by nonsteroidal anti-inflammatory drugs. *J Allergy Clin Immunol*. 1999;103(4):685–689.
26. Vidal C, Porras-Hurtado L, Cruz R, Quiralte J, Cardona V, Colas C, et al. Association of thromboxane A1 synthase

(TBXAS1) gene polymorphism with acute urticaria induced by nonsteroidal anti-inflammatory drugs. *J Allergy Clin Immunol*. 2013;132(4):989–991.

27. Fuerst D, Parmar S, Schumann C, Rudiger S, Boeck S, Heinemann V, et al. HLA polymorphisms influence the development of skin rash arising from treatment with EGF receptor inhibitors. *Pharmacogenomics*. 2012;13(13):1469–1476.

28. Steenholdt C, Enevold C, Ainsworth MA, Brynskov J, Thomsen OO, Bendtzen K. Genetic polymorphisms of tumour necrosis factor receptor superfamily 1b and fas ligand are associated with clinical efficacy and/or acute severe infusion reactions to infliximab in Crohn's disease. *Aliment Pharmacol Ther*. 2012;36(7):650–659.

29. Liebman HA. Thrombocytopenia in cancer patients. *Thromb Res*. 2014;133(suppl 2):S63–S69.

30. Arnold DM, Nazi I, Warkentin TE, Smith JW, Toltl LJ, George JN, et al. Approach to the diagnosis and management of drug-induced immune thrombocytopenia. *Transfus Med Rev*. 2013;27(3):137–145.

31. Lubenow N, Eichler P, Lietz T, Greinacher A. Lepirudin in patients with heparin-induced thrombocytopenia - results of the third prospective study (HAT-3) and a combined analysis of HAT-1, HAT-2, and HAT-3. Journal of thrombosis and haemostasis. *JTH*. 2005;3(11):2428–2436.

32. Cuker A. Heparin-induced thrombocytopenia: present and future. *J Thromb Thrombolysis*. 2011;31(3):353–366.

33. Potschke C, Selleng S, Broker BM, Greinacher A. Heparin-induced thrombocytopenia: further evidence for a unique immune response. *Blood*. 2012;120(20):4238–4245.

34. Gruel Y, Pouplard C, Lasne D, Magdelaine-Beuzelin C, Charroing C, Watier H. The homozygous FcgammaRI-IIa-158V genotype is a risk factor for heparin-induced thrombocytopenia in patients with antibodies to heparin-platelet factor 4 complexes. *Blood*. 2004;104(9):2791–2793.

35. Pamela S, Anna Maria L, Elena D, Giovanni M, Emanuele A, Silvia V, et al. Heparin-induced thrombocytopenia: the role of platelets genetic polymorphisms. *Platelets*. 2013;24(5):362–368.

36. Rollin J, Pouplard C, Gratacap MP, Leroux D, May MA, Aupart M, et al. Polymorphisms of protein tyrosine phosphatase CD148 influence FcgammaRIIA-dependent platelet activation and the risk of heparin-induced thrombocytopenia. *Blood*. 2012;120(6):1309–1316.

37. Rollin J, Pouplard C, Leroux D, May MA, Gruel Y. Impact of polymorphisms affecting the ACP1 gene on levels of antibodies against platelet factor 4-heparin complexes. *JTH*. 2013;11(8):1609–1611.

38. Karnes JH, Cronin RM, Rollin J, Teumer A, Pouplard C, Shaffer CM, et al. A genome-wide association study of heparin-induced thrombocytopenia using an electronic medical record. *Thromb Haemost*. 2015;113(4):772–781.

39. Gueant JL, Romano A, Cornejo-Garcia JA, Oussalah A, Chery C, Blanca-Lopez N, et al. HLA-DRA variants predict penicillin allergy in genome-wide fine-mapping genotyping. *J Allergy Clin Immunol*. 2015;135(1):253–259.

40. Huang CZ, Yang J, Qiao HL, Jia LJ. Polymorphisms and haplotype analysis of IL-4Ralpha Q576R and I75V in patients with penicillin allergy. *Eur J Clin Pharmacol*. 2009;65(9):895–902.

41. Huang CZ, Zou D, Yang J, Qiao HL. Polymorphisms of STAT6 and specific serum IgE levels in patients with penicillin allergy. *Int J Clin Pharmacol Ther*. 2012;50(7):461–467.

42. Ming L, Wen Q, Qiao HL, Dong ZM. Interleukin-18 and IL18 -607A/C and -137G/C gene polymorphisms in patients with penicillin allergy. *J Int Med Res*. 2011;39(2):388–398.

43. Ghattaoraya GS, Dundar Y, Gonzalez-Galarza FF, Maia MH, Santos EJ, da Silva AL, et al. A web resource for mining HLA associations with adverse drug reactions: HLA-ADR. *Database*. 2016:2016.

44. Illing PT, Vivian JP, Dudek NL, Kostenko L, Chen Z, Bharadwaj M, et al. Immune self-reactivity triggered by drug-modified HLA-peptide repertoire. *Nature*. 2012;486(7404):554–558.

45. Ostrov DA, Grant BJ, Pompeu YA, Sidney J, Harndahl M, Southwood S, et al. Drug hypersensitivity caused by alteration of the MHC-presented self-peptide repertoire. *Proc Natl Acad Sci USA*. 2012;109(25):9959–9964.

46. Hetherington S, Hughes AR, Mosteller M, Shortino D, Baker KL, Spreen W, et al. Genetic variations in HLA-B region and hypersensitivity reactions to abacavir. *Lancet*. 2002;359(9312):1121–1122.

47. Mallal S, Nolan D, Witt C, Masel G, Martin AM, Moore C, et al. Association between presence of HLA-B*5701, HLA-DR7, and HLA-DQ3 and hypersensitivity to HIV-1 reverse-transcriptase inhibitor abacavir. *Lancet*. 2002;359(9308):727–732.

48. Hung SI, Chung WH, Jee SH, Chen WC, Chang YT, Lee WR, et al. Genetic susceptibility to carbamazepine-induced cutaneous adverse drug reactions. *Pharmacogenet Genom*. 2006;16(4):297–306.

49. Hung SI, Chung WH, Liou LB, Chu CC, Lin M, Huang HP, et al. HLA-B*5801 allele as a genetic marker for severe cutaneous adverse reactions caused by allopurinol. *Proc Natl Acad Sci USA*. 2005;102(11):4134–4139.

50. Chung WH, Hung SI, Hong HS, Hsih MS, Yang LC, Ho HC, et al. Medical genetics: a marker for Stevens-Johnson syndrome. *Nature*. 2004;428(6982):486.

51. Donaldson PT, Daly AK, Henderson J, Graham J, Pirmohamed M, Bernal W, et al. Human leucocyte antigen class II genotype in susceptibility and resistance to co-amoxiclav-induced liver injury. *J Hepatol*. 2010;53(6):1049–1053.

52. Martin AM, Nolan D, James I, Cameron P, Keller J, Moore C, et al. Predisposition to nevirapine hypersensitivity associated with HLA-DRB1*0101 and abrogated by low CD4 T-cell counts. *AIDS*. 2005;19(1):97–99.

53. Chung WH, Chang WC, Lee YS, Wu YY, Yang CH, Ho HC, et al. Genetic variants associated with phenytoin-related severe cutaneous adverse reactions. *Jama*. 2014;312(5):525–534.

54. Carr DF, Chaponda M, Cornejo Castro EM, Jorgensen AL, Khoo S, Van Oosterhout JJ, et al. CYP2B6 c.983T>C polymorphism is associated with nevirapine hypersensitivity in Malawian and Ugandan HIV populations. *J Antimicrob Chemother.* 2014;69(12):3329–3334.

55. Yuan J, Guo S, Hall D, Cammett AM, Jayadev S, Distel M, et al. Toxicogenomics of nevirapine-associated cutaneous and hepatic adverse events among populations of African, Asian, and European descent. *AIDS.* 2011;25(10):1271–1280.

56. Zhang FR, Liu H, Irwanto A, Fu XA, Li Y, Yu GQ, et al. HLA-B*13:01 and the dapsone hypersensitivity syndrome. *N Engl J Med.* 2013;369(17):1620–1628.

57. Daly AK, Donaldson PT, Bhatnagar P, Shen Y, Pe'er I, Floratos A, et al. HLA-B*5701 genotype is a major determinant of drug-induced liver injury due to flucloxacillin. *Nat Genet.* 2009;41(7):816–819.

58. Mallal S, Phillips E, Carosi G, Molina JM, Workman C, Tomazic J, et al. HLA-B*5701 screening for hypersensitivity to abacavir. *N Engl J Med.* 2008;358(6):568–579.

59. Veenstra DL. The value of routine pharmacogenomic screening-Are we there yet? A perspective on the costs and benefits of routine screening-shouldn't everyone have this done? *Clin Pharmacol Ther.* 2016;99(2):164–166.

60. Mallal S, Phillips E. Introduction of pharmacogenetic screening to HIV clinical practice: potential benefits and challenges. *Eur Infect Dis.* June 1, 2007:13–18.

61. Phillips EJ. Classifying ADRs–does dose matter? *Br J Clin Pharmacol.* 2016;81(1):10–12.

62. Phillips EJ, Mallal SA. HLA and drug-induced toxicity. *Curr Opin Mol Ther.* 2009;11(3):231–242.

63. Phillips E, Mallal S. Successful translation of pharmacogenetics into the clinic: the abacavir example. *Mol Diagn Ther.* 2009;13(1):1–9.

64. Yip VL, Hawcutt DB, Pirmohamed M. Pharmacogenetic Markers of Drug Efficacy and Toxicity. *Clin Pharmacol Ther.* 2015;98(1):61–70.

65. Chen P, Lin JJ, Lu CS, Ong CT, Hsieh PF, Yang CC, et al. Carbamazepine-induced toxic effects and HLA-B*1502 screening in Taiwan. *N Engl J Med.* 2011;364(12):1126–1133.

66. Locharernkul C, Shotelersuk V, Hirankarn N. HLA-B* 1502 screening: time to clinical practice. *Epilepsia.* 2010;51(5):936–938.

67. Ko TM, Tsai CY, Chen SY, Chen KS, Yu KH, Chu CS, et al. Use of HLA-B*58:01 genotyping to prevent allopurinol induced severe cutaneous adverse reactions in Taiwan: national prospective cohort study. *Bmj.* 2015;351:h4848.

68. Saokaew S, Tassaneeyakul W, Maenthaisong R, Chaiyakunapruk N. Cost-effectiveness analysis of HLA-B*5801 testing in preventing allopurinol-induced SJS/TEN in Thai population. *Clin Chem Lab Med.* 2014;9(4):e94294.

69. Caudle KE, Rettie AE, Whirl-Carrillo M, Smith LH, Mintzer S, Lee MT, et al. Clinical pharmacogenetics implementation consortium guidelines for CYP2C9 and HLA-B genotypes and phenytoin dosing. *Clin Pharmacol Ther.* 2014;96(5):542–548.

70. Pavlos R, Mallal S, Ostrov D, Pompeu Y, Phillips E. Fever, rash, and systemic symptoms: understanding the role of virus and HLA in severe cutaneous drug allergy. *J Allergy Clin Immunol Pract.* 2014;2(1):21–33.

CHAPTER 6

Cutaneous Reactions to Drugs

STEPHEN J. LOCKWOOD, MD, MPH • ARTURO P. SAAVEDRA, MD, PHD

INTRODUCTION

Adverse drug reactions (ADRs) encompass the largest single category of adverse events experienced by hospitalized patients, accounting for about 18% of all injuries.[1] Approximately 700,000 emergency department visits and 120,000 hospitalizations per year are because of ADRs, costing the US healthcare system $3.5 billion annually.[2,3] ADRs are associated with increased prolonged hospitalizations, higher costs of care, and increased morbidity and mortality.[4,5] Complications related to medications include excessive bleeding, altered mental status, hypoglycemia, acute kidney injury, hypotension, respiratory complications, and severe allergic reactions. Cutaneous involvement in ADRs occurs often and may, in fact, be the presenting manifestation. Specifically, adverse cutaneous reactions to drugs occur in 2% of all individuals exposed to drugs, account for the majority (26%) of all ADRs presenting to emergency departments, and result in 0.1%–0.3% of all inpatient fatalities.[1,6]

An ADR is defined as an undesired or unintended response that occurs when a drug is administered for the appropriate indication. The adverse effect may be anticipated or unanticipated. The cause of the reaction is immunologic, toxic, or idiosyncratic. Nonimmunologic causes, such as dose-dependent reactions related to the pharmacokinetics of a drug, are common and more predictable. Cutaneous immunologic reactions to drugs (e.g., drug allergy), however, are more difficult to predict and can be subdivided into four main categories based on the Gell and Coombs classification system: (1) Type I reactions have an acute onset and are caused by IgE-mediated activation of both mast cells and basophils, resulting in urticaria, angioedema, and hemodynamic instability; (2) Type II reactions have a delayed onset and are caused by IgG antibody-mediated cell destruction, manifesting as bullous pemphigoid (BP) and pemphigus vulgaris (PV); (3) Type III reactions have a delayed onset and are caused by immune-complex deposition and complement activation, resulting in vasculitis or serum sickness–like reactions; (4) Type IV reactions have a delayed onset and are T cell–mediated, not only accounting for the common drug exanthems, such as the classic morbilliform rash, contact dermatitis, photosensitivity dermatitis, but also including rarer and more serious conditions such as Stevens-Johnson syndrome (SJS) and toxic epidermal necrolysis (TEN). Several other mechanisms underlying these reactions have been postulated and are further discussed in a separate chapter on the mechanisms of drug allergies.

There are several risk factors for developing an ADR, including the chemical composition and pharmacokinetics of the drug, route of exposure, dosage and duration, frequency of administration, patient gender (women are more frequently affected than men), genetic factors (human leukocyte antigen [HLA] type, drug metabolism, history of atopy), prior reaction(s) to a drug, medical comorbidities, immunosuppression, and other concurrent therapies. The most common medication classes implicated in drug allergy are penicillins, sulfonamides, and nonsteroidal antiinflammatory drugs (NSAIDs).

LYMPHOCYTIC AND EOSINOPHILIC EXANTHEMS

Morbilliform Exanthem Versus Drug Hypersensitivity

Exanthematous (morbilliform or maculopapular) eruptions are the classic and most common type of drug hypersensitivity reaction, accounting for about 95% of all drug-induced cutaneous reactions.[7] One to three weeks after drug exposure, a diffuse, symmetric, pruritic eruption of erythematous macules and papules with or without scale occurs over the trunk and upper extremities. If the offending drug is continued, the eruption may uncommonly progress to generalized exfoliative dermatitis.[8] Mucosal and visceral involvement is notably absent in classical exanthematous eruptions. Although rare, it is important to recognize that an exanthematous drug eruption may be the first indication of a more severe hypersensitivity reaction,

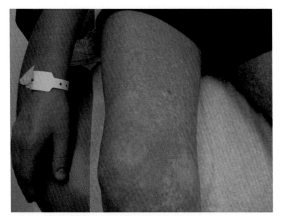

FIG. 6.1 **Morbilliform Exanthem.** Note the blanchable macules and papules reaching near confluence. The differential diagnosis includes a drug reaction and a viral etiology. Clinicopathologic correlation is always necessary to elicit the correct culprit. (Photo credit: Ellen Roh, MD, Massachusetts General Hospital, Harvard Medical School.)

such as drug rash with eosinophilia and systemic symptoms (DRESS), acute generalized exanthematous pustulosis (AGEP), SJS, or TEN, especially if the exanthema involves the face or oral, ocular, or genital mucosa. The most common medications implicated in exanthematous drug reactions include penicillins, sulfonamides, and phenytoin (Fig. 6.1).

Treatment of exanthematous eruptions is symptomatic. Management consists of topical corticosteroids and oral antihistamines. Commonly used sedating antihistamines include diphenhydramine or hydroxyzine 25 mg orally every 6 h. Cetirizine 10 mg once daily is a nonsedating antihistamine alternative. Potent (class I) topical steroids, including clobetasol 0.05% ointment, may be applied twice daily to the trunk and extremities, whereas sensitive areas of the face, axilla, inframammary region, and genitals should be treated with mild (class 4) topicals, such as hydrocortisone 2.5% cream. To avoid the effects of skin atrophy and other complications, such as dyspigmentation and infection, topical steroids should be limited to one to two times per day for no more than 3-week intervals. If possible, systemic steroid treatment should be avoided.

Drug-Induced Lichenoid Eruptions

Lichenoid drug eruption (also referred to as drug-induced lichen planus [LP]) is characterized by symmetrically distributed flat-topped erythematous to violaceous papules that often reach confluence on the trunk and extremities, resembling LP, but without the characteristic fine lacelike patterns (known as Wickham

striae) seen in classic LP. Furthermore, the lesional distribution of a lichenoid drug eruption differs from that of LP, usually affecting the extensor aspects of the extremities and dorsal hands.[9] Mucosal and nail involvement is rare. The eruption can occur months or years after administration of the offending drug. The classes of medications associated with lichenoid drug eruption include angiotensin converting enzyme (ACE) inhibitors, thiazide diuretics, antimalarials, anticonvulsants, penicillamine, ketoconazole, β blockers, NSAIDs, tumor necrosis factor (TNF)-α antagonists, and tyrosine kinase inhibitors.[10–13]

Histology of lichenoid drug eruption, as well as LP, reveals a nonspecific lichenoid interface dermatitis, basal keratinocyte apoptosis, and pigmentary incontinence.[14] Microscopic findings that are more typical of a lichenoid drug eruption include the presence of eosinophils and plasma cells, a deeper perivascular infiltrate, and a higher proportion of necrotic keratinocytes than seen in classic LP.[9,15] Direct immunofluorescence (DIF) demonstrates deposits of IgM, and less often IgG and IgA, at the dermal-epidermal junction.[16] Immunohistochemical staining is not routinely performed in the workup of a lichenoid skin eruption.

Treatment involves discontinuation of the offending medication. The majority of lichenoid drug eruptions resolve spontaneously over weeks to months after the drug is stopped. For patients who have extensive disease, pruritus, or persistent lesions, topical or systemic corticosteroids may be required. Clobetasol 0.05% twice daily for up to 4 weeks is recommended for patients with limited cutaneous disease. Patients with extensive or highly symptomatic disease benefit from systemic steroid therapy, such as prednisone 30–60 mg daily for 4 to 6 weeks. An oral retinoid, acitretin 25 mg daily for 6 to 12 weeks, is an alternative for patients who are intolerant or who, for medical reasons, cannot receive systemic corticosteroids.[17–20]

Symmetric Drug-Related Intertriginous and Flexural Exanthema

Symmetric drug-related intertriginous and flexural exanthema (SDRIFE) is a rare drug-induced cutaneous reaction that typically develops within hours to days after exposure to a drug. The clinical presentation is that of erythema, often sharply demarcated and resembling the shape of a "V," involving the gluteal, perianal, genital, or inguinal areas. Other flexural areas, such as the axillae, knees, or elbows, may also be affected. The eruption is usually mild or moderate in severity. Associated systemic symptoms, such as fever, are uncommon. Any signs of facial swelling, mucositis, or blistering should prompt immediate medical attention, because these may indicate a more severe hypersensitivity reaction, such as AGEP, DRESS, or SJS/TEN. The usual suspect medications in SDRIFE are antibiotics, including amoxicillin, ceftriazone, erythromycin, and clindamycin.[21] Other drugs reported implicated in SDRIFE are pseudoephedrine, valacyclovir, and iodinated contrast media.[22]

Treatment involves discontinuation of the offending medication. Management is largely symptomatic, involving antihistamines. Systemic corticosteroids are usually not required for cases of uncomplicated exanthematous drug eruptions.

NEUTROPHILIC EXANTHEMS
Acute Generalized Exanthematous Pustulosis

AGEP is a rare reaction that occurs after drug administration or infection and is characterized by the rapid appearance of hundreds to thousands of small nonfollicular subepidermal and intraepidermal sterile pustules on a background of erythema.[23,24] The eruption begins on the face or intertriginous areas and within 24 h disseminates diffusely, although delayed symptoms up to 3 weeks after drug exposure have been reported.[25] The pustular eruption is followed by postpustular desquamation. Severe cases of AGEP may present with atypical targetoid lesions and coalescent pustules, resulting in superficial erosions and widespread erythema, potentially resembling SJS/TEN.[26–29] In AGEP, however, involvement of mucous membranes is unusual and almost always limited to erosions on the lips (Fig. 6.2).

Cutaneous eruptions for longer than 2 weeks are unusual.[30] Fever and peripheral blood leukocytosis (>7000 neutrophils/mL) are typically present, with possible mild eosinophilia.[24] Visceral involvement is rare.[31] In a series of 97 cases of AGEP, the median time between drug exposure and development of symptoms was 1 day for antibiotics and 11 days for all other classes of drugs.[32] Antibiotics, particularly penicillins and macrolides, are implicated in 80% of cases.[24,32] AGEP has also been associated with several other drugs, including antimalarials and calcium channel blockers, among others.[24,33]

The estimated incidence of AGEP is one to five per million persons per year.[32,34–36] AGEP may occur at any age, although it most often affects middle-aged adults.[32] Both sexes are affected, with a slight female predominance.[32,37] The mortality rate in AGEP is around 5%.[38]

The pathologic mechanism of AGEP has not been extensively studied. AGEP is a T cell–mediated inflammatory disorder involving CD4+ T cells, cytotoxic CD8+

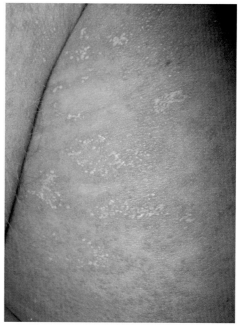

FIG. 6.2 **Acute Generalized Exanthematous Pustulosis.** The patient presented with pustules surrounded by intense erythema reaching near confluence. Notably, the patient experienced fever and leukocytosis after starting a cephalosporin. (Photo credit: Ellen Roh, MD, Massachusetts General Hospital, Harvard Medical School.)

T cells, and inflammatory chemokines and cytokines. CD4+ drug-specific T cells produce large amounts of interleukin 8 and granulocyte-macrophage colony-stimulating factor, both of which are involved in tissue accumulation of neutrophils.[39–41] T-helper 17 (Th17) cells contribute to the recruitment, activation, and migration of neutrophils in AGEP.[42,43]

Histologic examination of a skin biopsy is necessary to confirm the diagnosis and rule out other causes of pustular eruptions. Gram staining and culture of pustular exudate can be helpful to exclude a superficial skin infection. On histologic analysis, AGEP is characterized by a spongiotic subcorneal and/or intraepidermal pustule. Other features include extensive edema of the papillary dermis, keratinocyte necrosis, and dermal neutrophilic infiltrate with perivascular accentuation.[44,45] Eosinophils are typically present in the dermis and pustules.

Pustules can sometimes occur in patients with DRESS. However, unlike AGEP, DRESS is characterized by a long latency (2–6 weeks) between drug exposure and skin involvement, a more severe and prolonged clinical course, atypical lymphocytes and/or eosinophilia in peripheral blood, and visceral involvement (abnormal liver function tests in >90% of cases). Cases with features of both DRESS and AGEP have been described.[36,46,47]

Treatment of AGEP consists of withdrawal of the offending medication, topical corticosteroids, and antipyretics. Symptoms resolve in days. Older or immunocompromised individuals with a widespread eruption may still require hospitalization for fluid and electrolyte support.

Linear IgA Bullous Dermatosis

Linear IgA bullous dermatosis (LABD) is a rare, idiopathic or drug-induced autoimmune blistering disease of the subepidermis. The incidence of LABD ranges from 0.5 to 2.3 cases per million persons per year.[48] Idiopathic LABD and drug-induced LABD appear similar clinically.[49] Adults develop an abrupt onset of tense vesicles and bullae on the face, trunk, extensor surfaces, and buttocks.[48] In children, the most commonly affected body areas include the perineum, abdomen, and inner thighs.[50,51] Mucosal erosions or ulcers are a feature of both idiopathic and drug-induced LABD and occur in up to 80% of affected adults.[50,52] In some cases, LABD may appear like erythema multiforme (EM) or BP-like lesions.[53] Reports of LABD resulting in IgA nephropathy have been rarely described.[54] Histologically the disease is characterized by IgA antibody deposition along the dermoepidermal junction.

Vancomycin is implicated in most cases of drug-induced LABD. Other associated drug classes include antibiotics (amoxicillin-clavulanic acid), NSAIDs (naproxen, diclofenac), lithium, phenytoin, captopril, furosemide, interferon α, and cyclosporine.[48,55–57] LABD occurs within 1 month of administration of the drug. In cases in which multiple medications are suspected, drug-induced lymphocyte stimulation testing can help identify the culprit drug.[58] Withdrawal of the offending medication leads to complete resolution of disease.

Drug-Induced Sweet Syndrome

Sweet syndrome (also known as acute febrile neutrophilic dermatosis) is characterized by the rapid development of painful and erythematous cutaneous papules, plaques, and nodules. The upper extremities are preferentially affected, but lesions may also be widely distributed and involve the mucous membranes. Fever, peripheral leukocytosis, elevated erythrocyte sedimentation rate (ESR), anemia, and abnormal platelet counts are common. Musculoskeletal and ocular involvement has also been reported. Sweet syndrome

may occur idiopathically (classical Sweet syndrome) or in association with an underlying malignancy or drug exposure. Unlike the idiopathic or malignancy-associated variant, drug-induced Sweet syndrome almost never causes abnormal renal function.[59,60]

Several classes of drugs have been implicated in the development of Sweet syndrome, including antibiotics, antiepileptics, antihypertensives, antineoplastics, antipsychotics, contraceptives, diuretics, immunosuppressants, NSAIDs, retinoids, and colony-stimulating factors, among others.[59,61–66] Drug-induced Sweet syndrome typically begins within 2 weeks of exposure to a new medication and recurs if the drug is discontinued and restarted.[67,68]

Management of drug-induced Sweet syndrome includes discontinuation of the offending medication. Although spontaneous resolution of the disease has been reported after removal of the drug, systemic glucocorticoids (0.5–1 mg/kg per day) hasten the clinical response and are recommended as first-line agents for treatment.[69] The cutaneous lesions resolve within 2 weeks, and the course of prednisone can be tapered over 4 to 6 weeks.[70] Topical and/or intralesional corticosteroid injections may be considered as alternatives to systemic glucocorticoid therapy for patients with minimal body surface area (BSA) involvement (i.e., <5% BSA involvement).[69]

URITCARIA, ANGIOEDEMA, AND ANAPHYLAXIS

Type I IgE-mediated hypersensitivity reactions happen within minutes to hours after exposure to a drug. Classical urticarial lesions are painless erythematous plaques, which blanch with pressure and are intensely pruritic. The plaques may be circular, oval, or serpiginous, with a central pallor. Lesions are transient, appearing and disappearing within hours. A drug-induced vasculitis should be considered if lesions are painful or heal with residual bruising.

Pseudoallergic reactions are nonimmunologic in etiology and occur in some individuals who receive NSAIDs. The mechanism of pseudoallergic reactions may be caused by abnormalities in arachidonic acid metabolism, after inhibition of the cyclooxygenase 1 enzyme. Drug-induced urticaria may also result from activation of the complement cascade or immunologic derangements resulting in an increased production of bradykinin (Fig. 6.3).

Swelling of the lips and face represents angioedema, which is caused by edema of the deep dermis and subcutaneous tissues. ACE inhibitors are the leading cause of non-IgE drug-induced angioedema, which occurs in less than 1% of patients taking this class

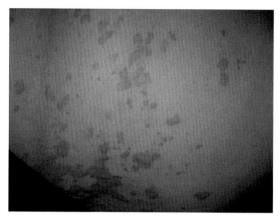

FIG. 6.3 **Urticaria.** The patient presents with polygonal and targetoid macules and papules that resolve within a day and heal without hyperpigmentation.

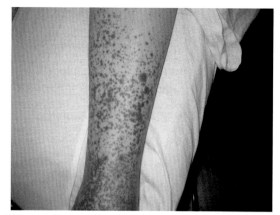

FIG. 6.4 **Drug-Induced Leukocytoclastic Vasculitis.** Note the pinpoint, hemorrhagic, nonblanchable purpura. The patient recovered within 6 days after withdrawal of allopurinol.

of medication.[71,72] Urticaria is usually absent in ACE inhibitor–induced angioedema. African-Americans and individuals older than 65 years seem to be more susceptible to developing drug-induced angioedema.[73] C1 esterase deficiency should be considered in cases of angioedema without urticaria when there is no suspected causal drug.

Although many cases of acute urticaria and angioedema resolve spontaneously, second-generation antihistamines are often given for symptomatic relief. Cetirizine 10 to 20 mg per day or levocetirizine 5 to 10 mg per day are reasonable nonsedating options. For severe urticaria, a combination of antihistamines and prednisone, 30 to 60 mg daily with a taper over 5 to 7 days, is recommended.

DRUG-INDUCED VASCULITIC REACTIONS

Hypersensitivity vasculitis is a Type III hypersensitivity reaction caused by drugs that act as soluble antigens, stimulating an immune response. The drug binds drug-specific IgG and forms immune complexes that activate the complement system and precipitate in various tissues, including blood vessels, joints, and renal glomeruli. Immune complement deposition results in an inflammatory response within tissues. Reexposure to similar or higher doses of the same drug causes a more rapid and severe immune response. ADRs account for 10% of cases of leukocytoclastic vasculitis.

Signs and symptoms of drug-induced vasculitis take 1 to 2 weeks to develop after drug exposure because significant amounts of antibody are required to generate antigen-antibody complexes. Patients may present with palpable purpura, fever, arthralgias, lymphadenopathy, headaches, abdominal pain, hematuria, peripheral neuropathy, elevated ESR, and sometimes reduced circulating serum complement levels. Hemorrhagic blisters, ulcers, and nodules may also be present. Laboratory testing for cutaneous vasculitis includes a complete blood count with differential and platelets, liver function tests, antinuclear antibody, blood urea nitrogen and creatinine, urinalysis with microscopy, and a fecal occult blood test (Fig. 6.4).

Hydralazine, minocycline, propylthiouracil, and levamisole-adulterated cocaine are most often implicated in cutaneous drug-induced vasculitis.[74] Penicillins, cephalosporins, sulfonamides (including loop and thiazide-type diuretics), phenytoin, and allopurinol have also been implicated.[75,76] Symptoms resolve with discontinuation of the drug. Steroids should be indicated for visceral involvement.

Tissue biopsy and DIF studies ought to be performed in all cases of suspected cutaneous vasculitis, particularly if a diagnosis of Henoch-Schönlein purpura (IgA vasculitis) is being considered.[77] Histopathology is most informative in certain conditions when skin biopsies are taken during the first 2 days of a cutaneous eruption. Pathology reveals blood vessel wall inflammation and damage. To meet strict criteria for a diagnosis of vasculitis, small vessels, arterioles, and venules must have at least two of the following three criteria: (1) angiocentric and/or angioinvasive inflammatory infiltrate, (2) fibrinoid necrosis of a vessel wall or lumen, and (3) destruction and/or disruption of vessel walls.[78] Histology can also rule out other competing diagnoses, such as polyarteritis nodosa and granulomatosis with polyangiitis (Wegener granulomatosis).

SEVERE ADVERSE DRUG REACTIONS
Erythema Multiforme

EM is characterized by an acute eruption with symmetric and bilateral targetoid lesions of concentric light and dark rings on the legs, palms, and soles. The incidence of EM has been estimated between 0.01% and 1.0% annually.[79] EM is often precipitated by infections (herpes simplex virus or *Mycoplasma pneumoniae*); however, there are reports of drug-induced EM.[80,81] Lesions appear within 72 h of drug exposure. Bullae and epidermal detachment involve less than 10% of the BSA. Morbidity is low with this condition, and lesions typically heal without complication after 2 weeks.

EM is a clinical diagnosis. Nonspecific laboratory findings include elevated white blood cell count, liver enzymes, and acute phase reactants.[79] Histopathology can help exclude other disorders with clinical features similar to those of EM. Microscopic features include papillary dermal edema, a dense dermal lymphohistiocytic infiltrate surrounding vessels, basal cell vacuolar degeneration, and keratinocyte necrosis.[82,83]

Drug Reaction With Eosinophilia and Systemic Symptoms

Unlike exanthematous eruptions, DRESS, also known as drug-induced hypersensitivity syndrome, is a rare, potentially life-threatening reaction presenting as a morbilliform rash with fever, malaise, lymphadenopathy, and hematologic derangements (eosinophilia >1500 mm^3, atypical lymphocytes, and transaminitis).[84-86] The rash starts as a morbilliform eruption on the face and upper body and then quickly progresses to diffuse, confluent erythematous plaques with perifollicular accentuation. The cutaneous eruption eventually involves >50% of the BSA and/or includes two or more of facial edema, infiltrated lesions, scaling, and purpura. Symmetric facial edema develops in approximately half of cases[87] (Fig. 6.5).

In 20%–30% of patients, erythema progresses to exfoliative dermatitis involving >90% of the BSA. Tense blisters or pustules can also develop. In contrast to SJS/, in which mucosal involvement includes desquamation of at least two sites in 90% of cases, inflammation and pain of mucous membranes is present in only up to half of patients with DRESS. It usually involves a single site (usually the mouth or pharynx) and does not progress to full-thickness ulceration.

The reaction starts 2 to 6 weeks after initiation of the drug. This latency between drug exposure and symptomatic onset is noticeably longer in DRESS than in most other cutaneous drug eruptions (4–9 days for morbilliform eruptions; 4–28 days for SJS/TEN). Liver

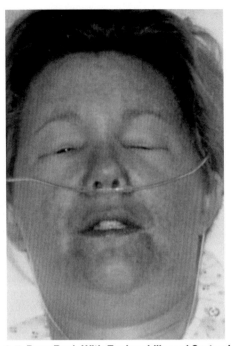

FIG. 6.5 **Drug Rash With Eosinophilia and Systemic Symptoms.** Note the morbilliform eruption on the trunk, which has progressed to diffuse confluent erythematous plaques on the patient's neck and face. The patient also exhibited facial edema and, on examination, had neck lymphadenopathy. The patient was taking phenytoin. (Photo credit: Ellen Roh, MD, Massachusetts General Hospital, Harvard Medical School.)

function impairment is generally mild and transient, but some patients develop a potentially life-threatening hepatitis. The kidneys, heart, and/or lungs may be affected, resulting in interstitial nephritis, pericarditis, and pulmonary infiltrates, respectively. Reactivation of herpesvirus infection concurrent with drug hypersensitivity is considered specific to DRESS.[88,89]

The incidence of DRESS is unknown. One prospective 7-year study in a West Indian general population estimated an annual incidence of less than 1% (0.9/100,000).[90] DRESS can occur in children, but most cases happen in adults without sex predilection.[91,92] DRESS has been associated with several different classes of medications, including sulfonamides, dapsone, vancomycin, minocycline, allopurinol, calcium channel blockers, and anticonvulsants.[87,93,94]

The proposed pathogenic mechanism for DRESS is an initial viral reactivation, which results in T cell expansion and cross-reaction with the drug. Tissue damage is caused by activated cytotoxic CD8$^+$ T lymphocytes

TABLE 6.1
European Registry of Severe Cutaneous Adverse Reactions (RegiSCAR) Scoring Classification System for DRESS

	SCORING SYSTEM FOR CLASSIFYING DRESS	
	SCORE	
Item	**Present**	**Absent**
Fever (≥101.3 F)	0	−1
Lymphadenopathy (two sites, >1 cm in size)	+1	0
Eosinophilia (>700) OR ≥10% in leukopenia	+1	0
Eosinophilia (>1500) OR ≥20% in leukopenia	+2	0
Atypical lymphocytes	+1	0
Rash ≥50% body surface area	+1	0
Rash suggestive of DRESS (≥2 of facial edema, infiltration, purpura, desquamation)	+1	0
Dermatopathology suggesting alternative diagnosis	−1	0
Visceral involvement (liver, kidney, muscle, heart, pancreas, other)	+1 (one organ) +2 (two or more organs)	0
Duration of disease ≥15 days	0	−1
Investigations for alternative causes (blood cultures, ANA, serology for HAV, HBV, HCV, mycoplasma, chlamydia)	+1 (if ≥3 tests done and all negative)	0
Total score <2: Excluded from DRESS 2 to 3: Possible DRESS 4 to 5: Probable DRESS ≥6: Definite DRESS		

DRESS, drug rash with eosinophilia and systemic symptoms; *HAV*, hepatitis A virus; *HBV*, hepatitis B virus; *HCV*, hepatitis C virus , *ANA*, antinuclear antibodies.
Adapted from Kardaun SH, Sidoroff A, Valeyrie-Allanore L, et al. Variability in the clinical pattern of cutaneous side-effects of drugs with systemic symptoms: does a DRESS syndrome really exist? *Br J Dermatol*. 2007;156:609–611.

directed against virus-related antigens.[95,96] Pharmacogenetic studies have demonstrated an association between different HLA haplotypes and increased risk for developing DRESS for some drugs.[97–100]

The most frequent pathologic findings in DRESS include atypical lymphocytes (activated CD8+ T cells) and an interface dermatitis involving the pilar units.[101] A variable combination of acanthosis, spongiosis, superficial dermal lymphocytic infiltrate, and eosinophils may be present.[102,103] Despite its name, peripheral eosinophilia is present in only 70% of DRESS cases (Table 6.1).

Patients with severe cutaneous reactions may need, in addition to prompt withdrawal of the offending medication, hospitalization and treatment for fluid and electrolyte imbalances. Patients with only modest transaminitis (<3 times the upper limit of normal) with no evidence of renal, pulmonary, or cardiac involvement can be symptomatically managed for pruritus with class II topical corticosteroids applied two to three times a day for 1 week.[104] Individuals with severe organ involvement of the lungs (interstitial pneumonitis/pleural effusion) or kidneys (acute interstitial nephritis) require systemic corticosteroids (prednisone 0.5–2 mg/kg) until clinical improvement and normalization of laboratory values. Once the condition has improved, prednisone should be slowly tapered over 8 to 12 weeks.[92,105] Patients with severe hepatocellular damage should be evaluated by a hepatologist. Other organs that may be involved by DRESS include the brain (encephalitis, meningitis), heart (myocarditis, pericarditis), pancreas, peripheral nerves, eyes (uveitis), gastrointestinal tract (erosions and bleeding), and thyroid (delayed autoimmune thyroiditis).[106]

There have been case reports of patients improving on intravenous immunoglobulin (IVIG) therapy; however, there are also reports of patients who experienced no beneficial effect and, in some cases, developed severe adverse events because of IVIG therapy.[107,108] Currently, we do not recommend the use of IVIG for the treatment of DRESS.

DRESS carries a 10% mortality rate if the reaction is severe, unrecognized, and untreated. Even with discontinuation of the offending medication, patients frequently experience relapses. In 10%–20% of cases a causal drug cannot be definitively established.[92,87]

Stevens-Johnson Syndrome and Toxic Epidermal Necrolysis

SJS and TEN are severe mucocutaneous reactions usually triggered by medications. Cutaneous findings occur approximately 1 to 3 weeks after drug exposure. A febrile prodrome typically precedes the cutaneous eruption. SJS and TEN are considered to be variants of the same disease continuum, distinguished by the percentage of BSA involvement. SJS is the less severe form, with epidermal detachment of <10% of the BSA, whereas TEN involves >30% of the BSA. SJS and TEN may overlap when 10%–30% of the body surface is involved. Both conditions present with mucosal lesions, blistering, erosions, extensive necrosis, and epidermolysis (Nikolsky sign) because of keratinocyte necrosis.[109,110] In both cases, the disease course is rapid and the prognosis is poor (Figs. 6.6 and 6.7).

The incidence of SJS/TEN is estimated at two to seven cases per million persons per year, with SJS occurring three times as often as TEN.[111–113] Individuals with human immunodeficiency virus infection have a 100-fold higher incidence of SJS/TEN than the general population.[114] SJS/TEN occurs in all age groups and is more common in women than in men, with a male to female ratio of 0.6.[115] The overall mortality rate is 5% for patients with SJS and 30% for those with TEN, with a combined total mortality of 20%–25%.

Medications are the leading trigger of SJS/TEN. Notably, the risk of developing SJS/TEN seems to be limited to the first 8 weeks after drug administration.[116] Medications implicated include allopurinol, aromatic anticonvulsants, antibacterial sulfonamides, lamotrigine, nevirapine, oxicam, and NSAIDs.[117,118] The drugs stimulate the immune system by directly binding to the major histocompatibility complex (MHC) I and the T cell receptors. Binding stimulates a clonal expansion of drug-specific cytotoxic T cells, which directly and indirectly contribute to keratinocyte necrosis.[119] The hallmark of SJS/TEN is partial- to full-thickness epidermal necrosis.[113]

The acute phase of SJS/TEN lasts between 1 and 2 weeks. Patients present with a viral-like prodrome of fever, malaise, progressive skin findings, and mucosal involvement. Mucosal involvement occurs in approximately 90% of cases and may precede or follow the cutaneous eruption.[120] The oral mucosa and vermilion border of the lips are invariably involved, with painful hemorrhagic erosions covered with a gray-white membrane. Conjunctival lesions are present in 85% of cases, ranging from asymptomatic hyperemia to keratitis, corneal erosions, and pseudomembrane formation. Erosions of the upper respiratory tract, gastrointestinal system, and urinary urethra may lead to respiratory compromise, impaired alimentation, and painful micturition, respectively.

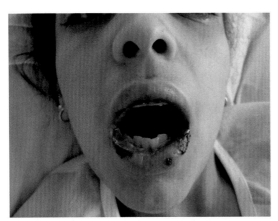

FIG. 6.6 Stevens-Johnson Syndrome. This patient presented with dysuria, conjunctivitis, and dysphagia, as well as with a viral prodrome of fever, arthritis, and malaise. She had been recently given trimethoprim-sulfamethoxazole for a urinary tract infection (Fig. 6.7).

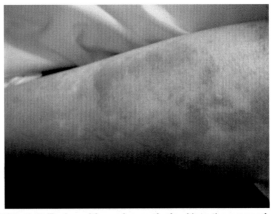

FIG. 6.7 Toxic epidermal necrolysis. Note the areas of dusky, violaceous discoloration with early blister formation and epidermal detachment. The condition evolved into full-thickness necrosis within 24 h.

Skin lesions in SJS/TEN classically start as ill-defined, coalescing erythematous purpuric macules, although many cases of SJS/TEN initially present with diffuse and painful erythema.[121,122] Lesions are symmetrically distributed and begin on the face and thorax before spreading to other body sites.[123] The scalp, palms, and soles are rarely involved.[124,125] As the disease progresses, vesicles and bullae develop and, within days, the skin sloughs, resulting in large, raw, painful areas of desquamation (Figure 6.7). At this stage, the appearance has been likened to that of extensive thermal injury.[126] Reepithelialization occurs over several weeks.[127]

Patients with SJS/TEN are at high risk of bacterial infection. Sepsis and septic shock, usually caused by *Staphylococcus aureus* and *Pseudomonas aeruginosa*, are the main causes of death in these patients. In a study of 179 patients with SJS/TEN, bacteremia was detected in 48 patients (27%).[128] Laboratory abnormalities, including a decreased white blood cell count and anemia, are common. Neutropenia is associated with a worse prognosis.[123,129]

SJS/TEN is a clinical diagnosis. There are no diagnostic pathologic criteria, and histologic findings are nonspecific. However, skin biopsy and immunofluorescence studies may be warranted to exclude other non-drug-related bullous and mucosal disorders, such as BP, PV, paraneoplastic pemphigus, and staphylococcal scalded skin syndrome.

Identification and early withdrawal of the causative drug is crucial to improved survival.[130] Assessment of drug causality is based on a detailed patient history and clinical judgment. An algorithm of drug causality for epidermal necrolysis (ALDEN) may aid the assessment of drug causality in patients presenting with SJS/TEN, particularly in those with multiple drug exposures.[116] Each potentially offending medication is assigned a score from −12 to +10 based on six criteria: (1) temporal delay from initial drug administration to onset of reaction (index day); (2) likelihood of drug still present in the body on the index day (i.e., drugs that have longer half-lives confer a worse prognosis); (3) previous history of exposure to the same drug (with or without a previous reaction); (4) presence of the drug beyond the progression phase of the disease; (5) drug known to cause SJS/TEN based on previous reports; and (6) presence or absence of other causes. The score is calculated as very probable (≥6), probable (4–5), possible (2–3), unlikely (0–1), and highly unlikely (≤0). In addition, a severity score has been developed to predict prognosis, known as the severity-of-illness score for TEN (SCORTEN; Table 6.2).

After discontinuation of the drug, patients should be admitted to the intensive care unit or burn unit,

particularly if ≥30% the BSA is involved. Supportive care includes fluid loss replacement, nutritional support, correcting acute kidney injury, wound care, and treating infections. All patients should have an ophthalmologic evaluation, and a gynecologic examination should be performed on female patients.

Beyond supportive care, no clear guidelines exist for systemic treatment. Immunosuppressive therapies, such as systemic corticosteroids, IVIG, cyclosporine, and anti-TNF monoclonal antibodies, have all been employed in clinical practice, but randomized controlled trials are lacking strong evidence. A mortality analysis of the RegiSCAR cohort and systemic review of case series have demonstrated no survival benefit from systemic corticosteroids in SJS/TEN.[115,131] Thalidomide is harmful and should not be used.[132]

DRUG-INDUCED ACANTHOLYTIC DISORDERS

Pemphigus

Pemphigus encompasses a group of rare life-threatening autoimmune blistering diseases, including PV, pemphigus foliaceus, IgA pemphigus, and paraneoplastic pemphigus. Pemphigus typically affects

---

TABLE 6.2
SCORTEN: Severity-of-Illness Score for Toxic Epidermal Necrolysis

Variables	Points
Age (≥40 years)	1
Heart rate (≥120 bpm)	1
BSA detachment >10% at day 1	1
Serum BUN >28 mg/dL	1
Serum bicarbonate level <20 meq/L	1
Serum glucose level >250 mg/dL	1
Cancer/hematologic malignancy	1
Score	**Mortality Rate (%)**
0–1	3
2	12
3	35
4	58
≥5	90

BSA, body surface area; *BUN*, blood urea nitrogen.
Adapted from Bastuji-Garin S, et al. *J Invest Dermatol* 2000;115(2): 149–153.

middle-aged adults and is characterized by acantholy-sis, resulting in intraepidermal mucosal and/or cutaneous blistering. Acantholysis is caused by the binding of autoantibodies to epithelial intercellular adhesion molecules.[133] The exact mechanism by which auto-antibodies bind is not clearly established. PV always manifests with mucosal involvement and variable cutaneous involvement. Autoantibodies against des-moglein 3 or both desmoglein 3 and desmoglein 1 are characteristic of PV. Pemphigus foliaceus involves cutaneous involvement with autoantibodies to des-moglein 1 only (Fig. 6.8).

Both PV and pemphigus foliaceus may be pre-cipitated by drugs. The most commonly implicated medications include penicillamine and other thiol compounds, such as captopril, or drugs that are metab-olized into thiols, such as piroxicam.[134] Penicillins, cephalosporins, enalapril, rifampin, and NSAIDs have all been reported as causal agents in drug-induced pemphigus.[135,136] Thiol drug–induced pemphigus may occur up to a year after drug administration. Sponta-neous remission after discontinuation of the drug is common.

The diagnosis of pemphigus requires clinical, histo-logic, and immunologic evidence. Although direct and indirect immunofluorescence (DIF and IIF) studies are occasionally negative in drug-induced pemphigus, an enzyme-linked immunosorbent assay (ELISA) is posi-tive in over 90% of cases for IgG antibodies to desmo-glein 1 or desmoglein 3.[136,137]

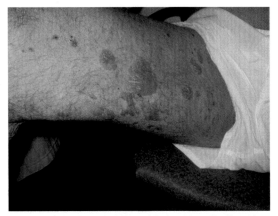

FIG. 6.8 Drug-Induced Pemphigus. Note the flaccid blisters, some with early rupture. The condition partially improved after the cessation of an angiotensin converting enzyme–inhibitor but the patient required systemic steroids for full remission.

The primary treatment objective for pemphigus is to decrease the synthesis of autoantibodies. This is often accomplished through the use of intravenous rituximab (1000 mg on day 1, day 15, and 6 months) and systemic corticosteroids (prednisone 1.0–2.0 mg/kg). Treatment should be initiated promptly to prevent further spread of disease. Blistering typically resolves within 3 weeks, and resolution of disease occurs within 6 to 8 weeks.[138] A slow tapering of predni-sone should be considered once no new lesions have formed for 1 week. Alternatively, steroids may be used in addition to steroid-sparing agents, such as azathioprine or mycophenolate. In the second approach, such agents are typically begun around the same time as prednisone, continued for 8 weeks after the discontinuation of the last prednisone dose, and then tapered over several weeks. Trials comparing the clinical effectiveness of these two approaches are currently lacking. Generally patient characteristics, contraindications to therapy, costs, and physician familiarity with these agents are important determi-nants in the decision of which approach is the most appropriate.

IVIG may also be an effective adjunct treatment, along with corticosteroids, for refractory pemphi-gus. Typical dosing of IVIG for pemphigus is 2 g/kg/ cycle over two to four consecutive days, with repeat cycles occurring in 4- to 6-week intervals.[139–141] Side effects of IVIG therapy include headache, abdomi-nal pain, increased blood pressure, aseptic menin-gitis, and rarely anaphylaxis in patients with IgA deficiency.[142]

Pemphigoid

Autoimmune BP can be precipitated by exposure to infections or drugs. The pathologic mechanism may be caused by antibody cross-reactivity with infectious agents or with drug antigens that reside in the epithe-lial basement membrane. Drug-induced BP is of two causes: (1) an acute, self-limited illness that resolves after withdrawal of the offending medication or (2) an autoimmune chronic pemphigoid that has merely been unmasked by administration of a drug.[143] Case-control studies have demonstrated a significant associa-tion between drug-induced BP and neuroleptics, loop diuretics (furosemide), and spironolactone.[144,145] Clin-ically the disease manifests with intense pruritus and inflammatory tense vesicles and bullae on the trunk and extremities of older adults. Bullae eventually rup-ture leaving behind wet surface erosions. Oral, nasal, ocular, pharyngeal, laryngeal, esophageal, anal, and genital lesions may be present. In some cases, patients can get an urticarial phase of BP in the setting of drug-induced BP (Fig. 6.9).

The workup of BP includes a biopsy of both lesional and perilesional tissue. Lesional tissue should be stored in formalin and processed for routine histologic examination with hematoxylin and eosin. Histologic findings in BP include supepidermal blistering with numerous eosinophils and a superficial inflammatory dermal infiltrate with variable numbers of eosinophils, neutrophils, and lymphocytes.[146] DIF of perilesional tissue (placed in Michel medium, not formalin) is more sensitive for the diagnosis than either IIF or ELISA and is the current gold standard.[147] DIF findings in BP include linear IgG and/or linear C3 staining along the basement membrane.[148] IIF and ELISA testing of serum to detect circulating basement membrane zone antibodies provide additional information to support the diagnosis, especially if the DIF is negative.

The initial treatment for BP consists of high-potency topical (clobetasol 0.05% cream) and systemic corticosteroids (prednisone 0.5–0.75 mg/kg per day). Other immunosuppressants are added as steroid-sparing agents to minimize the long-term negative effects of steroid treatment. These additional agents include mycophenolate mofetil, azathioprine, and methotrexate. Refractory cases of BP may require intravenous rituximab or IVIG. Disease remission may take years, and the disease is potentially fatal.

OTHER ADVERSE DRUG REACTIONS
Fixed Drug Eruption
Fixed drug eruptions account for about 20% of cutaneous drug eruptions and present clinically as acute-onset pruritic and erythematous well-demarcated macules or edematous plaques with or without vesicle or bullae formation. Lesions generally appear within minutes to hours after drug administration and most often affect the face, mouth, genitals, and acral areas.[149,150] Lesions recur in the same locations upon drug reexposure. Postinflammatory hyperpigmentation is a chronic feature. Systemic symptoms, such as fever, are typically absent. Diffuse eruptions over the body may mimic SJS/TEN; however, mucosal involvement in fixed drug eruptions is mild or absent and discontinuation of the offending medication results in rapid resolution within 1 to 2 weeks.[151] Histologically, these reactions are characterized by a predominantly lymphocytic lichenoid infiltrate and pigment incontinence; however, several atypical reaction patterns exist.[152,153]

Drugs commonly implicated include NSAIDs (naproxen, ibuprofen), acetaminophen, antibiotics (trimethoprim-sulfamethoxazole, penicillins, dapsone), antimalarials, and barbiturates.[151,154,155] Patch testing or a drug challenge may be performed to identify the causal drug when multiple medications are suspected.[155,156] The primary management of a fixed drug eruption involves discontinuing the offending medication. Symptoms of pruritus can often be managed with topical steroids and systemic antihistamines (Fig. 6.10).

Acneiform Eruptions
Acneiform eruptions are the classical adverse cutaneous reactions associated with all epidermal growth factor

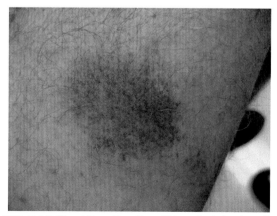

FIG. 6.10 **Fixed Drug Eruption.** This patient developed erythematous macules in a background of violaceous change within hours after the administration of trimethoprim sulfamethoxazole. The patient had a similar reaction in the past. (Photo credit: Evelyn Lilly, MD, Massachusetts General Hospital, Harvard Medical School.)

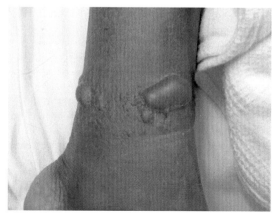

FIG. 6.9 **Bullous Pemphigoid.** Note the tense vesicles and bullae on the lower extremity. This patient also experienced intense pruritus.

receptor (EGFR) inhibitors: cetuximab, panitumumab, gefitinib, lapatinib. This class of medication is increasingly used in the treatment of advanced colorectal, pancreatic, lung, and head and neck cancers.[157–159] The cutaneous eruption occurs in about 80% of patients treated with EGFR inhibitors.[160] Although the reaction rarely poses a serious threat to a patient's long-term health, it can be cosmetically displeasing and result in pain, burning, and pruritus, which negatively affect the quality of life and adherence to cancer-related treatment protocols.[161,162]

EGFR-induced acneiform eruptions occur weeks to months after administration of the drug.[163] The areas affected most often include the face, especially the nose, nasolabial folds, cheeks, and perioral region. The upper trunk and neck are frequently involved.[164] Initial pustules are sterile, although secondary infections, usually by *S. aureus*, do occur.[165]

Treatment depends on the severity of the eruption and the clinical necessity to continue with anticancer therapy. Grading the severity of the eruption is important in guiding treatment and management. The National Cancer Institute Common Terminology Criteria for Adverse Events is used to assess cutaneous adverse reactions during cancer treatment.[166] Grade 1 eruptions involve <10% of the BSA and may or may not be associated with tenderness or pruritus. Grade 1 eruptions are treated with sunscreen, moisturizers, low-potency topical corticosteroids, and 1% clindamycin gel twice a day for 4 weeks.[167,168] Grade 2 eruptions involve 10%–30% of a patient's BSA. These eruptions are treated with low-potency topical corticosteroids twice a day on the face and neck, fluocinonide 0.05% cream twice a day on the chest and back for 4 weeks, and oral doxycycline or minocycline 100 mg twice a day for 4 to 6 weeks. Grade 3 and 4 eruptions involve >30% of the BSA and are associated with local cutaneous superinfection. In addition to oral antibiotics, patients with grade ≥3 eruptions may benefit from prednisone 0.5 mg/kg up to a maximum of 40 mg per day for 1 week.

Benefits of treatment with EGFR-inhibitor therapy should be reassessed and the medication dose lowered, interrupted, or even stopped depending on the clinical situation. If the eruption continues to be refractory to treatment, oral tetracycline may be discontinued and a trial of low-dose isotretinoin (20–30 mg per day) may be effective. Alternatively, intravenous antibiotics and systemic corticosteroids may be necessary.[169] Long-term sequelae of an acneiform eruption include telangiectasias, erythema, and postinflammatory hyperpigmentation.[170] Treatment with topical 4% hydroquinone may diminish the degree of hyperpigmentation.[171]

Acneiform eruptions also occur in people who have high levels of circulating corticosteroids in their blood or who have been using topical corticosteroids for prolonged periods of time. Steroid acne most often occurs on the face, neck, chest, back, and arms. The eruption present similarly to acne vulgaris, with monomorphous erythematous papules and comedones.

Acne-like dermatitis and folliculitis have also been reported in 25%–45% of organ-transplant patients taking sirolimus, a mammalian target of rapamycin inhibitor.[172–174] The eruption consists of erythematous papules and pustules and typically involves the face, trunk, and extremities. In contrast to acne vulgaris, comedones are usually absent in sirolimus-induced acneiform eruptions.[175] It has been postulated that the drug may have direct, toxic effects on the pilosebaceous unit or induce alterations in sebum production. The most likely explanation is that sirolimus inhibits the EGFR pathway, leading to hyperkeratosis, follicular plugging, and bacterial overgrowth.[174,176] The eruption can often be controlled with topical acne treatments, including topical antibiotics, benzoyl peroxide, and isotretinoin, but severe cases may require discontinuation of the drug[174,177] (Fig. 6.11).

Pigmentary Disorders

A variety of drugs are associated with cutaneous and mucous membrane hyperpigmentation.[178] Some examples of these medications include chemotherapeutic agents (bleomycin, cisplatin, fluorouracil), antimalarials (aminoquinolines), oral contraceptives, prostaglandin agonists, psychotropic medications (amitriptyline, chlorpromazine, thioridazine), amiodarone, minocycline, and topical tacrolimus. Heavy metals, such as arsenic, gold, iron, lead, mercury, and silver, can also cause hyperpigmentation of the skin. The clinical features vary depending on the type of medication involved. Hyperpigmentation usually fades with discontinuation of the drug, but the course can be prolonged over months to years in some cases and may be incomplete with permanent residual discoloration (Fig. 6.12).

Conversely, topical or intralesional corticosteroids may induce hypopigmentation, especially in dark-skinned individuals.[179,180] Patients treated with the EGFR inhibitor gefitinib, the tyrosine kinase inhibitor imatinib mesylate, pegylated interferon, topical imiquimod, and transdermal methylphenidate have also been reported to experience drug-induced leukoderma.[181–187]

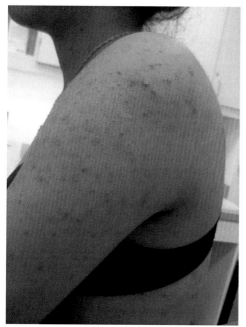

FIG. 6.11 **Steroid-Induced Acneiform Eruption.** Scattered monomorphous comedones and erythematous papules on the arm of a patient receiving prednisone. (Photo credit: Ellen Roh, MD, Massachusetts General Hospital, Harvard Medical School.)

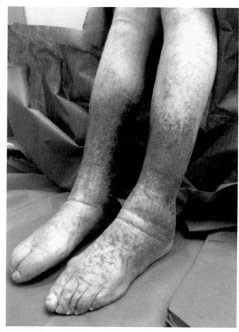

FIG. 6.12 **Drug-Induced Hyperpigmentation.** Note the bilateral and roughly symmetrical blue-black hyperpigmented patches with scale on the lower extremities. The pigmentation was nonblanching. This patient was administered minocycline. (Photo credit: Anar Mikailov, MD, Harvard Combined Residency in Dermatology, Boston, MA.)

Nail Disorders

Drug-induced nail changes occur with several different classes of drugs, often resulting in a wide array of clinical presentations, including reduced rate of nail growth, hyperpigmentation or hypopigmentation, onycholysis, transverse depressions of the nail plate (Beau lines), and pyogenic granulomas. Leukonychia is the most common pigmentary disorder of nails, presenting as white spots, lines, or complete nail whitening (leukonychia totalis).[188] Drug-induced leukonychia is usually caused by chemotherapy drugs (cyclophosphamide, vincristine, doxorubicin) or radiation but has also been reported after poisoning with sulfonamide drugs, pilocarpine, and arsenic.[189-194] Carbon monoxide poisoning, heart failure, Hodgkin disease, psoriasis, renal failure, and sickle cell anemia may all produce transverse bands of leukonychia.[195]

Drugs can also produce a hyperpigmentation of the nail. Activation of nail matrix melanocytes is associated with chemotherapy and immunosuppressive medications, such as doxorubicin, bleomycin, cyclophosphamide, 5-fluorouracil, hydroxyurea, infliximab,

methotrexate, and electron beam and radiation therapy.[195,196] Hyperpigmentation of the nail is usually slowly reversible over time, although some amount of discoloration may persist.[197]

Onycholysis, detachment of the overlying nail plate from the underlying nail bed, can be precipitated by drugs that damage the epithelium of the nail bed, causing loss of adhesion to the nail plate, or by the formation of a hemorrhagic blister on the nail bed. Taxanes (docetaxel/paclitaxel), anthracyclines (doxorubicin), and other immunosuppressants (rituximab), and more rarely retinoids, have been implicated in the formation of painful hemorrhagic blisters affecting the nail bed.[198-200]

Paronychia is usually caused by an infection of the periungual soft tissue. However, drug-induced paronychia with pseudopyogenic granuloma has also been reported. Paronychia presents with tender, erythematous, and swollen nail folds. Taxanes are a frequent cause of acute paronychia, but other drugs implicated in paronychia and pyogenic granulomas include systemic

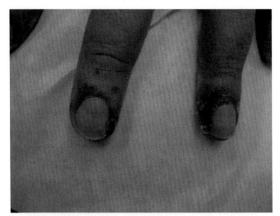

FIG. 6.13 **Paronychia.** Note the inflammation and desquamation along the proximal and lateral nail folds. Fingers are more often affected than toes. This reaction was caused by an epidermal growth factor receptor inhibitor. (Photo credit: Ellen Roh, MD, Massachusetts General Hospital, Harvard Medical School.)

and topical retinoids (isotretinoin, topical tretinoin), antiretrovirals (indinavir), EGFR inhibitors (gefitinib), etoposide, and capecitabine.[198,201] (Fig. 6.13)

Noncicatricial Alopecia

Drugs can cause hair loss either through inducing an abrupt cessation of mitotic activity in hair matrix cells (anagen effluvium) or by precipitating follicles into premature arrest (telogen effluvium). In anagen effluvium, hair loss occurs days to weeks after drug administration and cytotoxic agents (cyclophosphamide, doxorubicin, paclitaxel) are most commonly implicated. In telogen effluvium, hair loss occurs 2 to 4 months after administration of a drug. Medications associated with telogen hair loss include acitretin, isotretinoin, amantadine, amiodarone, anticonvulsants, lithium, captopril, cimetidine, colchicine, valproic acid, ketoconazole, and propranolol.[202]

Pruritus Without Rash

Pruritus without visible skin changes is a side effect of many medications. Retinoic acid can cause skin dryness, and doxycycline can cause irritation, both resulting in itch. Pruritus may occur after oral or parenteral opioid ingestion. Pruritus after intrathecal or epidural administration of opiates has been reported in 30%–100% of patients.[203] EGFR inhibitors, tyrosine kinase inhibitors, and proto-oncogene B-Raf and mitogen-activated kinase kinase (MEK) inhibitors have all been implicated in drug-induced pruritus.[204–206] Drug-induced cholestasis is another cause of generalized pruritus without a rash.[207]

Topical analgesics, such as paroxine, have been used successfully for symptomatic control. Oral hydroxyzine or diphenhydramine (25 mg three times daily) and pregabalin (25–75 mg daily) are medications that can serve as alternatives for pruritus that does not respond to initial treatments.[208,209] Ultraviolet B therapy is another therapeutic option for refractory cases.[210] Clinicians should always consider the possibility of lymphoma when evaluating patients with pruritus without an obvious rash.

REFERENCES

1. Budnitz DSPD, Weidenbach KN, Mendelsohn AB, Schroeder TJ, Annest JL. National surveillance of emergency department visits for outpatient adverse drug events. *JAMA.* 2006;296(15):1858–1866.
2. Leape LLBT, Laird N, Lawthers AG, et al. The nature of adverse events in hospitalized patients. Results of the Harvard Medical Practice Study II. *N Engl J Med.* 1991;324(6):377.
3. Aspden PWJ, Palugod RL, Bastien T. *Preventing Medication Errors.* Institute of Medicine of the National Academies; July 2006:2006.
4. Classen DCPS, Evans RS, Lloyd JF, Burke JP. Adverse drug events in hospitalized patients. Excess length of stay, extra costs, and attributable mortality. *JAMA.* 1997;277(4):301.
5. Phillips DPCN, Glynn LM. Increase in US medication-error deaths between 1983 and 1993. *Lancet.* 1998;351(9103):643.
6. Bigby MJS, Jick H, Arndt K. Drug-induced cutaneous reactions. A report from the Boston Collaborative Drug Surveillance Program on 15,438 consecutive inpatients, 1975 to 1982. *JAMA.* 1986;256(24):3358.
7. Bigby M. Rates of cutaneous reactions to drugs. *Arch Dermatol.* 2001;137(6):765–770.
8. Karakayli G, Beckham G, Orengo I, Rosen T. Exfoliative dermatitis. *Am Fam Physician.* 1999;59(3):625–630.
9. Van den Haute V, Antoine JL, Lachapelle JM. Histopathological discriminant criteria between lichenoid drug eruption and idiopathic lichen planus: retrospective study on selected samples. *Dermatologica.* 1989;179(1):10–13.
10. Antiga E, Melani L, Cardinali C, et al. A case of lichenoid drug eruption associated with sildenafil citratus. *J Dermatol.* 2005;32(12):972–975.
11. Asarch A, Gottlieb AB, Lee J, et al. Lichen planus-like eruptions: an emerging side effect of tumor necrosis factor-alpha antagonists. *J Am Acad Dermatol.* 2009;61(1):104–111.
12. Halevy S, Shai A. Lichenoid drug eruptions. *J Am Acad Dermatol.* 1993;29(2 Pt 1):249–255.
13. Vergara G, Silvestre JF, Betlloch I, Vela P, Albares MP, Pascual JC. Cutaneous drug eruption to infliximab: report of 4 cases with an interface dermatitis pattern. *Arch Dermatol.* 2002;138(9):1258–1259.

14. Sontheimer RD. Lichenoid tissue reaction/interface dermatitis: clinical and histological perspectives. *J Invest Dermatol*. 2009;129(5):1088–1099.

15. Lage D, Juliano PB, Metze K, de Souza EM, Cintra ML. Lichen planus and lichenoid drug-induced eruption: a histological and immunohistochemical study. *Int J Dermatol*. 2012;51(10):1199–1205.

16. Oliver GF, Winkelmann RK, Muller SA. Lichenoid dermatitis: a clinicopathologic and immunopathologic review of sixty-two cases. *J Am Acad Dermatol*. 1989;21(2 Pt 1):284–292.

17. Cribier B, Frances C, Chosidow O. Treatment of lichen planus. An evidence-based medicine analysis of efficacy. *Arch Dermatol*. 1998;134(12):1521–1530.

18. Laurberg G, Geiger JM, Hjorth N, et al. Treatment of lichen planus with acitretin. A double-blind, placebo-controlled study in 65 patients. *J Am Acad Dermatol*. 1991;24(3):434–437.

19. Le Cleach L, Chosidow O. Clinical practice. Lichen planus. *N Engl J Med*. 2012;366(8):723–732.

20. Cheng S, Kirtschig G, Cooper S, Thornhill M, Leonardi-Bee J, Murphy R. Interventions for erosive lichen planus affecting mucosal sites. *Cochrane Database Syst Rev*. 2012;(2). CD008092.

21. Häusermann P, Harr T, Bircher AJ. Baboon syndrome resulting from systemic drugs: is there strife between SDRIFE and allergic contact dermatitis syndrome? *Contact Dermatitis*. 2004;51(5–6):297–310.

22. Thyssen JP, Maibach HI. Drug-elicited systemic allergic (contact) dermatitis – update and possible pathomechanisms. *Contact Dermatitis*. 2008;59(4):195–202.

23. Halevy S. Acute generalized exanthematous pustulosis. *Curr Opin Allergy Clin Immunol*. 2009;9(4):322.

24. Roujeau JCB-SP, Bourseau C, Guillaume JC, et al. Acute generalized exanthematous pustulosis. Analysis of 63 cases. *Arch Dermatol*. 1991;127(9):1333.

25. Momin SBDRJ, Michaels B, Mobini N. Acute generalized exanthematous pustulosis: an enigmatic drug-induced reaction. *Cutis*. 2009;83(6):291.

26. Peermohamed SHR. Acute generalized exanthematous pustulosis simulating toxic epidermal necrolysis: a case report and review of the literature. *Arch Dermatol*. 2011;147(6):697–701.

27. Azib SFV, Fourrier F, Delaporte E, Staumont-Sallé D. Severe acute generalized exanthematous pustulosis with blistering mimicking toxic epidermal necrolysis, associated with a primary mumps infection. *Clin Exp Dermatol*. 2014;39(6):723–725.

28. van Hattem SBG, Kardaun SH. Severe flucloxacillin-induced acute generalized exanthematous pustulosis (AGEP), with toxic epidermal necrolysis (TEN)-like features: does overlap between AGEP and TEN exist? Clinical report and review of the literature. *Br J Dermatol*. 2014;171(6):1539.

29. SH K. Acute generalized exanthematous pustulosis (AGEP), presenting with toxic epidermal necrolysis-like features, due to morphine: a neglected culprit? *Eur J Dermatol*. 2011;21(3):427–428.

30. Treudler RGS, Gebhardt C, Simon JC. Prolonged course of acute generalized exanthematous pustulosis with liver involvement due to sensitization to amoxicillin and paracetamol. *Acta Derm Venereol*. 2009;89(3):314–315.

31. Hotz CV-AL, Haddad C, Bouvresse S, et al. Systemic involvement of acute generalized exanthematous pustulosis: a retrospective study on 58 patients. *Br J Dermatol*. 2013;169(6):1223.

32. Sidoroff ADA, Viboud C, Halevy S, et al. Risk factors for acute generalized exanthematous pustulosis (AGEP)-results of a multinational case-control study (EuroSCAR). *Br J Dermatol*. 2007;157(5):989.

33. Saissi EHB-SF, Jonville-Béra AP, Lorette G, Autret-Leca E. Centres Régionaux de Pharmacovigilance. Drugs associated with acute generalized exanthematous pustulosis. *Ann Dermatol Venereol*. 2003;130(6–7):612–618.

34. Sidoroff AHS, Bavinck JN, Vaillant L, Roujeau JC. Acute generalized exanthematous pustulosis (AGEP)–a clinical reaction pattern. *J Cutan Pathol*. 2001;28(3):113.

35. Ji YZGL, Qu HM, Zhou HB, Xiao T, Chen HD, Wei HC. Acute generalized exanthematous pustulosis induced by docetaxel. *Int J Dermatol*. 2011;50(6):763–765.

36. Son CHLC, Roh MS, Lee SK, Kim KH, Yang DK. Acute generalized exanthematous pustulosis as a manifestation of carbamazepine hypersensitivity syndrome. *J Investig Allergol Clin Immunol*. 2008;18(6):461–464.

37. Roujeau JCSR. Severe adverse cutaneous reactions to drugs. *N Engl J Med*. 1994;331(19):1272–1285.

38. JC R. Clinical heterogeneity of drug hypersensitivity. *Toxicology*. 2005;209:123–129.

39. Britschgi MSU, Schmid S, Depta JP, et al. T-cell involvement in drug-induced acute generalized exanthematous pustulosis. *J Clin Invest*. 2001;107(11):1433.

40. Britschgi M, von Greyerz S, Burkhart C, Pichler WJ. Molecular aspects of drug recognition by specific T cells. *Curr Drug Targets*. 2003;4(1):1–11.

41. Schmid SKP, Britschgi M, Steiner UC, et al. Acute generalized exanthematous pustulosis: role of cytotoxic T cells in pustule formation. *Am J Pathol*. 2002;161(6):2079.

42. Tokura YMT, Hino R. Psoriasis and other Th17-mediated skin diseases. *J UOEH*. 2010;32(4):317–328.

43. Kabashima RSK, Sawada Y, Hino R, Nakamura M, Tokura Y. Increased circulating Th17 frequencies and serum IL-22 levels in patients with acute generalized exanthematous pustulosis. *J Eur Acad Dermatol Venereol*. 2011;25(4):485–488.

44. Burrows NPRJR. Pustular drug eruptions: a histopathological spectrum. *Histopathology*. 1993;22(6):569–573.

45. Halevy SKS, Davidovici B, Wechsler J. EuroSCAR and RegiSCAR study group. The spectrum of histopathological features in acute generalized exanthematous pustulosis: a study of 102 cases. *Br J Dermatol*. 2010;163(6):1245–1252.

46. Teo WLPS, Koh HY. Allopurinol hypersensitivity syndrome with acute generalized exanthematous pustulosis manifestations. *Cutan Ocul Toxicol*. 2011;30(3):243–244.

47. Ben Salem CFN, Saidi W, Jeddi C, Ghariani N, Hmouda H, Bouraoui K. Acute generalized exanthematous pustulosis as a manifestation of anticonvulsant hypersensitivity syndrome. *Ann Pharmacother.* 2010;44(10):1681–1682.

48. Fortuna G, Marinkovich MP. Linear immunoglobulin A bullous dermatosis. *Clin Dermatol.* 2012;30(1):38–50.

49. Fortuna G, Salas-Alanis JC, Guidetti E, Marinkovich MP. A critical reappraisal of the current data on drug-induced linear immunoglobulin A bullous dermatosis: a real and separate nosological entity? *J Am Acad Dermatol.* 2012;66(6):988–994.

50. Wojnarowska F, Marsden RA, Bhogal B, Black MM. Chronic bullous disease of childhood, childhood cicatricial pemphigoid, and linear IgA disease of adults. A comparative study demonstrating clinical and immunopathologic overlap. *J Am Acad Dermatol.* 1988;19 (5 Pt 1):792–805.

51. Mintz EM, Morel KD. Clinical features, diagnosis, and pathogenesis of chronic bullous disease of childhood. *Dermatol Clin.* 2011;29(3):459–462. ix.

52. Chanal J, Ingen-Housz-Oro S, Ortonne N, et al. Linear IgA bullous dermatosis: comparison between the drug-induced and spontaneous forms. *Br J Dermatol.* 2013;169(5):1041–1048.

53. Kuechle MK, Stegemeir E, Maynard B, Gibson LE, Leiferman KM, Peters MS. Drug-induced linear IgA bullous dermatosis: report of six cases and review of the literature. *J Am Acad Dermatol.* 1994;30(2 Pt 1):187–192.

54. Kim JS, Choi M, Nam CH, et al. Concurrent drug-induced inear immunoglobulin A dermatosis and immunoglobulin A nephropathy. *Ann Dermatol.* 2015;27(3):315–318.

55. Ho JC, Ng PL, Tan SH, Giam YC. Childhood linear IgA bullous disease triggered by amoxicillin-clavulanic acid. *Pediatr Dermatol.* 2007;24(5):E40–E43.

56. Polat M, Lenk N, Kürekçi E, Oztaş P, Artüz F, Alli N. Chronic bullous disease of childhood in a patient with acute lymphoblastic leukemia: possible induction by a drug. *Am J Clin Dermatol.* 2007;8(6):389–391.

57. Kocyigit P, Akay BN, Karaosmanoglu N. Linear IgA bullous dermatosis induced by interferon-alpha 2a. *Clin Exp Dermatol.* 2009;34(5):e123–e124.

58. Tomida E, Kato Y, Ozawa H, et al. Causative drug detection by drug-induced lymphocyte stimulation test in drug-induced linear IgA bullous dermatosis. *Br J Dermatol.* 2015;175.

59. Walker DC, Cohen PR. Trimethoprim-sulfamethoxazole-associated acute febrile neutrophilic dermatosis: case report and review of drug-induced Sweet's syndrome. *J Am Acad Dermatol.* 1996;34(5 Pt 2):918–923.

60. Cohen PR, Kurzrock R. Sweet's syndrome and cancer. *Clin Dermatol.* 1993;11(1):149–157.

61. Rochet NM, Chavan RN, Cappel MA, Wada DA, Gibson LE. Sweet syndrome: clinical presentation, associations, and response to treatment in 77 patients. *J Am Acad Dermatol.* 2013;69(4):557–564.

62. White JM, Mufti GJ, Salisbury JR, du Vivier AW. Cutaneous manifestations of granulocyte colony-stimulating factor. *Clin Exp Dermatol.* 2006;31(2):206–207.

63. Juanola X, Nolla JM, Servitje O, Valverde J. Hydralazine induced lupus and Sweet's syndrome. *J Rheumatol.* 1991;18(6):948.

64. Thibault MJ, Billick RC, Srolovitz H. Minocycline-induced Sweet's syndrome. *J Am Acad Dermatol.* 1992;27 (5 Pt 2):801–804.

65. Arun B, Berberian B, Azumi N, Frankel SR, Luksenburg H, Freter C. Sweet's syndrome during treatment with all-trans retinoic acid in a patient with acute promyelocytic leukemia. *Leuk Lymphoma.* 1998;31(5–6):613–615.

66. Pintova S, Sidhu H, Friedlander PA, Holcombe RF. Sweet's syndrome in a patient with metastatic melanoma after ipilimumab therapy. *Melanoma Res.* 2013;23(6):498–501.

67. Kim MJ, Choe YH. EPONYM. Sweet syndrome. *Eur J Pediatr.* 2010;169(12):1439–1444.

68. Cohen PR. Sweet's syndrome – a comprehensive review of an acute febrile neutrophilic dermatosis. *Orphanet J Rare Dis.* 2007;2:34.

69. Cohen PR, Kurzrock R. Sweet's syndrome: a review of current treatment options. *Am J Clin Dermatol.* 2002;3(2):117–131.

70. von den Driesch P. Sweet's syndrome (acute febrile neutrophilic dermatosis). *J Am Acad Dermatol.* 1994;31(4). 535–556; quiz 557–560.

71. Messerli FHNJ. Vasopeptidase inhibition and angio-oedema. *Lancet.* 2000;356(9230):608.

72. Toh SRM, Houstoun M, Ross Southworth M, et al. Comparative risk for angioedema associated with the use of drugs that target the renin-angiotensin-aldosterone system. *Arch Intern Med.* 2012;172(20):1582.

73. Kostis JBKH, Rusnak J, Casale T, Kaplan A, Corren J, Levy E. Incidence and characteristics of angioedema associated with enalapril. *Arch Intern Med.* 2005;165(14):1637.

74. Pendergraft 3rd WF, Niles NJ. Trojan horses: drug culprits associated with antineutrophil cytoplasmic autoantibody (ANCA) vasculitis. *Curr Opin Rheumatol.* 2014;26(1):42–49.

75. Calabrese LHDG. Drug-induced vasculitis. *Curr Opin Rheumatol.* 1996;8(1):34.

76. Martinez-Taboada VMBR, Garcia-Fuentes M, Rodriguez-Valverde V. Clinical features and outcome of 95 patients with hypersensitivity vasculitis. *Am J Med.* 1997;102(2):186.

77. Hung SP, Yang YH, Lin YT, Wang LC, Lee JH, Chiang BL. Clinical manifestations and outcomes of Henoch-Schönlein purpura: comparison between adults and children. *Pediatr Neonatol.* 2009;50(4):162–168.

78. Carlson JANB, Chen KR. Cutaneous vasculitis update: diagnostic criteria, classification, epidemiology, etiology, pathogenesis, evaluation and prognosis. *Am J Dermatopathol.* 2005;27(6):504.

79. Huff JCWW, Tonnesen MG. Erythema multiforme: a critical review of characteristics, diagnostic criteria, and causes. *J Am Acad Dermatol.* 1983;8(6):763–775.

80. Roujeau JCSR. Severe adverse cutaneous reactions to drugs. *N Engl J Med.* 1994;331(19):1272.

81. Forman RKG, Shear NH. Erythema multiforme, Stevens-Johnson syndrome and toxic epidermal necrolysis in children: a review of 10 years' experience. *Drug Saf.* 2002;25(13):965.

82. Howland WWGL, Weston WL, Huff JC. Erythema multiforme: clinical, histopathologic, and immunologic study. *J Am Acad Dermatol.* 1984;10(3):438–446.

83. Ackerman ABPN, Clark WH. Erythema multiforme exudativum: distinctive pathological process. *Br J Dermatol.* 1971;84(6):554–566.

84. Bocquet HBM, Roujeau JC. Drug-induced pseudolymphoma and drug hypersensitivity syndrome (drug rash with eosinophilia and systemic symptoms: DRESS). *Semin Cutan Med Surg.* 1996;15(4):250.

85. Husain ZRB, Schwartz RA. DRESS syndrome: Part I. Clinical perspectives. *J Am Acad Dermatol.* 2013;68(5):693.

86. Kardaun SHSA, Valeyrie-Allanore L, Halevy S, Davidovici BB, Mockenhaupt M, Roujeau JC. Variability in the clinical pattern of cutaneous side-effects of drugs with systemic symptoms: does a DRESS syndrome really exist? *Br J Dermatol.* 2007;156(3):609.

87. Kardaun SHSP, Valeyrie-Allanore L, Liss Y, et al. RegiSCAR study group. Drug reaction with eosinophilia and systemic symptoms (DRESS): an original multisystem adverse drug reaction. Results from the prospective RegiSCAR study. *Br J Dermatol.* 2013;169(5):1071.

88. Descamps VVA, Edlinger C, Fillet AM, et al. Association of human herpesvirus 6 infection with drug reaction with eosinophilia and systemic symptoms. *Arch Dermatol.* 2001;137(3):301.

89. Kano YHK, Sakuma K, Shiohara T. Several herpesviruses can reactivate in a severe drug-induced multiorgan reaction in the same sequential order as in graft-versus-host disease. *Br J Dermatol.* 2006;155(2):301–306.

90. Muller PDP, Mahé A, Lamaury I, Salzer B, Deloumeaux J, Strobel M. Drug hypersensitivity syndrome in a West-Indian population. *Eur J Dermatol.* 2003;13(5):478–481.

91. Ahluwalia JAK, Perman MJ, Yan AC. Human herpesvirus 6 involvement in paediatric drug hypersensitivity syndrome. *Br J Dermatol.* 2015;172(4):1090–1095.

92. Cacoub PMP, Descamps V, Meyer O, Speirs C, Finzi L, Roujeau JC. The DRESS syndrome: a literature review. *Am J Med.* 2011;124(7):588.

93. Tennis PSR. Risk of serious cutaneous disorders after initiation of use of phenytoin, carbamazepine, or sodium valproate: a record linkage study. *Neurology.* 1997;49(2):542–546.

94. Guberman AHBF, Brodie MJ, Dooley JM, et al. Lamotrigine-associated rash: risk/benefit considerations in adults and children. *Epilepsia.* 1999;40(7):985.

95. Picard DJB, Descamps V, D'Incan M, et al. Drug reaction with eosinophilia and systemic symptoms (DRESS): a multiorgan antiviral T cell response. *Sci Transl Med.* 2010;2(46):46ra62.

96. Almudimeegh ARC, Ferrand H, Crickx B, Yazdanpanah Y, Descamps V. Drug reaction with eosinophilia and systemic symptoms, or virus reactivation with eosinophilia and systemic symptoms as a manifestation of immune reconstitution inflammatory syndrome in a patient with HIV? *Br J Dermatol.* 2014;171(4):895–898.

97. Phillips EJCW, Mockenhaupt M, Roujeau JC, Mallal SA. Drug hypersensitivity: pharmacogenetics and clinical syndromes. *J Allergy Clin Immunol.* 2011;127(suppl 3):S60–S66.

98. Hung SICW, Liou LB, Chu CC, et al. HLA-B*5801 allele as a genetic marker for severe cutaneous adverse reactions caused by allopurinol. *Proc Natl Acad Sci USA.* 2005;102(11):4134.

99. Cheng LXY, Qin CZ, Zhang W, Chen XP, Li J, Zhou HH. HLA-B*58:01 is strongly associated with allopurinol-induced severe cutaneous adverse reactions in Han Chinese patients: a multicentre retrospective case-control clinical study. *Br J Dermatol.* 2015;173(2):555–558.

100. Gonçalo MCI, Teixeira V, Gameiro AR, Brites MM, Nunes R, Martinho A. HLA-B*58:01 is a risk factor for allopurinol-induced DRESS and Stevens-Johnson syndrome/toxic epidermal necrolysis in a Portuguese population. *Br J Dermatol.* 2013;169(3):660.

101. Ortonne NV-AL, Bastuji-Garin S, Wechsler J, et al. Histopathology of drug rash with eosinophilia and systemic symptoms syndrome: a morphological and phenotypical study. *Br J Dermatol.* 2015;173(1):50.

102. Walsh SD-CS, Higgins E, Morris-Jones R, Bashir S, Bernal W, Creamer D. Drug reaction with eosinophilia and systemic symptoms: is cutaneous phenotype a prognostic marker for outcome? A review of clinicopathological features of 27 cases. *Br J Dermatol.* 2013;168(2):391–401.

103. Chi MHHR, Yang CH, Lin JY, et al. Histopathological analysis and clinical correlation of drug reaction with eosinophilia and systemic symptoms (DRESS). *Br J Dermatol.* 2014;170(4):866–873.

104. Uhara HSM, Kawachi S, Ashida A, Oguchi S, Okuyama R. Clinical course of drug-induced hypersensitivity syndrome treated without systemic corticosteroids. *J Eur Acad Dermatol Venereol.* 2013;27(6):722.

105. Funck-Brentano E, Duong TA, Bouvresse S, et al. Therapeutic management of DRESS: a retrospective study of 38 cases. *J Am Acad Dermatol.* 2015;72(2):246–252.

106. Cacoub P, Musette P, Descamps V, et al. The DRESS syndrome: a literature review. *Am J Med.* 2011;124(7):588–597.

107. Joly P, Janela B, Tetart F, et al. Poor benefit/risk balance of intravenous immunoglobulins in DRESS. *Arch Dermatol.* 2012;148(4):543–544.

108. Singer EM, Wanat KA, Rosenbach MA. A case of recalcitrant DRESS syndrome with multiple autoimmune sequelae treated with intravenous immunoglobulins. *JAMA Dermatol.* 2013;149(4):494–495.

109. Bastuji-Garin SRB, Stern RS, Shear NH, Naldi L, Roujeau JC. Clinical classification of cases of toxic epidermal necrolysis, Stevens-Johnson syndrome, and erythema multiforme. *Arch Dermatol.* 1993;129(1):92.

110. Roujeau JC. Stevens-Johnson syndrome and toxic epidermal necrolysis are severity variants of the same disease which differs from erythema multiforme. *J Dermatol.* 1997;24(11):726.

111. Chan HLSR, Arndt KA, Langlois J, Jick SS, Jick H, Walker AM. The incidence of erythema multiforme, Stevens-Johnson syndrome, and toxic epidermal necrolysis. A population-based study with particular reference to reactions caused by drugs among outpatients. *Arch Dermatol.* 1990;126(1):43.

112. Rzany BMM, Baur S, Schröder W, et al. Epidemiology of erythema exsudativum multiforme majus, Stevens-Johnson syndrome, and toxic epidermal necrolysis in Germany (1990–1992): structure and results of a population-based registry. *J Clin Epidemiol.* 1996;49(7):769.

113. Rzany BHO, Mockenhaupt M, Schröder W, Goerttler E, Ring J, Schöpf E. Histopathological and epidemiological characteristics of patients with erythema exudativum multiforme major, Stevens-Johnson syndrome and toxic epidermal necrolysis. *Br J Dermatol.* 1996;135(1):6.

114. Mittmann NKS, Koo M, Shear NH, Rachlis A, Rourke SB. Incidence of toxic epidermal necrolysis and Stevens-Johnson Syndrome in an HIV cohort: an observational, retrospective case series study. *Am J Clin Dermatol.* 2012;13(1):49–54.

115. Sekula PDA, Mockenhaupt M, Naldi L, et al. Comprehensive survival analysis of a cohort of patients with Stevens-Johnson syndrome and toxic epidermal necrolysis. *J Invest Dermatol.* 2013;133(5):1197–1204.

116. Sassolas BHC, Mockenhaupt M, Dunant A, et al. ALDEN, an algorithm for assessment of drug causality in Stevens-Johnson Syndrome and toxic epidermal necrolysis: comparison with case-control analysis. *Clin Pharmacol Ther.* 2010;88(1):60–68.

117. Mockenhaupt MVC, Dunant A, Naldi L, et al. Stevens-Johnson syndrome and toxic epidermal necrolysis: assessment of medication risks with emphasis on recently marketed drugs. The EuroSCAR-study. *J Invest Dermatol.* 2008;128(1):35.

118. Halevy SGP, Mockenhaupt M, Fagot JP, et al. Allopurinol is the most common cause of Stevens-Johnson syndrome and toxic epidermal necrolysis in Europe and Israel. *J Am Acad Dermatol.* 2008;58(1):25.

119. Ko TMCW, Wei CY, Shih HY, et al. Shared and restricted T-cell receptor use is crucial for carbamazepine-induced Stevens-Johnson syndrome. *J Allergy Clin Immunol.* 2011;128(6):1266–1276.

120. Letko EPD, Papaliodis GN, Daoud YJ, Ahmed AR, Foster CS. Stevens-Johnson syndrome and toxic epidermal necrolysis: a review of the literature. *Ann Allergy Asthma Immunol.* 2005;94(4):419.

121. Schwartz RAMP, Lee BW. Toxic epidermal necrolysis: Part I. Introduction, history, classification, clinical features, systemic manifestations, etiology, and immunopathogenesis. *J Am Acad Dermatol.* 2013;69(2):173. e171– e113.

122. Valeyrie-Allanore LRJ-C. In: *Epidermal Necrolysis (Stevens-Johnson Syndrome and Toxic Epidermal Necrolysis).* vol. 1. New York: McGrow-Hill Medical; 2012.

123. Roujeau JCCO, Saiag P, Guillaume JC. Toxic epidermal necrolysis (Lyell syndrome). *J Am Acad Dermatol.* 1990;23(6 Pt 1):1039.

124. Ramon Ruiz M. Acute disseminated epidermal necrosis types 1, 2, and 3: study of sixty cases. *J Am Acad Dermatol.* 1985;(4):13. 623.

125. Revuz JRJ, Guillaume JC, Penso D, Touraine R. Treatment of toxic epidermal necrolysis. Créteil's experience. *Arch Dermatol.* 1987;123(9):1156.

126. Lyell A. Toxic epidermal necrolysis: an eruption resembling scalding of the skin. *Br J Dermatol.* 1956;68(11):355.

127. Jordan MHLM, Jeng JG, Rees JM. Treatment of toxic epidermal necrolysis by burn units: another market or another threat? *J Burn Care Rehabil.* 1991;12(6):579.

128. de Prost NI-H-OS, Ta D, Valeyrie-Allanore L, et al. Bacteremia in Stevens-Johnson syndrome and toxic epidermal necrolysis: epidemiology, risk factors, and predictive value of skin cultures. *Medicine (Baltimore).* 2010;89(1):28–36.

129. Westly EDWH. Toxic epidermal necrolysis. Granulocytic leukopenia as a prognostic indicator. *Arch Dermatol.* 1984;120(6):721.

130. Garcia-Doval ILL, Bocquet H, Otero XL, Roujeau JC. Toxic epidermal necrolysis and Stevens-Johnson syndrome: does early withdrawal of causative drugs decrease the risk of death? *Arch Dermatol.* 2000;136(3):323.

131. Roujeau JCB-GS. Systematic review of treatments for Stevens-Johnson syndrome and toxic epidermal necrolysis using the SCORTEN score as a tool for evaluating mortality. *Ther Adv Drug Saf.* 2011;2(3):87.

132. Wolkenstein PLJ, Roujeau JC, Duguet C, et al. Randomised comparison of thalidomide versus placebo in toxic epidermal necrolysis. *Lancet.* 1998;352(9140):1586.

133. Sitaru CZD. Mechanisms of blister induction by autoantibodies. *Exp Dermatol.* 2005;14(12):861–875.

134. Brenner SB-GA, Ruocco V. Drug-induced pemphigus. *Clin Dermtol.* 1998;16(3):393.

135. Brenner SGI. Drug-induced pemphigus. *Clin Dermtol.* 2011;29(4):455.

136. Feng SZW, Zhang J, Jin P. Analysis of 6 cases of drug-induced pemphigus. *Eur J Dermatol.* 2011;21(5):696–699.

137. Joly PLN. Pemphigus group (vulgaris, vegetans, foliaceus, herpetiformis, brasiliensis). *Clin Dermatol.* 2011;29(4):432–436.

138. Harman KE, Albert S, Black MM. Dermatologists BAo. Guidelines for the management of pemphigus vulgaris. *Br J Dermatol.* 2003;149(5):926–937.

139. Herzog S, Schmidt E, Goebeler M, Bröcker EB, Zillikens D. Serum levels of autoantibodies to desmoglein 3 in patients with therapy-resistant pemphigus vulgaris successfully treated with adjuvant intravenous immunoglobulins. *Acta Derm Venereol.* 2004;84(1): 48–52.

140. Bystryn JC, Rudolph JL. IVIG treatment of pemphigus: how it works and how to use it. *J Invest Dermatol.* 2005;125(6):1093–1098.

141. Sami N, Qureshi A, Ruocco E, Ahmed AR. Corticosteroid-sparing effect of intravenous immunoglobulin therapy in patients with pemphigus vulgaris. *Arch Dermatol.* 2002;138(9):1158–1162.

142. Amagai M, Ikeda S, Shimizu H, et al. A randomized double-blind trial of intravenous immunoglobulin for pemphigus. *J Am Acad Dermatol.* 2009;60(4):595–603.

143. Smith EPTT, Meyer LJ, Zone JJ. Antigen identification in drug-induced bullous pemphigoid. *J Am Acad Dermatol.* 1993;29(5 Pt 2):879.

144. Bastuji-Garin SJP, Lemordant P, et al. French Study Group for Bullous Diseases. Risk factors for bullous pemphigoid in the elderly: a prospective case-control study. *J Invest Dermatol.* 2011;131(3):637.

145. Lloyd-Lavery ACC, Wojnarowska F, Taghipour K. The associations between bullous pemphigoid and drug use: a UK case-control study. *JAMA Dermatol.* 2013;149(1):58–62.

146. Schmidt E, della Torre R, Borradori L. Clinical features and practical diagnosis of bullous pemphigoid. *Dermatol Clin.* 2011;29(3):427–438. viii–ix.

147. Sárdy M, Kostaki D, Varga R, Peris K, Ruzicka T. Comparative study of direct and indirect immunofluorescence and of bullous pemphigoid 180 and 230 enzyme-linked immunosorbent assays for diagnosis of bullous pemphigoid. *J Am Acad Dermatol.* 2013;69(5):748–753.

148. Fleming TE, Korman NJ. Cicatricial pemphigoid. *J Am Acad Dermatol.* 2000;43(4). 571–591; quiz 591–574.

149. Brahimi N, Routier E, Raison-Peyron N, et al. A three-year-analysis of fixed drug eruptions in hospital settings in France. *Eur J Dermatol.* 2010;20(4):461–464.

150. Khaled A, Kharfi M, Ben Hamida M, et al. Cutaneous adverse drug reactions in children. A series of 90 cases. *Tunis Med.* 2012;90(1):45–50.

151. Cho YT, Lin JW, Chen YC, et al. Generalized bullous fixed drug eruption is distinct from Stevens-Johnson syndrome/toxic epidermal necrolysis by immunohistopathological features. *J Am Acad Dermatol.* 2014;70(3):539–548.

152. Shiohara T, Mizukawa Y. The immunological basis of lichenoid tissue reaction. *Autoimmun Rev.* 2005;4(4):236–241.

153. Agnew KL, Oliver GF. Neutrophilic fixed drug eruption. *Australas J Dermatol.* 2001;42(3):200–202.

154. Namazy JA, Simon RA. Sensitivity to nonsteroidal anti-inflammatory drugs. *Ann Allergy Asthma Immunol.* 2002;89(6). 542–550; quiz 550, 605.

155. Mahboob A, Haroon TS. Drugs causing fixed eruptions: a study of 450 cases. *Int J Dermatol.* 1998;37(11):833–838.

156. Shiohara T. Fixed drug eruption: pathogenesis and diagnostic tests. *Curr Opin Allergy Clin Immunol.* 2009;9(4):316–321.

157. Mendelsohn J, Baselga J. Epidermal growth factor receptor targeting in cancer. *Semin Oncol.* 2006;33(4):369–385.

158. Li S, Schmitz KR, Jeffrey PD, Wiltzius JJ, Kussie P, Ferguson KM. Structural basis for inhibition of the epidermal growth factor receptor by cetuximab. *Cancer Cell.* 2005;7(4):301–311.

159. Curry JL, Torres-Cabala CA, Kim KB, et al. Dermatologic toxicities to targeted cancer therapy: shared clinical and histologic adverse skin reactions. *Int J Dermatol.* 2014;53(3):376–384.

160. Pérez-Soler R, Delord JP, Halpern A, et al. HER1/EGFR inhibitor-associated rash: future directions for management and investigation outcomes from the HER1/EGFR inhibitor rash management forum. *Oncologist.* 2005;10(5):345–356.

161. Li T, Perez-Soler R. Skin toxicities associated with epidermal growth factor receptor inhibitors. *Target Oncol.* 2009;4(2):107–119.

162. Wagner LI, Lacouture ME. Dermatologic toxicities associated with EGFR inhibitors: the clinical psychologist's perspective. Impact on health-related quality of life and implications for clinical management of psychological sequelae. *Oncology (Williston Park).* 2007;21(11 Suppl 5):34–36.

163. Jacot W, Bessis D, Jorda E, et al. Acneiform eruption induced by epidermal growth factor receptor inhibitors in patients with solid tumours. *Br J Dermatol.* 2004;151(1):238–241.

164. Busam KJ, Capodieci P, Motzer R, Kiehn T, Phelan D, Halpern AC. Cutaneous side-effects in cancer patients treated with the antiepidermal growth factor receptor antibody C225. *Br J Dermatol.* 2001;144(6):1169–1176.

165. Lichtenberger BM, Gerber PA, Holcmann M, et al. Epidermal EGFR controls cutaneous host defense and prevents inflammation. *Sci Transl Med.* 2013;5(199):199ra111.

166. Chen AP, Setser A, Anadkat MJ, et al. Grading dermatologic adverse events of cancer treatments: the Common Terminology Criteria for Adverse Events Version 4.0. *J Am Acad Dermatol.* 2012;67(5):1025–1039.

167. Lacouture ME, Anadkat MJ, Bensadoun RJ, et al. Clinical practice guidelines for the prevention and treatment of EGFR inhibitor-associated dermatologic toxicities. *Support Care Cancer.* 2011;19(8):1079–1095.

168. Gutzmer R, Becker JC, Enk A, et al. Management of cutaneous side effects of EGFR inhibitors: recommendations from a German expert panel for the primary treating physician. *J Dtsch Dermatol Ges.* 2011;9(3):195–203.

169. E B, ME L. *The MASCC Textbook of Cancer Supportive Care and Survivorship.* New York: Springer; 2010.

170. Segaert S, Van Cutsem E. Clinical signs, pathophysiology and management of skin toxicity during therapy with epidermal growth factor receptor inhibitors. *Ann Oncol.* 2005;16(9):1425–1433.

171. Burtness B, Anadkat M, Basti S, et al. NCCN Task Force Report: management of dermatologic and other toxicities associated with EGFR inhibition in patients with cancer. *J Natl Compr Canc Netw.* 2009;7(suppl 1):S5–S21. quiz S22–S24.

172 Kahan BD. Efficacy of sirolimus compared with azathioprine for reduction of acute renal allograft rejection: a randomised multicentre study. The Rapamune US Study Group. *Lancet.* 2000;356(9225):194–202.

173. MacDonald AS. Rapamycin in combination with cyclosporine or tacrolimus in liver, pancreas, and kidney transplantation. *Transplant Proc.* 2003;35(suppl 3). 201S-208S.

174. Mahé E, Morelon E, Lechaton S, et al. Acne in recipients of renal transplantation treated with sirolimus: clinical, microbiologic, histologic, therapeutic, and pathogenic aspects. *J Am Acad Dermatol.* 2006;55(1):139–142.

175. Mahé E, Morelon E, Lechaton S, et al. Cutaneous adverse events in renal transplant recipients receiving sirolimus-based therapy. *Transplantation.* 2005;79(4):476–482.

176. Nomura M, He Z, Koyama I, Ma WY, Miyamoto K, Dong Z. Involvement of the Akt/mTOR pathway on EGF-induced cell transformation. *Mol Carcinog.* 2003;38(1):25–32.

177. Dereure O. Skin reactions related to treatment with anticytokines, membrane receptor inhibitors and monoclonal antibodies. *Expert Opin Drug Saf.* 2003;2(5):467–473.

178. Lerner EASA. Chemical and pharmacologic agents that cause hyperpigmentation or hypopigmentation of the skin. *Dermatol Clin.* 1988;6(2):327–337.

179. Schwartz CJS, Feinberg JS. Linear rays of hypopigmentation following intra-articular corticosteroid injection for post-traumatic degenerative joint disease. *Dermatol Online J.* 2012;18(5):11.

180. Shah CPRD, Garg SJ. Eyelid cutaneous hypopigmentation after sub-tenon triamcinolone injection after retinal detachment repair. *Retin Caes Brief Rep.* 2012;6(3):271–272.

181. Jalalat SZCP. Gefitinib-associated vitiligo: report in a man with parotid squamous cell carcinoma and review of drug-induced hypopigmentation. *Dermatol Online J.* 2013;19(10):20020.

182. Llamas-Velasco MFJ, Kutzner H, Steegmann JL, García-Diez A, Requena L. Hypopigmented macules secondary to imatinib for the treatment of chronic myeloid leukemia: a histopathologic and immunohistochemical study. *J Cutan Pathol.* 2014;41(5):417–426.

183. Aleem A. Hypopigmentation of the skin due to imatinib mesylate in patients with chronic myeloid leukemia. *Hematol Oncol Stem Cell Ther.* 2009;2(2):358–361.

184. Arya VBM, Girard L, Arya S, Valluri A. Vitiligo at Injection Site of PEG-IFN-α2a in two patients with chronic hepatitis C: case report and literature review. *Case Rep Dermatol.* 2010;2(2):156–164.

185. Burnett CTKD. Imiquimod-induced depigmentation: report of two cases and review of the literature. *Dermatol Surg.* 2012;38(11):1872–1875.

186. Li WXH, Ge L, Song H, Cao W. Induction of vitiligo after imiquimod treatment of condylomata acuminata. *BMC Infect Dis.* 2014;14:329.

187. Ghasri PGS, Saedi N, Ganesan AK. Chemical leukoderma after the application of a transdermal methylphenidate patch. *J Am Acad Dermatol.* 2012;66(6):e237–e238.

188. Grossman MSR. Leukonychia - review and classification. *Int J Dermatol.* 1990;29(535–541).

189. ES A. Images in clinical medicine - acquired leukonychia totalis. *N Engl J Med.* 2006;355: e2.

190. Antonarakis ES. Images in clinical medicine. Acquired leukonychia totalis. *N Engl J Med.* 2006;355(2):e2.

191. Chen GY, Chen W, Huang WT. Single transverse apparent leukonychia caused by 5-fluorouracil plus leucovorin. *Dermatology.* 2003;207(1):86–87.

192. Lehoczky O, Pulay T. Transverse leukonychia secondary to paclitaxel-carboplatin chemotherapy in a patient with ovarian cancer. *J Obstet Gynaecol.* 2002;22(6):694.

193. Saray Y, Seçkin D, Güleç AT, Akgün S, Haberal M. Nail disorders in hemodialysis patients and renal transplant recipients: a case-control study. *J Am Acad Dermatol.* 2004;50(2):197–202.

194. Daniel CR, Piraccini BM, Tosti A. The nail and hair in forensic science. *J Am Acad Dermatol.* 2004;50(2):258–261.

195. Piraccini BMAA. Drug-related nail disease. *Clin Dermatol.* 2013;31(5):618–626.

196. Jefferson J, Rich P. Melanonychia. *Dermatol Res Pract.* 2012;2012:952186.

197. Andre J, Lateur N. Pigmented nail disorders. *Dermatol Clin.* 2006;24:329–339.

198. Minisini AM, Tosti A, Sobrero AF, et al. Taxane-induced nail changes: incidence, clinical presentation and outcome. *Ann Oncol.* 2003;14(2):333–337.

199. Lau CP, Hui P, Chan TC. Docetaxel-induced nail toxicity: a case of severe onycholysis and topic review. *Chin Med J (Engl).* 2011;124(16):2559–2560.

200. Truchuelo M, Vano-Galvan S, Pérez B, Muñoz-Zato E, Jaén P. Unilateral taxane-induced onychopathy in a patient with a brain metastasis. *Dermatol Online J.* 2009;15(3):7.

201. Piraccini BM, Bellavista S, Misciali C, Tosti A, de Berker D, Richert B. Periungual and subungual pyogenic granuloma. *Br J Dermatol.* 2010;163(5):941–953.

202. JZ L. *Litt's Pocketbook of Drug Eruptions and Interactions.* 3rd ed. New York: The Parthenon Publishing Group; 2004.

203. Szarvas SHD, Murphy D. Neuraxial opioid-induced pruritus: a review. *J Clin Anesth.* 2003;15(3):234–239.

204. Joshi SSOS, Witherspoon JN, Rademaker A, et al. Effects of epidermal growth factor receptor inhibitor-induced dermatologic toxicities on quality of life. *Cancer.* 2010;116(391623).

205. Manousaridis IMS, Goerdt S, Leverkus M, Utikal J. Cutaneous side effects of inhibitors of the RAS/RAF/MEK/ERK signalling pathway and their management. *J Eur Acad Dermatol Venereol.* 2013;27(1):11–18.

206. Fischer ARA, Ensslin CJ, Wu S, Lacouture ME. Pruritus to anticancer agents targeting the EGFR, BRAF, and CTLA-4. *Dermatol Ther.* 2013;26(2):135–148.

207. Padda MSSM, Akhtar AJ, Boyer JL. Drug-induced cholestasis. *Hepatology.* 2011;53(4):1377–1387.

208. Russo GE, Spaziani M, Guidotti C, et al. [Pruritus in chronic uremic patients in periodic hemodialysis. Treatment with terfenadine (an antagonist of histamine H1 receptors)]. *Minerva Urol Nefrol.* 1986;38(4):443–447.

209. Rayner H, Baharani J, Smith S, Suresh V, Dasgupta I. Uraemic pruritus: relief of itching by gabapentin and pregabalin. *Nephron Clin Pract.* 2012;122(3–4):75–79.

210. Szepietowski JC, Schwartz RA. Uremic pruritus. *Int J Dermatol.* 1998;37(4):247–253.

CHAPTER 7

Basics of Skin Testing and Drug Challenges

MIGUEL A. PARK, MD • SARA M. MAY, MD

KEY POINTS

- During the evaluation of adverse drug reactions, the clinical history must be reviewed before performing skin testing.
- Skin testing should only be performed for reactions that are consistent with drug allergy.
- Skin testing should be performed by trained personnel who can treat systemic reactions if needed.

SKIN TESTING

During the evaluation of adverse drug reactions, the clinical history must be reviewed before performing skin testing. Skin testing should only be performed for reactions that are consistent with drug allergy. These reactions can be immediate or delayed, but both are due to immune mechanisms to be defined as drug allergy.[1-3] In general, immediate reactions occur within 1 hour of the first dose during the treatment course and may be an IgE-mediated reaction.[1,2,4,5] Nonimmediate also termed delayed reactions are typically due to T cell–mediated reactions and usually develop days into the treatment course.[1-3] Guidelines established in the United States (US) recommend skin prick testing (SPT) and intradermal (ID) testing, also termed intracutaneous testing for immediate reactions and delayed reading of ID testing for delayed reactions. European guidelines are similar but advocate for patch testing to evaluate for delayed reactions and for severe reactions such as Stevens-Johnson syndrome (SJS) and many others.[1,3,6,7] Patch testing will be discussed in another chapter. Throughout this chapter, information and recommendations of skin testing will be discussed based on literature for adult patients but can be extrapolated to children as well.[7]

Skin testing should be performed by trained personnel who can treat systemic reactions if needed. The procedure is performed in a standardized fashion following a set protocol.[1,2,6,7] In general, skin testing should be performed at least 4–6 weeks after the reaction to limit false-negative testing.[2] Preferably, testing is done on healthy individuals in an outpatient setting but can be performed on hospitalized patients including critically ill patients if needed.[1,8-17] Systemic reactions are rare (72 reactions per 100,000 penicillin and antibiotic skin tests) with most reactions being mild.[1,6,16,18-23] Penicillin skin testing has been shown to be safe in pregnant patients and children,[22-27] but reactions occur more frequently with ID testing than prick testing.[18] Even though skin testing is safe, risks of the procedure must be communicated to the patient. Consent should be obtained before testing in addition to review of any contraindications and precautions (Table 7.1) in performing the test.

Unfortunately, the diagnostic value of skin testing is not known for many drugs because of various reasons.[2,7] Therefore, if drug allergy testing with nonirritating concentrations leads to positive reactions, the patient is considered to be sensitized and allergic. If testing is negative, allergy has not been completely ruled out and the patient should undergo drug challenge to confirm testing results.[1,2,7,28] That being said, literature for evaluation of immediate reactions toward penicillin, platinum salt-based chemotherapy drugs, and neuromuscular blocking agents has shown good sensitivity and predictive values.[2,7]

Ideally, skin testing is performed with commercially available testing reagents.[1] However, as discussed in Chapter 10, many reagents are not available for commercial purchase. If commercial reagents are not available, then testing should be performed with the intravenous (IV) drug when possible. Ease of obtaining IV formulations varies between countries.[2,7] In addition, some IV formulations require dilution in sterile water for stability, and sterile water can lead to irritant reactions. If only oral formulations are available, testing can be performed

TABLE 7.1
Contraindications to Skin Testing for Evaluation of Immediate Drug Reactions

CONTRAINDICATIONS	
Incorrect diagnostic modality	History of severe blistering skin reactions[a]
	Cytotoxic reactions
	Immune complex–mediated reactions
	Delayed-type hypersensitivity reactions
	Vasculitic reactions
	DRESS
	Pulmonary drug hypersensitivity
	Drug-induced granulomatous disease
	Immunogenic hepatitis
PRECAUTIONS	
Risk of anaphylaxis	Uncontrolled asthma
	Severely reduced lung function
	History of recent life-threatening reaction
Skin reactivity	Recent systemic reaction[b]
	Dermatographism
	Urticaria
	Cutaneous mastocytosis

DRESS, drug related eosinophilia with systemic symptoms.
[a]Severe blister reaction such as Stevens-Johnson syndrome, toxic epidermal necrolysis, etc.
[b]Systemic allergic reaction less than 4–6 weeks before testing can lead to reduced skin reactivity.

TABLE 7.2
Drugs That Have Antihistamine Properties and Can Inhibit the Wheal and Flare Response During Skin Testing Must be Held Before Testing.

Drug Class	Days To Hold
First-generation antihistamines (H1)	2–3[a]
Second-generation antihistamines (H1)	2–3[b]
H2 blockers	Days to
Antidepressants (TCA)	7
Topical steroids	14–21
Prednisone	0[c]
Omalizumab	90

H1, histamine 1 receptor; *H2*, histamine 2 receptor; *TCA*, tricyclic antidepressants.
[a]Hydroxyzine 5 days and Cyproheptadine 9 days.
[b]Loratadine 7 days at 40 mg per day dosing.
[c]Studies have shown doses of prednisone 20–30 mg per day for certain durations not effecting reactivity.

by dissolving the drug in 0.9% normal saline after removal of protective coating. Unfortunately, many oral formulations contain inactive fillers that have a potential to cause irritating reactions. It is also important to note the ability of the drug to dissolve into solution to elicit an accurate testing concentration.[7,29] The concentration used for testing should always be the highest concentration that does not lead to direct irritation. If this concentration is not known, testing should be performed on healthy controls at the same time.[1,7]

Before the procedure, medications that inhibit histamine must be stopped at various days to limit false-negative results (Table 7.2).[30–42] Antihistamines can reduce skin reactivity for up to 9 days, but most for only 2 or 3 days (Table 7.2). For simplicity and to reduce the risk of false-negative testing, holding antihistamines for 1 week before testing should be considered. Similarly, antidepressants with H1 antagonism such as tricyclic antidepressants (TCA's) should be stopped 1 week

before testing if safe to do so in the patient. Selective serotonin reuptake inhibitors (SSRIs) do not affect skin reactivity. Topical steroids should not be used at testing site for 1 week.[36] In addition, histamine 1 mg/mL for prick testing and 0.1 mg/mL for intradermal testing is placed to confirm skin reactivity.[19,43] Normal saline is used for negative controls in both testing procedures.[1]

SPT is an effective initial test for evaluating drug hypersensitivity because of ease of performing the test, comfort for the patient, cost, and quick results.[2,19] Testing is done on the volar aspect of the forearm via pricking through a drop of the drug, but this area of testing may lead to a smaller wheal and flare response.[44–46] After 15 min, the test is read to confirm that positive and negative controls are accurate and if any of the drugs produced positive readings.[47] To interpret the test, the superior reporting method, compared with other methods, is measuring the largest diameter of the wheal and flare and perpendicular to that diameter recording all measurements (i.e., 5 × 5 mm wheal, 15 × 15 mm flare).[1,48,49]If positive readings are recorded, the patient is considered sensitized, and no further testing is performed. If SPT is negative, then ID testing is performed to the right of negative prick results.[1,19] A hypodermic needle is used to introduce the drug just under the epidermis eliciting a 3 × 3 mm wheal.[1,50] This generally requires about 0.02 mL of the drug.[19,50] Intradermal testing is the best procedure for diagnosing drug allergy with increased sensitivity and more reproducibility.[6,48,51–56] Unfortunately, what constitutes a positive ID test result is not standardized. Most aller-gists use a wheal greater than 3 mm larger in diameter than the negative control with surrounding erythema as a cutoff for a positive test.[19] The manufacturer of Pre-Pen recommends a wheal of 5 mm or greater with flare be considered positive.[50] Due to this controversy, appli-cation of ID testing in duplicate should be considered.

β-Lactam Antibiotics

Penicillin antibiotics

Penicillin skin testing is the most dependable method to evaluate for IgE-mediated reactions toward peni-cillin and should be performed to evaluate for drug allergy.[1,2,7,57] It is the only drug allergy evaluation that should be performed electively because of improved clinical outcomes and is cost-effective.[1,8–17]

The native penicillin drug is converted to a major determinant (benzylpenicilloyl) and minor determi-nants (penicilloate, penilloate, and native drug peni-cillin).[58] Testing for penicillin should include these in addition to amoxicillin. However, because of commer-cial availability, penicillin skin testing in the United States generally includes only the major determinant purchased as Pre-PEN and one minor determinant (penicillin G). The remaining two minor determinants cannot be purchased for testing. Table 7.3 outlines pen-icillin testing reagents, but detailed information regard-ing these will be covered in Chapter 10. The negative predictive value (NPV) for penicillin skin testing with the major and all minor determinants is near 100% and, the positive predictive value (PPV) is between 40% and 100%.[1,55,59] Testing with the major determinant and only penicillin G can miss 10%–20% of sensitized patients.[1,55,59,60] However, whether sensitivity to only penicillioate and penilloate represents clinical allergy to penicillin is not known. Reaction rates to penicillin challenges are similar in patients with negative test-ing with benzylpenicilloyl-polylysine and penicillin G compared with patients tested with all penicillin determinants.[1,55,59–61]

Some patients may only be sensitized to the syn-thetic penicillin antibiotics.[1,62] In Europe this is more common than in the United States.[7,63] If evaluation is negative in these patients, a drug challenge is required because of unknown NPV and PPV.[1] Allergy literature published in Europe documents good sensitivity and predictive values with synthetic penicillin testing.[2,7] The ideal testing concentration is unknown, but rec-ommendations for nonirritating concentrations are available (Table 7.3) including for reactions toward amoxicillin–clavulanic acid that could be directed at clavulanic acid.[24,64,65]

TABLE 7.3
Concentrations for Skin Testing to Penicillin and Related Compounds

Drug Name	Testing Concentrations (United States)
MAJOR PENICILLIN DETERMINANT	
(Penicilloyl-polylysine)	6×10^{-5} M
MINOR PENICILLIN DETERMINANTS	
Penicilloate[a]	0.01 M
Penilloate[a]	0.01 M
Penicillin G	10,000 U/mL
SYNTHETIC PENICILLINS	
Amoxicillin[b]	4 mg/mL
Ampicillin[b]	NA
Clavulanic acid[c]	20 mg/mL

[a]Not available commercially in the United States and made together as minor determinant mixture.
[b]Unable to obtain intravenous formulation in the United States and therefore, tablets must be used. Higher concentrations than 4 mg/mL tend not to dissolve.
[c]Test using amoxicillin–clavulanic acid under the trade name Aug-mentin because clavulanic acid cannot be purchased individually.

TABLE 7.4
Cross-reactivity Between Synthetic Penicillin Antibiotics and Other Cephalosporins Based on Identical R-Groups.

Synthetic Penicillin	Cephalosporin Cross-reactivity
Amoxicillin	Cefadroxil, cefprozil, cefatrizine
Ampicillin	Cephalexin, cefaclor, cephradine, cephaloglycin, and loracarbef

Cephalosporin antibiotics

Cephalosporin allergic reactions are less common than penicillin.[1] Cross-reactivity between penicillin and ceph-alosporin antibiotics is always a concern and will be addressed in detail in subsequent chapters. It is thought that the cross-reactivity between cephalosporins is related to the R-group side chains, and patients should be able to tolerate cephalosporins with different R-groups,[1] especially if skin testing yielded negative results toward the alternative drug.[66] That being said, patients sensi-tive to amoxicillin or ampicillin should avoid specific cephalosporins because of increased risk of cross-reac-tivity (Table 7.4).[1] The NPV and PPV for cephalosporin SPT are unknown and therefore patients with negative testing should undergo a drug challenge. Ideal testing concentrations are not known and differ between the US and European drug allergy guidelines (Table 7.5).[1,7] In general, 10-fold dilutions produce a nonirritating testing concentration (Table 7.5).[1] European guidelines recommend skin prick and intradermal (SPT and ID) testing of cephalosporins be conducted at concentrations of 2 mg/mL, but other studies have recommended higher testing concentrations (Table 7.5).[7,71,72] In addition, European guidelines recommend skin testing patients to the major and minor determinants of penicillin, amoxicillin, suspected cephalosporin, leading to hypersensitivity reaction, and cephalosporins with similar side chains.[7,57] In the United States, testing to the minor determinants is not the standard of care for evaluation of these patients because cross-reactivity is unlikely related to the minor determinants of penicillin.

Monobactam antibiotics

There is no cross-reactivity between penicillin and aztreonam,[73] which is the only monobactam antibiotic available in the United States. However, aztreonam and ceftazidime have a risk of cross-reaction, and sensitized patients should avoid both drugs. Skin testing can be performed with aztreonam diluted in normal saline to a concentration of 2 mg/mL (Table 7.5), but as with most drugs there is no standardized skin testing procedure for aztreonam allergy evaluation.[1,7]

Carbapenem antibiotics

Theoretical risk of cross-reactivity between these drugs and penicillin exists. However, four studies (528 patients) have shown minimal sensitivity toward carbapenems in penicillin SPT-positive patients.[73,74] There is no standardized skin testing procedure for evaluation of carbapenem allergy,[1] but nonirritating concentrations have been determined (Table 7.5).[3,73] In patients with confirmed penicillin allergy via skin testing or unknown penicillin allergy, a carbapenem most likely can be given as a graded challenge safely if needed.[1] If SPT for carbapenem antibiotics is available and results are negative, carbapenem antibiotics can be given in typical fashion without graded challenge.[73]

Non-β-Lactam Antibiotics

Testing is performed with commercially available drugs and ideally with drugs that can be delivered intravenously as described earlier in this chapter. The value of skin testing with these antibiotics is not known.[7] Therefore, skin testing should only be done if the drug is needed and not performed on an elective basis.[1]

Skin testing is not validated, and therefore a positive test is suggestive of drug hypersensitivity, but a negative test does not rule out hypersensitivity and challenge is needed.[1]

Macrolide antibiotics

Skin testing sensitivity and specificity is variable depending on the study.[63,69] In addition, different studies have shown different concentrations that are nonirritating and have been used during evaluation (Table 7.5).[67–69]

Quinolone antibiotics

Hypersensitivity reactions are increasing toward quinolone antibiotics.[1] Evaluation with SPT is controversial with risk of false-positive tests because of irritation. Some authors have found nonirritating concentrations listed in Table 7.5,[3,63,67] but this is not consistent throughout the literature. Please refer Chapter 13 for details.

Sulfonamide antibiotics

Sulfonamide antibiotics tend to lead to a morbilliform or maculopapular eruption with fever, but many other clinical symptoms can be seen with these drugs.[1] IgE-mediated reactions toward sulfonamide antibiotics are quite rare, but have been reported. These rare cases can be evaluated with SPT at 0.8 mg/mL concentration (Table 7.5).[67]

Other antibiotics

Testing with gentamicin and tobramycin (aminoglycoside antibiotics) can be performed, but testing should not be performed with streptomycin (Table 7.5).[67,75] Reactions toward vancomycin are generally not IgE mediated, but skin testing can be useful, keeping in mind the risk of direct mast cell activation (Table 7.5).[1] Testing for clindamycin hypersensitivity is not recommended because one study showed nearly 30% of patients with negative skin testing reacted to oral challenge.[70] Nonirritating concentrations have been reported for doxycycline SPT and ID testing (Table 7.5).[6]

Aspirin and Nonsteroidal Drugs

Several distinct phenotypes have been formulated to describe specific clinical reactions based on symptoms and mechanism eliciting the reaction toward this drug class. Only one of these categories describes reactions that may be related to IgE antibodies and drug specific, but skin testing has not been carefully evaluated for these reactions.[1,7]

TABLE 7.5

Nonirritating Concentrations for Skin Test Evaluation Toward Multiple Antibiotics Compared With US Guidelines, European Guidelines, and Other Specific Studies Discussed in the Text.

Category of Drug	Name of Drug	US Guidelines	Dilution	European Guidelines	Other
Penicillins	Nafcillin	25 µg/mL	1:10,000	20 mg/mL[a]	
	Ticarcillin	20 mg/mL	1:10	20 mg/mL[a]	
Cephalosporins	Cefepime			2 mg/mL	2 mg/mL[3]
	Cefotaxime	10 mg/mL	1:10	2 mg/mL	20 mg/mL[3]
	Cefuroxime	10 mg/mL	1:10	2 mg/mL	20 mg/mL[3]
	Cefazolin	33 mg/mL	1:10	2 mg/mL	20 mg/mL[3]
	Ceftazidime	10 mg/mL	1:10	2 mg/mL	20 mg/mL[3]
	Ceftriaxone	10 mg/mL	1:10	2 mg/mL	20 mg/mL[3]
Carbapenems	Imipenem	0.5 mg/mL	1:10		Imipenem/cilastatin 0.1–1 mg/mL
	Meropenem	1 mg/mL	1:50		1 mg/mL
Monobactam	Aztreonam				2 mg/mL
Quinolones[b]	Levofloxacin	25 µg/mL	1:1000		5 mg/mL SPT, 0.05 mg/mL ID
	Ciprofloxacin				2 mg/mL SPT, 0.006 mg/mL ID
	Moxifloxacin				1.6 mg/mL SPT, 0.004 or 0.16 mg/mL ID
Aminoglycosides	Gentamicin	4 mg/mL	1:10		4 mg/mL
	Tobramycin	4 mg/mL	1:10		4 mg/mL
Macrolides[c]	Azithromycin	10 µg/mL	1:10,000		250 mg/mL SPT, 0.01 mg/mL ID
	Erythromycin	50 µg/mL	1:1000		500 mg/mL SPT, 0.01 mg/mL ID
	Clarithromycin				50 mg/mL or 250 mg/mL SPT, 0.01 mg/mL or 0.05 mg/mL
Tetracycline	Doxycycline				20 mg/mL skin prick 2 mg/mL ID
Other	Clindamycin[d]	15 mg/mL	1:10	NA	NA
	Sulfamethoxazole				0.8 mg/mL
	Vancomycin	5 µg/mL	1:10,000		0.1 mg/mL

[a]European guidelines recommend skin testing for "other penicillins" to be conducted at 20 mg/mL and therefore no specific recommendations for these two drugs.

[b]Listed concentrations for prick test only, intradermal testing ranges from 1:100 to 1:1000 dilutions to obtain nonirritating concentrations. Levofloxacin can be made with 1:1000 dilutions from purchased 25 mg/mL drug. Moxifloxacin 0.016 mg/mL is made from 1:100 dilution of 1.6 mg/mL purchased drug.[63,67]

[c]Concentrations outlined in US guidelines can be prepared with commercially available drugs in the US.[67] Other nonirritating concentrations are prepared using drugs that are not commercially available in the United States.[68] A final study used different concentrations for clarithromycin testing utilizing IV formulation.[69]

[d]Skin testing for clindamycin hypersensitivity does not appear to be useful with many false negative tests.[70]

TABLE 7.6
Skin Prick and Intradermal Skin Testing Concentrations That Have Been Shown to be Nonirritating for the Evaluation of Drug Hypersensitivity to Platinum Based Chemotherapeutic Agents.

Platinum Salts	Skin Prick (mg/mL)	Intradermal (mg/mL)
Carboplatin	10	5 mg/mL
Oxaliplatin	5 mg/mL	5 mg/mL
Cisplatin	1	1 mg/mL

TABLE 7.7
Nonirritating Concentrations That Have Been Reported in the Literature for Skin Prick and Intradermal Testing to Heparin, Iodinated Contrast, Monoclonal Drugs and Corticosteroids.

MISCELLANEOUS MEDICATIONS		
Drug Name	Skin Prick (mg/mL)	Intradermal (mg/mL)
Heparin[a]	Undiluted	1:10 dilution (serial)
Iodinated contrast	Undiluted	1:10 dilution
Adalimumab	50	5
Etanercept	25	5
Infliximab	10	10
Omalizumab	0.0125	0.0125
Methylprednisolone	2 and 20	0.2 and 2
Triamcinolone	4 and 40	0.4 and 4

[a]Heparin skin testing should include heparins from various classes (i.e., unfractionated, low molecular weight, etc.) and intradermal tests should start at a 1:1000 dilution and if negative proceed to 1:100 dilution and finally 1:10 dilution due to risk of irritant reactions.[7,79]

Chemotherapy Drugs

Drug hypersensitivity reactions occur and may be toward the drug or toward excipients.[1] Drugs in the taxane family tend to lead to reactions from direct mast cell stimulation, but medications that are platinum compounds can lead to hypersensitivity reactions. Therefore, skin prick testing for platinum-based medications is useful and should be repeated before each dose (Table 7.6).[1,76–78] In addition, skin testing to asparaginase specifically is recommended before treatment because 43% of patients are likely to develop sensitivity after the fourth dose.[1]

Biologics and Monoclonal Antibodies

Reactions to biologics and monoclonal antibodies occur and some may be immune mediated. Unfortunately, only a very small percentage of the drugs that are being used have published nonirritating concentrations for skin testing (Table 7.7).[1,80–82] In these studies, only a small number of controls were available for evaluation of nonirritating concentrations.

Perioperative Drugs (Including Local Anesthetics)

IgE antibodies to medications used in the perioperative arena have been identified and include many antibiotics discussed earlier in this chapter.[1] Medications that can induce hypersensitivity reactions include induction agents, neuromuscular blocking agents, opiates, latex, and chlorhexidine in addition to antibiotics.[1] In the United States, antibiotics are more likely to cause reactions, and neuromuscular blocking agents are the main culprits in Europe. Fortunately, many multicenter studies have been conducted in Europe for the evaluation of perioperative hypersensitivity reactions, and therefore nonirritating concentrations for skin testing is known (Table 7.8).[7] Skin testing with opiates can be performed if needed, but interpretation of testing results is difficult because of direct mast cell activation (Table 7.8).[1] Reactions toward local anesthetics are very rarely due to IgE-mediated reactions, but skin testing can be done (Table 7.8).[1,7] If SPT is negative, there are limited data to suggest ID testing improves results, and drug allergy guidelines in the United States recommend directly performing a challenge.[1]

Radiocontrast Media

There are differing opinions about reactions toward radiocontrast media between drug allergy specialists in the United States and Europe. In the United States, reactions are thought to be primarily due to direct mast cell activation, but in Europe, IgE-mediated reactions are thought to occur. See the chapter on Radiocontrast reactions for more details. Therefore, skin testing may be useful, particularly in those patients with reactions that occur despite premedication (Table 7.7).[1,2,7,92]

Corticosteroids

Hypersensitivity reactions toward corticosteroids are rare, and some may be related to preservatives and therefore skin testing should be conducted using the parent drugs and excipients (Table 7.7).[1,7]

TABLE 7.8
Nonirritating Concentrations for Skin Prick and Intradermal Testing to Medications Used in the Perioperative Arena Including Local Anesthetics.

Drug	Skin Prick (mg/mL)	Intradermal (mg/mL)
INDUCTIVE AGENT		
Thiopental	25	2.5
Propofol	10	1
Ketamine	10	1
Etomidate	2	0.2
SEDATIVE		
Midazolam	5	0.5
OPIOID		
Fentanyl	0.05	0.005
Alfentanil	0.5	0.05
Sufentanil	0.005	0.0005
Remifentanil	0.05	0.005
Morphine	1	0.01
MUSCLE RELAXER/NEUROMUSCULAR BLOCKADE		
Atracurium	1	0.01
Cisatracurium	2	0.02
Mivacurium	0.2	0.002
Rocuronium	10	0.05
Vecuronium	4	0.4
Pancuronium	2	0.2
Suxamethonium	10	0.1
LOCAL ANESTHETICS		
Any[a]	Undiluted	1:10 Dilution
OTHER		
Chlorhexidine	5	0.002

[a]Must preform using anesthetics without vasoconstricting agents.

Heparins

Heparins are commonly used for anticoagulation in both prophylaxis and treatment. These medications are divided into four groups (unfractionated heparins, low-molecular-weight heparins, semisynthetic heparinoid, and synthetic pentasaccharide).[79] Immune-mediated reactions toward heparin medications occur with cell-mediated reactions being the most common. These reactions typically manifest as pruritic erythematous lesions at injection sites.[79] Even though immune-mediated reactions are rare, IgE-mediated reactions including anaphylaxis have been reported.[79,83] European allergists consider skin testing for hypersensitivity reactions toward heparin has good sensitivity and predictive values.[2,7] Testing should include medications from all four of the different classes (Table 7.6).[7] Similar to all other drug allergy evaluation, SPT should be conducted first. Undiluted concentrations have been found to be nonirritating. If SPT is negative, ID testing starting at 1:1000 dilution with serial ID testing to maximal testing concentration of 1:10 should be conducted (Table 7.7).[79,83] ID testing with undiluted heparin medications leads to irritant reactions. If SPT and ID testing at 1:10 dilution are negative, patient is considered not sensitized. To demonstrate tolerance of these medications, a subcutaneous drug challenge should be performed to the desired medication.[79]

DRUG CHALLENGES

Drug challenge is the gold standard in determining the culprit medication suspected in the adverse drug reaction[1] and/or to determine the tolerance of medication. Drug challenge is also known by the following terms in the literature: drug provocation test, test dose, graded challenge, and graded dose challenge. The purpose of a drug challenge differs slightly based on the different practice guidelines for drug allergies. The practice parameters by the Joint Task Force of the American Academy of Allergy, Asthma and Immunology (AAAAI), the American College of Allergy, Asthma and Immunology (ACAAI), and the Joint Council of Allergy, Asthma and Immunology (JCAAI) define the purpose of a drug challenge is to identify a drug that is unlikely to cause an allergic reaction.[2] For example, in a patient with a history of penicillin allergy but a negative penicillin skin test, a drug challenge with penicillin would be appropriate to confirm that it is safe to administer penicillin in the future. An exception to this purpose may be in aspirin-exacerbated respiratory disease (AERD). In AERD, a drug challenge is considered to confirm the diagnosis of AERD. The Drug Allergy Interest Group/European Network for Drug Allergy of the European Academy of Allergy and Clinic Immunology guidelines differ slightly by including the additional purpose of a drug challenge, that is, to establish the culprit medication suspected in the previous adverse drug reaction[1] and not just to confirm the diagnosis of AERD. Hence, drug challenges are used to identify safe medication but, in some special cases, to identify the culprit medication that may have caused

TABLE 7.9
Example of an Immediate Adverse Reaction Drug Challenge Protocol

Drug	Doses	Cumulative Doses	Time Interval	Vitals: Blood Pressure, Peak Flow
Amoxicillin: target dose of 500 mg	5 mg (1:100)	5 mg	30 min	BP; peak flow
	50 mg (1:10)	55 mg	30 min	BP; peak flow
	500 mg (1:1)	560 mg[a]	30 min	BP; peak flow

[a]The cumulative dose maybe greater than the target dose.

the previous adverse drug reaction or as part of evaluation and confirmation of a disease such as AERD. Both practice guidelines agree that a drug challenge is contraindicated in the cases of suspected previous life-threatening adverse drug reactions such as SJS, toxic epidermal necrolysis, drug reaction with eosinophilia and systemic symptoms, vasculitis, and acute generalized exanthematous pustulosis.

During discussion of drug challenges, it is important to delineate the differences between a drug challenge and induction of tolerance, also termed desensitization. Induction of tolerance alters the immune system to enable the patient to tolerate the medication and is indicated for a medication that is suspected in the previous adverse drug reaction. This is only recommended if the drug is medically indicated and no alternative drug is available.[2] Drug challenges, as noted above, are indicated for the situation in which the probability of the medication that is medically indicated has a low chance of an adverse drug reaction.[2] Both drug challenges and induction of tolerance are administered in increasing doses. However, the literature is unclear about the number of steps that delineates between a drug challenge and the induction of tolerance. It has been suggested that four or more steps in the administration of increasing doses may induce tolerance.[2]

As noted above, drug challenges are performed when the probability of the adverse drug reaction is low. Under these circumstances, several studies have shown that drug challenges are safe.[84–86] A drug challenge should only be done in a medical facility with trained professionals who are equipped to treat any life-threatening reaction such as anaphylaxis. Drug challenges can be administered orally or by IV. Most drug challenges are conducted in a nonblinded fashion. However, because up to 41% of healthy volunteers can have subjective and objective evidence of possible adverse reaction to placebo,[87,88] a single blinded or double-blinded with placebo may be needed. For a thorough risk assessment of the likelihood of an adverse drug reaction, patient's current state of health must be addressed before the procedure.

No standardized protocol exists for drug challenges. If an immediate drug adverse reaction is of concern, the starting dose can range from 1:1000 to the full therapeutic dose. Subsequent doses are increased by 10-fold every 30 min to 1 h depending on the clinical situation, severity of the previous adverse reaction, and risk of adverse reaction.[1,89] This process continues until the therapeutic dose has been given. However, a full therapeutic dose challenge is also appropriate in certain clinical situations such as in a patient with a history of penicillin allergy and negative penicillin skin test. The optimal time interval between doses for immediate adverse drug reaction is also unclear but, in general, seems to range from 30 min to 1 h; however, the intervals between doses may be affected by the route of administration (oral vs. IV) and the bioavailability of the medication (see Table 7.9 for examples).

For delayed adverse reactions, the optimal drug challenge protocols have not been defined. Several examples have been described in the literature with significant variation. For example, in the study of Caubet JC et al.,[90] after an oral drug challenge was completed for an immediate adverse reaction (150% of therapeutic dose if intradermal skin test negative vs. 50% of therapeutic dose followed by 100% of therapeutic dose if skin test positive), the patients were given therapeutic doses for 2 day at home. In the study of Ponvert C et al.,[91] the patients were prescribed the full therapeutic dose to be taken at home for 5–7 days. Hence, depending on the previous adverse reaction and risk of an adverse reaction to the drug to be challenged, it may be prudent to observe the first therapeutic dose under medical supervision and then continue the challenge at home for 3–7 days with close phone or face-to-face follow-up (see Table 7.10 for an example).

In conclusion, drug challenge is safe in the appropriate patient and a valuable diagnostic tool in the evaluation of drug allergy.

TABLES 7.10
Example of a Delayed Adverse Reaction Drug Challenge Protocol

Drug	Doses	Time	Follow-Up Phone Call or Face to Face Visit
Amoxicillin: target dose of 500 mg	500 mg	Day 1	In office supervision
	500 mg twice a day	Day 2–3 or 7	Follow-up phone call or face to face visit

REFERENCES

1. Joint Task Force on Practice Parameters, American Academy of Allergy, Asthma and Immunology, American College of Allergy, Asthma and Immunology, Joint Council of Allergy, Asthma and Immunology. Drug allergy: an updated practice parameter. *Ann Allergy Asthma Immunol.* 2010;105(4):259–273.
2. Demoly P, Adkinson NF, Brockow K, et al. International consensus on drug allergy. *Allergy.* 2014;69(4):420–437.
3. Romano A, Caubet JC. Antibiotic allergies in children and adults: from clinical symptoms to skin testing diagnosis. *J Allergy Clin Immunol Pract.* 2014;2(1):3–12.
4. Bircher AJ, Scherer Hofmeier K. Drug hypersensitivity reactions: inconsistency in the use of the classification of immediate and nonimmediate reactions. *J Allergy Clin Immunol.* 2012;129(1):263–264. Author reply 265–266.
5. Romano A, Torres MJ, Castells M, Sanz ML, Blanca M. Diagnosis and management of drug hypersensitivity reactions. *J Allergy Clin Immunol.* 2011;127(suppl 3):S67–S73.
6. Brockow K, Romano A, Blanca M, Ring J, Pichler W, Demoly P. General considerations for skin test procedures in the diagnosis of drug hypersensitivity. *Allergy.* 2002;57(1):45–51.
7. Brockow K, Garvey LH, Aberer W, et al. Skin test concentrations for systemically administered drugs – an ENDA/EAACI drug allergy interest group position paper. *Allergy.* 2013;68(6):702–712.
8. Sade K, Holtzer I, Levo Y, Kivity S. The economic burden of antibiotic treatment of penicillin-allergic patients in internal medicine wards of a general tertiary care hospital. *Clin Exp Allergy.* 2003;33(4):501–506.
9. MacLaughlin EJ, Saseen JJ, Malone DC. Costs of beta-lactam allergies: selection and costs of antibiotics for patients with a reported beta-lactam allergy. *Arch Fam Med.* 2000;9(8):722–726.
10. Kwan T, Lin F, Ngai B, Loeb M. Vancomycin use in 2 ontario tertiary care hospitals: a survey. *Clin Invest Med.* 1999;22(6):256–264.
11. Lee CE, Zembower TR, Fotis MA, et al. The incidence of antimicrobial allergies in hospitalized patients: implications regarding prescribing patterns and emerging bacterial resistance. *Arch Intern Med.* 2000;160(18):2819–2822.
12. Macy E, Contreras R. Health care use and serious infection prevalence associated with penicillin "allergy" in hospitalized patients: a cohort study. *J Allergy Clin Immunol.* 2014;133(3):790–796.
13. Picard M, Begin P, Bouchard H, et al. Treatment of patients with a history of penicillin allergy in a large tertiary-care academic hospital. *J Allergy Clin Immunol Pract.* 2013;1(3):252–257.
14. del Real GA, Rose ME, Ramirez-Atamoros MT, et al. Penicillin skin testing in patients with a history of beta-lactam allergy. *Ann Allergy Asthma Immunol.* 2007;98(4):355–359.
15. Frigas E, Park MA, Narr BJ, et al. Preoperative evaluation of patients with history of allergy to penicillin: comparison of 2 models of practice. *Mayo Clin Proc.* 2008;83(6):651–662.
16. Nadarajah K, Green GR, Naglak M. Clinical outcomes of penicillin skin testing. *Ann Allergy Asthma Immunol.* 2005;95(6):541–545.
17. Park M, Markus P, Matesic D, Li JT. Safety and effectiveness of a preoperative allergy clinic in decreasing vancomycin use in patients with a history of penicillin allergy. *Ann Allergy Asthma Immunol.* 2006;97(5):681–687.
18. Valyasevi MA, Maddox DE, Li JT. Systemic reactions to allergy skin tests. *Ann Allergy Asthma Immunol.* 1999;83(2):132–136.
19. Bernstein IL, Li JT, Bernstein DI, et al. Allergy diagnostic testing: an updated practice parameter. *Ann Allergy Asthma Immunol.* 2008;100(3 suppl 3):S1–S148.
20. Sullivan TJ, Wedner HJ, Shatz GS, Yecies LD, Parker CW. Skin testing to detect penicillin allergy. *J Allergy Clin Immunol.* 1981;68(3):171–180.
21. Macy E, Richter PK, Falkoff R, Zeiger R. Skin testing with penicilloate and penilloate prepared by an improved method: amoxicillin oral challenge in patients with negative skin test responses to penicillin reagents. *J Allergy Clin Immunol.* 1997;100(5):586–591.
22. Fox SJ, Park MA. Penicillin skin testing is a safe and effective tool for evaluating penicillin allergy in the pediatric population. *J Allergy Clin Immunol Pract.* 2014;2(4):439–444.
23. Macy E. Penicillin skin testing in pregnant women with a history of penicillin allergy and group B streptococcus colonization. *Ann Allergy Asthma Immunol.* 2006;97(2):164–168.
24. Ponvert C, Perrin Y, Bados-Albiero A, et al. Allergy to beta-lactam antibiotics in children: results of a 20-year study based on clinical history, skin and challenge tests. *Pediatr Allergy Immunol.* 2011;22(4):411–418.
25. Pichichero ME, Pichichero DM. Diagnosis of penicillin, amoxicillin, and cephalosporin allergy: reliability of examination assessed by skin testing and oral challenge. *J Pediatr.* 1998;132(1):137–143.

26. Atanaskovic-Markovic M, Velickovic TC, Gavrovic-Jankulovic M, Vuckovic O, Nestorovic B. Immediate allergic reactions to cephalosporins and penicillins and their cross-reactivity in children. *Pediatr Allergy Immunol.* 2005;16(4):341–347.

27. Ponvert C, Le Clainche L, de Blic J, Le Bourgeois M, Scheinmann P, Paupe J. Allergy to beta-lactam antibiotics in children. *Pediatrics.* 1999;104(4):e45.

28. Mirakian R, Ewan PW, Durham SR, et al. BSACI guidelines for the management of drug allergy. *Clin Exp Allergy.* 2009;39(1):43–61.

29. Romano A, Gueant-Rodriguez RM, Viola M, et al. Diagnosing immediate reactions to cephalosporins. *Clin Exp Allergy.* 2005;35(9):1234–1242.

30. Cook TJ, MacQueen DM, Wittig HJ, Thornby JI, Lantos RL, Virtue CM. Degree and duration of skin test suppression and side effects with antihistamines. A double blind controlled study with five antihistamines. *J Allergy Clin Immunol.* 1973;51(2):71–77.

31. dos Santos RV, Magerl M, Mlynek A, Lima HC. Suppression of histamine- and allergen-induced skin reactions: comparison of first- and second-generation antihistamines. *Ann Allergy Asthma Immunol.* 2009;102(6):495–499.

32. Rao KS, Menon PK, Hilman BC, Sebastian CS, Bairnsfather L. Duration of the suppressive effect of tricyclic antidepressants on histamine-induced wheal-and-flare reactions in human skin. *J Allergy Clin Immunol.* 1988;82(5 Pt 1):752–757.

33. Miller J, Nelson HS. Suppression of immediate skin tests by ranitidine. *J Allergy Clin Immunol.* 1989;84(6 Pt 1):895–899.

34. Kupczyk M, Kuprys I, Gorski P, Kuna P. The effect of montelukast (10 mg daily) and loratadine (10 mg daily) on wheal, flare and itching reactions in skin prick tests. *Pulm Pharmacol Ther.* 2007;20(1):85–89.

35. White M, Rothrock S, Meeves S, Liao Y, Georges G. Comparative effects of fexofenadine and montelukast on allergen-induced wheal and flare. *Allergy Asthma Proc.* 2005;26(3):221–228.

36. Pipkorn U, Hammarlund A, Enerback L. Prolonged treatment with topical glucocorticoids results in an inhibition of the allergen-induced weal-and-flare response and a reduction in skin mast cell numbers and histamine content. *Clin Exp Allergy.* 1989;19(1):19–25.

37. Des Roches A, Paradis L, Bougeard YH, Godard P, Bousquet J, Chanez P. Long-term oral corticosteroid therapy does not alter the results of immediate-type allergy skin prick tests. *J Allergy Clin Immunol.* 1996;98(3):522–527.

38. Corren J, Shapiro G, Reimann J, et al. Allergen skin tests and free IgE levels during reduction and cessation of omalizumab therapy. *J Allergy Clin Immunol.* 2008;121(2):506–511.

39. Almind M, Dirksen A, Nielsen NH, Svendsen UG. Duration of the inhibitory activity on histamine-induced skin weals of sedative and non-sedative antihistamines. *Allergy.* 1988;43(8):593–596.

40. Hill 3rd SL, Krouse JH. The effects of montelukast on intradermal wheal and flare. *Otolaryngol Head Neck Surg.* 2003;129(3):199–203.

41. Saarinen JV, Harvima RJ, Horsmanheimo M, Harvima IT. Modulation of the immediate allergic wheal reaction in the skin by drugs inhibiting the effects of leukotriene C4 and prostaglandin D2. *Eur J Clin Pharmacol.* 2001;57(1):1–4.

42. Slott RI, Zweiman B. A controlled study of the effect of corticosteroids on immediate skin test reactivity. *J Allergy Clin Immunol.* 1974;54(4):229–234.

43. Aas K, Belin L. Standardization of diagnostic work in allergy. *Int Arch Allergy Appl Immunol.* 1973;45(1):57–60.

44. Nelson HS, Knoetzer J, Bucher B. Effect of distance between sites and region of the body on results of skin prick tests. *J Allergy Clin Immunol.* 1996;97(2):596–601.

45. Roovers MH, Gerth van Wijk R, Dieges PH, van Toorenenbergen AW. Phazet skin prick tests versus conventional prick tests with allergens and histamine in children. *Ann Allergy.* 1990;64(2 Pt 1):166–169.

46. Antico A, Di Berardino L. Prilotest, an innovative disposable skin puncture test: qualitative aspects. *Allerg Immunol (Paris).* 1994;26(8):297–301.

47. Aas K. Some variables in skin prick testing. *Allergy.* 1980;35(3):250–252.

48. Vanto T. Efficiency of different skin prick testing methods in the diagnosis of allergy to dog. *Ann Allergy.* 1983;50(5):340–344.

49. Oppenheimer J, Nelson HS. Skin testing. *Ann Allergy Asthma Immunol.* 2006;96(2 suppl 1):S6–S12.

50. PRE-PEN Procedure: skin testing dosage and technique. https://penallergytest.com/procedure/.

51. Langley JM, Halperin SA, Bortolussi R. History of penicillin allergy and referral for skin testing: evaluation of a pediatric penicillin allergy testing program. *Clin Invest Med.* 2002;25(5):181–184.

52. Saxon A, Adelman DC, Patel A, Hajdu R, Calandra GB. Imipenem cross-reactivity with penicillin in humans. *J Allergy Clin Immunol.* 1988;82(2):213–217.

53. Anderson JA, Adkinson Jr NF. Allergic reactions to drugs and biologic agents. *JAMA.* 1987;258(20):2891–2899.

54. Saxon A, Beall GN, Rohr AS, Adelman DC. Immediate hypersensitivity reactions to beta-lactam antibiotics. *Ann Intern Med.* 1987;107(2):204–215.

55. Sogn DD, Evans 3rd R, Shepherd GM, et al. Results of the national institute of allergy and infectious diseases collaborative clinical trial to test the predictive value of skin testing with major and minor penicillin derivatives in hospitalized adults. *Arch Intern Med.* 1992;152(5):1025–1032.

56. Indrajana T, Spieksma FT, Voorhorst R. Comparative study of the intracutaneous, scratch and prick tests in allergy. *Ann Allergy.* 1971;29(12):639–650.

57. Blanca M, Romano A, Torres MJ, et al. Update on the evaluation of hypersensitivity reactions to betalactams. *Allergy.* 2009;64(2):183–193.

58. Levine BB, Redmond AP. Minor haptenic determinant-specific reagins of penicillin hypersensitivity in man. *Int Arch Allergy Appl Immunol.* 1969;35(5):445–455.

59. Gadde J, Spence M, Wheeler B, Adkinson Jr NF. Clinical experience with penicillin skin testing in a large inner-city STD clinic. *JAMA.* 1993;270(20):2456–2463.

60. Solley GO, Gleich GJ, Van Dellen RG. Penicillin allergy: clinical experience with a battery of skin-test reagents. *J Allergy Clin Immunol.* 1982;69(2):238–244.

61. Green GR, Rosenblum AH, Sweet LC. Evaluation of penicillin hypersensitivity: value of clinical history and skin testing with penicilloyl-polylysine and penicillin G. A cooperative prospective study of the penicillin study group of the american academy of allergy. *J Allergy Clin Immunol.* 1977;60(6):339–345.

62. Blanca M, Vega JM, Garcia J, et al. Allergy to penicillin with good tolerance to other penicillins; study of the incidence in subjects allergic to beta-lactams. *Clin Exp Allergy.* 1990;20(5):475–481.

63. Solensky R, Khan DA. Evaluation of antibiotic allergy: the role of skin tests and drug challenges. *Curr Allergy Asthma Rep.* 2014;14(9). 459–014–0459-z.

64. Sanchez-Morillas L, Perez-Ezquerra PR, Reano-Martos M, Laguna-Martinez JJ, Sanz ML, Martinez LM. Selective allergic reactions to clavulanic acid: a report of 9 cases. *J Allergy Clin Immunol.* 2010;126(1):177–179.

65. Torres MJ, Ariza A, Mayorga C, et al. Clavulanic acid can be the component in amoxicillin-clavulanic acid responsible for immediate hypersensitivity reactions. *J Allergy Clin Immunol.* 2010;125(2):502–505.e2.

66. Romano A, Gaeta F, Valluzzi RL, et al. IgE-mediated hypersensitivity to cephalosporins: cross-reactivity and tolerability of alternative cephalosporins. *J Allergy Clin Immunol.* 2015;136(3):685–691.e3.

67. Empedrad R, Darter AL, Earl HS, Gruchalla RS. Nonirritating intradermal skin test concentrations for commonly prescribed antibiotics. *J Allergy Clin Immunol.* 2003;112(3):629–630.

68. Seitz CS, Brocker EB, Trautmann A. Suspicion of macrolide allergy after treatment of infectious diseases including helicobacter pylori: results of allergological testing. *Allergol Immunopathol (Madr).* 2011;39(4):193–199.

69. Mori F, Barni S, Pucci N, et al. Sensitivity and specificity of skin tests in the diagnosis of clarithromycin allergy. *Ann Allergy Asthma Immunol.* 2010;104(5):417–419.

70. Notman MJ, Phillips EJ, Knowles SR, Weber EA, Shear NH. Clindamycin skin testing has limited diagnostic potential. *Contact Dermatitis.* 2005;53(6):335–338.

71. Testi S, Severino M, Iorno ML, et al. Nonirritating concentration for skin testing with cephalosporins. *J Investig Allergol Clin Immunol.* 2010;20(2):171–172.

72. Romano A, Gaeta F, Valluzzi RL, et al. Diagnosing nonimmediate reactions to cephalosporins. *J Allergy Clin Immunol.* 2012;129(4):1166–1169.

73. Gaeta F, Valluzzi RL, Alonzi C, Maggioletti M, Caruso C, Romano A. Tolerability of aztreonam and carbapenems in patients with IgE-mediated hypersensitivity to penicillins. *J Allergy Clin Immunol.* 2015;135(4):972–976.

74. Solensky R, Mendelson LM. Drug allergy and anaphylaxis. In: *Pediatric Allergy: Principles and Practice.* 2nd ed. Saunders Elsevier; 2010:616.

75. Sanchez-Borges M, Thong B, Blanca M, et al. Hypersensitivity reactions to non beta-lactam antimicrobial agents, a statement of the WAO special committee on drug allergy. *World Allergy Organ J.* 2013;6(1). 18–4551-6-18.

76. Garufi C, Cristaudo A, Vanni B, et al. Skin testing and hypersensitivity reactions to oxaliplatin. *Ann Oncol.* 2003;14(3):497–498.

77. Markman M, Zanotti K, Peterson G, Kulp B, Webster K, Belinson J. Expanded experience with an intradermal skin test to predict for the presence or absence of carboplatin hypersensitivity. *J Clin Oncol.* 2003;21(24):4611–4614.

78. Leguy-Seguin V, Jolimoy G, Coudert B, et al. Diagnostic and predictive value of skin testing in platinum salt hypersensitivity. *J Allergy Clin Immunol.* 2007;119(3):726–730.

79. Bircher AJ, Harr T, Hohenstein L, Tsakiris DA. Hypersensitivity reactions to anticoagulant drugs: diagnosis and management options. *Allergy.* 2006;61(12):1432–1440.

80. Lieberman P, Rahmaoui A, Wong DA. The safety and interpretability of skin tests with omalizumab. *Ann Allergy Asthma Immunol.* 2010;105(6):493–495.

81. Vultaggio A, Matucci A, Nencini F, et al. Anti-infliximab IgE and non-IgE antibodies and induction of infusion-related severe anaphylactic reactions. *Allergy.* 2010;65(5):657–661.

82. Benucci M, Manfredi M, Demoly P, Campi P. Injection site reactions to TNF-alpha blocking agents with positive skin tests. *Allergy.* 2008;63(1):138–139.

83. Bottio T, Pittarello G, Bonato R, Fagiolo U, Gerosa G. Life-threatening anaphylactic shock caused by porcine heparin intravenous infusion during mitral valve repair. *J Thorac Cardiovasc Surg.* 2003;126(4):1194–1195.

84. Kao L, Rajan J, Roy L, Kavosh E, Khan DA. Adverse reactions during drug challenges: a single US institution's experience. *Ann Allergy Asthma Immunol.* 2013;110(2):86–91.e1.

85. Iammatteo M, Blumenthal KG, Saff R, Long AA, Banerji A. Safety and outcomes of test doses for the evaluation of adverse drug reactions: a 5-year retrospective review. *J Allergy Clin Immunol Pract.* 2014;2(6):768–774.

86. Aun MV, Bisaccioni C, Garro LS, et al. Outcomes and safety of drug provocation tests. *Allergy Asthma Proc.* 2011;32(4):301–306.

87. Aberer W, Kranke B. Provocation tests in drug hypersensitivity. *Immunol Allergy Clin North Am.* 2009;29(3):567–584.

88. Reidenberg MM, Lowenthal DT. Adverse nondrug reactions. *N Engl J Med.* 1968;279(13):678–679.

89. Romano A, Viola M, Gueant-Rodriguez RM, Gaeta F, Valluzzi R, Gueant JL. Brief communication: tolerability of meropenem in patients with IgE-mediated hypersensitivity to penicillins. *Ann Intern Med.* 2007;146(4):266–269.

90. Caubet JC, Kaiser L, Lemaitre B, Fellay B, Gervaix A, Eigenmann PA. The role of penicillin in benign skin rashes in childhood: a prospective study based on drug rechallenge. *J Allergy Clin Immunol.* 2011;127(1):218–222.

91. Ponvert C, Weilenmann C, Wassenberg J, et al. Allergy to betalactam antibiotics in children: a prospective follow-up study in retreated children after negative responses in skin and challenge tests. *Allergy.* 2007;62(1):42–46.

92. Brockow K, Christiansen C, Kanny G, et al. Management of hypersensitivity reactions to iodinated contrast media. *Allergy.* 2005;60(2):150–158.

CHAPTER 8

In Vitro and In Vivo Tests for Drug Hypersensitivity Reactions

JUSTIN GREIWE, MD • JONATHAN A. BERNSTEIN, MD

KEY POINTS

- Accurate identification of the culprit agent associated with an ADR can have far-reaching economic and health effects, emphasizing the need for simple and reliable diagnostic tests.
- The combination of skin testing if available, followed by an oral challenge is generally considered the gold standard for diagnostic testing of an immediate drug allergy.
- DPT is not without risks and should be performed under the supervision of experienced personnel.
- More research is needed to developed better methods of identifying the cause of allergic drug reactions.

INTRODUCTION

The ability to evaluate and accurately identify the responsible agent in an adverse drug reaction (ADR) is an essential skill for any allergist/clinical immunologist. ADRs can be broadly divided into two types: Type A and Type B. Type A are more common and predictable, resulting from the known pharmacologic properties of a drug (i.e., heart racing from β-agonists, oral thrush with inhaled glucocorticoids, or nephrotoxicity with aminoglycosides). Type B include drug hypersensitivity reactions (DHRs), which occur less frequently, are mostly unpredictable, and often occur in predisposed patients (i.e., anaphylaxis from β-lactam antibiotics, Stevens-Johnson syndrome [SJS] with trimethoprim-sulfamethoxazole). DHRs are classified as either allergic (5%–10% of ADRs) or nonallergic.[1] Allergic DHRs may be classified by the Gell-Coombs classification system, which includes IgE mediated (Type I), cytotoxic (Type II), immune complex mediated (Type III), and cellular mediated (Type IV). In contrast, nonallergic DHRs do not have a demonstrable immune mechanism and are most commonly associated with agents such as nonsteroidal antiinflammatory drugs (NSAIDs), radiocontrast media (RCM), and opioids.[2,3]

The importance of appropriately characterizing ADRs cannot be overstated, especially in patients with a history of multiple drug "allergies," because often these reactions are not true DHRs, but rather Type A reactions incorrectly labeled as allergy. Misdiagnosis of true drug allergy has major economic and health impacts on our society when one considers the magnitude of patients with a history of drug allergy. For example, analysis of Kaiser Permanente electronic medical records data from 2,375,424 patients found that 478,283 (20.1%) of its health plan members had at least one reported "drug allergy," and 49,582 (2.1%) were found to have multiple drug allergy syndrome, defined by three or more unrelated drug class "allergies."[4] Demographic data from this cohort revealed an association with older overweight females, a history of anxiety, and high rates of healthcare and medication usage.[4]

Patients with multiple drug allergies are difficult to manage, leading to the use of alternative agents that may be more expensive, less efficacious, and/or have more side effects. A penicillin allergy label, for example, is the most common drug "allergy" listed in medical records during hospital admissions. This label has been connected to longer hospital stays, more broad-spectrum antibiotic use, and increased prevalence of *Clostridium difficile*, methicillin-resistant *Staphylococcus aureus*, and vancomycin-resistant *Enterococcus* infections.[5] After an IgE-mediated allergic reaction to penicillin, the chance of having a positive response to penicillin skin testing diminishes with time. By some estimates, the response rate decreases by 10% per year. Therefore, an estimated 50% of patients who had immediate reactions to penicillin will have a negative skin test after 5 years, and 75%–80% will be negative at 10 years.[6] In fact, most patients carrying a label of "drug allergy" do not have true hypersensitivity and may be needlessly avoiding medications. To investigate the reliability of patient-reported penicillin allergies, one prospective observational cohort study enrolled 150 emergency department (ED) patients with a self-reported penicillin allergy and found more than 90% of these patients had negative penicillin major and minor determinant skin testing.[7] The negative skin test findings resulted in ED physicians changing their clinical decision on which antibiotic they would have used, resulting in decreased use of broader-spectrum, more expensive antibiotics. These findings are consistent with previous reports from other non-ED patient populations, which also found high false-positive rates (>85%) of self-reported penicillin allergy.[8-12]

There are a number of challenges associated with managing patients with DHRs, including the lack of reliable diagnostic testing. The variability of clinical reactions to drugs experienced by patients coupled with the difficulty in differentiating adverse versus immunologically mediated drug reactions by physicians frequently results in misclassification of drug reactions. Symptoms that suggest the absence of a true drug allergy frequently are mild and nonspecific, typically occurring in response to multiple unrelated medications without obvious objective findings. In contrast, patients who have a history of a true allergic drug reaction to one agent may subsequently develop fear and anxiety related to taking all medications.

Accurate identification of the culprit agent associated with an ADR can have far-reaching economic and health effects, emphasizing the need for simple and reliable diagnostic tests. Appropriate evaluation of DHRs includes a detailed clinical history and physical examination, followed by one or more of the following procedures: skin prick testing (SPT) and in appropriate cases intracutaneous testing (ICT), in vitro testing, and, when applicable, a drug provocation test.[13] A thorough and focused assessment using this algorithmic approach often provides much needed clarity related to the responsible drug and underlying mechanism. However, medical history, especially in patients with multiple drug allergies, is often unreliable and confusing because patients frequently have poor recollection of the reaction and surrounding events. Although there are a broad spectrum of diagnostic modalities available to evaluate DHRs, not all of these tests are clinically accessible or well standardized. Various tests have been developed to confirm or exclude biochemical or immunologic reactions associated with DHRs (Table 8.1).[14] This chapter will summarize the utility of these in vivo and in vitro tests for use in the clinical setting.

SKIN TESTING

The most valuable test for detecting IgE-mediated drug reactions is immediate hypersensitivity skin testing. The combination of skin testing followed by an oral challenge is generally considered the gold standard for diagnostic testing of an immediate drug allergy. Cutaneous testing involves SPT and when possible ICT using nonirritating dilutions of the drug. SPT to drugs that cause direct mast cell activation (i.e., vancomycin, opiates) leads to false-positive results, making testing impractical for these agents. Typically, an epicutaneous SPT is applied first because it is considered more specific and safer, followed by more sensitive ICT if necessary. Skin testing to penicillin using a defined hapten coupled to polylysine, which is commercially available, has been extensively studied, and the current scientific

TABLE 8.1
Diagnostic Testing for Drug Hypersensitivity Reactions

Immune Reaction (Gell and Coombs Classification)	Laboratory Tests
Type I (IgE mediated)	Skin testing, serum RIA, ELISA, or FEIA, serum tryptase
Type II (cytotoxic)	Direct or indirect Coombs test
Type III (immune complex)	ESR, CRP, immune complexes, complement studies, antinuclear antibody, antihistone antibody, tissue biopsy for immunofluorescence studies
Type IV (delayed, cell mediated)	Patch testing, lymphocyte transformation test

ELISA, enzyme-linked immunosorbent assay; *FEIA*, fluorescent enzyme immunoassay; *RIA*, radioimmunoassay.
Adapted or reprinted with permission from Adverse Drug Reactions: Types and Treatment Options. *Am Fam Physician*. November 1, 2003;68(9) Copyright © 2003 American Academy of Family Physicians. All Rights Reserved.

evidence supports its use. Although in vivo testing to muscle relaxants/neuromuscular blocking agents (NMBA), local anesthetics, and high-molecular-weight agents such as insulin, vaccines, streptokinase, polyclonal or monoclonal antibodies, and latex have also been well described, standardized skin test reagents for these drugs are not commercially available.[15–18] A positive SPT in these scenarios suggests that the patient may have an IgE-mediated allergy to these medications; however, a positive skin test reaction should always be correlated with the patient's reaction history. The negative predictive value of skin testing is only useful with penicillin because the specificity of this test has been sufficiently determined (Table 8.2).[15,18–27]

DRUG PROVOCATION TESTING

Current options for drug testing are often limited and not sufficiently sensitive or specific; therefore, DPT remains the only reliable way to confirm clinical sensitivity to medications in many scenarios. However, DPT is not without risks and should only be administered by trained personnel in either an outpatient or inpatient setting, depending on the severity of the initial reaction with emergency therapy (e.g., epinephrine) readily available. Drug provocation testing should be considered on a case by case basis after taking into account the risk–benefit ratio, potential contraindications, and the values and wishes of the patient. In situations where skin testing is available and is negative, the drug can be administered as a single dose or beginning with a small test dose (e.g., 5 mg) followed by a full dose after 30 min. When skin testing is not readily available, the drug can be administered at incrementally increasing doses referred to as a graded challenge. Certain types of drug reactions are inappropriate and/or contraindicated for DPT, including severe anaphylaxis, toxic epidermal necrolysis (TEN), SJS, drug hypersensitivity syndromes (DRESS), acute generalized exanthematous pustulosis, drug-induced autoimmune disease, and systemic vasculitis. Despite its limitations, DPT is currently considered to be the "gold standard" diagnostic approach for establishing or excluding a diagnosis of a DHR and for helping to clarify the clinical relevance of in vivo and in vitro testing methods.[13] This holds true even for penicillin testing because there are reports of positive DPT despite negative in vivo and in vitro testing. The utility of DPT is especially apparent for medications where there is no reliable in vivo or in vitro testing or where testing has very low sensitivity (i.e., antibiotics such as sulfonamides, quinolones, and macrolides, as well as corticosteroids and NSAIDs).[28]

IN VITRO DIAGNOSTIC TESTING

Because drug hypersensitivity testing is an expansive topic covering various classes of medications, this review will focus on antibiotics, specifically in vitro testing for Type B ADRs of Gell-Coombs Type I and IV. As mentioned, the lack of accurate and comprehensive biologic testing for antibiotics results in physicians prescribing more expensive and often

---

TABLE 8.2			
Cutaneous Testing of Immediate Drug Allergy			
Medication	**Sensitivity**	**Specificity**	**NPP**
Penicillin (PPL + MDM)	70%[19]	97%–100%[19]	97%–99%[20,21]
Cephalosporin	30.7%–69.7%[22]		
Muscle relaxants/NMBA	94%–97%[15,23]	>95%[15]	
Latex	SPT 96%/ICT: 93%[18]	SPT: 100%/ICT: 96%[18]	

ICT, intracutaneous testing; *MDM*, minor determinants mixture (benzylpenicillin, sodium benzylpenicillinoate, and benzylpenicilloic acid); *NMBA*, neuromuscular blocking agents (most common cause of perioperative anaphylaxis); *PPL*, penicillin major determinant (benzylpenicilloyl poly-L-lysine); Important to consider SPT and ICT to amoxicillin when appropriate because patients with selective side chain–mediated reactions to amoxicillin will be missed by PPL and MDM testing. Similarly, negative penicillin cutaneous testing does not exclude a cephalosporin allergy because sIgE may be directed against unique side chains rather than the β-lactam ring.[25] In penicillin-allergic patients, ≤5% will cross-react to first-generation cephalosporins and <2% for third- and fourth-generation cephalosporins.[26,27] Some cephalosporins share a side chain with other β-lactams (i.e., cephalexin and ampicillin) and therefore may cross-react.[19,26] Latex: ideal diagnostic accuracy safely achieved with nonammoniated latex at 100 μg/mL for skin prick test and 1 μg/mL for ICT.

less effective medications. Creating simple, reliable serum tests that pose no risk to the patient to correctly identify culprit agents would be especially useful in cases where patients have received multiple antibiotics simultaneously or in cases of severe, life-threatening antibiotic allergy where skin testing and/or DPT are not possible or contraindicated.[29] Furthermore, in vitro test results are not affected by most concomitant drug treatments such as antihistamines and are not limited by the patient's skin condition (i.e., dermatographism or extensive dermatitis). Thus in theory, in vitro testing offers many advantages, but in clinical practice its utility is limited because of lack of sensitivity. With the advent of anti-IgE monoclonal antibodies (e.g., omalizumab) for treatment of allergic asthma and chronic urticaria, specific IgE in vitro assays would have no utility in patients treated with this medication.

MEDIATORS OF AN ALLERGIC REACTION

In a DHR, well-characterized bioactive mediators are released during both the acute and late-phase response that can be readily measured in the serum, plasma, urine, and skin. Mediators that can be useful for the diagnosis of an immediate reaction include histamine, proteases, TNF-α, prostaglandin D2, leukotriene C4 (LTC4), platelet-activating factor, pro-inflammatory cytokines, and chemokines.[30] It is important to note that these mediators are often more accurate when drawn during the active phase of a reaction. Ultimately, IgE-mediated activation of mast cells or basophils is a pivotal step in the allergic cascade that is amplified by the recruitment of effector cells such as eosinophils and Th2 lymphocytes.

Measuring Histamine and Histamine Metabolites

Histamine, which is stored mainly in mast cells and basophil granules, is a prominent mediator of allergic inflammation. Histamine is a principal component in acute anaphylaxis but needs to be collected within the first hour because of its short half-life (20 min).[31] Because of their rapid metabolism, histamine metabolites (N-methylhistamine and N-methylimidazoleacetic acid) are typically measured in a 24-h urine sample as an indirect method for assessing histamine release. Plasma histamine is not used reliably in clinical practice because of its inadequate sensitivity (61%–92%) and a specificity of 51%–91% and has therefore been replaced by serum tryptase as a means to confirm mast cell activation related to an IgE-mediated reaction.[29]

Serum Tryptase

Tryptase is a preformed mediator comprising of an immature α monomer isoform and a mature β heterotetramer isoform. β-Tryptase is rapidly released on mast cell activation; however, no commercial test is currently available to measure the mature tryptase form specifically. Therefore, clinically, total tryptase is determined by immunoassay; however, it must be drawn as early as possible (30–120 min) but within 4–6 h after a reaction because of its short half-life and should be compared with a baseline level measured at least 24 h after resolution of anaphylactic symptoms.[32] Obtaining a tryptase level during the acute phase of a DHR is a useful method for confirming mast cell–mediated reaction with a sensitivity of 30%–94.1% and a specificity of 92.3%–94.4%.[29]

IN VITRO TESTING FOR SPECIFIC IGE-MEDIATED AND NON-IGE-MEDIATED REACTIONS

Immunoassays for the detection of serum drug-specific IgE (sIgE) antibodies are the most widely available in vitro test currently in use. In vitro testing for IgE is available for only a limited number of drugs and is based on the quantification of drug antigen (hapten-carrier conjugate) and IgE antibody binding. There are several immunoassay methods available including radioimmunoassay (RIA), enzyme-linked immunosorbent assay (ELISA), and fluorescent enzyme immunoassay (FEIA). FEIAs (i.e., Immuno-CAP Phadia, Uppsala, Sweden) and RIAs analogous to radioallergosorbent testing are the most commonly used tests. Each test has its advantages and disadvantages; however, the main barrier to their universal application is that only a limited number of drugs are able to form adducts used for testing. While β-lactams, NMBA, and some NSAIDs are able to form hapten-carrier conjugates, penicillin forms adducts readily and therefore is the model drug for in vitro testing.[33,34] While serum sIgE testing has been a useful tool in diagnosing aeroallergen and food allergies with relatively high positive predictive values,[35] most drug-sIgE testing has not been appropriately clinically validated (Table 8.3). These tests have reasonably high specificity but consistently poor sensitivity because the immunogenic determinants of many drugs are undefined, making the predictive value of in vitro testing poor.[36] Sensitivity of testing depends on the drug involved and the test being used (Table 8.4).[29,37–42] As mentioned, these tests are not useful for patients with suspected DHRs taking omalizumab.

TABLE 8.3
FEIA ImmunoCAP Drug–Specific IgE Assays Available for Commercial and Research Purposes[a]

DRUG-SPECIFIC IGE ASSAYS THAT ARE COMMERCIALLY AVAILABLE FROM THERMO FISHER SCIENTIFIC, UPPSALA, SWEDEN		
Penicilloyl G	Penicilloyl V	Ampicilloyl and amoxicilloyl determinants
Cefaclor	Chlorhexidine	Chymopapain
(Bovine) gelatin	Morphine	Human, bovine, and porcine insulin
Pholcodine	Suxamethonium	
DRUG-SPECIFIC IGE ASSAYS FOR RESEARCH PURPOSES ONLY AVAILABLE FROM THERMO FISHER SCIENTIFIC SPECIAL ALLERGEN SERVICE		
Adrenocorticotropic hormone	Atracurium	Bacitracin
Carboplatin	Cefamandole	Cefoxitin
Cefotaxime	Cisplatinum	Mepivacaine
Methylprednisolone-21-succinate	Protamine	Rocuronium
Oxaliplatin	Penicillin minor determinants (e.g., penicillanyl)	
Propyphenazone	Nafamostat (4-guanidinobenzoic acid)	
Tetanus toxoid		

[a]The majority of these assays have not been adequately clinically validated.
Adapted from Uyttebroek, AP, Sabato V, Bridts CH, Ebo DG. In vitro diagnosis of immediate IgE-mediated drug hypersensitivity warnings and (unmet) needs. *Immunol Allergy Clin North Am*. August 2014;34(3):681–689.
FEIA, fluorescent enzyme immunoassay.

TABLE 8.4
Sensitivity and Specificity of In Vitro Testing in Determining Drug-Specific IgE Antibodies

Immunoassay Methods	RAST-RIA (Sensitivity/Specificity)	CAP-FEIA
β-lactams	42.9%–75%/66.7%–83.3%[37] 48%–50%/95%[38] 42.9%–75%/67.7%–83.3%[29] PPV: 38.5% NPV: 81.5%[37]	0%–25%/83.3%–100%[37] 54%/95%–100%[39] 0%–50%[29] PPV: 45.5% NPV: 77.1%[37]
Aminopenicillins (amoxicillin)	28.6%–64.3%/72.7%–100%[37]	58%–68%/96%–100%[40]
Cefaclor[a]	40%/75%[37]	6.7%/75%[37]
Rocuronium		68%/93%[41] 83%–92%[29]
Suxamethonium		60%/100%[41] 44%[29]
Morphine		88%/100%[41] 78%–84%[29]
Pholcodine		86%/100%[41]
Chlorhexidine (with+ST)		91.6%/100%[42]
Fluoroquinolones	31.6%–54.6%[29]	
Cetuximab		68%–92%/90%–92%[29]
Infliximab		26%/90%[29]

[a]Cefaclor is the only commercially available serum sIgE test for cephalosporin allergy. Testing for other cephalosporins is used for research purposes only.
CAP, capture assay; *FEIA*, fluorescent enzyme immunoassay; *RAST*, radioallergosorbent testing; *RIA*, radioimmunoassay; *ST*, skin testing.

Cross-linking of neighboring IgE/high-affinity IgE receptor (FcεRI) complexes expressed on the membranes of basophils and mast cells causes a cascade of biochemical reactions, leading to the immediate release of various preformed mediators (histamine, PAF, and tryptase) and followed quickly by newly synthesized mediators such as leukotrienes, prostaglandins, and cytokines. While the signs and symptoms of an IgE-mediated drug reaction are a direct consequence of this sequence of events, mediator release is not specific to the IgE-mediated pathway. A number of medications including opioids, NMBAs, iodinated contract media, quinolones, and vancomycin cause direct mast cell activation, leading to release of the abovementioned mediators. Traditional sIgE assays fail to capture this subset of immediate DHRs, highlighting the need for additional cellular tests to accurately encompass non-IgE-mediated DHR mechanisms. A number of cellular assays (i.e., mediator release assays, basophil activation test [BAT]) attempt to mimic in vivo IgE-mediated cell activation and mediator release but have the advantage of not relying on hapten-carrier conjugates.[29] However, these tests require fresh blood, and it is unclear how other medications/treatments may influence their results.[29]

Mediator Release Assays (Histamine and CysLTs)

Even though basophils represent less than 0.5% of total leukocytes in peripheral blood, these cells have been found to be important as tissue mast cells in mediating the allergic response.[43] In an attempt to exploit their pivotal role, a number of in vitro tests have focused on measuring activation of circulating basophils. The first attempt to measure basophil functional responses was the histamine release assay. Both histamine and sulfidoleukotriene release assays measure the mediator histamine and LTC4, respectively, in the supernatant, on cell activation with the suspected drug.[44] These tests are not widely used clinically because they are not considered reliable because of their low sensitivity and specificity. A histamine release assay that uses a rat basophil leukemic cell line to measure β-hexosaminidase as a marker for histamine release has also been used for research purposes but has not been well studied as a clinical assay for evaluating IgE-mediated drug reactions. This has led to the development of more accurate testing using flow cytometry.

Basophil Activation Test

The BAT measures drug-induced activation of basophils by flow cytometry, which detects surface expression of activation markers such as CD63 or CD203c.[45] The use of BAT has focused on a limited number of drugs to date, including β-lactams and NMBA.[46] While not routinely used in clinical practice, this test can be helpful for assessing cases of multiple drug allergies or situations where cross-reactivity between related drugs needs to be examined, as more than one drug can be tested at a time.[47] BAT has also been shown to be a useful adjunctive test when cutaneous and/or serum sIgE testing results are equivocal or ambiguous. For β-lactams, sensitivity ranges between 22% and 55% and specificity between 79% and 100%, whereas NMBA sensitivity ranges between 36% and 86% with specificity between 81% and 100%, and NSAID sensitivity ranges between 17% and 70% with specificity between 40% and 100%.[25,34,47] Basophil activation testing has also been found to be useful for diagnosing IgE-mediated allergy to pyrazolones, fluoroquinolones, and RCM. In addition, BAT has been recommended before in vivo testing in cases of life-threatening reactions or high-risk patients.[29]

ASSESSING T CELL–MEDIATED DRUG ALLERGY

Type IV delayed DHRs to medications are T cell–mediated responses that have varied clinical presentations. Type IV DHRs range in severity from mild cutaneous reactions without systemic involvement to severe, potentially life-threatening cutaneous reactions often with multisystem involvement. Drug-induced hypersensitivity syndrome (DIHS) include SJS/TEN and DRESS/drug-hypersensitivity induced syndrome (DHIS). These reactions often manifest weeks after uncomplicated treatment with a drug. In vivo tests such as patch testing and in vitro tests such as lymphocyte transformation tests (LTTs) and enzyme-linked immunosorbent spot assays (ELISpot) have shown some potential for identifying patients with true immunologically mediated delayed reactions to a specific drug. However, the sensitivity of these tests varies considerably and is typically determined by the type of delayed reaction and the suspected drug being tested.[25]

Patch Testing

Typically, Type IV reactions present as an allergic contact dermatitis to a topical medication, which can be confirmed by patch testing. A patch test is considered positive if erythema, induration, and a vesiculopapular eruption at the site of the patch develops 48–96 h after application. However, lack of standardization of reagent concentrations may limit its clinical utility.

According to the most recent practice parameter, drug patch testing may be useful for certain types of cutaneous drug reactions, including maculopapular exanthems, acute generalized exanthematous pustulosis, and fixed drug eruptions, but generally is not helpful for identifying culprit drug responsible for SJS or urticarial eruptions.[48] Unlike serologic testing, patch testing results can be very subjective and therefore requires an experienced clinician to apply and interpret. In addition, several of the antigens used in patch testing are relatively potent, and sensitization through the patch test procedure itself is possible.[49] As more antigens are added to patch testing panels, there is also concern that some of these low-molecular-weight compounds have the potential for toxicity.[50] The sensitivity of patch testing varies considerably but is generally <70% with higher sensitivities reported for acute generalized exanthematous pustulosis, abacavir hypersensitivity syndrome (HSS), carbamazepine SJS/DRESS, and fixed drug eruptions.[25]

Intracutaneous Testing With Delayed Readings

ICT with delayed readings has also been studied in the diagnosis of Type IV delayed DHRs. Parenterally available drugs are ideal candidates for this testing, and the procedure mimics ICT for IgE-mediated reactions with the exception that readings should be performed 24 h after the application of the highest nonirritating concentration of the drug. While some studies have shown higher sensitivity for ICT with delayed readings compared with patch testing for delayed reactions, neither test is sensitive enough for determining whether oral provocation to the concerning drug is appropriate.[51] In nonsevere delayed reactions to drugs, ICT with delayed readings are the most sensitive skin tests, especially for β-lactam antibiotics, RCM, and heparin, but may also be useful for some biologic agents.[52] Despite their limitations, both patch and ICT with delayed readings have the advantage of being able to be performed on multiple drugs simultaneously, and/or on structurally related medications, that may have been given concurrently when the patient developed a DHR.[25]

Human Leukocyte Antigen Typing for Drug Hypersensitivity Screening

Human leukocyte antigen (HLA) refers to a complex of genes on chromosome 6 that are involved in a variety of immunologic actions. Studies have found that HLA typing is a useful in vitro assay that can help identify individual risk of a DHR before a drug is administered. This test requires isolation of DNA from the peripheral blood mononuclear cells to perform a reverse sequence–specific oligonucleotide–polymerase chain reaction. A classic example where HLA typing has been successful is with abacavir, which is a nucleoside reverse transcriptase inhibitor indicated for treatment of HIV. Patients being considered for this treatment are at increased risk for a number of Type IV reactions including severe hypersensitivity reactions, SJS/TEN, and DRESS/DIHS if they express the HLA-B*5701 allele.[29] Subsequently, several other drugs have demonstrated strong associations with specific HLA class I and II alleles, including allopurinol, carbamazepine, lamotrigine, phenobarbital, phenytoin, sulfamethoxazole, and nevirapine.[29] These associations have resulted in recommendations to prescreen patients for specific HLA phenotypes before prescribing. Before HLA typing had developed, abacavir was associated with a drug hypersensitivity syndrome in 5%–8% of mainly Caucasian patients characterized by fever, malaise, and rash with a more severe reaction upon reexposure.[25] With more experience and improved technology, other HLA-drug associations have been discovered, but their application into valid testing has not been as successful as for abacavir screening. Carbamazepine-induced SJS/TEN DHR was found to be associated with HLA-B*1502 in the Han Chinese population where this allele has a prevalence of 10%–15%.[53] Currently, the FDA has recommended routine HLA-B*1502 screening in high-risk individuals of Southeast Asian origin before using this medication.[25] The HLA-B*58:01 allele is associated with allopurinol-induced DRESS and SJS/TEN in the Han Chinese as well, prompting the American College of Rheumatology to recommend screening patients of this origin for this phenotype before starting this medication.[29]

Lymphocyte Transformation Testing

LTT is another in vitro alternative test that was developed to assess whether a patient has developed drug-specific T cells as a marker of sensitization. LTT has a higher sensitivity than skin testing for diagnosing Type IV reactions with a sensitivity ranging from 27% to 88.8% and specificity from 63% to 100% depending on the inciting drug.[29] β-Lactams have been more extensively studied with a sensitivity and specificity ranging from 58% to 88.8% and 85%–100%, respectively.[29] Sensitivity also depends on the type of reaction, with lower sensitivities reported in CD8+ T cell–mediated reactions.[54] While LTT is an alternative to traditional patch testing, it often provides inconsistent results when compared with patch testing and until sensitivity is improved, should only be used in conjunction with other tests. Because of its low sensitivity, the clinical applicability of LTT is questionable, specifically when applied to severe cutaneous ADRs. In scenarios where SJS/TEN or DRESS/DHIS is suspected, even if LTT is negative, patients are typically advised to avoid the suspected drug, class of drugs, or multiple drugs that might have caused the reaction.

Enzyme-Linked Immunosorbent Spot Assays

Similar to LTT, the antibody-based ELISpot assay has been used primarily in research settings to help identify various Type IV delayed HSRs.[25] This test quantifies the number of cytokine-secreting T cells in relation to exposure to pharmacologic concentrations of the suspected drug or drug metabolite. The anticytokine antibody used depends greatly on the cytokine being detected. For example, IFNγ for abacavir HSS and β-lactam reactions and granulysin or granzyme B for severe cutaneous reactions such as SJS/TEN. The sensitivity of ELISpot for β-lactam reactions ranges from 13% to 91%.[25,29]

Combining Tests to Increase Sensitivity

Standard in vitro and skin testing for delayed-type DHRs including SJS/TEN are notoriously inaccurate, leading some clinicians to consider combined testing to increase accuracy. Porebski et al. analyzed 15 patients with SJS/TEN and demonstrated that LTT and ELISpot used in isolation had a sensitivity of 27% and 33%, respectively, while testing of granulysin expression on CD4[+] T cells in conjunction with granzyme B and IFNγ production by ELISpot provided a sensitivity of 80% and specificity of 95%.[55,56]

Adachi et al. evaluated several types delayed DHRs by performing side-by-side comparisons of LTT and BAT. They observed that samples that yielded positive results for LTT and BAT did not overlap, suggesting that the two analyses might negate each assay's false-negative results. Combined sensitivity was found to be higher compared with the sensitivity for the individual assays. The negative predictive value for BAT and LTT was 14.7% and 28.2%, respectively, whereas it was 96.4% when these assays were used in combination.[56,57]

SKIN BIOPSY

Obtaining a skin biopsy can be helpful in complex cases where multiple medications are involved, especially when there is extensive skin involvement and no obvious temporal relationship is identified. While a biopsy has the potential to help clarify whether a drug-induced eruption is contributing to the skin reaction, there are no absolute histologic criteria for identifying the specific cause of these eruptions nor does it always differentiate DHRs from other cutaneous drug reactions.[58]

CONCLUSION

Choosing the appropriate diagnostic test in a patient who has experienced a possible Type I or Type IV allergic drug reaction can be challenging. A comprehensive clinical history and appropriate phenotyping are essential for establishing the correct diagnosis and provide the framework necessary to accurately risk stratify the allergic patient and help guide choice of diagnostic tests. Accurate identification of true medication allergies can have far-reaching economic and health effects highlighting the importance of developing and validating simple and reliable in vitro testing. Algorithmically, if a patient presents with drug allergy, it is important to differentiate clinically whether it is IgE mediated versus cellular in nature.[29] Immediate skin prick and if indicated ICT to the suspected agent should be performed.[29] If the history is concerning for a severe reaction, then obtaining a specific IgE test to the drug and/or performing a BAT if available may be considered before skin testing. If a cell-mediated reaction is suspected, then patch testing or late reading IC testing can be performed.[29] An LTT can also be performed if available with preference for this in vitro test in patients with a history of a severe cell-mediated reaction.[29] Technologic advances in this field have the potential to lower costs while reducing morbidity and mortality associated with severe ADRs. Increasing the sensitivity of in vitro testing can provide clinicians with a safe and efficient way to screen, evaluate, and diagnose their patients with drug allergies. Despite the advantages of in vitro testing, there are various limitations that prevent these tests from gaining mainstream acceptance, including limited commercial availability of well-validated standardized drug-specific tests. Most in vitro testing lacks sensitivity and therefore should not be performed in isolation to establish the correct diagnosis. The level of evidence based on the GRADE method is B for serum tryptase, 24 h urine histamine and its metabolites, cellular phenotypic analysis in skin biopsies, sIgE by ImmunoCAP, BAT, and HLA allele determination. However, for all other assays discussed in this chapter the level of evidence is much lower.[29] Therefore, more research to address this gap in knowledge is required, with a focus on appropriate validation of in vitro and in vivo drug testing in patients with well-characterized ADRs.

ABBREVIATIONS

ADRs   Adverse drug reactions
BAT   Basophil activation testing
DHR   Drug hypersensitivity syndrome
DPT   Drug provocation testing
DRESS   Drug reaction with eosinophilia and systemic symptoms
ED   Emergency department
ELISA   Enzyme-linked immunosorbent assay
FEIA   Fluorescent enzyme immunoassay
HLA   Human leukocyte antigen
HSS   Hypersensitivity syndrome
ICT   Intracutaneous testing
LTT   Lymphocyte transformation test
NMBA   Neuromuscular blocking agents
RIA   Radioimmunoassay
sIgE   Specific IgE
SJS   Stevens-Johnson syndrome
SPT   Skin prick testing
TEN   Toxic epidermal necrolysis

CONFLICT OF INTEREST

Dr. Greiwe is a speaker for Mylan pharmaceutical. Dr. Bernstein is an investigator, consultant, and speaker for Novartis, Genentech, Shire, CSL Behring, Sanofi, AZ, and BI; consultant for Flint Hills Resources; and Editor in Chief for the Journal of Asthma.

REFERENCES

1. Johansson SG, Bieber T, Dahl R, et al. Revised nomenclature for allergy for global use: Report of the Nomenclature Review Committee of the World Allergy Organization, October 2003. *J Allergy Clin Immunol.* May 2004;113(5):832–836.
2. Kowalski ML, Asero R, Bavbek S, et al. Classification and practical approach to the diagnosis and management of hypersensitivity to nonsteroidal anti-inflammatory drugs. *Allergy.* October 2013;68(10):1219–1232.
3. Brockow K, Christiansen C, Kanny G, et al. Management of hypersensitivity reactions to iodinated contrast media. *Allergy.* February 2005;60(2):150–158.
4. Macy E, Ho NJ. Multiple drug intolerance syndrome: prevalence, clinical characteristics, and management. *Ann Allergy Asthma Immunol.* February 2012;108(2):88–93.
5. Macy E, Contreras R. Health care use and serious infection prevalence associated with penicillin "allergy" in hospitalized patients: A cohort study. *J Allergy Clin Immunol.* March 2014;133(3):790–796.
6. Arroliga ME, Pien L. Penicillin allergy: consider trying penicillin again. *Cleve Clin J Med.* April 2003;70(4):313–314. 317-8, 320-1.7.
7. Raja AS, Lindsell CJ, Bernstein JA, Codispoti CD, Moellman JJ. The use of penicillin skin testing to assess the prevalence of penicillin allergy in an emergency department setting. *Ann Emerg Med.* July 2009;54(1):72–77.
8. Gadde J, Spence M, Wheeler B, et al. Clinical experience with penicillin skin testing in a large inner-city STD clinic. *JAMA.* 1993;270:2456–2463.
9. Lin R. A perspective on penicillin allergy. *Arch Intern Med.* 1992;152:930–937.
10. del Real GA, Rose ME, Ramirez-Atamoros MT, et al. Penicillin skin testing in patients with a history of beta-lactam allergy. *Ann Allergy Asthma Immunol.* 2007;98:355–359.
11. Stember RH. Prevalence of skin test reactivity in patients with convincing, vague, and unacceptable histories of penicillin allergy. *Allergy Asthma Proc.* 2005;26:59–64.
12. Whitmore SE. How predictive is a history of penicillin allergy? *JAMA.* 2001;286:1174–1175.
13. Aberer W, Bircher A, Romano A, et al. Drug provocation testing in the diagnosis of drug hypersensitivity reactions: general considerations. *Allergy.* 2003;58:854–863.
14. Riedl MA, Casillas Adrian M. Adverse drug reactions: types and treatment options. *Am Fam Physician.* November 1, 2003;68(9):1781–1791.
15. Moneret-Vautrin DA, Kanny G. Anaphylaxis to muscle relaxants: rational for skin tests. *Allerg Immunol (Paris).* September 2002;34(7):233–240.
16. Moscicki RA, Sockin SM, Corsello BF, Ostro MG, Bloch KJ. Anaphylaxis during induction of general anesthesia: subsequent evaluation and management. *J Allergy Clin Immunol.* 1990;86:325–332.
17. Patterson R, DeSwarte RD, Greenberger PA, et al. Drug allergy and protocols for management of drug allergies. *Allergy Proc.* September–October 1994;15(5):239–264.
18. Hamilton RG, Adkinson Jr NF. Natural rubber latex skin testing reagents: safety and diagnostic accuracy of nonammoniated latex, ammoniated latex, and latex rubber glove extracts. *J Allergy Clin Immunol.* 1996;98:872–883.
19. Kränke B, Aberer W. Skin testing for IgE-mediated drug allergy. *Immunol Allergy Clin North Am.* 2009;29:503–516.
20. Sogn DD, Evans 3rd R, Shepherd GM, Casale TB, Condemi J, Greenberger PA, et al. Results of the National Institute of Allergy and Infectious diseases collaborative clinical trial to test the predictive value of skin testing with major and minor penicillin derivatives in hospitalized adults. *Arch Intern Med.* 1992;152:1025–1032.
21. Fox S, Park MA. Penicillin skin testing in the evaluation and management of penicillin allergy. *Ann Allergy Asthma Immunol.* 2011;106:1–7.

22. Blanca M, Romano A, Torres MJ, Férnandez J, Mayorga C, Rodriguez J, et al. Update on the evaluation of hypersensitivity reactions to betalactams. *Allergy.* 2009;64:183–193.

23. Mertes PM, Aimone-Gastin I, Guéant-Rodriguez RM, Mouton-Faivre C, Audibert G, O'Brien J, et al. Hypersensitivity reactions to neuromuscular blocking agents. *Curr Pharm Des.* 2008;14:2809–2825.

24. Khan DA, Solensky R. Drug allergy. *J Allergy Clin Immunol.* 2010;125(suppl 2):S126–S137.

25. Rive CM, Bourke J, Phillips EJ. Testing for Drug Hypersensitivity Syndromes. *Clin Biochem Rev.* February 2013;34(1):15–38.

26. Torres MJ, Blanca M. The complex clinical picture of beta-lactam hypersensitivity: penicillins, cephalosporins, monobactams, carbapenems, and clavams. *Med Clin North Am.* 2010;94:805–820.

27. Greenberger PA. Chapter 30: Drug allergy. *Allergy Asthma Proc.* 2012;33(suppl 1):S103–S107.

28. Bousquet PJ, Gaeta F, Bousquet-Rouanet L, Lefrant JY, Demoly P, Romano A. Provocation tests in diagnosing drug hypersensitivity. *Curr Pharm Des.* 2008;14:2792–2802.

29. Mayorga C, Celik G, Rouzaire P, Whitaker P, et al. In vitro tests for drug hypersensitivity reactions: an ENDA/EAACI Drug Allergy Interest Group position paper. *Allergy.* August 2016;71(8):1103–1134.

30. Sanz ML, Gamboa PM, Garia-Figueroa BE, Ferrer M. In vitro diagnosis of anaphylaxis. *Chem Immunol Allergy.* 2010;95:125–140.

31. Berroa F, Lafuente A, Javaloyes G, Ferrer M, Moncada R, Goikoetxea MJ, et al. The usefulness of plasma histamine and different tryptase cut-off points in the diagnosis of peranaesthetic hypersensitivity reactions. *Clin Exp Allergy.* 2014;44:270–277.

32. Schwartz LB, Yunginger JW, Miller J, Bokhari R, Dull D. Time course of appearance and disappearance of human mast cell tryptase in the circulation after anaphylaxis. *J Clin Invest.* May 1989;83(5):1551–1555.

33. Gómez E, Torres MJ, Mayorga C, Blanca M. Immunologic evaluation of drug allergy. *Allergy Asthma Immunol Res.* 2012;4:251–263.

34. Mayorga C, Sanz ML, Gamboa PM, García BE, Caballero MT, García JM, et al. In vitro diagnosis of immediate allergic reactions to drugs: an update. *J Investig Allergol Clin Immunol.* 2010;20:103–109.

35. Sampson HA. Update on food allergy. *J Allergy Clin Immunol.* 2004;113:805–819.

36. Gruchalla RS, Sullivan TJ. In vivo and in vitro diagnosis of drug allergy. *Immunol Allergy Clin North Am.* 1991;11:595–610.

37. Fontaine C, Mayorga C, Bousquet PJ, Arnoux B, Torres MJ, Blanca M, et al. Relevance of the determination of serum-specific IgE antibodies in the diagnosis of immediate β-lactam allergy. *Allergy.* 2007;62:47–52.

38. García JJ, Blanca M, Moreno F, et al. Determination of IgE antibodies to the benzylpenicilloyl determinant: a comparison of the sensitivity and specificity of three radio allegro sorbent test methods. *J Clin Lab Anal.* 1997;11:251–257.

39. Guéant JL, Guéant-Rodriguez RM, Viola M, Valluzzi RL, Romano A. IgE-mediated hypersensitivity to cephalosporins. *Curr Pharm Des.* 2006;12:3335–3345.

40. Blanca M, Mayorga C, Torres MJ, et al. Clinical evaluation of Pharmacia CAP System RAST FEIA amoxicilloyl and benzylpenicilloyl in patients with penicillin allergy. *Allergy.* 2001;56:862–870.

41. Ebo DG, Venemalm L, Bridts CH, et al. Immunoglobulin E antibodies to rocuronium: a new diagnostic tool. *Anesthesiology.* 2007;107:253–259.

42. Garvey LH, Kroigaard M, Poulsen LK, Skov PS, Mosbech H, Venemalm L, et al. IgE-mediated allergy to chlorhexidine. *J Allergy Clin Immunol.* 2007;120:409–415.

43. Boumiza R, Debard AL, Monneret G. The basophil activation test by flow cytometry: recent developments in clinical studies, standardization and emerging perspectives. *Clin Mol Allergy.* 2005;3:9.

44. De Week AL, Sanz ML, Gamboa PM, Aberer W, Sturm G, Bilo MB, et al. Diagnosis of immediate-type beta-lactam allergy in vitro by flow-cytometric basophil activation test and sulfidoleukotriene production: a multicenter study. *J Investig Allergol Clin Immunol.* 2009;19(2):91–109.

45. Leysen J, Sabato V, Verweij MM, De Knop KJ, Bridts CH, De Clerck LS, et al. The basophil activation test in the diagnosis of immediate drug hypersensitivity. *Expert Rev Clin Immunol.* 2011;7:349–355.

46. Sanz ML, Gamboa PM, Mayorga C. Basophil activation tests in the evaluation of immediate drug hypersensitivity. *Curr Opin Allergy Clin Immunol.* August 2009;9(4):298–304.

47. Hausmann OV, Gentinetta T, Bridts CH, Ebo DG. The basophil activation test in immediate-type drug allergy. *Immunol Allergy Clin North Am.* 2009;29:555–566.

48. Solensky R, Khan DA. Joint task force on practice parameters. American Academy of Allergy, Asthma and Immunology. American College of Allergy, Asthma and Immunology. Joint Council of Allergy, Asthma and Immunology Drug allergy: an updated practice parameter. *Ann Allergy Asthma Immunol.* 2010;105:259–273. The clinical usefulness of drug patch testing.

49. Sieben S, Kawakubo Y, Al Masaoudi T, Merk HF, Blömeke B. Delayed-type hypersensitivity reaction to paraphenylenediamine is mediated by 2 different pathways of antigen recognition by specific alphabeta human T-cell clones. *J Allergy Clin Immunol.* June 2002;109(6):1005–1011.

50. HF1 M, Abel J, Baron JM, Krutmann J. Molecular pathways in dermatotoxicology. *Toxicol Appl Pharmacol.* March 15, 2004;195(3):267–277.

51. Barbaud A, Reichert-Penetrat S, Tréchot P, Jacquin-Petit MA, Ehlinger A, Noirez V, et al. The use of skin testing in the investigation of cutaneous adverse drug reactions. *Br J Dermatol.* 1998;139:49–58.

52. Barbaud A. Skin testing and patch testing in non-IgE-mediated drug allergy. *Curr Allergy Asthma Rep.* June 2014;14(6):442.

53. Pavlos R, Mallal S, Phillips E. HLA and pharmacogenetics of drug hypersensitivity. *Pharmacogenomics.* 2012;13:1285–1306.

54. Naisbitt DJ, Nattrass RG, Ogese MO. In vitro diagnosis of delayed-type drug hypersensitivity. *Immunol Allergy Clin N Am.* 2014;34:691–705. http://dx.doi.org/10.1016/j.iac.2014.04.009.

55. Porebski G, Pecaric-Petkovic T, Groux-Keller M, Bosak M, Kawabata TT, Pichler WJ. In vitro drug causality assessment in Stevens–Johnson syndrome—alternatives for lymphocyte transformation test. *Clin Exp Allergy J Br Soc Allergy Clin Immunol.* 2013;43:1027–1037.

56. Schrijvers R, Gilissen L, Mirela Chiriac A, Demoly P. Pathogenesis and diagnosis of delayed-type drug hypersensitivity reactions, from bedside to bench and back. *Clin Transl Allergy.* 2015;5:31.

57. Adachi T, Takahashi H, Funakoshi T, Hirai H, Hashiguchi A, Amagai M, et al. Comparison of basophil activation test and lymphocyte transformation test as diagnostic assays for drug hypersensitivity. *Clin Transl Allergy.* 2014;4:P30.

58. Solensky R, Khan DA. Joint Task Force on Practice Parameters. American Academy of Allergy, Asthma and Immunology. American College of Allergy, Asthma and Immunology. Joint Council of Allergy, Asthma and Immunology Drug allergy: an updated practice parameter. *Ann Allergy Asthma Immunol.* 2010;105:259–273.

CHAPTER 9

Drug Desensitization

KAREN S. HSU BLATMAN, MD

KEY POINTS

- Adverse drug reactions are impediments to standard, first-line treatments for various medical conditions.
- Rapid drug desensitization is a way to safely administer an essential drug in incremental doses until a full therapeutic dose is tolerated.
- Desensitization is a procedure that results in a temporary tolerance to a drug that has caused a hypersensitivity reaction.

Adverse drug reactions are impediments to standard, first-line treatments for various medical conditions. Rapid drug desensitization is a way to safely administer an essential drug in incremental doses until a full therapeutic dose is tolerated. Desensitization is a procedure that results in a temporary tolerance to a drug that has caused a hypersensitivity reaction.

Experience with antibiotic desensitizations was first published in 1985 by Wendel et al., which described a case series of successful penicillin desensitization in 15 pregnant women with histories of penicillin hypersensitivity reactions.[1] Typically, the decision to undergo desensitization for antibiotics is made with an infectious disease consultant, to determine the best therapy for the patient. The desensitization process has now been successfully used in patients with hypersensitivity reactions to various other medications, including aspirin, chemotherapy, and monoclonal antibodies. The medication can be administered either orally or intravenously. If the adverse drug reactions are consistent with a Type I hypersensitivity reaction and the offending drug is the ideal plan with no reasonable alternatives, then rapid drug desensitization may be the best choice for treatment.

Because the target cells of desensitizations are mast cells and possibly basophils, reactions amenable to desensitization typically occur during or within 1 h after completion of administration. These symptoms and/or signs include flushing, pruritus, urticaria, angioedema, bronchospasm, light-headedness, and/or hypotension, hypoxia, syncope, nausea, and/or vomiting. Severe back, pelvic, and chest pains have also been described by patients who experience acute infusion reactions.[2] Some delayed drug reactions (i.e.,

sulfamethoxazole/trimethoprim) have been amenable to desensitization.[3] Delayed Type IV reactions have been further subdivided into subcategories a, b, c, and d. Type IVa represents a tuberculin reaction or contact dermatitis.[4] Type IVb represents exanthems or macular/papular reactions with eosinophilia occurring 24–48 h or later after the infusion. In 2014, the allergy research group at the Mayo Clinic reported the largest case series of successful rapid administration of trimethoprim–sulfamethoxazole in patients without HIV and a history of sulfonamide Type IVb delayed reactions.[3] Type IVc and Type IVd are consistent with Stevens-Johnson syndrome/toxic epidermal necrolysis and acute generalized exanthematous pustulosis (AGEP), respectively, and patients presenting with these syndromes would not be candidates for desensitization.[5]

With other drug infusion reactions (either Type I or Type IV), where we do not fully understand the mechanism, patients have been able to be desensitized to the drug. One drug with multiple possible mechanisms for an adverse drug reaction is rituximab.[6]

Immediate adverse drug reactions typically result from sudden activation of mast cells and/or basophils, which release inflammatory mediators; they can be both IgE-mediated and non-IgE-mediated reactions. For an IgE-mediated reaction, the given drug or drug–protein complex is recognized by IgE antibodies.[7] Drug-specific IgE antibodies occupy surface receptors on mast cells and basophils throughout the body. If the mast cells and basophils are then sensitized, encountering the same drug the next time can cause cross-linking of the receptors, which activate the cells. The cells release mediators, such as histamine, tryptase, prostaglandins, and leukotrienes, resulting in allergic symptoms.

Examples of drugs known to cause IgE-mediated reactions include penicillins,[1] cephalosporins,[8] and platinum-based chemotherapy drugs (e.g., carboplatin).[9]

Non-IgE-mediated immediate reactions (such as taxanes) can present clinically similar to IgE-mediated reactions. However, the exact mechanism of the non-IgE immediate reactions is still unclear. For example, non-IgE-mediated reactions to paclitaxel often happen on a first dose.[10] One hypothesis for this reaction is due to complement activation by a vehicle such as Cremophor (polyethoxylated castor oil), as paclitaxel is solubilized in Cremophor.

Aspirin and other nonsteroidal antiinflammatory drugs can also cause a range of adverse reactions, including exacerbation of respiratory disease, anaphylaxis, and urticaria and angioedema. The mechanism is typically related to aberrant arachidonic acid metabolism, but sometimes it may be related to IgE.[11] There are several published aspirin desensitization protocols.[12-14] Until 1999, the oral desensitization protocol for aspirin exacerbated respiratory disease (AERD) would take 3 days.[13] Then, leukotriene receptor antagonists, such as montelukast, came to the US market. Pretreatment with one of the leukotriene receptor antagonists decreased the severity of the respiratory reactions during the desensitizations.[13] Most recently, Dr. Chen with Dr. Khan published a shorter desensitization protocol for patients with AERD,[14] which decreased the time between doses from 3-h intervals to hourly intervals, starting with 40 mg dose and proceeding to 81 mg, 120 mg, 162 mg, and 325 mg. This protocol allowed aspirin oral desensitizations to be completed in 1–2 days.[14] For patients presenting with anaphylaxis, urticaria, or angioedema, the initial dose may be much lower (such as 1 mg), and desensitization may be harder to achieve.[15]

Certain types of adverse drug reactions are not good candidates for desensitization. Examples of Gel-Coombs Type II and Type III hypersensitivity reactions include serum sickness, hemolytic anemias, drug-induced interstitial nephritis, pneumonitis, hepatitis, vasculitis, and blood cell dyscrasias.[2] Certain cutaneous reactions, which are non–mast cell mediated, are absolute contraindications for desensitization.[5] In these situations, there is high risk that even small doses of the implicated drug may induce recurrent, irreversible desquamative reactions. These include exfoliative dermatitis syndromes and dermatoses with mucous membrane lesions: Stevens-Johnson syndrome, toxic epidermal necrolysis, drug reaction with eosinophilia and systemic syndrome, fixed drug eruption, erythema multiforme, bullous dermatitis, and AGEP.[2]

A known adverse reaction may mimic a hypersensitivity reaction. Liposomal doxorubicin is known to cause palmoplantar erythrodysesthesia ("hand-foot" syndrome), stomatitis, and/or a diffuse follicular eruption with an intertriginous distribution.[16,17] Patients can initially notice painful erythema affecting their palms and soles. In a study by Kim et al., severe skin toxicity associated with liposomal doxorubicin occurred infrequently when lower initial doses were administered. When skin reactions occurred, it was early in treatment and improved with dose reduction.[16]

POSSIBLE MECHANISMS

The mechanism of desensitization is still not fully understood. In vitro studies have demonstrated that subthreshold doses of antigen can render mast cells and basophils unresponsive to activation by that specific antigen but still be responsive to other activating stimuli.[18,19] Subthreshold doses of antigen may result in monomeric binding to the IgE receptor, leading to internalization of the antigen–receptor complex, so that the cell does not become activated. In vitro rapid desensitization of human mast cells induces decreased levels of signal-transducing molecules, such as syk.[20]

Research from Sancho-Serra et al. at the Brigham and Women's Hospital suggested that low doses of antigen might induce rearrangement of the cell membrane in the antigen-sensitized mast cells, preventing the internalization of the antigen/IgE and protecting against anaphylaxis.[21] Their research investigated the molecular mechanisms underlying specific mast cell desensitization using an in vitro model of antigen-specific, rapid mast cell/IgE desensitization in the presence of physiologic levels of calcium.[21] In this in vitro model of mast cell desensitization, double doses of antigen provided the best inhibition of mast cell mediators, including granule mediators, leukotrienes, and prostaglandins. This provided the basis for a modified human rapid desensitization protocol that has been used successfully at our institution.[22] In addition, the in vitro model provided evidence of lack of delayed mediator release, providing grounds for safety and lack of delayed reactions in human protocols.

IgE and IgG antibodies specific to the antigen increase after desensitization, as in the case of penicillin desensitization.[23] The increased IgG titer may neutralize drug epitopes and serve as a "blocking" function for IgE-mediated reactions.

In a mouse model of rapid antigen desensitization, the transcription factor STAT 6 was shown to be necessary for desensitization.[24] Based on in vitro observations by Morales, twofold or threefold dose escalation at each time interval has been more successful than a tenfold dose escalation.[24] STAT-6-deficient mast cells can release mediators during the early phase but cannot release late-phase mediators and cannot be desensitized to antigens.[25]

Aydogan et al. report a case where a patient with an anaphylaxis-like reaction to rituximab on first exposure was subsequently and successfully desensitized to rituximab.[26] In patients with allergic rhinitis, allergen-specific immunotherapy has been used for almost a century as a desensitization strategy. The induction of peripheral T cell tolerance through the generation of allergen-specific T regulatory cells presents a key step in successful allergen immunotherapy. In the report, Aydogan demonstrated an increase in $CD4^+CD25^+$ and CD4CD25FoxP3 Treg cells in the patient after desensitization.[26]

DESENSITIZATION PROCESS

Grading the patient's severity of the initial reaction can be helpful in determining the type of setting for desensitization, outpatient infusion center versus in the hospital or intensive care unit. Brown et al.[27] has described a useful anaphylaxis grading system, dividing hypersensitivity into grade 1 through 3 reactions. Grade 1 reactions are strictly cutaneous reactions. Grade 2 reactions include symptoms that involve respiratory, cardiovascular, or gastrointestinal involvement. Grade 3 reactions include either hypotension or hypoxia, loss of consciousness, and cardiovascular collapse. At the Brigham and Women's Hospital, most of the desensitizations are done in an ambulatory center, reserving a bed in the intensive care unit only for patients with a history of a grade 3 reaction. If the patient does well during the first desensitization, the patient may often be moved to the ambulatory infusion center for his or her next desensitization. If nursing staff is available, then desensitizations could also be done on a general medical floor in the hospital. We also do the majority of our aspirin desensitizations for patients with AERD in the outpatient clinic. Informed consent must be obtained before each desensitization. The potential risks and benefits of the process must be reviewed with the patient before each desensitization.

After the desensitization protocol is designed by the team and if the patient has reactions during desensitization, the protocol will typically be adjusted with additional steps and/or added premedication. High-risk patients are considered ones with an initial reaction involving hypotension, oxygen desaturation, or cardiovascular collapse. β-Blockers and ACE inhibitors are risk factors for poor response to epinephrine during treatment for anaphylaxis, so they should be avoided during desensitizations. Morphine derivatives can promote mast cell degranulation during desensitization.

PRETREATMENT

Pretreatment regimens are aimed at preventing or minimizing breakthrough reactions during the rapid drug desensitization. The regimens vary by protocol. Many protocols include H_1 and H_2 antihistamines in the premedication regimen. Others include steroids. At our institution, we no longer add steroid premedication because it does not seem to prevent anaphylaxis or death and is consistent with findings on use of dexamethasone with platinum agents in the FDA Adverse Event Reporting System, AERS.[28] Using premedication is not consistent among all protocols. Herrero et al. support avoiding premedication altogether, so it does not mask early signs of anaphylaxis.[29]

In another case series, Breslow et al. found that adding oral aspirin 325 mg and oral montelukast 10 mg prophylactically helped patients tolerate subsequent desensitizations, particularly those with complaints of flushing or bronchospasm. The benefit is mostly seen in patients with skin and respiratory symptoms, which suggests a dominant role for prostaglandins and leukotrienes in these acute reactions.[30] Breslow reported that some patients who had previously failed methylprednisolone pretreatments, developed mild or no reaction after montelukast and aspirin pretreatment. If flushing occurred during the initial reaction, then aspirin 325 mg premedication is routinely added to the premedication regimen. If bronchospasm occurred during the initial reaction, then montelukast is routinely added as a premedication.

In another report about carboplatin desensitization, Ojaimi et al. present the added benefit of omalizumab, a recombinant humanized monoclonal antibody, which binds to the FceR binding domain of soluble IgE and blocks the interaction with its receptors on mast cells and basophils.[31] After three doses of omalizumab, Ojaimi reported the patient was successfully desensitized to carboplatin. After nine doses of omalizumab treatment, the patient's skin test became negative, along with a decrease in total serum IgE. It is one of few reported cases of the use of omalizumab to overcome IgE-mediated drug allergy. For patients who fail standard desensitization protocols to a preferred medication, this may be an option.

1) Fill in the orange boxes (dose, volume and final rate of infusion) **to set the total dose and** target concentration **desired.**
(For chemotherapy desensitizations, use 75-80 mL/hr as the final rate of infusion)
For "repeat dosing" medications such as antibiotics, the calculated **standard time of infusion** should be close to standard infusion times.

2) The **Time (min)** for steps 1-11 may be adjusted if the patient has a history of reactions during a previous desensitization. *Our standard protocol is 15 min per step.*

3) If more solution is needed in order to "prime the pump" *but not be infused,* enter the **additional** desired volume per bag (rarely needed):

Additional volume (*not infused*):

Name of Medication: _____ *(enter here)*

Target Dose (mg)	750
Standard volume per bag (mL)	250
Final rate of infusion (mL/hr)	80
Calculated target concentration (mg/mL)	3
Standard time of infusion (minutes)	187.5

				Total mg per Bag	Amount of Bag Infused (mL)
Solution 1	250	mL of	0.030 mg/mL	7.500	9.25
Solution 2	250	mL of	0.300 mg/mL	75.000	18.75
Solution 3	250	mL of	2.976 mg/mL	744.098	250.00

*** PLEASE NOTE *** The total volume and dose dispensed are more than the final dose given to patient because the initial solutions are *not completely infused*

Step	Solution	Rate (mL/hr)	Time (min)	Volume Infused per Step (mL)	Dose Administered With This Step (mg)	Cumulative Dose (mg)
1	1	2.0	15	0.50	0.0150	0.0150
2	1	5.0	15	1.25	0.0375	0.0525
3	1	10.0	15	2.50	0.0750	0.1275
4	1	20.0	15	5.00	0.1500	0.2775
5	2	5.0	15	1.25	0.3750	0.6525
6	2	10.0	15	2.50	0.7500	1.4025
7	2	20.0	15	5.00	1.5000	2.9025
8	2	40.0	15	10.00	3.0000	5.9025
9	3	10.0	15	2.50	7.4410	13.3435
10	3	20.0	15	5.00	14.8820	28.2254
11	3	40.0	15	10.00	29.7639	57.9893
12	3	80.0	174.375	232.50	692.0107	750.0000
	Total time (min) =		339.375	= 5.66 hr		

FIG. 9.1 BWH desensitization protocol template, 12 steps.

The Brigham and Women's Hospital/Dana Farber Cancer Institute desensitization program produced a 12-step standard protocol in which unresponsiveness to a triggering antigen dose was achieved by delivering doubling doses of antigen at fixed time intervals (see Fig. 9.1).[22] The protocol is based on three solutions administered sequentially starting with the solutions containing a 1/100 dilution, then a 1/10 dilution and an undiluted dose of any medication. Patients who react to the protocol starting with the 1/100 dilution may start with a bag containing 1/1000 dilution, which created a four-bag protocol. For those who will continue to receive the offending drug after desensitization, it is also important to match the concentration (hence the bag volume) of the strongest solution (typically the last bag) to the concentration typically administered to nonallergic patient. If the patient is not going to have continued exposure after the initial desensitization, such as in the case of chemotherapy or monoclonal antibodies, then the patient will need to be desensitized for each drug exposure. Each desensitization protocol is customized to the specific dose, so that the patient will receive his or her full therapeutic dose. Various protocols using similar methodology have been successfully applied to monoclonal antibodies, including infliximab, trastuzumab, and rituximab.[32]

BREAKTHROUGH REACTIONS DURING DESENSITIZATION

In a large series of desensitizations to chemotherapy described at our institution, most reactions were mild cutaneous reactions, and patients were able to complete the desensitizations.[22] Risk of anaphylaxis remains, so medications such as epinephrine, antihistamines, and bronchodilators are at the bedside. As soon as the reaction is noted, the infusion is stopped and treatment appropriately with antihistamines, steroids, and albuterol as needed. Severe reactions may require epinephrine. The physician may request a serum tryptase to be drawn at the time of the reaction although the results will not be available for a couple of days. Once the reaction is resolved, the infusion is restarted at the point of interruption or one step prior. For protocol modifications, we add either premedications or schedule medications in between steps. For example, if a patient had a cutaneous reaction at step 12, then typically an antihistamine will be added either between finishing step 10 or before initiating step 11. Alternatively, a step could be added between step 11 and step 12. Aspirin and montelukast to block prostaglandins and leukotrienes can be used at the time of reactions (unpublished data).

OUTCOMES

In the largest case series of rapid desensitizations to chemotherapeutic agents,[22] 67% proceeded without an acute infusion reaction, while 27% had only mild reactions. Six percent were characterized as severe reactions; however, there were no intubations or deaths. One reaction during desensitization required epinephrine treatment. All patients in the case series received their full target dose. For patients who received multiple desensitizations, most reactions occurred during the first five desensitizations (94.8%), and the majority of the reactions occurred during the first two desensitizations (61%). A follow-up study by Brennan et al. that focused on monoclonal antibodies also showed a high success rate, with 104 of 105 desensitizations successfully completed.[32] In that series, acute infusion reactions

happened during 29% of desensitizations. Of those, 27 were mild reactions, one moderate reaction, and two severe reactions. Epinephrine use is reserved for patients with hypotension and/or desaturation or anaphylaxis during the course of the desensitizations. Between September 2012 and April 2014, only 2 patients of 1635 desensitizations required epinephrine (unpublished data).

Allergic reactions to medications remain an important barrier to care. Rapid drug desensitizations are proved to be a safe and effective way for patients to receive their first-line drug therapies when no comparable alternative is available. It is critical to remember that the desensitization procedure does not eliminate or cure the IgE-mediated drug allergy. Although the molecular basis of rapid desensitizations is still not completely understood, an in vitro mast cell model has shown evidence of profound inhibitory mechanisms of mast cell activation during desensitization, which correlates with the success of these desensitization protocols. Further studies in the field will lead to a better understanding of mechanisms behind rapid drug desensitization and further reduce risk.

REFERENCES

1. Wendel GD, Stark BJ, Jamison RB, Molina RD, Sullivan TJ. Penicillin allergy and desensitization in serious infections during pregnancy. *N Engl J Med.* 1985;312(19):1229–1232. http://dx.doi.org/10.1056/nejm198505093121905.
2. Cernadas JR, Brockow K, Romano A, et al. General considerations on rapid desensitization for drug hypersensitivity - a consensus statement. *Allergy.* 2010;65(11):1357–1366. http://dx.doi.org/10.1111/j.1398-9995.2010.02441.x.
3. Pyle RC, Butterfield JH, Volcheck GW, et al. Successful outpatient graded administration of trimethoprim-sulfamethoxazole in patients without HIV and with a history of sulfonamide adverse drug reaction. *J Allergy Clin Immunol Prac.* 2014;2(1):52–58. http://dx.doi.org/10.1016/j.jaip.2013.11.002.
4. Celik C, Pichler W, Adkinson Jr NF. Drug allergy. In: Adkinson Jr NF, Bochner B, Busse W, Holgate S, Lemanske Jr R, Simons FE, eds. *Middleton's Allergy Principles & Practice.* 7th ed. Mosby Elsevier; 2017:1274–1295.
5. Drug allergy: An updated practice parameter. *Ann Allergy Asthma Immunol.* 2010;105(4):259–273.e78. http://dx.doi.org/10.1016/j.anai.2010.08.002.
6. Levin A, Otani I, Lax T, Hochberg E, Banerji A. Reactions to rituximab in an outpatient infusion center: a 5-year review. *J Allergy Clin Immunol Prac.* 2017;5(1):107–113.e1. http://dx.doi.org/10.1016/j.jaip.2016.06.022.
7. Stone S, Phillips E, Wiese M, Heddle R, Brown S. Immediate-type hypersensitivity drug reactions. *Br J Clin Pharmacol.* 2014;78(1):1–13. http://dx.doi.org/10.1111/bcp.12297.

8. Romano A, Gaeta F, Valluzzi R, et al. IgE-mediated hypersensitivity to cephalosporins: cross-reactivity and tolerability of alternative cephalosporins. *J Allergy Clin Immunol.* 2015;136(3):685–691.e3. http://dx.doi.org/10.1016/j.jaci.2015.03.012.

9. Lee C, Matulonis U, Castells M. Carboplatin hypersensitivity: a 6-h 12-step protocol effective in 35 desensitizations in patients with gynecological malignancies and mast cell/IgE-mediated reactions. *Gynaecol Oncol.* 2004;95(2):370–376. http://dx.doi.org/10.1016/j.ygyno.2004.08.002.

10. Szebeni J, Alving C, Muggia F. Complement activation by cremophor EL as a possible contributor to hypersensitivity to paclitaxel: an in vitro study. *Jnci (J Natl Cancer Inst).* 1998;90(4):300–306. http://dx.doi.org/10.1093/jnci/90.4.300.

11. Picaud J, Beaudouin E, Renaudin J, et al. Anaphylaxis to diclofenac: nine cases reported to the Allergy Vigilance Network in France. *Allergy.* 2014;69(10):1420–1423. http://dx.doi.org/10.1111/all.12458.

12. Kowalski M, Makowska J, Blanca M, et al. Hypersensitivity to nonsteroidal anti-inflammatory drugs (NSAIDs) - classification, diagnosis and management: review of the EAACI/ENDA# and GA2LEN/HANNA*. *Allergy.* 2011;66(7):818–829. http://dx.doi.org/10.1111/j.1398-9995.2011.02557.x.

13. Stevenson DD, White AA. Aspirin desensitization in aspirin-exacerbated respiratory disease: consideration of a new oral challenge protocol. *J Allergy Clin Immunol Prac.* 2015;3(6):932–933. http://dx.doi.org/10.1016/j.jaip.2015.07.006.

14. Chen JR, Buchmiller BL, Khan DA. An hourly dose-escalation desensitization protocol for aspirin-exacerbated respiratory disease. *J Allergy Clin Immunol Prac.* 2015;3(6):926–931. http://dx.doi.org/10.1016/j.jaip.2015.06.013. e1.

15. Page N, Schroeder W. Rapid desensitization protocols for patients with cardiovascular disease and aspirin hypersensitivity in an era of dual antiplatelet therapy. *Ann Pharmacother.* 2006;41(1):61–67. http://dx.doi.org/10.1345/aph.1h437.

16. Kim RJ, Peterson G, Kulp B, Zanotti KM, Markman M. Skin toxicity associated with pegylated liposomal doxorubicin (40 mg/m^2) in the treatment of gynecologic cancers. *Gynaecol Oncol.* 2005;97(2):374–378. http://dx.doi.org/10.1016/j.ygyno.2004.12.057.

17. Lotem M, Hubert A, Lyass O, et al. Skin toxic effects of polyethylene glycol–coated liposomal doxorubicin. *Arch Dermatol.* 2000;(12):136. http://dx.doi.org/10.1001/archderm.136.12.1475.

18. Pruzansky JJ, Patterson R. Desensitization of human basophils with suboptimal concentrations of agonist. Evidence for reversible and irreversible desensitization. *Immunology.* November 1988;65(3):443–447.

19. MacGlashan Jr D, Lichtenstein LM. Basic characteristics of human lung mast cell desensitization. *J Immunol.* July 15, 1987;139(2):501–505.

20. MacGlashan D, Miura K. Loss of syk kinase during IgE-mediated stimulation of human basophils. *J Allergy Clin Immunol.* 2004;114(6):1317–1324. http://dx.doi.org/10.1016/j.jaci.2004.08.037.

21. Sancho-Serra M, del C, Simarro M, Castells M. Rapid IgE desensitization is antigen specific and impairs early and late mast cell responses targeting FcεRI internalization. *Eur J Immunol.* 2011;41(4):1004–1013. http://dx.doi.org/10.1002/eji.201040810.

22. Castells MC, Tennant NM, Sloane DE, et al. Hypersensitivity reactions to chemotherapy: outcomes and safety of rapid desensitization in 413 cases. *J Allergy Clin Immunol.* 2008;122(3):574–580. http://dx.doi.org/10.1016/j.jaci.2008.02.044.

23. Naclerio R, Mizrahi E, Adkinson Jr N. Immunologic observations during desensitization and maintenance of clinical tolerance to penicillin. *J Allergy Clin Immunol.* 1983;71(3):294–301. http://dx.doi.org/10.1016/0091-6749(83)90083-0.

24. Morales AR, Shah N, Castells M. Antigen-IgE desensitization in signal transducer and activator of transcription 6-deficient mast cells by suboptimal doses of antigen. *Ann Allergy Asthma Immunol.* 2005;94:575–580. http://dx.doi.org/10.1016/S1081-1206(10)61136-2.

25. Malaviya R, Uckun FM. Role of STAT6 in IgE receptor/fcepsilonRI-mediated late phase allergic responses of mast cells. *J Immunol.* 2002;168(1):421–426.

26. Aydogan M, Yologlu N, Gacar G, Uyan ZS, Eser I, Karaoz E. Successful rapid rituximab desensitization in an adolescent patient with nephrotic syndrome: increase in number of treg cells after desensitization. *J Allergy Clin Immunol.* 2013;132(2):478–480. http://dx.doi.org/10.1016/j.jaci.2013.02.004.

27. Brown SGA. Clinical features and severity grading of anaphylaxis. *J Allergy Clin Immunol.* 2004;114(2):371–376. http://dx.doi.org/10.1016/j.jaci.2004.04.029.

28. Sakaeda T. Platinum agent-induced hypersensitivity reactions: data mining of the public version of the FDA adverse event reporting system, AERS. *Int J Med Sci.* 2011:332. http://dx.doi.org/10.7150/ijms.8.332.

29. Herrero T, Tornero P, Infante S, et al. Diagnosis and management of hypersensitivity reactions caused by oxaliplatin. *J Investiga Allergol Clin Immunol.* 2006;16(5):327–330.

30. Breslow RG, Caiado J, Castells MC. Acetylsalicylic acid and montelukast block mast cell mediator–related symptoms during rapid desensitization. *Ann Allergy Asthma Immunol.* 2009;102(2):155–160. http://dx.doi.org/10.1016/s1081-1206(10)60247-5.

31. Ojaimi S, Harnett PR, Fulcher DA. Successful carboplatin desensitization by using omalizumab and paradoxical diminution of total IgE levels. *J Allergy Clin Immunol Prac.* 2014;2(1):105–106. http://dx.doi.org/10.1016/j.jaip.2013.08.009.

32. Brennan PJ, Bouza TR, Hsu FI, Sloane DE, Castells MC. Hypersensitivity reactions to mAbs: 105 desensitizations in 23 patients, from evaluation to treatment. *J Allergy Clin Immunol.* 2009;124(6):1259–1266. http://dx.doi.org/10.1016/j.jaci.2009.09.009.

CHAPTER 10

Penicillins

ERIC MACY, MS, MD

KEY POINTS

- Most penicillin-associated adverse drug reactions are not immunologically mediated or reproducible on rechallenge.
- Most individuals with benign histories of penicillin "allergy" can have their clinical tolerance of penicillins verified by a single-dose oral amoxicillin challenge.
- Only a small minority will have true IgE-mediated penicillin allergy or a clinically significant T cell–mediated delayed-type hypersensitivity.

INTRODUCTION

The literature on penicillin-associated adverse drug reactions has evolved dramatically over the past 74 years. The cumulative literature is very confusing, often apparently contradictory, and almost impossible to reconcile in its entirety.[1] Non-IgE immunologically mediated reactions and even nonimmunologically mediated reactions are commonly referred to as "allergy," which adds to the confusion in both patients and many physicians. Given this, it is not surprising that current penicillin hypersensitivity testing practices vary widely.[2] Life-threatening IgE-mediated anaphylaxis and serum sickness–like reactions after penicillin use are much rarer today than they were 60+ years ago.[3] Anaphylaxis was reported in 2007 to occur only in 1 of 50,000 to 100,000 exposures, although these estimates have wide confidence intervals.[4,5] What remains is a fear of high rate of penicillin-associated anaphylaxis that still drives policy and practice patterns. The FDA still will not allow the production of penicillin skin testing reagents in facilities used to produce other injectable medications for the fear of sensitizing individuals or causing anaphylaxis in unsuspecting recipients of penicillin-contaminated products. Data on other penicillin-associated severe adverse reactions, including serious cutaneous adverse drug reactions (SCARs), hepatitis, and nephritis, are not well known. A recent review of an integrated allergy repository of a large health system found a prevalence of toxic epidermal necrolysis/Stevens-Johnson syndrome (SJS/TEN) of 375 patients per million, but more data are still needed.

Penicillin, in 2017, is still the most commonly reported drug intolerance. Paradoxically, the greatest current risk to the vast majority of individuals with a penicillin "allergy" is not anaphylaxis or some other serious immunologically mediated adverse reaction with reexposure to a penicillin, but continued avoidance of penicillins when they are clinically indicated.

The current reference standard when studying the epidemiology of clinically significant penicillin-associated, or other, adverse drug reactions is what is reported in the drug "allergy" field of the electronic health record (EHR) after exposure. If there is no notation made in the EHR, then any adverse reaction that may have occurred cannot affect future antibiotic choice, and an inaccurate notation in the EHR will greatly reduce future penicillin exposure. Only a small minority of individuals with a penicillin "allergy" notation in their EHR will have a clinically significant acute-onset IgE-mediated allergy with another penicillin exposure. Only a small minority will have a clinically significant delayed-onset T cell–mediated hypersensitivity reaction with another penicillin exposure. An unconfirmed penicillin "allergy" notation in the EHR is not benign.[6] Individuals with an active, but inaccurate, penicillin "allergy" suffer with significantly higher rates of serious antibiotic resistant infections; are given clindamycin, fluoroquinolones, vancomycin, and third- or higher-generation cephalosporins more frequently, all of which are associated with increased morbidity, compared with a penicillin, when a penicillin is the antibiotic of choice; and spend more time in the hospital.[6]

In 2014, the Choosing Wisely campaign of the American Board of Internal Medicine recommended physicians, "Don't overuse non-beta lactam antibiotics in patients with a history of penicillin allergy, without an appropriate evaluation."[7] In 2016, penicillin allergy testing was recognized by the Centers for

Disease Control and Prevention (CDC), the Infectious Diseases Society of America (IDSA), and the Society for Healthcare Epidemiology of America (SHEA) as an important part of an antibiotic stewardship program.[8,9]

Currently, about 6.8% of the US population that uses healthcare has a penicillin intolerance noted in the EHR.[10] Women are more likely to have a penicillin "allergy," in part, because they are more likely to seek healthcare, more likely to be prescribed antibiotics, and report new penicillin "allergies" at higher rates than men after all exposures.[11] In typical hospitalized populations, the prevalence of penicillin "allergy" is about 9.9% because the prevalence of a penicillin "allergy" record rises with increasing age, and very few individuals either have their penicillin intolerance confirmed, as a clinically significant IgE-mediated allergy or T cell–mediated delayed-type hypersensitivity, or removed.

In 2015 there were only about 20,000 doses of penicilloyl-polylysine (Pre-Pen), the major penicillin skin testing determinant, sold in the United States, and as of April 2016 sales were only about 5000 doses per month. Given that there are about 21.6 million penicillin-"allergic" individuals in the Unites States currently, skin testing for penicillin allergy alone is not making much of an impact.

The rate of positive penicillin skin test results in individuals with a history of penicillin intolerance has fallen markedly over the past 25 years.[12,13] The safety and efficacy of using a direct oral challenge to verify acute clinical tolerance in individuals with benign index reactions associated with penicillin exposures is now well established.[14–16]

THE EARLY PENICILLIN HYPERSENSITIVITY OBSERVATIONS

Penicillin was one of the first widely available antibiotics, coming into use in the early 1940s. It is remarkably nontoxic to humans, but its immunogenicity, particularly in its early, relatively impure, versions, can be significant. The description of the first use of penicillin in the United States, 5000 U given intravenously every 4 h to a female with β-hemolytic streptococcal sepsis at Yale-New Haven Hospital, on March 14, 1942, is instructive. "We discussed what to do with the pungent, brown-red powder. 'We decided to dissolve it in saline and pass it through an E.K. Seitz [asbestos] filter pad to sterilize it' wrote Dr. Tager in 1976."[17] Pure penicillin in solution is colorless. In 1943, it was reported that almost 16% of 209 soldiers treated with the earliest batches of penicillin in army

hospitals had urticaria eruptions.[18] Acute-onset urticaria rashes were noted after 0.5%–5.7% of penicillin exposures, depending on the underlying infection by 1946, along with multiple cases of serum sickness–like reactions.[19] Skin testing using native penicillin to evaluate the risk of immunologically mediated reexposure reactions was reported by 1948.[20] By 1956, the two most feared parenteral penicillin-associated adverse drug reactions were delayed-onset serum sickness, often resulting in hospitalization, occurring after 1%–5% of courses, and fatal anaphylaxis, with an estimated annual incidence of 100 cases occurring in the United States in 1952.[3] This high level of fatal anaphylaxis lead virtually all individuals with any rash after any penicillin use in the 1950s to be told never to be exposed to any penicillin again because they could "die." This fear has influenced future generations of physicians and is still present to some degree today. By 1961, the immunochemistry of penicillin metabolites able to haptenate serum protein sulfhydryl and amino groups was worked out well.[21] A polylysine synthetic peptide, with most of the lysines bound to a benzylpenicilloyl moiety, penicilloyl-polylysine (PPL) (Fig. 10.1), was shown to work well as a skin test reagent to evaluate penicillin allergy and not induce new sensitization.[22]

PENICILLIN SPECIFIC T CELLS RESPONSIBLE FOR DELAYED-ONSET PENICILLIN HYPERSENSITIVITY

By 2000, small numbers of individuals with delayed-onset penicillin-associated rashes had been studied with patch testing and in vitro leukocyte transformation tests.[23] These studies support a T cell–mediated pathologic mechanism. In 2009, amoxicillin-specific circulating T cells were reported to be present in 20 (91%) of 22 patients with maculopapular rashes associated with amoxicillin use, but not in 11 control patients with other drug-associated maculopapular rashes, 15 control patients with verified IgE-mediated penicillin allergy, or in 20 healthy control subjects.[24] T cell–mediated delayed hypersensitivity to penicillins can result in a variety of rash morphologies including maculopapular rashes, localized or systemic erythematous eruptions, and rarely acute generalized exanthematous pustulosis or fixed drug eruptions.[24–27] These reactions can start in less than 24 h after exposure but more typically occur 2–5 days into therapy.[28] Most of these T cell–mediated reactions are benign and self-limiting if the penicillin is stopped. Itching can be treated with antihistamines, and a short course of systemic corticosteroids is often given.

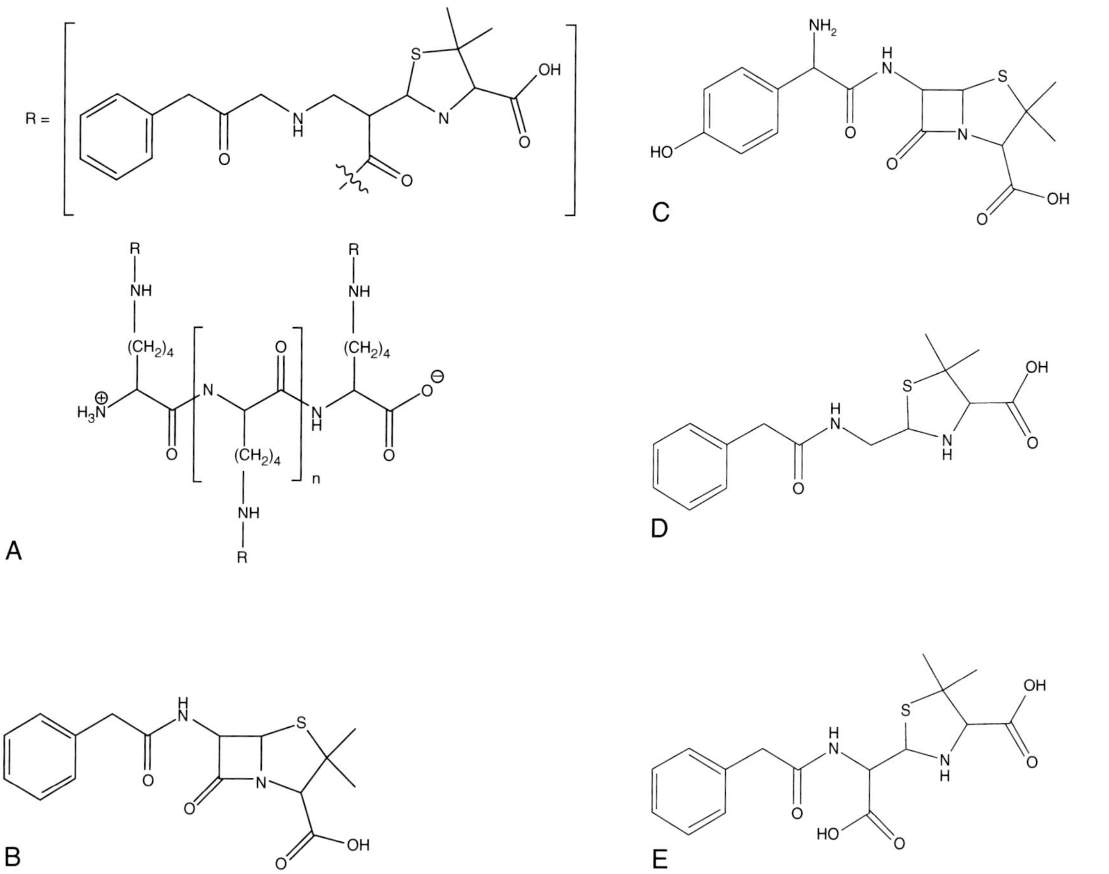

FIG. 10.1 **(A)** Penicilloyl-polylysine; **(B)** Penicillin; **(C)** Amoxicillin; **(D)** Penilloate; **(E)** Penicilloate.

ANTIPENICILLIN IGG AND SERUM SICKNESS–LIKE REACTIONS

Penicillin-associated serum sickness typically occurs 6–21 days after exposure because it takes this long to generate new antipenicillin IgG.[29] The time to onset can be much quicker, occurring in hours, if there are significant levels of preformed antipenicillin IgG present. Serum sickness–like reactions are typically self-limiting, clearing within 1–2 weeks, although rare cases can last longer. A decrease in C3, C4, and total hemolytic complement is a confirmatory laboratory finding, but often absent. Treatment with a tapering course of corticosteroids can help mitigate symptoms in severe cases.[30]

OTHER SERIOUS PENICILLIN-ASSOCIATED ADVERSE REACTIONS

Piperacillin use has been associated with hemolytic anemia.[31] Outpatient *Clostridium difficile* rates fall when all outpatient antibiotic usage falls in a population, with the greatest impact seen when there is less overall penicillin usage.[32] Penicillins cause much less acute renal toxicity compared with certain cephalosporins and carbapenems.[33] Penicillin-associated interstitial nephritis is currently rarely reported.[34] Acute renal injury has been associated with piperacillin/tazobactam use, occurring in up to 10% of courses, but with no difference in frequency noted between intermittent and extended infusions.[35] T cells appear to be responsible for some penicillin-induced liver injury.[36] Both amoxicillin-specific and clavulanic acid–specific T cells have been identified in rare cases. Penicillins are rarely uniquely associated with TEN or SJS. In the Han Chinese and in other non-Japanese Asians, the presence of the HLA-A2 allele is associated with a midlevel, 5- to 10-fold, increased risk for TEN or SJS occurring after aminopenicillin exposure.[37]

WHY PENICILLIN "ALLERGY" IS STILL SO COMMON

Penicillins are still one of the most widely used classes of antibiotics, with most of the exposures now to oral amoxicillin and amoxicillin/clavulanate. There is a certain predictable rate of new drug intolerances reported in the EHR after all therapeutic antibiotic use. For penicillins, the rate can be as high as 1% per course for males and 2% per course for females, depending on how long after the exposure the EHR is surveyed.[11,38] Individuals with any drug "allergies" are more likely to report new drug "allergies" with all drug exposures.[11] Penicillins, like all antibiotics, are widely overused.[39] Penicillins are frequently given to individuals with viral upper respiratory infection symptoms. Urticaria and other rashes are commonly associated with viral infections. The prevalence of penicillin "allergy" in over 11,000 individuals seen in an Allergy Department was noted to be three times higher in those with chronic urticaria, and the prevalence of chronic urticaria was noted to be three times higher in the same cohort in individuals with a history of penicillin "allergy."[40]

In 2013, a French study of a group of 184 individuals with documented active Epstein-Barr virus (EBV) infections reported that 34 (18.5%) had rashes, and the probability of having received any antibiotic, penicillin, amoxicillin, or amoxicillin plus clavulanate was not significantly different between those with and without rashes.[41] In the patients without rashes, 63% were exposed to an antibiotic versus 50% in those with a rash. In 2013, an Israeli study noted than in a group of 238 children with documented acute EBV infections, 173 (72.7%) were mistreated with antibiotics, and there was a no significant difference in the rash rate between those mistreated and untreated, 32.9% versus 23.1%.[42] What is interesting is that even in these cohorts where EBV was such a significant diagnostic consideration that EBV testing was performed, over 60% still received inappropriate antibiotic therapy.

In 2010, a Swiss study reported on 88 children, who presented to an emergency department with delayed-onset urticarial or maculopapular rashes, occurring during or within 3 days of empiric beta-lactam therapy. Most, 87.5% had been given amoxicillin or amoxicillin-clavulanic acid. All were subsequently oral challenged with the culprit antibiotic and tested for evidence of an acute viral infection. There were only 6 (6.8%) children who were oral challenge positive and 54 (65.9%) of the oral challenge negative children were viral study positive.[15]

Aged injectable penicillins are apparently more immunologically sensitizing.[43] The lower use of injectable penicillins over the past several decades in primary care has probably contributed to fewer individuals with significant immunologic sensitization. Individuals with any drug "allergies" are more likely to report new drug "allergies" with all drug exposures.[11]

Because of all of the above factors, penicillin "allergies" tend to accumulate in the population over time.

PENICILLIN BIOCHEMISTRY AND EARLY PENICILLIN SKIN TEST STUDIES

Penicillins are bactericidal antibiotics that disrupt bacterial cell walls by preventing cross-linking.[44] Because of this mechanism of action, they are also able to bind to lysine and cysteine residues on human serum proteins and function as haptens.[21] Human serum albumin is the protein most affected by amoxicillin with the lysine residues 190 and 199 the most haptenated.[45] A metabolite of the β-lactam core structure of penicillins, penicilloyl, is the major antigenic determinant. Commercially available penicilloyl-polylysine (PPL) is a multivalent antigen with 12–15 penicilloyl moieties coupled to a synthetic peptide consisting of about 20 lysine residues with an average molecular weight of about 7500 (Fig. 10.1). Historically, a variety of minor determinants, including native penicillin, penicilloate, penilloate, and native amoxicillin (Fig. 10.1), have also been used for penicillin skin testing, typically at 0.01 M.[46] These small molecules need to quickly haptenate interstitial fluid proteins to trigger mast cells sensitized with antipenicillin IgE. Their current clinical utility is minimal, except in high-risk cases with a recent history of anaphylaxis or shortness of breath, acutely associated with a penicillin exposure.[16] PPL, supplied as a 6×10^{-5} M solution, stable at room temperature, has been sold in the United States as Pre-Pen since July 1974, with several periods of unavailability from October 2000 until November 2001 and again from October 2004 until December 2009. This serial unavailability led to several classes of allergy/immunology fellows having essentially no experience with penicillin skin testing during their training.

In 1962, it was reported that 75% of 86 individuals who had a history of an adverse reaction associated with a penicillin use were skin test positive to PPL as compared with 3% of 1317 control individuals without a history of penicillin intolerance.[47]

In 1963, a study using PPL to skin test 1022 US Navy recruits noted that 15 (35%) of 43 individuals with a history of a reaction after a 1.2 million unit injection of benzathine penicillin G had a positive PPL skin test result compared with 58 (6.8%) of 825 who tolerated the prophylactic penicillin injection.[48] In the

868 individuals with a previous penicillin exposure, 73 (8.4%) were skin test positive compared with 4 (3%) of the 125 with no previous exposure to a penicillin.

In 1964, a multicenter US clinical trial of individuals seen in venereal disease clinics reported on 1003 patients, with a history of penicillin allergy compared with 12,559 controls subjects seen in the same clinics without a history of penicillin allergy.[49] They noted positive skin test results using only PPL in 396 (39.4%) of the cases and in 775 (6.2%) of the controls. The authors commented that there were no episodes of anaphylaxis or life-threatening penicillin-associated adverse reactions requiring hospitalization in the test-negative individuals after penicillin therapy, when they expected to see four such cases based on previous experience, or about 1 for every 3000 individuals treated with a parenteral penicillin.

The first collaborative clinical trial on penicillin skin testing, published in 1977, noted that 326 (19%) of 1718 positive history individuals were skin test positive, 254 (78%) at least to PPL, and the remaining 72 (22%) only to native penicillin G.[50] It is also of interest that 86 (7%) of the 1229 history negative, control, individuals tested also recorded positive skin test results to at least one of the two reagents, again the majority positive to PPL. In the 346 test-negative individuals challenged with a therapeutic course of a penicillin, 10 (3%) noted a reaction, but only a minority of these reactions were acute onset.

In the second collaborative clinical trial on penicillin skin testing, published in 1992, this time using PPL, native benzylpenicillin, benzylpenicilloate, and benzylpenicilloyl-*N*-propylamine, among those who completed the protocol, 566 (78%) of the 726 with a history of penicillin intolerance were test negative versus 570 (95%) of the 600 without a history of penicillin intolerance.[51] Only 15 (9%) of the 167 skin test positive individuals reacted only to benzylpenicilloate or benzylpenicilloyl-*N*-propylamine.

These five classic studies over three decades showed numerous positive skin test results in individuals with no history of penicillin intolerance, most of the skin test positive individuals were positive to PPL, and there was a falling rate of positive skin test results to PPL in individuals with a history of penicillin "allergy." The false-positive result rate noted with penicillin skin testing in individuals with a history of penicillin "allergy" was started to be noted. A small number of penicillin "allergy" history positive and skin test positive subjects have been exposed to therapeutic doses of penicillins over the years, without undergoing desensitization, and many did not have any acute adverse reaction.[15,50,52,53]

PENICILLIN ALLERGY TESTING TODAY

Box 10.1 outlines those questions that need to be addressed when evaluating a penicillin or any other drug "allergy" testing protocol.[54] Box 10.2 outlines those essential elements of a drug intolerance history that will influence the diagnostic approach.[54] Penicillin skin testing results, particularly when done with lax criteria for a positive result, correlate poorly with the current reference standard, an oral challenge with a therapeutic dose. Penicillin allergy testing should only be performed on individuals with a history of anaphylaxis, hives, other benign rashes, gastrointestinal symptoms, headaches, other benign symptoms, or unknown reactions associated with the previous use of a penicillin class antibiotic. If there has been no exposure to a penicillin, then testing for penicillin allergy is not indicated, and it is accepted to use penicillins therapeutically, if clinically indicated. Penicillin allergy testing is also not indicated, or useful, if there is concern about a cephalosporin or other nonpenicillin β-lactam

---

BOX 10.1

Nine Essential Questions Needed to Evaluate the Safety, Efficacy, and Clinical Utility of Penicillin Allergy Testing Protocols

1. What is the baseline incidence of new penicillin intolerance reports after therapeutic penicillin use in the population of interest?
2. What is the false-positive rate of any testing, skin testing or in vitro testing, used before administering the reference standard for acute penicillin tolerance, an oral challenge with a therapeutic dose?
3. What is the adverse reaction rate associated with any skin testing used?
4. What is the serious oral challenge reaction rate?
5. How long does the testing procedure take and how much does it cost?
6. What is the incidence of new penicillin intolerance reports after therapeutic penicillin use in test-negative individuals?
7. In individuals with new penicillin intolerance reports, what is the new IgE-mediated resensitization rate?
8. How does the penicillin allergy testing protocol alter the spectrum of antibiotics used in the tested subjects?
9. How does the penicillin allergy testing protocol affect overall healthcare utilization and morbidity in tested subjects?

> **BOX 10.2**
> **The Three Essential Elements of a Drug Intolerance Entry in the Electronic Health Record**
>
> 1. Date of the index adverse reaction
> 2. Time to onset of the index adverse reaction after the first dose of the last course
> 3. Specific clinical characteristics of the index adverse reaction (note one or more of the following in as much detail as possible)
>   a. Anaphylaxis or shortness of breath
>   b. Hives
>   c. Other benign rashes
>   d. Gastrointestinal symptoms
>   e. Other benign symptoms
>   i. Headaches
>   ii. Cough
>   iii. Others
>   iv. Unknown
>   f. SCARs (serious cutaneous adverse drug reactions) or other serious systemic symptoms
>   i. DRESS (drug reaction with eosinophilia and systemic symptoms)
>   ii. SJS (Stevens-Johnson syndrome)
>   iii. TEN (toxic epidermal necrolysis)
>   iv. Hepatitis
>   v. Nephritis
>   vi. Hemolytic anemia
>   vii. Other severe symptoms
>   1. Angioedema
>   2. Tendon rupture
>   3. Others

intolerance. Do not test for penicillin allergy or rechallenge any individuals with any the following extremely rare events associated with a penicillin exposure: any SCAR, including a drug reaction with eosinophilia and systemic symptoms (DRESS), TEN, and SJS; serious hepatitis; hemolytic anemia; or interstitial nephritis, given our current state of knowledge outside of a clinical trial.

THE SAFETY AND CURRENT INDICATIONS FOR A DIRECT ORAL CHALLENGE TO VERIFY ACUTE PENICILLIN TOLERANCE

The current reference standard test to determine acute penicillin tolerance is an oral challenge with a therapeutic dose of penicillin.[14] Any clinically significant IgE-mediated penicillin allergy would result in hives or some other objective systemic allergic reaction starting within 1 h of such an exposure. Any clinically significant underlying antipenicillin T cell–mediated hypersensitivity would result in a delayed-onset rash within the next 5 days. Any clinically significant propensity to develop an IgG-mediated serum sickness because of preformed antipenicillin IgG would result in delayed-onset rash, fever, and possibly joint pain over the next 2 days. Penicillin skin testing is essentially done to minimize the number of serious acute IgE-mediated oral challenge reactions and is not very clinically useful in identifying T cell–mediated or IgG-mediated reactions. The history of the index reaction to the penicillin guides the diagnostic approach. Individuals with a history of hives, other benign rashes, gastrointestinal upset, headaches, mild drug fevers without any other systemic symptoms, other benign symptoms, or an unknown history all can undergo direct oral amoxicillin challenge with 1 h of observation. The Australasian Society of Clinical Immunology and Allergy adopted this approach in their 2016 consensus statement on the assessment of patients with penicillin allergy.[55]

In 2016, a landmark Canadian study evaluated 818 sequential unselected children with a history of amoxicillin "allergy" manifest primarily by rashes associated with amoxicillin use with direct oral amoxicillin challenge.[16] Anaphylaxis was not excluded per protocol, but none of the children presented with a history of anaphylaxis. The oral amoxicillin challenge was delivered in two steps: weight adjusted 50 mg/kg to a maximum of 1.5 g, 10% (55–150 mg) as a first dose and then 20 min later the remaining 90% (545–1350 mg), with 1 h of observation after the second dose. There were only 17 (2.1%) children who had an acute reaction, all mild, and 31 (3.8%) who developed delayed-onset reactions, again all mild. The 17 acute challenge positive children were then penicillin skin tested 2–3 months later with PPL and benzylpenicillin and only 1 (5.6%) was positive.

Challenge with oral amoxicillin 250 mg, with 1 h of observation, is adequate to determine acute penicillin tolerance.[14,56] Amoxicillin is used because there are rare individuals with clinically IgE-mediated allergy specifically directed at the amoxicillin side chain, and amoxicillin accounts for the vast majority of all penicillin class antibiotic exposures in both North America and Europe. The oral amoxicillin dose may be adjusted down, typically to about 125 mg, for individuals under age 4. An oral amoxicillin challenge in properly selected individuals is a safe procedure. There were no cases of fatal anaphylaxis associated with oral amoxicillin use in a population exposed to 100 million treatment courses over a 35-year period.[4]

When performing oral amoxicillin challenges, it is necessary to have trained individuals in attendance, able to treat mild reactions with antihistamines and any signs or symptoms of systemic anaphylaxis with intramuscular epinephrine. The risks associated with a direct oral amoxicillin challenge in properly selected patients are in line with the risks associated with oral food challenges and are much lower than the risks associated with aspirin desensitizations done for nonsteroidal antiinflammatory drug–associated respiratory disease, procedures commonly done in the outpatient setting. Delayed reactions can be reported by the patient from home if they occur and then treated if needed. Subjective reactions are often more common than objective reactions during acute oral challenges, and it is important to document objective signs of an IgE-mediated allergy before calling a challenge positive.[56]

PENICILLIN SKIN TESTING BEFORE ORAL CHALLENGE

If there is a history of anaphylaxis or shortness of breath associated with the first dose of the last penicillin exposure, the probability of having positive allergy testing approximately doubles, with higher rates again noted if the time since the index reaction is shorter.[12] There may be decay of true IgE-mediated allergy to penicillin over time, although the kinetics of this process is not well established.[1] Much of the European literature on penicillin allergy testing comes from national centers that concentrate on studying the most severe reactions, often soon after their anaphylaxis episodes.[1] This helps explain the very high rate of positive test and challenge results they note, which are not seen in the general population.

I recommend that individuals with any history of anaphylaxis or shortness of breath associated with their last penicillin exposure undergo penicillin skin testing before the oral amoxicillin challenge, if they are skin test negative. Both puncture and intradermal skin testing should be done with 6×10^{-5} M PPL. The use of native penicillin and other minor determinants is optional, and the additional risk of false-positive skin testing must be weighed against the small potential benefit of fewer oral challenge reactions. Puncture testing should always be done before intradermal testing to identify those rare individuals who are extremely allergic to penicillin. Intradermal testing should be done with 0.01–0.02 mL of PPL. Both puncture and intradermal testing should be read at 20 min, and the mean diameter of the wheal needs to be greater than or equal to 5 mm with flare greater than wheal for a positive

result.[46,56,57] Skin test negative individuals then need to have an oral amoxicillin 250 mg challenge with 1 h of observation to confirm both acute and delayed tolerance.

The amount of PPL used and the size of the skin test result are considered to be positive matters significantly because too low of a threshold will result in many more false-positive skin test results, increased patient morbidity, and the additional time and expense of unneeded oral desensitization procedures. In the military recruit study from 1963, 0.05–0.07 mL of 6×10^{-5} M PPL was used, with 8 mm of wheal considered positive.[48] In the venereal disease study from 1964, 0.05 mL of 6×10^{-5} M PPL was used, with 12 mm of wheal considered positive.[49] In the first collaborative clinical trial in 1977, 0.01–0.03 mL of 6×10^{-5} M PPL was used, and a wheal at least three times the size of the control wheal was considered positive.[50] In the second collaborative clinical trial in 1992, 0.01 mL of 1×10^{-6} M PPL (octa-benzylpenicilloyl-octalysine, MW about 3800) was used, with a class I (4–6 mm) wheal considered positive.[51] In the Pre-Pen package insert, a bleb of 3 mm is recommended, assuming the volume is not specified, and a positive result is considered to be at least 5–15 mm or more of wheal with flare greater than wheal.[57] If only 3 mm of wheal is considered a positive result, then females are much more likely to be falsely labeled as skin test positive.[58] The major risk of too low of a threshold for a positive test result is not anaphylaxis from an oral challenge, but continued unnecessary avoidance of penicillins when clinically indicated. Penicillin allergy testing can be safely done in the outpatient setting, in children and pregnant women, and throughout the hospital.[37,59–68] Single nucleotide polymorphisms of HLA-DRA and ZNF300 correlate with skin test positivity to amoxicillin and other penicillins but interestingly not to cephalosporins.[69]

Adverse Reactions Associated With Penicillin Skin Testing

The risk of skin testing associated adverse reactions depends highly on the pretest probability of penicillin-associated anaphylaxis occurring with subsequent penicillin exposures. The greatest risk is when there has been recently well-documented penicillin-associated anaphylaxis or shortness of breath. In a group of 1710 individuals who were penicillin allergy tested at the Mayo Clinic between 1992 and 1999, there were systemic reactions associated with skin testing noted in 2.3% of the test positive subjects and in 0.12% of all subjects tested.[70] A French group in 2006, who used very high concentrations of amoxicillin and ampicillin, up to 25 mg/mL, for intradermal testing, reported much higher rates of serious acute adverse reactions: 13 (8.8%) of 147 (14.7%) skin test positive individuals of a total of 998 tested.[71] This was a relatively unique cohort tested at a specialized national drug allergy center and included a very high fraction of individuals with relatively recent index reactions of anaphylaxis. More recent studies have noted extremely low rates of skin testing–associated adverse reactions.[56] The take-home lessons are to always perform puncture testing before intradermal testing in high-risk individuals, never use more than 0.02 mL of 0.01 M penicillin minor determinant skin test reagents, and do not perform any intradermal testing on individuals with any positive puncture test results.

COMMERCIALLY AVAILABLE ANTIPENICILLIN IGE BLOOD ALLERGY TESTS ARE NOT CURRENTLY CLINICALLY USEFUL

The currently commercially available antipenicillin IgE blood allergy tests are not useful in identifying skin test negative individuals who will have positive oral challenges.[72] In a prospective convenience sample of 150 individuals with a history of penicillin allergy, 6 (4%) had positive penicillin skin test results, 4 (2.7%) had positive antipenicillin IgE blood allergy test results, and 3 (2%) individuals had negative skin test results and positive oral challenge results. None of the oral challenge positive individuals was antipenicillin IgE blood allergy test positive.[73] Using antipenicillin IgE blood allergy tests, particularly in individuals with high total IgE levels, can result in significantly more individuals falsely being given a diagnosis of penicillin allergy and then needlessly avoiding penicillins, with its attendant morbidity, partially because of false identification of IgE directed against phenylethylamine with a benzyl group.[74]

RESENSITIZATION

About 3% of all subsequent therapeutic courses of penicillin class antibiotics in penicillin allergy test negative individuals will result in a new entry in the drug intolerance field of the EHR.[50,53] Developing a new clinically significant IgE-mediated penicillin allergy after a negative penicillin allergy test is still very rare. In 2003 we reported that only about 1 of 33 penicillin-"allergic" individuals who were initially penicillin skin test negative, had received at least one course of a therapeutic penicillin, and noted a new adverse reaction were then penicillin skin test positive on retesting.[75]

DESENSITIZATION

If an individual is penicillin allergy test positive and needs penicillin for a life-threatening infection, then oral desensitization is a safe and effective way to proceed.[76] Oral penicillin desensitization can be safely performed in the outpatient clinic or in a nonmonitored hospital bed. When performing an oral penicillin desensitization, it is necessary to have trained individuals in attendance, able to treat mild reactions with antihistamines and any signs or symptoms of systemic anaphylaxis with intramuscular adrenaline. See Table 10.1 for a standard 12-step oral penicillin desensitization protocol. The starting oral dose of 0.25 mg is about three times the amount of penicillin in an intradermal skin test using 0.02 mL of 3.725 mg/mL, or 0.01 M, penicillin G. An oral penicillin desensitization, with a final dose of at least 500 mg, should be performed before the use of any parenteral penicillin. If an oral challenge is performed, and an individual has an acute objective reaction and a therapeutic penicillin is acutely needed, after the challenge reaction has been treated and the patient stabilized, it is accepted to proceed immediately with the therapeutic penicillin use because the individual has essentially been acutely

TABLE 10.1		
12-Step Oral Penicillin Desensitization Protocol Based on a 500 mg Final Penicillin Therapeutic Dose		
Step	**Dose (mg)**	**Time (min)**
1	0.25	0
2	0.5	15
3	1.0	30
4	2.0	45
5	4.0	60
6	8.0	75
7	15.625	90
8	31.25	105
9	62.5	120
10	125	135
11	250	150
12	500	165

Total time = 180 min (3 h).

If a parenteral penicillin is needed, administer it half an hour after the completion of the oral desensitization protocol and then observe at least 1 h after the parenteral dose. Never allow more than three half-lives of the penicillin to expire before additional penicillin dosing to maintain desensitization.

desensitized. If the penicillin allergy testing is done in advance of need, and more than five half-lives of the penicillin have passed, then repeat the penicillin skin testing before any future therapeutic penicillin exposure. If the skin testing is negative on retesting, give an oral challenge again. If the repeat penicillin skin testing is positive, then proceed directly with a 12-step oral penicillin desensitization.

CONCLUSIONS

Most penicillin-associated adverse drug reactions are not immunologically mediated or reproducible on rechallenge. Most individuals with benign histories of penicillin "allergy" can have their clinical tolerance of penicillins verified by a single-dose oral amoxicillin challenge. Only a small minority will have true IgE-mediated penicillin allergy or a clinically significant T cell–mediated delayed-type hypersensitivity. An unverified penicillin "allergy" is a worldwide public health risk and malady.[77-79] Avoiding β-lactam antibiotics in patients with β-lactam "allergies" results in more clinical therapeutic failures.[80] Most patients believe drug challenges are useful and would recommend similar challenges to others.[81] Multiple step challenges do not appear to confer any added safety over single test doses.[82] There will be new penicillin-associated adverse reactions associated with about 3% of all future therapeutic penicillin exposures in oral challenge negative individuals, but only a small minority of these new reactions will be immunologically mediated. Avoiding unnecessary penicillin use is still essential to help reduce future reactions. All individuals with an unverified penicillin "allergy" should undergo confirmatory testing, with the greatest benefit seen in those using the most healthcare.

REFERENCES

1. Joint Task Force on Practice Parameters; American Academy of Allergy, Asthma, and Immunology; American College of Allergy, Asthma, and Immunology; Joint Council of Allergy, Asthma, and Immunology. Drug allergy: an updated practice parameter. *Ann Allergy Asthma Immunol.* 2010;105. 259–273e1-78.
2. Gerace KS, Karlin E, Mckinnon E, Phillips E. Varying penicillin allergy testing practices in the United States: a time for consensus. *J Allergy Clin Immunol Pract.* 2015;3:791–793.
3. Feinberg SM, Feinberg AR. Allergy to penicillin. *JAMA.* 1956;160:778–779.
4. Lee P, Shanson D. Results of a UK survey of fatal anaphylaxis after oral amoxicillin. *J Antimicrobial Chemotherapy.* 2007;60:1172–1179.
5. Johannes CB, Ziyadeh N, Seeger JD, et al. Incidence of allergic reactions associated with antibacterial use in a large, managed care organization. *Drug Saety.* 2007;30:705–713.
6. Macy E, Contreras R. Healthcare utilization and serious infection prevalence associated with penicillin "allergy" in hospitalized patients: a cohort study. *J Allergy Clin Immunol.* 2014;133:790–796.
7. http://www.choosingwisely.org/aaaai-releases-second-list-of-tests-and-procedures-that-are-overused-to-diagnose-and-treat-allergies-asthma-and-immunologic-diseases/.
8. http://www.cdc.gov/getsmart/week/downloads/getsmart-penicillin-factsheet.pdf.
9. Barlam TF, Cosgrove SE, Abbo LM, et al. Implementing an antibiotic stewardship program: guidelines by the infectious diseases Society of America and the Society for Healthcare Epidemiology of America. *Clin Infect Dis.* 2016;62(10):e51–e77. http://dx.doi.org/10.1093/cid/ciw118.
10. Macy E, Contreras R. Adverse reactions associated with oral and parenteral cephalosporin use: a retrospective population-based analysis. *J Allergy Clin Immunol.* 2015;135:745–752.e5.
11. Macy E, Ho NJ. Multiple drug intolerance syndrome: prevalence, clinical characteristics, and management. *Ann Allergy Asthma Immunol.* 2012;108:88–93.
12. Macy E, Schatz M, Lin C, Poon KWT. The falling rate of positive penicillin skin tests from 1995 to 2007. *Perm J.* 2009;13:12–18.
13. Harandian F, Pham D, Ben-Shoshan M. Positive penicillin allergy testing results: a systematic review and meta-analysis of papers published from 2010 through 2015. *Postgrad Med.* 2016. http://dx.doi.org/10.1080/00325481.2106.1191319.
14. Bousquet PJ, Pipet A, Bousquet-Rouanet L, Demoly P. Oral challenges are needed in the diagnosis of β-lactam hypersensitivity. *Clin Exp Allergy.* 2008;38:185–190.
15. Caubet JC, Kaiser L, Lemaitre B, et al. The role of penicillin in benign skin rashes in childhood; a prospective study based on drug rechallenge. *J Allergy Clin Immunol.* 2011;127:218–222.
16. Mill C, Primeau MH, Medoff E, et al. Assessing the diagnostic properties of a graded oral provocative challenge for the diagnosis of immediate and nonimmediate reactions to amoxicillin in children. *JAMA Pediatr.* 2016;170:e160033.
17. Grossman CM. The first use of penicillin in the United States. *Ann Intern Med.* 2008;149:135–136.
18. Criep LH. Allergy to penicillin. *JAMA.* 1944;126:429–430.
19. Gordon EJ. Delayed serum sickness reaction to penicillin. *JAMA.* 1946;131:727–730.
20. Farrington J, Riley K, Olansky S. Untoward reactions and cutaneous testing in penicillin therapy. *South Med J.* 1948;4:614–620.
21. Parker CW, Shapiro J, Kern M, Eisen HN. Hypersensitivity to penicillenic acid derivatives in human beings with penicillin allergy. *J Exp Med.* 1962;115:821–838.

22. Levine BB, Redmond AP, Voss HE. Penicilloyl-polylysine skin tests and allergies. *JAMA.* 1966;197:313–322.

23. Schnyder B, Pichler WJ. Skin and laboratory tests in amoxicillin- and penicillin-induced morbilliform skin eruption. *Clin Exp Allergy.* 2000;30:590–595.

24. Rozieres A, Hennino A, Rodet K, et al. Detection and quantification of drug-specific T cells in penicillin allergy. *Allergy.* 2009;64:534–542.

25. Andre MC, Silva R, Filipe PL, Lopes A, de Almeida LMS. Systemic contact allergy to penicillin after prick and intradermal tests. *Ann Allergy Asthma Immunol.* 2011;106:174–175.

26. Bommarito L, Zisa G, Delrosso G, Farinelli P, Galimberti M. A case of acute generalized exanthemetous pustulosis due to amoxicillin-clavulanate with multiple positivity to beta-lactam patch testing. *Eur Ann Allergy Clin Immunol.* 2013;45:178–180.

27. Chaabane A, Fredj NB, Chadly Z, Boughattas NA, Aouam K. Fixed drug eruption; a selective reaction to amoxicillin. *Therapie.* 2013;68:183–185.

28. Barbaud AM, Bene MC, Schmutz JL, et al. Role of delayed cellular hypersensitivity and adhesion molecules in amoxicillin-induced morbilliform rashes. *Arch Dermatol.* 1997;133:481–486.

29. Clark BM, Kotti GH, Shah AD, Conger NG. Severe serum sickness reaction to oral and intramuscular penicillin. *Pharmacotherapy.* 2006;26:705–708.

30. Tatum AJ, Ditto AM, Patterson R. Severe serum sickness-like reaction to oral penicillin drugs: three case reports. *Ann Allergy Asthma Immunol.* 2001;86:330–334.

31. Arndt PA. Drug-induced immune hemolytic anemia: the last 30 years of changes. *Immunohematology.* 2014;30:44–54.

32. Dantes R, Hicks LA, Cohen J, et al. Association between outpatient antibiotic prescribing practices and community-associated *Clostridium difficile* infection. *Open Forum Infect Dis.* 2015;2:ofv113. http://dx.doi.org/10.1093/ofid/ofv113.

33. Tune BM. Nephrotoxicity of beta-lactam antibiotics: mechanisms and strategies for prevention. *Pediatr Nephrol.* 1997;11:768–772.

34. Maxwell D, Szwed JJ, Wahle W, Kleit SA. Ampicillin nephropathy. *JAMA.* 1974;230:586–587.

35. McCormick H, Tomaka N, Baggett S, et al. Comparison of acute renal injury associated with intermittent and extended infusion piperacillin/tazobactam. *Am J Health-Syst Pharm.* 2015;72(suppl 1):s25–s30.

36. Kim SH, Saide K, Farrell J, et al. Characterization of amoxicillin- and clavulanic acid-specific T cells in patients with amoxicillin-clavulanate-induced liver injury. *Hepatology.* 2015;62:887–899.

37. Stern RS. Exanthematous drug eruptions. *N Engl J Med.* 2012;366:2492–2501.

38. Macy E, Poon KWT. Self-reported antibiotic allergy incidence and prevalence: age and sex effects. *Am J Med.* 2009;122:778.e1–e7.

39. Lee GC, Reveles KR, Attridge RT, et al. Outpatient antibiotic prescribing in the United States: 2000 to 2010. *BMC Medicine.* 2014;12:96.

40. Silverman S, Localio R, Apter AJ. Association between chronic urticaria and self-reported penicillin allergy. *Ann Allergy Asthma Immunol.* 2016;116:317–320.

41. Hocqueloux L, Guinard J, Buret J, Causse X, Guigon A. Do penicillins really increase the frequency of a rash when given during Epstein-Barr virus primary infection? *CID.* 2013;57:1661–1662.

42. Chovel-Sella A, Tov AB, Lahav E, et al. Incidence of rash after amoxicillin treatment in children with infectious mononucleosis. *Pediatrics.* 2013;131:e1424–e1427.

43. Neftel KA, Walti M, Schulthess HK, Gubler J. Adverse reactions following intravenous penicillin-G relate to degradation of the drug in vitro. *Klinische Wochenschrift.* 1984;62:25–29.

44. Yocum RR, Waxman DJ, Rasmussen JR, Strominger JL. Mechanism of penicillin action: penicillin and substrate bind covalently to the same active site serine in two bacterial D-alanine carboxypeptidases. *Proc Natl Acad Sci USA.* 1979;76:2730–2734.

45. Ariza A, Garzon D, Abanades DR, et al. Protein haptenation by amoxicillin: high resolution mass spectrometry analysis and identification of target proteins in serum. *J Proteomics.* 2012;77:504–520.

46. Macy E, Richter PK, Falkoff R, Zeiger RS. Skin testing with penicilloate and penilloate prepared by an improved method: amoxicillin oral challenge in patients with negative skin test responses to penicillin reagents. *J Allergy Clin Immunol.* 1997;100:586–591.

47. Medical News. Skin test developed to test allergy to penicillin. *JAMA.* 1962;182:37–38.

48. Rytel MW, Klion FM, Arlander TR, Miller LF. Detection of penicillin hypersensitivity with penicilloyl-polylysine. *JAMA.* 1963;186:894–898.

49. Brown BC, Price EV, Moore MB. Penicilloyl-polylysine as an intradermal test of penicillin sensitivity. *JAMA.* 1964;189:599–604.

50. Green GR, Rosenblum AH, Sweet LC. Evaluation of penicillin hypersensitivity: value of clinical history and skin testing with penicilloyl-polylysine and penicillin G. *J Allergy Clin Immunol.* 1977;60:339–345.

51. Sogn DD, Evans III R, Shepherd GM, et al. Results of the National Institute of Allergy and Infectious Diseases collaborative clinical trial to test the predictive value of skin testing with major and minor penicillin derivatives in hospitalized adults. *Arch Intern Med.* 1992;152:1025–1032.

52. Macy E, Burchette RJ. Oral antibiotic adverse reactions after penicillin testing: multi-year follow-up. *Allergy.* 2002;57:1151–1158.

53. Macy E, Ho NJ. Adverse reactions associated with therapeutic antibiotic use after penicillin skin testing. *Perm J.* 2011;15:31–37.

54. Blumenthal KG, Park MA, Macy EM. Redesigning the allergy module of the electronic health record. *Ann Allergy Asthma Immunol.* June 14, 2016. pii:S1081-1206(16)30267-8.

55. ASCIA Penicillin allergy consensus statement. http://www.allergy.org.au/members .

56. Macy E, Ngor EW. Safely diagnosing clinically significant penicillin allergy using only penicilloyl-poly-lysine, penicillin, and oral amoxicillin. *J Allergy Clin Immunol Pract.* 2013;1:258–263.

57. http://www.pre-pen.com/PrePen_Package_Insert.pdf.

58. Park M, Matesic D, Markus PJ, Li JT. Female sex as a risk factor for penicillin allergy. *Ann Allergy Asthma Immunol.* 2007;99:54–58.

59. Macy E, Roppe L, Schatz M. Routine penicillin skin testing in hospitalized patients with a history of penicillin allergy. *Perm J.* 2004;8:20–24.

60. Macy E. Penicillin skin testing in pregnant women with a history of penicillin allergy and group B streptococcus colonization. *Ann Allergy Asthma Immunol.* 2006;97:164–168.

61. Fox SJ, Park MA. Penicillin skin testing is a safe and effective tool for evaluating penicillin allergy in the pediatric population. *J Allergy Clin Immunol Pract.* 2014;2:439–444.

62. Philipson EH, Lang DM, Gordon SJ, Burlingame JM, Emery SP, Arroliga ME. Management of group B streptococcus in pregnant women with penicillin allergy. *J Reprod Med.* 2007;52:480–484.

63. Cook DJ, Barbara DW, Singh KE, Dearani JA. Penicillin skin testin in cardiac surgery. *J Thorac Cardiovasc Surg.* 2014;147:1931–1935.

64. Raja AS, Lindsell CJ, Bernstein JA, Codispoti CD, Moellman JJ. The use of penicillin skin testing to assess the prevalence of penicillin allergy in an emergency department setting. *Ann Emerg Med.* 2009;54:72–77.

65. Arroliga ME, Radojicic C, Gordon SM, et al. A prospective observational study of the effect of penicillin skin testing on antibiotic use in the intensive care unit. *Infect Control Hosp Epidemiol.* 2003;24:347–350.

66. Wall GC, Peters L, Leaders CB, Wille JA. Pharmacist-managed service providing penicillin allergy skin tests. *Am J Health-Syst Pharm.* 2004;61:1271–1275.

67. Frigas E, Park MA, Narr BJ, et al. Preoperative evaluation of patients with history of allergy to penicillin: comparison of 2 models of practice. *Mayo Clin Proc.* 2008;83:651–657.

68. Rimawi RH, Cook PP, Gooch M, et al. The impact of penicillin skin testing on clinical practice and antimicrobial stewardship. *J Hosp Med.* 2013;8:341–345.

69. Gueant LJ, Romano A, Cornejo-Garcia JA, et al. HLA-DRA variants predict penicillin allergy in genome-wide fine-mapping genotyping. *J Allergy Clin Immunol.* 2015;135:253–259.

70. Valyasevi MA, Van Dellen RG. Frequency of systemic reactions to penicillin skin tests. *Ann Allergy Asthma Immunol.* 2000;85:363–365.

71. Minh HCB, Bousquet PJ, Fontaine C, Kvedariene V, Demoly P. Systemic reactions during skin tests with lactams; a risk factor analysis. *J Allergy Clin Immunol.* 2006;117:466–468.

72. Decuyper II , Ebo DG, Uyttebroek AP, et al. Quantification of specific IgE antibodies in immediate drug hypersensitivity: More shortcomings than potentials? *Clinica Chimica Acta.* 2016;460:184–189.

73. Macy E, Goldberg B, Poon KWT. Use of commercial anti-penicillin-IgE FEIAs to diagnose penicillin allergy. *Ann Allergy Asthma Immunol.* 2010;105:136–141.

74. Johansson SGO, Adedoyin J, van Hage M, Gronneberg R, Nopp A. False-positive penicillin immunoassay: an unnoticed common problem. *J Allergy Clin Immunol.* 2013;132:235–237.

75. Macy E, Mangat R, Burchette RJ. Penicillin skin testing in advance of need: Multiyear follow-up in 568 test result-negative subjects exposed to oral penicillins. *J Allergy Clin Immunol.* 2003;111:1111–1115.

76. Stark BJ, Earl HS, Gross GN, Lumry WR, Goodman EL, Sullivan TJ. Acute and chronic desensitization of penicillin-allergic patients using oral penicillin. *J Allergy Clin Immunol.* 1987;79:523–532.

77. van Dijk SM, Gardarsdottir H, Wassenberg MWM, Oosterheert JJ, de Groot MCH, Rockmann H. The high impact of penicillin allergy registration in hospitalized patients. *J Allergy Clin Immunol Pract.* 2016;4(5).

78. Solensky R. Penicillin allergy as a public health measure. *J Allergy Clin Immunol.* 2014;133:797–798.

79. Lang DM. The malady of penicillin allergy. *Ann Allergy Asthma Immunol.* 2016;116:269–270.

80. Jeffres MN, Narayanan PP, Shuster JE, Schramm GE. Consequences of avoiding β-lactams in patients with β-lactams allergies. *J Allergy Clin Immunol.* 2016;137:1148–1153.

81. Gomes ER, Kvedariene V, Demoly P, Bousquet PJ. Patients' satisfaction with diagnostic drug provocation tests and perception of its usefulness. *Int Arch Allergy Immunol.* 2011;156:333–338.

82. Iammatteo M, Blumenthal KG, Saff R, Long AA, Banerji A. Safety and outcomes of test doses for the evaluation of adverse drug reactions: a 5-year retrospective review. *J Allergy Clin Immunol Pract.* 2014;2:768–774.

CHAPTER 11

Cephalosporin Allergy

ANTONINO ROMANO, MD • ROCCO LUIGI VALLUZZI, MD •
FRANCESCO GAETA, MD, PHD

KEY POINTS

- Cephalosporins are among the most commonly used antibiotics in the treatment of routine infections, and their use is increasing.
- Cephalosporins can cause a range of hypersensitivity reactions, from mild, delayed-onset maculopapular exanthemas to life-threatening anaphylaxis.
- Structures of the R1 and R2 side chains are immunologically important and similarities in these structures may determine cross-reactivity among cephalosporins and even between penicillins and cephalosporins.

INTRODUCTION

Cephalosporins are among the most commonly used antibiotics in the treatment of routine infections, and their use is increasing.[1-4] In particular, cephalosporins represented 11.4% of all antibiotic outpatient prescriptions in Europe in 2009.[1]

Cephalosporins can cause a range of hypersensitivity reactions, from mild, delayed-onset maculopapular exanthemas to life-threatening anaphylaxis.[5-10] According to Johansson et al.,[11] only when a definite immunologic mechanism has been demonstrated—either antibody mediated or T cell mediated—these reactions should be classified as allergic. The latter ones can be further classified according to the Coombs and Gell classification system into four types: I (mediated by drug-specific IgE antibodies), II (cytotoxic), III (mediated by drug-specific IgG or IgM antibodies), and IV (mediated by drug-specific T lymphocytes).

Clinically, hypersensitivity reactions to cephalosporins can be classified as immediate or nonimmediate according to the time interval between the last drug administration and their onset.[12] Immediate reactions occur within the first hour after the last drug administration and may be induced by an IgE-mediated mechanism.[12,13] Nonimmediate reactions are those occurring at least 1 h after the initial drug administration in sensitized patients, but usually after several hours or even days,[12,13] and are often associated with a delayed IgG-mediated or T cell—dependent mechanism.[12-15]

This chapter takes into account exclusively IgE- and T cell—mediated reactions.

CEPHALOSPORIN ALLERGENIC DETERMINANTS

Cephalosporins share the four-membered β-lactam ring with penicillins but differ in that the five-membered thiazolidine ring of penicillin is replaced by a six-membered sulfur-containing dihydrothiazine ring (Fig. 11.1). Other differences concern their two side-chain structures (R1 and R2) and the chemistry of their degradation and transformation. Under physiologic conditions, the cephalosporin β-lactam ring opens, and its carbonyl moiety binds a protein, forming the cephalosporoyl determinant,[16] which tends to undergo extensive fragmentation, probably including the cleavage of the dihydrothiazine ring.[17-19] Cephalosporin side-chain structures usually survive such fragmentation and may be responsible for sensitization.[20-24] In fact, it has been demonstrated that antibodies to structures of the R1 side chain are immunologically important and that similarities or identities in such structures may determine a cross-reactivity among cephalosporins and even between penicillins and cephalosporins.[20,21,23,24] Specifically, Antunez et al.[23] performed in vitro studies in cephalosporin-allergic subjects, demonstrating that the side chain at the R1 position is crucial for recognition. In effect, cross-reactivity among cefuroxime, ceftriaxone, cefotaxime, cefodizime, and ceftazidime, as well as between cefaclor and cephalexin and between these two aminocephalosporins and aminopenicillins (e.g., ampicillin and amoxicillin), has been observed.[8,23,25-28] Indeed, cefuroxime, ceftriaxone, cefotaxime, and cefodizime, together with cefepime, share a methoxyimino group in their R1 side chains (Fig. 11.2).[29,30] Moreover, ceftriaxone, cefotaxime,

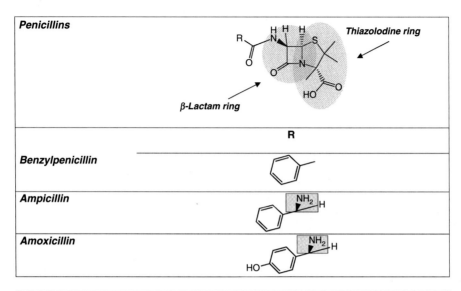

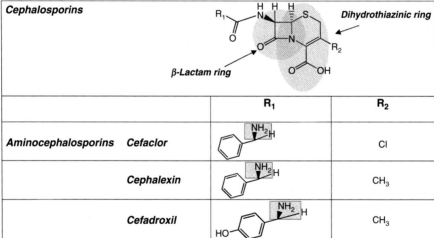

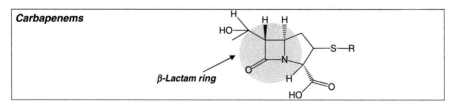

FIG. 11.1 Chemical structures of penicillins, cephalosporins, carbapenems, and aztreonam, with the amino group of ampicillin, amoxicillin, and aminocephalosporins highlighted in gray.

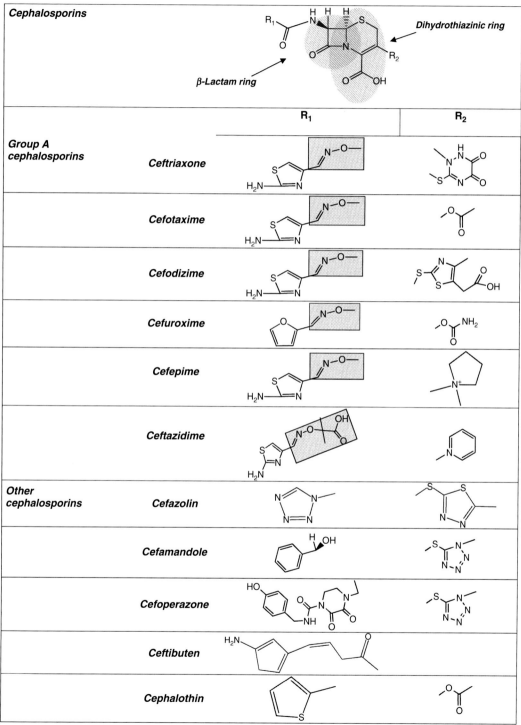

FIG. 11.2 Chemical structures of cephalosporins, with the methoxyimino group and the alkoxyimino group highlighted in gray.

cefodizime, and cefepime have an identical R1 side chain (Fig. 11.2). Ceftazidime has an R1 side chain that is slightly different from those of the aforementioned cephalosporins. Specifically, the ceftazidime R1 side chain has an alkoxyimino group that has greater steric hindrance than the methoxyimino moiety (Fig. 11.2).[29] Cefaclor and cephalexin share identical R1 side chains that contain an amino group and are identical or similar to those of ampicillin and amoxicillin (Fig. 11.1).

Less frequently, R2 side chains also play a role in sensitization, and cross-reactivity among cephalosporins may be influenced by R2 side-chain recognition.[20,31] In one study concerning 102 cephalosporin-allergic subjects,[28] one participant had reacted to cefoperazone and was skin-test positive to both cefoperazone and cefamandole, which share an identical R2 side chain with an N-methyl-tetrazole-thiol group (Fig. 11.2). In another study,[8] however, no significant cross-reactivity between cefotaxime and cephalothin was found, despite identical R2 side chains (Fig. 11.2).

Other specificities of antibody reactivity against cephalosporin molecules are possible. Small moieties shared by cephalosporins and penicillins can also be recognized. In one in vitro study,[32] a population of IgE antibodies toward a methylene group present in cephalothin and benzylpenicillin side chains (Figs. 11.1 and 11.2) was identified in the sera of allergic patients. In addition to the methylene group, recognition regarded neighboring structures, including the amide group, and extended weakly to the β-lactam ring.

In subjects with immediate hypersensitivity to cefaclor, in vitro studies[33] have demonstrated an IgE antibody reactivity with the entire molecule, specifically with both ends of the cefaclor molecule, i.e., the side-chain group (R1 substituent) and the ring structures with the attached R2 group (Fig. 11.1). In this regard, there are cases of immediate hypersensitivity to cephalosporins, such as cefazolin,[34-38] cefuroxime,[39,40] cefixime,[41] ceftriaxone,[42,43] ceftazidime,[44] cefodizime,[45] ceftibuten,[46] and cefepime,[47] in which selective responses have been confirmed by the negativity of skin tests (STs), serum-specific IgE assays (SsIgEs), and controlled challenges with other β-lactams, including alternative cephalosporins. These cases may be explained by the last of the aforesaid patterns of reactivity.

In cephalosporin-allergic subjects, the selective recognition by IgE antibodies of the β-lactam ring seems to be very rare. In one study concerning 98 cephalosporin-allergic subjects,[48] which assessed cross-reactivity between cephalosporins and other β-lactam classes, only one subject was ST positive to all the β-lactams tested, including aztreonam, imipenem-cilastatin, and meropenem; therefore, his IgE antibodies were probably directed against the β-lactam ring, which is shared by all β-lactams.

CLINICAL MANIFESTATIONS

Immediate Reactions

Immediate reactions are usually manifested as urticaria, angioedema, conjunctivitis, rhinitis, bronchospasm, gastrointestinal symptoms, and anaphylactic shock.

As far as anaphylactic reactions to cephalosporins are concerned, some authors suggest that they are rare.[5,7,9,49] Specifically, Tejedor Alonso et al.[49] analyzed the incidence of anaphylaxis among hospitalized patients, reporting four anaphylactic reactions to cephalosporins (two to cefazolin, one to cefotaxime, and one to ceftriaxone) in 104,350 patients. A study[9] investigated the incidence of new reports of cephalosporin-associated "allergy" among all members of the Kaiser Permanente Southern California health plan, from January 1, 2010, through December 31, 2012. There were 622,456 members exposed to 901,908 courses of oral cephalosporins and 326,867 members exposed to 487,630 courses of parenteral cephalosporins over the 3-year study period. Physician-documented cephalosporin-associated anaphylaxis occurred with five oral exposures (95% CI, 1/1,428,571 to 1/96,154) and eight parenteral exposures (95% CI, 1/200,000 to 1/35,971). However, an increasing number of anaphylactic reactions, particularly to ceftriaxone, cefuroxime, cefaclor, and cefazolin, have been reported in the last decade, especially in Europe.[23,26,38,50-56] Specifically, one European study[52] analyzed 333 cases of drug-induced anaphylaxis collected by 59 allergists of the Allergy Vigilance Network from 2002 to 2010 and found that cephalosporins were responsible for 41 cases (12.3%). The most involved cephalosporins were cefuroxime (15 cases) and ceftriaxone (7 cases).

Nonimmediate Reactions

The most common nonimmediate reactions to cephalosporins are maculopapular exanthemas and delayed-appearing urticaria/angioedema;[10,57-60] more rarely, fixed drug eruption, bullous exanthemas, erythema multiforme, exfoliative dermatitis, vasculitis, acute generalized exanthematous pustulosis (AGEP), drug reactions (or rash) with eosinophilia and systemic symptoms (DRESS, also called drug-induced hypersensitivity syndrome—DiHS), Stevens-Johnson syndrome (SJS), and toxic epidermal necrolysis (TEN) can be elicited.[10,59-63]

Regarding SJS/TEN, Papay et al.[61] conducted an analysis to identify drugs that were most associated with these syndromes in the US Food and Drug Administration Adverse Event Reporting System database. Fifty drugs were identified as being associated with SJS/TEN. This included 12 "highly suspect" drugs and 36 "suspect" drugs; 13 of the latter were cephalosporins, mainly ceftriaxone, cefuroxime, ceftazidime, and cephalexin.

DIAGNOSIS

The diagnosis of cephalosporin allergy is based on clinical histories, physical examinations (if signs or symptoms are still present), STs, patch tests (PTs), in vitro tests, and challenges or drug provocation tests (DPTs).

Clinical History

The history of a drug reaction should ascertain the following: the agent responsible for the reaction and the indication for its use; the signs and symptoms involved, to detect severe reactions, such as anaphylaxis and SJS/TEN; the dose and route of the drug concerned; other concurrent medications, especially if they were new or temporary; the timing of the onset of the reaction (from the precipitating dose, as well as from the initiation of the course of therapy); any treatment given and response to such treatment (including the duration of the reaction); and any prior or subsequent history of exposure to the same drug or structurally similar drugs, with or without reactions.[10] However, the identification of a nonimmediate reaction is sometimes difficult because of the heterogeneity of the clinical manifestations, mainly cutaneous symptoms, which can be quite similar to the symptoms of infectious diseases. Moreover, these reactions may be favored by a concomitant viral infection, such as those caused by the human immunodeficiency virus, cytomegalovirus, human herpesvirus 6, or Epstein-Barr virus.[64,65]

Immediate Reactions
Skin testing

According to the European guidelines,[66,67] suspect cephalosporins diluted in normal saline should be employed in skin testing, in addition to the classic penicillin reagents (penicilloyl-poly-L-lysine—PPL, minor determinant mixture—MDM, and benzylpenicillin) and amoxicillin (Fig. 11.3).

In effect, even though STs with cephalosporins are not as well validated as those with penicillins, several studies have demonstrated their usefulness in the diagnosis of immediate reactions to the responsible compounds.[23,26,28,38,48,50,55,68] Specifically, in three European studies involving adults,[26] both children and adults,[23] and children[50] with immediate reactions to cephalosporins, the rates of positive responses to cephalosporin STs were 69.7% (53 of 76 subjects), 30.7% (39 of 127), and 72.1% (31 of 43), respectively. In these studies,[23,26,50] a cephalosporin concentration of 2 mg/mL was used. A European position paper,[69] however, taking into account the results of some studies[58,70,71] stated that "… for cefuroxime, ceftriaxone, cefotaxime, ceftazidime, cefazolin, cephalexin, cefaclor, and cefatrizine, but not cefepime, concentrations up to 20 mg/mL are probably also not irritant and might improve the sensitivity without affecting the specificity." In this regard, a study[38] diagnosed an IgE-mediated hypersensitivity to cefazolin in 19 of 66 cefazolin-exposed patients who had experienced a perioperative anaphylaxis; 12 patients had a positive intradermal test (IDT) at a concentration of up to 2 mg/mL and additional 7 (27%) had positive IDTs at 20 mg/mL.

For injectable cephalosporins, the intravenous form under sterile conditions is used, whereas for noninjectable cephalosporins, the powder contained in capsules or obtained by removing the external layer of tablets with a scalpel can be used. After weighing the powder, solutions are prepared under a laminar flow and sterilized by filtration through single-use devices, as previously described.[26]

The reliability of STs in patients with immediate reactions to cephalosporins is confirmed by the fact that physicians who have performed challenges with cephalosporins to which patients were positive elicited immediate urticarial or anaphylactic reactions.[39,41,43,72] In one study by Yoon et al.,[73] however, 74 (5.2%) of 1421 patients displayed positive responses to preoperative cephalosporin STs at a concentration of 2 mg/mL, but none of them had immediate hypersensitivity reactions after a surgical prophylaxis with the same (or a different) cephalosporin, which was ST positive. Moreover, four patients who suffered generalized urticaria and itching after the cephalosporin administration had negative STs for the corresponding drug.

On the other hand, negative responses to STs with the suspect cephalosporins suggest that the patient does not have specific IgE antibodies to the cephalosporin concerned in its native state. However, the patient could still have IgE antibodies against a metabolite or metabolite—protein complex, and the negative predictive value of cephalosporin skin testing is not well defined. For example, in a study of 76 adults with immediate reactions to cephalosporins,[26] 8 of 13 subjects with negative allergy tests agreed to undergo challenges with the suspect drug,

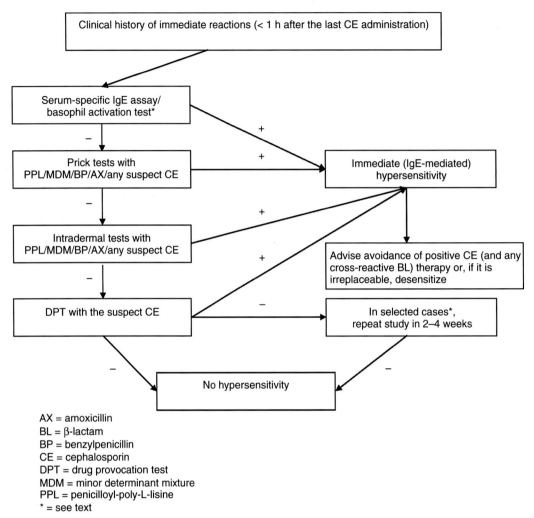

FIG. 11.3 Algorithm for the diagnosis of immediate hypersensitivity reactions to cephalosporins.

AX = amoxicillin
BL = β-lactam
BP = benzylpenicillin
CE = cephalosporin
DPT = drug provocation test
MDM = minor determinant mixture
PPL = penicilloyl-poly-L-lisine
* = see text

and two reacted. Another study[53] assessed 89 adults with suspect perioperative cefuroxime-associated hypersensitivity reactions by performing STs at concentrations up to 0.5 mg/mL, in vitro tests (i.e., cefuroxime SsIgE and histamine release test), and challenges. In this study,[53] 23 (25.8%) of the 89 patients were diagnosed with hypersensitivity to cefuroxime defined as a positive challenge, or, if it was not performed, at least two other positive tests. Specifically, eight patients (34.8%) were positive only on the challenge.

In vitro tests

According to the European guidelines,[66,67,74] in vitro tests are complementary to STs. Moreover, these guidelines[66,67,74] suggest performing in vitro tests before STs in subjects with histories of severe anaphylaxis to reduce the risk of systemic reactions to STs.

The main in vitro tests for evaluating immediate reactions to β-lactams are SsIgEs and flow cytometric basophil activation tests (BATs). The former ones are not commonly used because they are less sensitive than STs and not widely available.[23,26,66] The only commercially available immunoassay is for cefaclor (Immuno-CAP, Thermo Fisher Scientific, Uppsala, Sweden). In three studies,[28,50,51] however, this test proved to be less sensitive than STs, confirming their positivity only in 6 of 12, 3 of 18, and 2 of 8 cephalosporin-allergic subjects, respectively.

Only a few studies have performed investigational assays for IgE to cephalosporins other than cefaclor in samples larger than 20 patients with immediate reactions, who have also undergone cephalosporin STs,[23,26,53] demonstrating that SsIgEs were less sensitive than STs. In these studies,[23,26,53] nevertheless, a few subjects with negative STs and positive SsIgEs were found.

In some studies,[56,75,76] the BAT has been performed for evaluating immediate reactions to cephalosporins, such as cefuroxime, cefazolin, and cefaclor, showing a sensitivity lower than that of STs. The BAT is not widely available, and additional comprehensive studies in large samples are required to further validate the technique and provide a definitive assessment of its sensitivity.

It should be noted that SsIgE and BAT sensitivity decreases more rapidly than that of STs,[77] although lengthy persistence of specific IgE antibodies to cefaclor has been reported.[78]

Drug provocation tests

According to the recommendations of both the American[79] and European[80] guidelines, in selected cases displaying negative results in allergy tests, a DPT with the implicated cephalosporin can be done to establish a firm diagnosis.

It is important to note that negative ST results should be interpreted in light of the time elapsed since the subject's last exposure to the drug

In fact, literature data indicate that in subjects with immediate reactions to β-lactams, STs tend to be positive the less time has elapsed since the clinical reaction.[26,50,68,81] Cephalosporin allergy may be lost over time, as with penicillin allergy.[82] One study[27] evaluated 72 patients with an IgE-mediated hypersensitivity to cephalosporins prospectively over 5 years of follow-up. STs and SsIgEs were repeated 1 year after the first evaluation and, in case of persistent positivity, 3 and 5 years later. Forty-five (62.5%) of the seventy-two subjects became negative; one was lost to follow-up. Therefore, in subjects with immediate reactions to cephalosporins who present negative STs when evaluated more than 6 months after their immediate reactions, the pathogenic mechanism can be clarified by performing challenges with suspect cephalosporins and, in case of negative responses, by administering a full therapeutic course. However, it is advisable to retest such patients after 4 weeks to exclude a possible resensitization after loss of sensitivity.[26,66,67] In fact, resensitization—diagnosed on the basis of renewed ST positivity—has been described in patients retested about 1 month after either positive challenges or negative ones, whether the latter were followed or not by full therapeutic courses.[26,50,68,81]

In particular, Moreno et al.[81] diagnosed an IgE-mediated hypersensitivity to cephalosporins in 59 subjects on the basis of ST positivity; 9 of them were diagnosed with such hypersensitivity in the reevaluation performed 3 weeks after the first negative allergy work-up, including DPTs. In summary, resensitization is possible, although the rate at which this occurs and whether this represents true clinical allergy are not defined.

Nonimmediate Reactions
In vivo testing
The manner in which nonimmediate reactions are evaluated differs significantly between the United States and Europe. In the former, PTs and delayed-reading IDTs are not widely performed. Instead, the most common approach is to diagnose nonimmediate reactions to drugs based on signs and symptoms.[83] In patients with severe reactions, such as TEN, SJS, DRESS/DiHS, and AGEP, cephalosporins are simply avoided. If the nonimmediate reaction involved hives or angioedema, the patient may be evaluated for IgE-mediated allergy to the cephalosporin that caused the reaction, as well as the cephalosporin that is needed in the immediate future. If the patient's past reaction did not involve hives or angioedema and was mild (e.g., maculopapular rash), then a graded challenge to the required cephalosporin can be performed.[10]

The European guidelines[15,67] recommend assessing nonimmediate reactions to β-lactams by both PTs and delayed-reading IDTs. PTs with the suspect β-lactams are usually performed first (i.e., before IDTs) at a concentration of 5% in petrolatum; if positive, IDTs may be avoided.

Delayed-reading IDTs with β-lactams have a higher sensitivity than PTs, with a similar specificity.[58,84,85]

Fig. 11.4 shows an algorithm for in vivo evaluation of mild nonimmediate reactions to cephalosporins, such as urticarial eruptions, angioedematous manifestations, and maculopapular rashes, lasting a few days. This algorithm includes STs with the classic benzylpenicillin reagents, ampicillin, amoxicillin, and the suspect cephalosporin. The aforesaid reagents are tested up to the highest concentrations recommended for evaluating immediate reactions. However, STs with PPL and MDM are scarcely useful in evaluating nonimmediate reactions to β-lactams, especially cephalosporins.[58,84,85] Moreover, delayed-reading IDTs are negative in most patients who experienced mild nonimmediate reactions to cephalosporins.[58] Therefore, considering that

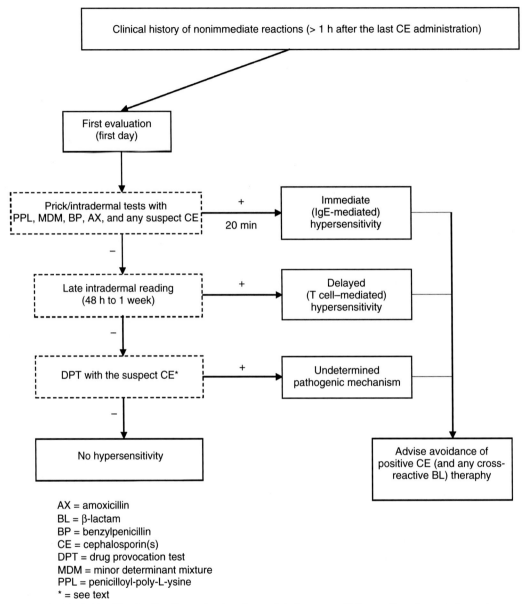

AX = amoxicillin
BL = β-lactam
BP = benzylpenicillin
CE = cephalosporin(s)
DPT = drug provocation test
MDM = minor determinant mixture
PPL = penicilloyl-poly-L-ysine
* = see text

FIG. 11.4 Algorithm for the diagnosis of nonimmediate hypersensitivity reactions to cephalosporins.

IDTs are more sensitive than PTs, the latter may be avoided in such patients.[86]

Subjects who are negative in all of the above tests could undergo DPTs with the suspect cephalosporin. According to the European guidelines,[15,67] an initial dose of one-hundredth of the therapeutic one can be administered. In cases with negative results, 3 days to 1 week later (depending on the time interval between the drug intake and the index adverse reaction), a dose of one-tenth should be given and, if the result is again negative, after the previous time interval, a full dose.

A negative result may not preclude a nonimmediate reaction with a full therapeutic treatment. Indeed, studies of penicillin reactions have documented that some delayed reactions develop only after several days of a full therapeutic dose or in the presence of a concomitant viral infection.[87,88] Thus, there may be certain drug reactions that cannot be elicited with any challenge protocol and will only recur if the drug is subsequently used.[89] However, a multicenter study performed on subjects with either immediate or nonimmediate reactions to β-lactams,[90] mostly penicillins, demonstrated that the negative predictive value of DPTs with single doses of the suspect β-lactam was 94.1%; specifically, 111 of 118 patients tolerated therapeutic courses, with the suspect β-lactams found negative in allergy work-ups.

This algorithm does not advise retesting subjects who had nonimmediate reactions and present negative results in delayed-reading IDTs. In fact, unlike IgE-mediated hypersensitivity, delayed hypersensitivity to β-lactams seems to be a persistent condition.[15]

Regarding severe nonimmediate reactions, in a multicenter study of subjects with these reactions,[62] PTs were first performed with drugs diluted to 1% in petrolatum, and if the results were negative, they were repeated with the drug diluted to 30%. PTs were positive in 46 of 72 patients with DRESS (including two subjects who had reacted to ceftriaxone), 26 of 45 with AGEP (including one subject who had reacted to ceftriaxone), and 4 of 17 with SJS/TEN, with only one recurrence of AGEP. One study[60] evaluated 91 subjects with nonimmediate reactions to cephalosporins, including 2 with DRESS, by performing only PTs with the drugs diluted to 10% in petrolatum. Four patients (4.4%) displayed positive results: one had experienced a DRESS associated with ceftriaxone therapy and three had a maculopapular rash; two of them had reacted to cefoxitin and one to cefazolin.

As far as mild cutaneous reactions to cephalosporins are concerned, in a Finnish study,[57] 12 (4.1%) of the 290 patients with such reactions, mostly exanthemas, were positive to cephalosporin PTs: 4 of 10 to ceftriaxone, 4 of 29 to cefuroxime, 3 of 173 to cephalexin, and 1 of 51 to cefadroxil. Only 1 of the 75 negative patients who underwent DPTs reacted (to cefadroxil). For PTs the drugs were diluted to 20% or 30% in petrolatum and/or normal saline. Another study[58] evaluated 105 adults with mild nonimmediate reactions to cephalosporins according to the European guidelines.[15,67] Six subjects (5.7%) presented positive responses to delayed-reading IDTs with the responsible compounds (three to ceftriaxone, two to cephalexin, and one to cefaclor); three of them were also PT positive (two to ceftriaxone and one to cephalexin). Another patient, who had experienced a local reaction to intramuscular cefodizime, presented an immediate-reading IDT positivity to it. Of the 98

negative subjects, 86 accepted challenges with the suspect cephalosporins and tolerated them.

In vitro tests

According to a European position paper,[74] the lymphocyte transformation test (LTT) and the enzyme-linked immunosorbent spot (ELISpot) assay can be used for evaluating nonimmediate reactions to β-lactams. The LTT measures the proliferation of drug-specific T cells on stimulation with suspect drugs, whereas the ELISpot determines the number of cells that release relevant cytokines and cytotoxic markers after their activation by the culprit drugs or their metabolites. However, very few studies have assessed small samples of subjects with nonimmediate reactions to cephalosporins, such as ceftriaxone, cefuroxime, ceftazidime, and cefazolin, by performing these tests with positive results.[91–93] In particular, Tanvarasethee et al.[93] evaluated 25 patients with maculopapular exanthemas associated with ceftriaxone (20 subjects) or ceftazidime (5 subjects) treatments by performing STs and ELISpot assays for the analysis of IFN-γ-releasing (or IL-5- or IL-10-releasing) cells. The combination of IFN-γ and IL-5 ELISpot assays was more sensitive than STs to diagnose cephalosporin allergy (40% vs. 8%, $P = .008$). Nevertheless, neither American[79] nor European[15,67] guidelines currently recommend this testing.

Moreover, the LTT and its variants are still rather complex procedures, which require skilled personnel and specific experience[94]; thus, they are not routinely used. In any case, to increase their clinical applicability, large-scale studies are needed.

ADMINISTRATION OF ALTERNATIVE β-LACTAMS, INCLUDING CEPHALOSPORINS, IN SUBJECTS ALLERGIC TO CEPHALOSPORINS

Only two studies administered alternative β-lactams that were found to be negative in allergy tests in samples of larger than 20 cephalosporin-allergic subjects.[23,48] In one Spanish study,[23] 2 of the 24 cephalosporin-allergic subjects were positive to penicillin determinants, whereas 22 were negative to them and tolerated benzylpenicillin challenges. Another study[48] evaluated 98 subjects with an IgE-mediated hypersensitivity to cephalosporins, mostly ceftriaxone, ceftazidime, and cefotaxime, by performing STs and SsIgE with penicillins, as well as STs with aztreonam, imipenem/cilastatin, and meropenem. Positive results to penicillins were displayed by 25 subjects (25.5%), including one positive to all reagents tested and another positive to aztreonam. An additional subject, who had experienced an anaphylactic reaction to both ceftazidime and aztreonam, was ST positive to both these β-lactams, which share an identical side chain (Figs. 11.1 and 11.2). Negative subjects, including 10 additional ceftazidime-allergic patients, underwent challenges with amoxicillin, aztreonam, imipenem/cilastatin, and meropenem: only one reacted to imipenem/cilastatin, experiencing an urticarial reaction.

Regarding the administration of alternative cephalosporins to cephalosporin-allergic subjects, a few studies evaluated such subjects using SsIgE and STs with penicillin reagents, as well as with different cephalosporins, including those responsible.[23,25-27,95] Three patterns of reactivity were observed: cross-reactivity with penicillins, cross-reactivity with cephalosporins other than those responsible, and selective reactivity to responsible cephalosporins. In these studies,[23,25-27,95] however, cephalosporin-allergic subjects did not undergo challenges, with alternative cephalosporins found negative in allergy tests. A study[28] assessed 102 cephalosporin-allergic adults by performing SsIgE with cefaclor and STs with different cephalosporins. On the basis of the results of both allergy tests, subjects were classified into four groups: group A (73 subjects), positive to one or more of ceftriaxone, cefuroxime, cefotaxime, cefepime, cefodizime, and ceftazidime; group B (13 subjects), positive to aminocephalosporins (i.e., cephalexin, cefaclor, and cefadroxil); group C (7 patients), positive to cephalosporins other than those belonging to the aforementioned groups; and group D (9 participants), positive to cephalosporins belonging to two different groups. The last group of subjects displayed different patterns of positivity, most of which cannot be explained by either similar or identical side chains or by the common β-lactam ring. These cases suggest that coexisting sensitivities are possible, and thus the risk of positive allergy test responses with alternative cephalosporins is not connected only with the structural similarities among their side-chain determinants.

In this study,[28] group A subjects underwent challenges with cefaclor, cefazolin, and ceftibuten; group B participants with cefuroxime axetil, ceftriaxone, cefazolin, and ceftibuten; and group C and D subjects with some of the aforementioned cephalosporins selected on the basis of their patterns of positivity. A total of 326 challenges with alternative cephalosporins (ceftibuten in 101, cefazolin in 96, cefaclor in 82, and cefuroxime axetil and ceftriaxone in 22 subjects) were well tolerated. Therefore, in assessing subjects with an IgE-mediated hypersensitivity to cephalosporins, negative results in skin testing with alternative β-lactams, including cephalosporins other than those responsible, seem to be a reliable indicator of tolerability.

Similar studies in large samples of subjects with a T cell—mediated hypersensitivity to cephalosporins are lacking.

In rare cases, a patient requires the same cephalosporin or an alternative β-lactam, to which there is evidence of IgE-mediated allergy. A formal desensitization protocol should be performed in this situation.[79,96]

ABBREVIATIONS

AGEP   Acute generalized exanthematous pustulosis
BAT   Basophil activation test
DiHS   Drug-induced hypersensitivity syndrome
DPT   Drug provocation test
DRESS   Drug reaction with eosinophilia and systemic symptoms
ELISpot   Enzyme-linked immunosorbent spot
IDT   Intradermal test
LTT   Lymphocyte transformation test
MDM   Minor determinant mixture
PPL   Penicilloyl-poly-L-lysine
PT   Patch test
SJS   Stevens-Johnson syndrome
SsIgE   Serum-specific IgE assay
ST   Skin test
TEN   Toxic epidermal necrolysis

REFERENCES

1. Versporten A, Coenen S, Adriaenssens N, et al. European surveillance of antimicrobial consumption (ESAC): outpatient cephalosporin use in Europe (1997-2009). *J Antimicrob Chemother.* 2011;66(Suppl. 6):vi25–35.
2. Vaz LE, Kleinman KP, Raebel MA, et al. Recent trends in outpatient antibiotic use in children. *Pediatrics.* 2014;133:375–385.
3. Muraki Y, Yagi T, Tsuji Y, et al. Japanese antimicrobial consumption surveillance: first report on oral and parenteral antimicrobial consumption in Japan (2009-2013). *J Glob Antimicrob Resist.* 2016;7:19–23.
4. Lin H, Dyar OJ, Rosales-Klintz S, et al. Trends and patterns of antibiotic consumption in Shanghai municipality, China: a 6 year surveillance with sales records, 2009-14. *J Antimicrob Chemother.* 2016;71:1723–1729.
5. Kelkar PS, Li JT-C. Cephalosporin allergy. *N Engl J Med.* 2001;345:804–809.
6. Romano A, Torres MJ, Namour F, et al. Immediate hypersensitivity to cephalosporins. *Allergy.* 2002;57(Suppl. 72):52–57.
7. Madaan A, Li JT-C. Cephalosporin allergy. *Immunol Allergy Clin N Am.* 2004;24:463–476.
8. Guéant JL, Guéant-Rodríguez RM, Viola M, Valluzzi RL, Romano A. IgE-mediated hypersensitivity to cephalosporins. *Curr Pharm Des.* 2006;12:3335–3345.

9. Macy E, Contreras R. Adverse reactions associated with oral and parenteral use of cephalosporins: a retrospective population-based analysis. *J Allergy Clin Immunol.* 2015;135:745–752.e5.

10. Romano A. Cephalosporin allergy: clinical manifestations and diagnosis. In: Post TW, ed. *UpToDate.* 2017. Waltham, MA.

11. Johansson SG, Bieber T, Dahl R, et al. Revised nomenclature for allergy for global use: report of the Nomenclature Review Committee of the World Allergy Organization. *J Allergy Clin Immunol.* October 2003;2004(113):832–836.

12. Romano A, Torres MJ, Castells M, Sanz ML, Blanca M. Diagnosis and management of drug hypersensitivity reactions. *J Allergy Clin Immunol.* 2011;127:S67–S73.

13. Demoly P, Adkinson NF, Brockow K, et al. International consensus on drug allergy. *Allergy.* 2014;69:420–437.

14. Pichler WJ. Delayed drug hypersensitivity reactions. *Ann Intern Med.* 2003;139:683–693.

15. Romano A, Blanca M, Torres MJ, et al. Diagnosis of non-immediate reactions to beta-lactam antibiotics. *Allergy.* 2004;59:1153–1160.

16. Feinberg JG. Allergy to antibiotics. I. Fact and conjecture on the sensitizing contaminants of penicillins and cephalosporins. *Int Arch Allergy.* 1968;33:439–443.

17. Newton GGF, Hamilton-Miller JMT. Cephaloridine: chemical and biochemical aspects. *Postgrad Med J.* 1967;43(Suppl. 1):10–17.

18. Hamilton-Miller JMT, Newton GGF, Abraham EP. Products of aminolysis and enzymic hydrolysis of the cephalosporins. *Biochem J.* 1970;116:371–384.

19. Hamilton-Miller JM, Richards E, Abraham EP. Changes in proton-magnetic-resonance spectra during aminolysis and enzymic hydrolysis of cephalosporins. *Biochem J.* 1970;116:385–395.

20. Baldo BA. Penicillins and cephalosporins as allergens–structural aspects of recognition and cross-reactions. *Clin Exp Allergy.* 1999;29:744–749.

21. Blanca M, Mayorga C, Torres MJ, et al. Side-chain-specific reactions to betalactams: 14 years later. *Clin Exp Allergy.* 2002;32:192–197.

22. Sánchez-Sancho F, Perez-Inestrosa E, Suau R, et al. Synthesis, characterization and immunochemical evaluation of cephalosporin antigenic determinants. *J Mol Recognit.* 2003;16:148–156.

23. Antunez C, Blanca-Lopez N, Torres MJ, et al. Immediate allergic reactions to cephalosporins: evaluation of cross-reactivity with a panel of penicillins and cephalosporins. *J Allergy Clin Immunol.* 2006;117:404–410.

24. Romano A, Gaeta F, Arribas Poves MF, Valluzzi RL. Cross-reactivity among beta-lactams. *Curr Allergy Asthma Rep.* 2016;16:24.

25. Romano A, Mayorga C, Torres MJ, et al. Immediate allergic reactions to cephalosporins: cross-reactivity and selective responses. *J Allergy Clin Immunol.* 2000;106:1177–1183.

26. Romano A, Guéant-Rodriguez RM, Viola M, Amoghly F, Gaeta F, Guéant JL. Diagnosing immediate reactions to cephalosporins. *Clin Exp Allergy.* 2005;35:1234–1242.

27. Romano A, Gaeta F, Valluzzi RL, Zaffiro A, Caruso C, Quaratino D. Natural evolution of skin-test sensitivity in patients with IgE-mediated hypersensitivity to cephalosporins. *Allergy.* 2014;69:806–809.

28. Romano A, Gaeta F, Valluzzi RL, et al. IgE-mediated hypersensitivity to cephalosporins: cross-reactivity and tolerability of alternative cephalosporins. *J Allergy Clin Immunol.* 2015;136:685–691.e3.

29. Hasdenteufel F, Luyasu S, Renaudin JM, Trechot P, Kanny G. Anaphylactic shock associated with cefuroxime axetil: structure-activity relationships. *Ann Pharmacother.* 2007;41:1069–1072.

30. Hasdenteufel F, Luyasu S, Hougardy N, et al. Structure-activity relationships and drug allergy. *Curr Clin Pharmacol.* 2012;7:15–27.

31. Baldo BA, Pham NH. Allergenic significance of cephalosporin side chains. *J Allergy Clin Immunol.* 2015;136:1426–1428.

32. Zhao Z, Baldo BA, Rimmer J. β-Lactam allergenic determinants: fine structural recognition of a cross-reacting determinant on benzylpenicillin and cephalothin. *Clin Exp Allergy.* 2002;32:1644–1650.

33. Pham NH, Baldo BA. β-Lactam drug allergens: fine structural recognition patterns of cephalosporin-reactive IgE antibodies. *J Mol Recognit.* 1996;9:287–296.

34. Igea JM, Fraj J, Davila I, Cuevas M, Cuesta J, Hinojosa M. Allergy to cefazolin: study of in vivo cross reactivity with other betalactams. *Ann Allergy.* 1992;68:515–519.

35. Warrington RJ, McPhillips S. Independent anaphylaxis to cefazolin without allergy to other β-lactam antibiotics. *J Allergy Clin Immunol.* 1996;98:460–462.

36. Weber EA. Cefazolin specific side chain hypersensitivity. *J Allergy Clin Immunol.* 1996;98:849–850.

37. Pipet A, Veyrac G, Wessel F, et al. A statement on cefazolin immediate hypersensitivity: data from a large database, and focus on the cross-reactivities. *Clin Exp Allergy.* 2011;41:1602–1608.

38. Uyttebroek AP, Decuyper II, Brids CH, et al. Cefazolin hypersensitivity: toward optimized diagnosis. *J Allergy Clin Immunol Pract.* 2016;4:1232–1236.

39. Marcos Bravo C, Luna Ortiz I, Gonzalez Vazquez R. Hypersensitivity to cefuroxime with good tolerance to other betalactams. *Allergy.* 1995;50:359–361.

40. Romano A, Quaratino D, Venuti A, Venemalm L, Mayorga C, Blanca M. Selective type-1 hypersensitivity to cefuroxime. *J Allergy Clin Immunol.* 1998;101:564–565.

41. Gaig P, San Miguel MM, Enrique E, García-Ortega P. Selective type-1 hypersensitivity to cefixime. *Allergy.* 1999;54:901–902.

42. Romano A, Piunti E, Di Fonso M, Viola M, Venuti A, Venemalm L. Selective immediate hypersensitivity to ceftriaxone. *Allergy.* 2000;55:415–416.

43. Demoly P, Messaad D, Sahla H, Hillaire-Buys D, Bousquet J. Immediate hypersensitivity to ceftriaxone. *Allergy.* 2000;55:418–419.

44. Romano A, Di Fonso M, Artesani MC, Viola M, Adesi FB, Venuti A. Selective immediate hypersensitivity to ceftazidime. *Allergy.* 2001;56:84–85.

45. Romano A, Viola M, Guéant-Rodriguez RM, Valluzzi RL, Guéant JL. Selective immediate hypersensitivity to cefodizime. *Allergy.* 2005;60:1545–1546.

46. Atanasković-Marković M, Cirković Velicković T, Gavrović-Jankulović M, Ivanovski P, Nestorović B. A case of selective IgE-mediated hypersensitivity to ceftibuten. *Allergy.* 2005;60:1454.

47. Moreno E, Dávila I, Laffond E, et al. Selective immediate hypersensitivity to cefepime. *J Invest Allergol Clin Immunol.* 2007;17:52–54.

48. Romano A, Gaeta F, Valluzzi RL, Caruso C, Rumi G, Bousquet PJ. IgE-mediated hypersensitivity to cephalosporins: cross-reactivity and tolerability of penicillins, monobactams, and carbapenems. *J Allergy Clin Immunol.* 2010;126:994–999.

49. Tejedor Alonso MA, Moro MM, Hernández JE, et al. Incidence of anaphylaxis in hospitalized patients. *Int Arch Allergy Immunol.* 2011;156:212–220.

50. Romano A, Gaeta F, Valluzzi RL, Alonzi C, Viola M, Bousquet PJ. Diagnosing hypersensitivity reactions to cephalosporins in children. *Pediatrics.* 2008;122:521–527.

51. Novembre E, Mori F, Pucci N, Bernardini R, Romano A. Cefaclor anaphylaxis in children. *Allergy.* 2009;64:1233–1235.

52. Renaudin JM, Beaudouin E, Ponvert C, Demoly P, Moneret-Vautrin DA. Severe drug-induced anaphylaxis: analysis of 333 cases recorded by the allergy vigilance network from 2002 to 2010. *Allergy.* 2013;68:929–937.

53. Christiansen IS, Krøigaard M, Mosbech H, Skov PS, Poulsen LK, Garvey LH. Clinical and diagnostic features of perioperative hypersensitivity to cefuroxime. *Clin Exp Allergy.* 2015;45:807–814.

54. Sachs B, Fischer-Barth W, Merk HF. Reporting rates for severe hypersensitivity reactions associated with prescription-only drugs in outpatient treatment in Germany. *Pharmacoepidemiol Drug Saf.* 2015;24:1076–1084.

55. Kuhlen Jr JL, Camargo Jr CA, Balekian DS, et al. Antibiotics are the most commonly identified cause of perioperative hypersensitivity reactions. *J Allergy Clin Immunol Pract.* 2016;4:697–704.

56. Kim SY, Kim JH, Jang YS, et al. The basophil activation test is safe and useful for confirming drug-induced anaphylaxis. *Allergy Asthma Immunol Res.* 2016;8:541–544.

57. Lammintausta K, Kortekangas-Savolainen O. The usefulness of skin tests to prove drug hypersensitivity. *Br J Dermatol.* 2005;152:968–974.

58. Romano A, Gaeta F, Valluzzi RL, et al. Diagnosing nonimmediate reactions to cephalosporins. *J Allergy Clin Immunol.* 2012;129:1166–1169.

59. Drago F, Cogorno L, Agnoletti AF, Ciccarese G, Parodi A. A retrospective study of cutaneous drug reactions in an outpatient population. *Int J Clin Pharm.* 2015;37:739–743.

60. Pinho A, Coutinho I, Gameiro A, Gouveia M, Gonçalo M. Patch testing – a valuable tool for investigating non-immediate cutaneous adverse drug reactions to antibiotics. *J Eur Acad Dermatol Venereol.* 2017;31:280–287.

61. Papay J, Yuen N, Powell G, Mockenhaupt M, Bogenrieder T. Spontaneous adverse event reports of Stevens-Johnson syndrome/toxic epidermal necrolysis: detecting associations with medications. *Pharmacoepidemiol Drug Saf.* 2012;21:289–296.

62. Barbaud A, Collet E, Milpied B, et al. A multicentre study to determine the value and safety of drug patch tests for the three main classes of severe cutaneous adverse drug reactions. *Br J Dermatol.* 2013;168:555–562.

63. Lin YF, Yang CH, Sindy H, et al. Severe cutaneous adverse reactions related to systemic antibiotics. *Clin Infect Dis.* 2014;58:1377–1385.

64. Shiohara T, Kano Y. A complex inter-action between drug allergy and viral infection. *Clin Rev Allergy Immunol.* 2007;33:124–133.

65. White KD, Chung WH, Hung SI, Mallal S, Phillips EJ. Evolving models of the immunopathogenesis of T cell-mediated drug allergy: the role of host, pathogens, and drug response. *J Allergy Clin Immunol.* 2015;136:219–234.

66. Torres MJ, Blanca M, Fernandez J, et al. Diagnosis of immediate allergic reactions to beta-lactam antibiotics. *Allergy.* 2003;58:961–972.

67. Blanca M, Romano A, Torres MJ, et al. Update on the evaluation of hypersensitivity reactions to betalactams. *Allergy.* 2009;64:183–193.

68. Pichichero ME, Pichichero DM. Diagnosis of penicillin, amoxicillin, and cephalosporin allergy: reliability of examination assessed by skin testing and oral challenge. *J Pediatr.* 1998;132:137–143.

69. Brockow K, Garvey LH, Aberer W, et al. Skin test concentrations for systemically administered drugs – an ENDA/EAACI Drug Allergy Interest Group position paper. *Allergy.* 2013;68:702–712.

70. Empedrad R, Darter AL, Earl HS, Gruchalla RS. Nonirritating intradermal skin test concentrations for commonly prescribed antibiotics. *J Allergy Clin Immunol.* 2003;112:629–630.

71. Testi S, Severino M, Iorno ML, et al. Nonirritating concentration for skin testing with cephalosporins. *J Investig Allergol Clin Immunol.* 2010;20:171–172.

72. Audicana M, Bernaola G, Urrutia I, et al. Allergic reactions to betalactams: studies in a group of patients allergic to penicillin and evaluation of cross-reactivity with cephalosporin. *Allergy.* 1994;49:108–113.

73. Yoon SY, Park SY, Kim S, et al. Validation of the cephalosporin intradermal skin test for predicting immediate hypersensitivity: a prospective study with drug challenge. *Allergy.* 2013;68:938–944.

74. Mayorga C, Celik G, Rouzaire P, et al. In vitro tests for drug hypersensitivity reactions: an ENDA/EAACI Drug Allergy Interest Group position paper. *Allergy.* 2016;71:1103–1134.

75. Torres MJ, Padial A, Mayorga C, Fernández T, et al. The diagnostic interpretation of basophil activation test in immediate allergic reactions to betalactams. *Clin Exp Allergy.* 2004;34:1768–1775.

76. Uyttebroek AP, Sabato V, Cop N, et al. Diagnosing cefazolin hypersensitivity: lessons from dual-labeling flow cytometry. *J Allergy Clin Immunol Pract.* 2016;4:1243–1245.

77. Fernández TD, Torres MJ, Blanca-López N, et al. Negativization rates of IgE radioimmunoassay and basophil activation test in immediate reactions to penicillins. *Allergy.* 2009;64:242–248.

78. Bernardini R, Novembre E, Lombardi E, Pucci N, Rossi ME, Vierucci A. Long persistence of IgE antibody to cefaclor. *Allergy.* 2000;55:984–985.

79. Solensky R, Khan DA, Bernstein IL, et al. Drug allergy: an updated practice parameter. *Ann Allergy Asthma Immunol.* 2010;105:259–273.

80. Aberer W, Bircher A, Romano A, et al. Drug provocation testing in the diagnosis of drug hypersensitivity: general considerations. *Allergy.* 2003;58:854–863.

81. Moreno E, Laffond E, Muñoz-Bellido F, et al. Performance in real life of the European network on drug allergy algorithm in immediate reactions to beta-lactam antibiotics. *Allergy.* 2016;71:1787–1790.

82. Blanca M, Torres MJ, García JJ, et al. Natural evolution of skin test sensitivity in patients allergic to beta-lactam antibiotics. *J Allergy Clin Immunol.* 1999;103:918–924.

83. Romano A, Warrington R. Antibiotic allergy. *Immunol Allergy Clin N Am.* 2014;34:489–506, vii.

84. Torres MJ, Sánchez-Sabaté E, Álvarez J, et al. Skin test evaluation in nonimmediate allergic reactions to penicillins. *Allergy.* 2004;59:219–224.

85. Romano A, Gaeta F, Valluzzi RL, Caruso C, Rumi G, Bousquet PJ. The very limited usefulness of skin testing with penicilloyl-polylysine and the minor determinant mixture in evaluating nonimmediate reactions to penicillins. *Allergy.* 2010;65:1104–1107.

86. Romano A, Caubet JC. Antibiotic allergies in children and adults: from clinical symptoms to skin testing diagnosis. *J Allergy Clin Immunol Pract.* 2014;2:3–12.

87. Blanca-López N, Zapatero L, Alonso E, et al. Skin testing and drug provocation in the diagnosis of nonimmediate reactions to aminopenicillins in children. *Allergy.* 2009;64:229–233.

88. Hjortlund J, Mortz CG, Skov PS, Bindslev-Jensen C. Diagnosis of penicillin allergy revisited: the value of case history, skin testing, specific IgE and prolonged challenge. *Allergy.* 2013;68:1057–1064.

89. Schnyder B, Pichler WJ. Nonimmediate drug allergy: diagnostic benefit of skin testing and practical approach. *J Allergy Clin Immunol.* 2012;129:1170–1171.

90. Demoly P, Romano A, Botelho C, et al. Determining the negative predictive value of provocation tests with beta-lactams. *Allergy.* 2010;65:327–332.

91. Hari Y, Frutig-Schnyder K, Hurni M, Yawalkar N, Zanni MP, Schnyder B, et al. T cell involvement in cutaneous drug eruptions. *Clin Exp Allergy.* 2001;31:1398–1408.

92. Polak ME, Belgi G, McGuire C, et al. In vitro diagnostic assays are effective during the acute phase of delayed-type drug hypersensitivity reactions. *Br J Dermatol.* 2013;168:539–549.

93. Tanvarasethee B, Buranapraditkun S, Klaewsongkram J. The potential of using enzyme-linked immunospot to diagnose cephalosporin-induced maculopapular exanthems. *Acta Derm Venereol.* 2013;93:66–69.

94. Pichler WJ, Tilch J. The lymphocyte transformation test in the diagnosis of drug hypersensitivity. *Allergy.* 2004;59:809–820.

95. Romano A, Quaratino D, Aimone-Gastin I, et al. Cephalosporin allergy: characterization of unique and cross-reacting cephalosporin antigens. *Int J Immunopathol Pharmacol.* 1997;10(Suppl. 2):187–191.

96. Cernadas JR, Brockow K, Romano A, et al. General considerations on rapid desensitization for drug hypersensitivity - a consensus statement. *Allergy.* 2010;65:1357–1366.

CHAPTER 12

Macrolide Allergy

MERIN KURUVILLA, MD

KEY POINTS

- Macrolide hypersensitivity is clearly overestimated and but rarely reproduced by oral challenge.
- On the basis of DPT results in the literature, 90% of these patients are unnecessarily avoiding these antibiotics.
- While skin or in vitro testing may be an adjunctive strategy to verify tolerance, they have little value as a diagnostic tool.
- Drug provocation testing is the most important diagnostic tool in management and should be considered based on a favorable risk–benefit assessment.

INTRODUCTION

Macrolides are a group of related compounds that have a lactone ring (14–16 atoms) bonded to one or more deoxy sugar molecules. They are classified according to the number of carbon atoms in their lactone ring: 14 membered (erythromycin, troleandomycin, roxithromycin, dirithromycin, and clarithromycin), 15 membered (azithromycin), and 16 membered (spiramycin, rokitamycin, josamycin, and midecamycin).

On the basis of their biochemical and immunologic properties, macrolide antibiotics are considered low-risk medications in the context of allergic reactions.[1] They have relatively low potential to induce hypersensitivity reactions and are generally regarded as innocuous antibiotics. Older reports define incidence of allergic reactions in as few as 0.5% patients.[2]

However, parallel to the increasing use of macrolide antibiotics, allergic reactions to this drug group have been increasingly reported over the past 10 years.[57] Azithromycin, in particular, is overprescribed for upper respiratory tract infections. Various factors contribute to this, especially the perceived low adverse effect profile.[3]

More recent reports describe hypersensitivity reactions to macrolides occurring in 0.4%–3% of treatments[4] and drug rash in approximately 6% of pediatric cases.[5] Currently, macrolide antibiotics are associated with allergy population prevalence rates of approximately 1 in 200 or greater.[1]

Clarithromycin was the most common cause of reactions reported (63.6%) among non-β-lactam (non-BL) antibiotic allergic reactions in children.[6] Similarly, macrolides were the most common non-BL antibiotics causing reactions in other pediatric studies.[7,8]

CLINICAL MANIFESTATIONS

Our understanding of macrolide allergy is limited by the sparsity of published literature. These are mostly limited to case reports or small series of patients. Underlying immunologic mechanisms have rarely been evaluated because of the paucity of cases described. Furthermore, diagnostic workup is not completely validated.

Broadly, clinical manifestations can be categorized as immediate reactions (IRs; within 1 h, IgE mediated) versus nonimmediate reactions (NIRs; delayed onset, T cell mediated).

IMMEDIATE REACTIONS

Several clinical observations support the importance of IgE-mediated allergy. Acute urticaria is the most frequent clinical manifestation of macrolide allergy.[4,9–13]

There have been occasional descriptions of severe anaphylactic reactions to clarithromycin[14] and telithromycin,[15] associated with Kounis syndrome in one report.[16]

Other systemic manifestations include bronchospastic reactions.[17] Evidence of occupational asthma with spiramycin was found in 4 of 51 (7.8%) employees of a pharmaceutical company, with variable results on skin testing.[18,19]

NONIMMEDIATE REACTIONS
Maculopapular Exanthema

Macrolide-induced delayed skin reactions most commonly present as maculopapular exanthema (MPE).[20] These can occur independently or may appear only in the presence of a concurrent infection (such as when ampicillin is prescribed during mononucleosis). Three separate cases of azithromycin-induced rash have been described in the setting of infectious mononucleosis, akin to those reported with the use of other antibiotics.[21] The mechanism is thought to be virus-induced immune dysregulation or altered drug metabolism secondary to Epstein-Barr virus (EBV).

Allergic Contact Dermatitis

Contact dermatitis to topical erythromycin is extremely rare. While initially thought to be nonsensitizing, in the mid-1990s, three cases of sensitization to erythromycin base were reported.[22-24]

Occupational allergic contact dermatitis (ACD) has also been reported in pharmaceutical workers who handle azithromycin during its formulation. Almost all of these workers presented features of airborne contact dermatitis.[25] In addition, azithromycin in eye solutions have been implicated in the pathogenesis of contact dermatitis in nonoccupational settings.[26]

Fixed Drug Eruption

Apart from urticaria and MPEs, among more specific skin eruptions, episodes of fixed drug eruption (FDE) have been most often described. There have been several case reports of clarithromycin- and erythromycin-induced FDE.[27-30] A T cell–mediated pathogenic mechanism has been demonstrated in some patients on the basis of positive patch test responses in some cases. Both positive skin tests on unaffected skin and falsely negative skin tests in former lesional skin have been reported.[28-30] Oral provocation testing has been uniformly positive in all reports.

Acute Generalized Exanthematous Pustulosis

Severe cutaneous reactions have been rarely reported with macrolides. Acute generalized exanthematous pustulosis induced by azithromycin has been described in two separate reports.[31,32]

Symmetric Drug-Related Intertriginous and Flexural Exanthema

Systemic allergic dermatitis affecting the major flexures has been reported with erythromycin and roxithromycin,[33] as well as clarithromycin.[34] Patch test results have been variable.

Drug Reaction With Eosinophilia and Systemic Symptoms

Sporadic pediatric reports of azithromycin-induced drug reaction with eosinophilia and systemic symptoms (DRESS) exist, in the context of acute EBV infection.[35,36] There has only been one adult case of definite DRESS syndrome associated with azithromycin exposure.[37]

Stevens-Johnson Syndrome/Toxic Epidermal Necrolysis

The literature describes only four cases of Stevens-Johnson syndrome (SJS) attributed to azithromycin to date.[38] In one of these pediatric cases, azithromycin was the apparent trigger of SJS, although herpes simplex virus reactivation was demonstrated a month later.[39] Similarly, there has been a solitary report linking clarithromycin with the development of toxic epidermal necrolysis (TEN) in a patient who previously tolerated roxithromycin.[40] The first reported case of roxithromycin causing TEN was recently published.[41]

Eosinophilic Pneumonia

Although macrolides rarely provoke drug-induced lung disease, clarithromycin does have the potential to cause eosinophilic pneumonia.[42,43] Symptoms and lung infiltrates were resolved on drug discontinuation in both cases.

Vasculitic Syndromes

A vasculitic rash was reproduced by clarithromycin as well as azithromycin in one case[44]; and two other reported cases of leukocytoclastic vasculitis due to clarithromycin have been described.[45,46] Drug-induced Henoch-Schonlein purpura is a common association in adults. Cases, although infrequent, have been reported secondary to macrolide antibiotics, including midecamycin, erythromycin, and spiramycin.[47]

Vasculitic syndromes have been reported more frequently with immunosuppressant macrolides, which will be discussed later in this chapter.

DIAGNOSIS

Macrolides are frequently used empirically for respiratory infections, and the most common scenario triggering a label of macrolide allergy is the development of a delayed rash during therapy. It becomes difficult to distinguish between a true drug eruption versus a viral exanthema, especially because the literature provides little guidance regarding a validated diagnostic pathway for macrolide allergies.

Hypersensitivity reactions to macrolides can be assessed with the diagnostic algorithm shown in Fig. 12.1.

SKIN TESTING

Reported allergy to macrolides is occasionally corroborated by skin tests, possibly because of low molecular

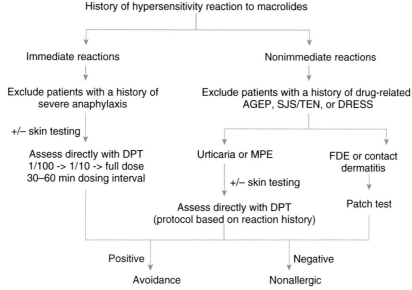

FIG. 12.1 Algorithm for the diagnosis of allergic reactions to macrolides. In the rare setting of anaphylaxis and a positive skin test, drug provocation test would not be performed. *AGEP*, acute generalized exanthematous pustulosis; *DPT*, drug provocation test; *DRESS*, drug reaction with eosinophilia and systemic symptoms; *FDE*, fixed drug eruption; *MPE*, maculopapular exanthema; *SJS*, Stevens-Johnson syndrome; *TEN*, toxic epidermal necrolysis.

weight and/or implication of drug metabolites.[11] The literature has consistently demonstrated the futility of macrolide skin testing in the evaluation of possible hypersensitivity, being compounded by high rates of false-positive as well as false-negative results.

The few cases described with probable IgE-mediated hypersensitivity, as determined by positive skin prick test (SPT) responses and suggestive symptoms have mostly been attributed to spiramycin.[48] In a series of 21 patients with spiramycin and erythromycin allergy who underwent skin tests, 17 patients also had drug provocation tests (DPTs). The three patients with positive DPT to spiramycin demonstrated positive skin tests to both macrolides tested.[49] In contrast, among five patients with immediate-onset cutaneous eruptions (one related to erythromycin and four secondary to spiramycin), none had a positive SPT response. However, sensitization was proved by oral challenges in every case.[50]

A patient in the literature with roxithromycin immediate hypersensitivity demonstrated positive skin prick testing to roxithromycin in glycerin (30 mg/mL), and also to erythromycin and clarithromycin at unknown concentrations.[12] Five healthy individuals did not present positive prick test reactions to any of the tested macrolides.

Skin tests have sometimes been used in diagnosing clarithromycin allergy, but they have not been validated in terms of specificity and sensitivity. A concentration of 0.01 mg/mL of azithromycin and 0.05 mg/mL for erythromycin has been suggested as non-irritating based on serial 10-fold dilutions in healthy subjects.[51] However, a study evaluating nonirritant intradermal concentrations in 61 healthy adults found a more than 10-fold discrepancy for previous known concentrations for azithromycin.[52] Furthermore, interindividual variability of the skin test results for azithromycin was more than 100-fold.

Additional studies investigating nonirritant intradermal test (IDT) concentrations for diagnosing clarithromycin allergy have shown a high rate of false-positive tests in the pediatric population. A study comparing IDTs with DPT data across 64 pediatric patients demonstrated a sensitivity of 75%, but a positive predictive value of 33% for ID testing to clarithromycin.[53] The 0.5 mg/mL dilution was established as the nonirritating threshold concentration for IDTs in this study. Another study demonstrated that IDTs even with 1:100,000 dilutions of clarithromycin might produce false-positive test results during childhood.[54] However, the investigators used a lyophilized form of an injectable clarithromycin, which is not available in the United States.

Intradermal skin tests with late reading might be useful in the evaluation of NIRs if they are performed

TABLE 12.1
Nonirritating Skin Test Concentrations of Macrolide antibiotics

Antibiotic	Full-strength Concentration, (mg/mL)	Maximum Skin Prick Test Concentration, (mg/mL)	Maximum Intradermal Test Concentration, (mg/mL)
Roxithromycin	30 mg/mL	Full strength[12]	N/A
Erythromycin	50 mg/mL	Full strength	10 mg/mL[51]
Azithromycin	100 mg/mL	Full strength	0.01 mg/mL[51]
Clarithromycin[a]	50 mg/mL	Full strength	0.5 mg/mL[53] 0.05 mg/mL[55]

[a]Parenteral Preparations not Available in the United States

in concentrations proved to be nonirritant. However, the predictive values of this testing is unknown.

Overall, skin testing to macrolides appears to have limited diagnostic potential. The highest published nonirritant concentrations for individual macrolide antibiotics are outlined in Table 12.1.

PATCH TESTING

Positive responses to patch tests at concentrations up to 10% of crushed tablets in petrolatum have been described in subjects with NIRs (for example, FDEs and contact dermatitis) to erythromycin and azithromycin.[25,30]

On the other hand, macrolides were tested in 130 patients with delayed cutaneous ADRs, but no positive patch test reactions were observed.[56]

IN VITRO TESTING FOR SPECIFIC IGE

Clinically validated tests for drug-specific IgE are difficult to develop, and there is very limited evidence available for IgE testing of macrolides.

An immediate IgE-dependent hypersensitivity has been shown with erythromycin in a unique case with positive skin test as well as specific IgE assays, based on sepharose-radioimmunoassay.[10] Similarly, there appeared to be reasonable concordance between skin test and serum IgE results in a pediatric study.[57]

OTHER FORMS OF IN VITRO TESTING

Lymphocyte transformation test (LTT) and basophil histamine release test are not validated and have been rarely investigated for macrolide hypersensitivity.[58] While positive LTTs were noted historically with spiramycin,[48] basophil activation test and LTT were negative in all tested subjects to erythromycin, azithromycin, and clarithromycin, in a study.[59]

DRUG PROVOCATION TESTING

Oral provocation tests are usually necessary to establish or exclude the diagnosis of hypersensitivity to macrolide antibiotics. Several recent studies have confirmed the safety of DPTs in children who developed a benign rash without signs of severity. With low probability medications, the suggested reexposure method in patients with a history of an immediate hypersensitivity reaction is either a graded or full-dose DPT.[1]

DPTs appear to be especially useful and safe with macrolide antibiotics compared with other drug classes.[60,61] Using DPT, studies of patients with suspected macrolide allergy have shown confirmation rates of only 7.5%–13.7%.[29,59] Furthermore, reactions provoked by oral challenge have been typically mild and easily reversible.

Of 107 oral DPTs 8 were positive (7.5%) in a cohort with clinical histories of suspected macrolide hypersensitivity.[20] Seven patients reacted to spiramycin and one to roxithromycin; IDTs with spiramycin at the concentration of 10 mg/mL were positive in only four of these seven patients. The original reactions were mainly mucocutaneous manifestations (MPE, urticaria, and angioedema). The authors were unable to discern any relationship between a particular clinical presentation and positivity to oral DPTs.

Similarly, only 4 of 64 (6%) children reporting drug reactions to clarithromycin had a confirmed diagnosis following stepwise allergological evaluation.[53] These studies mirror the findings of Seitz et al., who examined the results of allergy testing in a large cohort of 125 patients with suspected macrolide allergy, and prove that 87.2% of patients in their series were unnecessarily labeled as allergic to macrolides.[59] In that series too, the description of the initial rash was sometimes not the rash produced by drug provocation. Notably, four patients developed exanthema during challenges

TABLE 12.2
In Vivo and In Vitro Evaluations of Macrolide Allergy

Study Population	Positive Skin Prick Test Results	Positive Intradermal Test Results	Positive Drug Provocation Tests
Pediatric cohort (n = 45)[54]	0/45 (0%)	9/20 (45%) to clarithromycin	2/45 (4.4%) to clarithromycin despite negative skin testing
Adult/pediatric cohort (n = 107)[20]	Not reported	Not reported	8/107 (7.5%)
Pediatric cohort (n = 77)[57]	1/58 (1.7%) to clarithromycin; 1/19 (5%) to azithromycin	6/58 (10%) to clarithromycin; 8/19 (42%) to azithromycin	2/51 (3.9%) to clarithromycin despite negative skin testing
Pediatric cohort (n = 64)[53]	0/64 (0%) at 50 mg/mL clarithromycin	9/64 (14%) at 0.5 mg/mL clarithromycin	4/64 (6%)—two immediate and two delayed reactions
Adult cohort (n = 125)[59]	0/125 (0%) at full strength erythromycin, clarithromycin, azithromycin	0/53 (0%) with IRs, and 1/72 (1.3%) with NIR (delayed positive IDT) to erythromycin, clarithromycin, and azithromycin (0.01 mg/mL)	0/47 (0%) with IRs and 4/66 (6%) with NIRs
Pediatric cohort (n = 54)[62]	Not reported	Not performed	3/54 (6.8%)

IDT, intradermal test; *IR*, immediate reaction; *NIR*, nonimmediate reaction.

despite negative skin tests. Likewise, only 2 of 45 patients in a pediatric cohort developed urticaria during DPTs.[54]

While most of the data available for macrolide allergy pertain to clarithromycin, a study suggested that azithromycin appears to be more allergenic. Barni et al.[57] retrospectively reviewed the charts of 77 children with a history of hypersensitivity to clarithromycin or azithromycin. Patients were investigated with skin tests, specific IgE to both drugs and, if necessary, oral DPT. Positive results to skin tests and/or DPT with the suspect drug confirmed the diagnosis in 15.5% (9/58) of reactions to clarithromycin and in 47.4% (9/19) of reactions to azithromycin (P = .004). Most of these labels were based on skin testing: 7/9 with clarithromycin and all of the azithromycin cases. It is important to note that this is only one study and results may have been influenced by geographic differences, as well as the potential for false-positive reactions with macrolide skin testing.

History of Delayed Reactions
It is well documented that some NIRs appear only after a treatment for several days at full therapeutic dosage. A 5-day DPT has been described in the diagnosis of NIRs to clarithromycin in a pediatric cohort.[54] No reactions were reported.

See Table 12.2 for summarization of in vitro and in vivo evaluation of macrolide allergy.

DESENSITIZATION PROTOCOLS
Descriptions of macrolide desensitization are confined to a few case reports, mostly in adults. Clarithromycin desensitization was first reported in an adult female with remote histories of anaphylaxis to erythromycin and bronchospasm to roxithromycin.[63] Neither skin testing nor DPT was performed. No adverse drug reactions were recorded. A successful 14-step desensitization to clarithromycin was subsequently performed in a patient with clinical reactions and positive IDTs to both clarithromycin and azithromycin.[64] In a pediatric patient with recurrent diffuse urticarial rash in response to intravenous clarithromycin, an oral desensitization protocol was executed uneventfully[65] despite failed desensitization with azithromycin.

CROSS-REACTIVITY
The preponderance of evidence suggests that there is no cross-reactivity between subgroups of macrolides.

The only structural differences between macrolide subgroups are confined to the side chains. It has been hypothesized that side chain similarity may confer predisposition toward cross-reactivity. A patient with immediate hypersensitivity to roxithromycin demonstrated positive skin prick testing to erythromycin and clarithromycin.[12] These macrolides have a similar chemical structure comprising a 14-membered carbon ring, compared with 15-membered (azithromycin) and

16-membered macrolides (spiramycin). In the case series describing contact dermatitis to azithromycin, two subjects showed cross-reactivity on patch testing with azithromycin intermediates, including erythromycin.[25] Similar findings were noted in another patient with clinical reactions as well as positive skin tests to both clarithromycin as well as azithromycin.[64] Conversely, in another case of immediate urticaria due to spiramycin with positive SPT results, the patient tolerated clarithromycin and erythromycin.[65]

Although these reports may represent true-positive cross-reactivity, allergy testing for macrolides has clearly not been standardized, and definitive conclusions are difficult. Furthermore, this concept of cross-reactivity based on carbon ring structure is contradicted by other case reports. Igea et al. reported selective clarithromycin allergy reproduced by oral challenge, with tolerance of erythromycin.[66] Reports of cross-reactivity among macrolides on the basis of patch test results have also been variable in cases of FDE.[27,30]

In any case, the pattern of cross-reactivity appears to be complex and difficult to predict. Should concern exist for cross-reactivity, a graded challenge to the desired macrolide may be an option to rule out sensitization.

HYPERSENSITIVITY REACTIONS TO IMMUNOSUPPRESSANT MACROLIDES

Although commonly thought of as a class of antibiotics, there are also nonantibiotic macrolides such as tacrolimus, everolimus, and sirolimus. These are used for the prevention and treatment of acute rejection after solid organ transplantation and hematopoietic stem cell transplantation. Allergy to sirolimus and other mTOR inhibitors has been previously reported with hypersensitivity reactions such as angioedema, dyspnea, and hypoxia.[67] Noninfectious pneumonitis is a known class effect of immunosuppressant macrolides, found in 13.5%–25% of cases in the everolimus efficacy trials.[68] There are no data on skin testing in these patients or other diagnostic investigations.

While poor understanding exists between the cross-reactivity among nonantibiotic and antibiotic macrolides, at least one hypersensitivity reaction has been described with use of tacrolimus in a clarithromycin-allergic patient.[69]

CONCLUSION

Macrolide hypersensitivity is clearly overestimated and rarely reproduced by oral challenge. On the basis of DPT results in the literature, 90% of these patients are unnecessarily avoiding these antibiotics. While skin or in vitro testing may be an adjunctive strategy to verify tolerance, they have little value as a diagnostic tool. DPT is the most important diagnostic tool in management and should be considered based on a favorable risk–benefit assessment.

REFERENCES

1. Macy E. Practical management of patients with a history of immediate hypersensitivity to common non-beta-lactam drugs. *Curr Allergy Asthma Rep.* 2016;16:4.
2. Reynolds JEF. *Martindale. The Extra Pharmacopoeia.* London: The Pharmaceutical Press; 1993:179–224.
3. Nambudiri VE. More than skin deep—the costs of antibiotic overuse: a teachable moment. *JAMA Intern Med.* 2014;174(11):1724–1725.
4. Araújo L, Demoly P. Macrolides allergy. *Curr Pharm Des.* 2008;14(27):2840–2862.
5. Harris JA, Kolokathis A, Campbell M, Cassell GH, et al. Safety and efficacy of azithromycin in the treatment of community-acquired pneumonia in children. *Pediatr Infect Dis J.* 1998;17(10):865–871.
6. Guvenir H, Dibek Misirlioglu E, Capanoglu M, Vezir E, et al. Proven non-β-lactam antibiotic allergy in children. *Int Arch Allergy Immunol.* 2016;169(1):45–50.
7. Kavadas FD, Kasprzak A, Atkinson AR. Antibiotic skin testing accompanied by provocative challenges in children is a useful clinical tool. *Allergy Asthma Clin Immunol.* 2013;9(1):22.
8. Arikoglu T, Aslan G, Batmaz SB, Eskandari G, et al. Diagnostic evaluation and risk factors for drug allergies in children: from clinical history to skin and challenge tests. *Int J Clin Pharm.* 2015;37(4):583–591.
9. López Serrano C, Quiralte Enríquez J, Martínez Alzamora F. Urticaria from erythromycin. *Allergol Immunopathol (Madr).* 1993;21(6):225–226.
10. Pascual C, Crespo JF, Quiralte J, Lopez C, et al. In vitro detection of specific IgE antibodies to erythromycin. *J Allergy Clin Immunol.* 1995;95(3):668–671.
11. Jorro G, Morales C, Brasó JV, Peláez A. Anaphylaxis to erythromycin. *Ann Allergy Asthma Immunol.* 1996;77(6):456–458.
12. Kruppa A, Scharffetter-Kochanek K, Krieg T, Hunzelmann N. Immediate reaction to roxithromycin and prick test cross sensitization to erythromycin and clarithromycin. *Dermatology.* 1998;196:335–336.
13. Gurvinder SK, Tham P, Kanwar AJ. Roxithromycin induced acute urticaria. *Allergy.* 2002;57(3):262.
14. Ben-Shoshan M, Moore A, Primeau MN. Anaphylactic reaction to clarithromycin in a child. *Allergy.* 2009;64(6):962–963.
15. Bottenberg MM, Wall GC, Hicklin GA. Apparent anaphylactoid reaction after treatment with a single dose of telithromycin. *Ann Allergy Asthma Immunol.* 2007;98(1):89–91.

16. Bilgin M, Akyel A, Doğan M, Sunman H, et al. Acute coronary syndrome secondary to clarithromycin: the first case and review of the literature. *Turk Kardiyol Dern Ars.* 2014;42(5):461–463.

17. Gangemi S, Ricciardi L, Fedele R, Isola S, et al. Immediate reaction to clarithromycin. *Allergol Immunopathol (Madr).* 2001;29(1):31–32.

18. Malo JL, Cartier A. Occupational asthma in workers of a pharmaceutical company processing spiramycin. *Thorax.* 1988;43:371–377.

19. Malet A, Amat P, Valero A, Bescós M, et al. Occupational hypersensitivity to spiramycin. Report of a case. *Allergol Immunopathol.* 1992;20(3):127–130.

20. Benhamed S, Scaramuzza C, Messaad D, Sahla H, et al. The accuracy of the diagnosis of suspected macrolide antibiotic hypersensitivity: results of a single-blinded trial. *Allergy.* 2004;59(10):1130–1133.

21. Banerjee I, Mondal S, Sen S, Tripathi SK, et al. Azithromycin-induced rash in a patient of infectious mononucleosis – a case report with review of literature. *J Clin Diagn Res.* 2014;8(8):HD01–HD02.

22. Martins C, Freitas JD, Gonçalo M, Gonçalo S. Allergic contact dermatitis from erythromycin. *Contact Dermatitis.* 1995;33:360.

23. Valsecchi R, Pansera B, Reseghetti A. Contact allergy to erythromycin. *Contact Dermatitis.* 1996;34(6):428.

24. Fernandez Redondo V, Casas L, Taboada M, Toribio J. Systemic contact dermatitis from erythromycin. *Contact Dermatitis.* 1994;30:43–44.

25. Milkovic-Kraus S, Macan J, Kanceljak-Macan B. Occupational allergic contact dermatitis from azithromycin in pharmaceutical workers: a case series. *Contact Dermatitis.* 2007;56(2):99–102.

26. Flavia Monteagudo Paz A, Francisco Silvestre Salvador J, Latorre Martínez N, Cuesta Montero L, et al. Non-occupational allergic contact dermatitis caused by azithromycin in an eye solution. Allergic contact dermatitis caused by azithromycin in an eye drop. *Contact Dermatitis.* 2011;64(5):300–301.

27. Rosina P, Chieregato C, Schena D. Fixed drug eruption from clarithromycin. *Contact Dermatitis.* 1998;38 (105).

28. Hamamoto Y, Ohmura A, Kinoshita E, Muto M. Fixed drug eruption due to clarithromycin. *Clin Exp Dermatol.* 2001;26(1):48–49.

29. Malkarnekar SB, Naveen L. Fixed drug eruption due to clarithromycin. *J Res Pharm Pract.* 2013;2(4):169–171.

30. San Pedro de Saenz B, Gómez A, Quiralte J, Florido JF, et al. FDE to macrolides. *Allergy.* 2002;57(1):55–56.

31. da Cunha Filho RR, Bordignon SC, Cassol M, Rastelli GJ. Acute generalized exanthematous pustulosis by azithromycin. *Int J Dermatol.* 2015;54(6):e247–e249.

32. Trevisi P, Patrizi A, Neri I, Farina P. Toxic pustuloderma associated with azithromycin. *Clin Exp Dermatol.* 1994;19:280–281.

33. Amichai B, Grunwald MH. Baboon syndrome following oral roxithromycin. *Clin Exp Dermatol.* 2002;27(6):523.

34. Can C, Yazicioglu M, Ozdemir PG, Kilavuz S, et al. Symmetrical drug-related intertriginous and flexural exanthema induced by two different antibiotics. *Allergol Immunopathol (Madr).* 2014;42(2):173–175.

35. Bauer KA, Brimhall AK, Chang TT. Drug reaction with eosinophilia and systemic symptoms (DRESS) associated with azithromycin in acute Epstein-Barr virus infection. *Pediatric Dermatol.* 2011;28(6):741–743.

36. Schmutz JL, Trechot P. DRESS associated with azithromycin in a child. *Ann Dermatol Venereol.* 2013;140(1):75.

37. Sriratanaviriyakul N, Nguyen LP, Henderson MC, Albertson TE. Drug reaction with eosinophilia and systemic symptoms syndrome (DRESS) syndrome associated with azithromycin presenting like septic shock: a case report. *J Med Case Rep.* 2014;8:332.

38. Nappe TM, Goren-Garcia SL, Jacoby JL. Stevens-Johnson syndrome after treatment with azithromycin: an uncommon culprit. *Am J Emerg Med.* 2016;34(3):676.e1–3.

39. Aihara Y, Ito S, Kobayashi Y, Aihara M. Stevens–Johnson syndrome associated with azithromycin followed by transient reactivation of herpes simplex virus infection. *Allergy.* 2004;59(1):118.

40. Khaldi N, Miras A, Gromb S. Toxic epidermal necrolysis and clarithromycin. *Can J Clin Pharmacol.* 2005;12(3):e264–e268.

41. Das S, Mondal S, Dey JK. Roxithromycin-induced toxic epidermal necrolysis. *Ther Drug Monit.* August 2012;34(4):359–362.

42. Ohnishi H, Abe M, Yokoyama A, Hamada H, et al. Clarithromycin induced eosinophilic pneumonia. *Intern Med.* 2004;43(3):231–235.

43. Terzano C, Petroianni A. Clarithromycin and pulmonary infiltration with eosinophilia. *BMJ.* 2003;326(7403):1377–1378.

44. Park HY, Park SB, Jang KT, Koh WJ. Leukocytoclastic vasculitis associated with macrolide antibiotics. *Intern Med.* 2008;47(12):1157–1158.

45. Gavura SR, Nusinowitz S. Leukocytoclastic vasculitis associated with clarithromycin. *Ann Pharmacother.* 1998;32:543–545.

46. De Vega T, Blanco S, Lopez C, Pascual E, et al. Clarithromycin-induced leukocytoclastic vasculitis. *Eur J Clin Microbiol Infect Dis.* 1993;12:563.

47. Valero PI, Calvo CJ, Hortelano ME, et al. Schönlein–Henoch purpura associated with spiramycin and with important digestive manifestations. *Rev Esp Enferm Dig.* 1994;85:47–49.

48. Halpern B, Amache N. Diagnosis of drug allergy in vitro with the lymphocyte transformation test. *J Allergy.* 1967;40(3):168–181.

49. Demoly P, Benahmed S, Sahla H, Messaad D, et al. Allergy to macrolides. *Presse Med.* 2000;29(6):294–298.

50. Igea JM, Quirce S, de la Hoz B, Fraj J, et al. Adverse cutaneous reactions to macrolides. *Ann Allergy.* 1991;66:216–218.

51. Empedrad R, Darter AM, Earl HS, Gruchalla RS. Nonirritating intradermal skin test concentrations for commonly prescribed antibiotics. *J Allergy Clin Immunol.* 2003;112:629–630.

52. Won HK, Yang MS, Song WJ, Chang YS, et al. Determining non-irritating concentration for intradermal skin test with commonly prescribed antibiotics in Korean adults. *J Allergy Clin Immunol.* 2016;137(2):AB36.

53. Mori F, Barni S, Pucci N, Rossi E, et al. Annals of allergy. *Asthma Immunol.* 2010;104(5):417–419.

54. Cavkaytar O, Karaatmaca B, Yilmaz EA, Sekerel BE, et al. Testing for clarithromycin hypersensitivity: a diagnostic challenge in childhood. *J Allergy Clin Immunol.* 2016;4(2):330–332.

55. Brož P, Harr T, Hecking C, Grize L, et al. Nonirritant intradermal skin test concentrations of ciprofloxacin, clarithromycin, and rifampicin. *Allergy.* 2012;67(5):647–652.

56. Lammintausta K, Kortekangas-Savolainen O. The usefulness of skin tests to prove drug hypersensitivity. *Br J Dermatol.* 2005;152(5):968–974.

57. Barni S, Butti D, Mori F, Pucci N, et al. Azithromycin is more allergenic than clarithromycin in children with suspected hypersensitivity reaction to macrolides. *J Investig Allergol Clin Immunol.* 2015;25:128–132.

58. Chia FL, Thong BY. Macrolide allergy: which tests are really useful? *Allergol Immunopathol (Madr).* 2011;39(4):191–192.

59. Seitz CS, Bröcker EB, Trautmann A. Suspicion of macrolide allergy after treatment of infectious diseases including *Helicobacter pylori*: results of allergological testing. *Allergol Immunopathol (Madr).* 2011;39(4):193–199.

60. Na HR, Lee JM, Jung JW, Lee SY. Usefulness of drug provocation tests in children with a history of adverse drug reaction. *Korean J Pediatr.* 2011;54(7):304–309.

61. Messaad D, Sahla H, Benahmed S, Godard P, et al. Drug provocation tests in patients with a history suggesting an immediate drug hypersensitivity reaction. *Ann Intern Med.* 2004;140(12):1001–1006.

62. Luu NN, DesRoches A, Primeau M. Drug provocation test (DPT) in patients with a history of macrolide allergy. *J Allergy Clin Immunol.* 2016;117(2):S224.

63. Holmes NE, Hodgkinson M, Dendle C, Korman TM. Report of oral clarithromycin desensitization. *Br J Clin Pharmacol.* 2008;66(2):323–324.

64. Swamy N, Laurie SA, Ruiz-Huidobro E, Khan DA. Successful clarithromycin desensitization in a multiple macrolide-allergic patient. *Ann Allergy Asthma Immunol.* 2010;105(6):489–490.

65. Sánchez-Morillas L, Laguna-Martínez JJ, Reaño-Martos M, Rojo-Andrés E, et al. Hypersensitivity to spiramycin with good tolerance of other macrolides. *J Investig Allergol Clin Immunol.* 2007vol. 17(6):413–423.

66. Igea JM, Lazaro M. Hypersensitivity reaction to clarithromycin. *Allergy.* 1998;53(1):107–109.

67. Andersen LK, Jensen JE, Bygum A. Second episode of near-fatal angioedema in a patient treated with everolimus. *Ann Allergy Asthma Immunol.* 2015;115(2):152–153.

68. White DA, Schwartz LH, Dimitrijevic S, Scala LD, et al. Characterization of pneumonitis in patients with advanced non-small cell lung cancer treated with everolimus. *J Thorac Oncol.* 2009;4(11):1357–1363.

69. Riley L, et al. Cross-sensitivity reaction between tacrolimus and macrolide antibiotics. *Bone Marrow Transplant.* 2000;25:907–908.

FURTHER READING

1. Misirlioglu ED, Toyran M, Capanoglu M, Kaya A, et al. Negative predictive value of drug provocation tests in children. *Pediatr Allergy Immunol.* 2014;25(7):685–690.

CHAPTER 13

Quinolone Allergy

INMACULADA DOÑA, MD, PHD • ESTHER BARRIONUEVO, MD, PHD • MARÍA I. MONTAÑEZ, PHD • TAHIA D. FERNÁNDEZ, PHD[a] • MARÍA J. TORRES, MD, PHD[a]

KEY POINTS

- Fluoroquinolones (FQs) are generally safe and well-tolerated antibiotics; however, adverse effects have been reported.
- The incidence of hypersensitivity reactions to FQs has been rising, and they are now the most frequent non-β-lactam antibiotics involved in drug hypersensitivity.
- A precise diagnosis can be difficult because history is often unreliable and test reagents are not standardized. Drug provocation testing (DPT) is generally accepted as the gold standard.
- Skin tests have a low sensitivity and high rate of false-positive results.
- There are currently no validated commercial in vitro tests for the evaluation of FQ allergy.

INTRODUCTION

Quinolones represent an important category of antibiotics, the most relevant members of which are the FQs, a group of synthetic antibiotics with a wide range of activities against both gram-negative and gram-positive bacteria. Ciprofloxacin is the most frequently used FQ worldwide.[1]

Although FQs are generally safe and well-tolerated antibiotics, adverse effects have been reported involving hypersensitivity and phototoxicity. In the last few decades, there has been an increase in the incidence of hypersensitivity reactions to FQs,[2] some of which have been severe, including anaphylactic reactions, acute exanthematic reactions, and toxic epidermal necrolysis (TEN).[3]

CLASSIFICATION AND CHEMICAL STRUCTURE

The basic quinolone structure is shown in Table 13.1. It consists of a bicyclic aromatic core displaying the R1-substituted nitrogen at the 1 position, the ketone group at the C4 position, and a carboxylic group at the C3 position.[4] The atom attached at the 8 position can be a carbon, in the case of true quinolones, or a nitrogen, in which case the structure formed is a naphthyridone, although both structures are considered quinolone agents. The analogs have different substituents

at the C2, C6, C7, or C8 positions. These structural differences modify their antibacterial activity, half-life, and toxicity. Quinolones are classified into four generations with different antibacterial spectra (Table 13.1). The first generation includes nalidixic acid and cinoxacin, which have a gram-negative spectrum. The addition of a fluorine atom at C6 and a dialkylamino substituent at C7 yields FQs corresponding to the second, third, and fourth generations, with an extended antibacterial spectrum covering gram-negative and gram-positive bacteria.[4]

EPIDEMIOLOGY AND RISK FACTORS

Although hypersensitivity reactions to FQs are considered unusual,[5] their incidence has been rising, and FQs are now the most frequent non-β-lactam antibiotics involved in drug hypersensitivity[2,5,6] and the third leading cause of confirmed hypersensitivity to drugs.[2] This is likely because of their increased prescription and the introduction of moxifloxacin,[5] which has been shown to be the most frequent cause of FQ reactions.[7] Most hypersensitivity reactions to FQs are immediate reactions (IRs), which are IgE mediated, being severe in 70% of cases.[7-9] Although less common, delayed reactions (DRs), which are T cell–dependent reactions, have also been reported.[10-16]

Considering risk factors, 21% of penicillin allergic patients have been reported to develop allergy to non-β-lactam antibiotics such as FQ, compared with just

---

[a] Both have contributed equally to the work.

TABLE 13.1
Basic Structure of Quinolone Antibacterial Agents and Classification by Generation

Basic Structure	CLASSIFICATION OF QUINOLONES			
	1st Generation	**2nd Generation**	**3rd Generation**	**4th Generation**
	Cinoxacin	Lomefloxacin	Levofloxacin	Gemifloxacin
	Nalidixic acid	Enoxacin	Gatifloxacin	Moxifloxacin
		Ciprofloxacin	Sparfloxacin	Trovafloxacin
		Norfloxacin	Pazufloxacin	Clinafloxacin
		Ofloxacin	Temafloxacin	Sitafloxacin
			Grepafloxacin	Ulifloxacin
			Tosufloxacin	Besifloxacin

X= H Quinolone
X= F Fluoroquinolone

A= N, CH or CR$_4$

1% of those who were not penicillin allergic. In fact, a previous diagnosis of IR to β-lactam antibiotics has been shown to be a strong risk factor for developing FQ allergy (odds ratio [OR], 23.654; 95% confidence interval [CI], 1.529–365.853; P = .024). It is unclear whether this is because of an inherent predisposition to developing an allergy or because patients diagnosed as allergic to β-lactams are more likely to be prescribed FQs.[7]

Moxifloxacin has been shown to be the most common culprit for IR and has been shown to increase the odds of suffering a reaction by fourfold, compared with other drugs (OR, 4.20; 95% CI, 3.19–5.55).[17] However, ciprofloxacin has been associated with a higher risk of developing severe cutaneous DR (OR, 6.9; 95% CI, 1.8–27)[18] compared with other drugs and norfloxacin, ofloxacin, and ciprofloxacin with a high risk of acute generalized exanthematous pustulosis (AGEP) (OR, 33; 95% CI, 8.5–127)[19] compared with other FQs.

CLINICAL SYMPTOMS

Allergic reactions to FQs can be classified as either IR, appearing within 1 h after drug intake, or DR, appearing more than 1 h after drug intake.[20]

Immediate Reactions

Most published studies reporting IR after FQ administration are case reports or short series.[3,19,21–25] Symptoms experienced by patients comprise anaphylaxis (32.8%–42.1% of cases), anaphylactic shock (13%–26.3%), and urticaria, which can be accompanied by angioedema (31.6%–85%).[6,9,26–28] The FQs most frequently involved include ciprofloxacin (23.2%–43.7%), moxifloxacin (15.4%–63.2%), and levofloxacin (7.9%–38.5%).[6,9,26–28]

Delayed Reactions

DRs to FQs are less frequent than IRs, and most published studies are case reports or short series.[10–15,19,26,28,29] Maculopapular exanthema (MPE), fixed drug eruption (FDE), and photoallergy are the most commonly reported reactions,[12,20,26,28] although other less frequent entities, such as AGEP,[12,19] Steven-Johnson syndrome, and TEN,[13–15] have been described. The most frequent FQ involved in DR is ciprofloxacin, followed by moxifloxacin, ofloxacin, and levofloxacin.[12,26,28]

DIAGNOSIS

Diagnostic procedures in FQ hypersensitivity may include patient history, skin testing (ST), in vitro testing, and DPT.[30,31,33] However, a precise diagnosis can be difficult as history is often unreliable because different drugs are often taken simultaneously and test reagents are not standardized, either for in vitro testing or for ST; therefore DPT is generally accepted as the gold standard.[13,31,32]

Clinical History

Diagnostic evaluation is based on a detailed description of the symptoms, which can be obtained from the patient, the family in the case of children and when patients are unable to do so themselves, from clinical reports. However, a precise clinical history can be difficult to obtain, especially when the reaction occurred a long time ago. It is important to register the time interval between drug administration and the onset of the reaction and a detailed description of the symptomatology. The first is needed to classify the reaction as IR or DR and the second to define the type of reaction. It is also necessary to take into account the dose of the drug and the route of administration and, if required, to assess tolerance to the same drug and others belonging to the same pharmacologic group.

Other data that must be registered in the clinical history are previous episodes of hypersensitivity induced by the same drug or others belonging to the same group, how long the patient was taking the culprit drug before the reaction occurred, and the treatment received to resolve the reaction, as well as age, gender, atopy, underlying diseases, other drugs usually taken by the patient, and allergies to other drugs.[33]

Skin Tests

For IR, the procedure generally begins with a skin prick test, and if negative, intradermal test (IDT). However, for diagnosing hypersensitivity reactions to FQs there is controversy regarding the utility of ST because of a low sensitivity and high rate of false-positive results. In a study performed in patients with suspected IR to FQ, 56% of cases had a positive ST; however, only 14.8% of these showed a positive DPT (sensitivity 8.2%). The ST specificity was 46.5% and the positive and negative predictive values were 14.8% and 95.2%, respectively.[34] However, in another study, ST showed a sensitivity of 71% and a specificity of 86%, with positive and negative predictive values of 50% and 94%, respectively.[28] Other studies suggest that ST is not valid because it can induce both false-negative[6,32] and false-positive results.[13,29,32,35] The reasons for these false-positive results are not completely clear, but they could be due to the capacity of some FQs to induce direct histamine release by mast cells.[9] To avoid false-positive results, some authors have determined optimal, nonirritating FQ test concentrations by performing IDT in a group of healthy, nonallergic subjects.[19] However, other authors have been unable to establish an ideal non-irritant concentration for IDT.[3,6,22–26] Because of this controversy, we do not recommend ST for assessing FQ hypersensitivity.

The evaluation of DR is usually performed by delayed-reading IDT and patch tests (PTs).[30] When photoallergic or phototoxic reactions are suspected, photopatch tests with ultraviolet A light exposure can be performed.[36] Moreover, scarification of the skin before photopatch testing to enhance drug penetration has been suggested to increase sensitivity.[19] Concerning DR, as with IR, studies of the role of PT or IDT have shown contradictory results. Sensitivity ranges widely depending on the symptomatology of the reaction, diagnostic test used (IDT or PT), drug concentration, drug vehicle used in PT (petrolatum, dimethylsulfoxide, etc.), and if the test is only performed on unaffected skin (or previously affected skin in FDE). Other factors that can contribute to low ST sensitivity in DR include whether it is performed during the refractory period (2 weeks after the resolution of the reaction), sensitization to FQ metabolites rather than to the native drug, and the limited skin penetration capacity of the drug.[37] Regarding IDT, 80% of FQ allergic subjects have been reported to give positive test results, although the possibility of an irritant response was not ruled out.[28] IDT has been shown to be positive in 60% of cases with urticaria or MPE 24 h after FQ administration, 66.6% of which were ultimately confirmed as allergic.[28]

Results vary with regards to PT: some authors have found positive PT in 50% of DRs,[12,19] whereas others found no positive results.[26] In a study of six patients with MPE and AGEP related to ciprofloxacin, moxifloxacin, and norfloxacin, positive PTs to ciprofloxacin were observed in three patients[12]; in another study, PTs were shown to be positive for more than 50% of AGEP cases.[19] There is currently one report of a positive PT in a patient with FDE related to ciprofloxacin, which was performed in lesional skin.[16] No positive PTs could be obtained in another study of 37 patients with FDE.[26]

In vitro tests

There are currently no validated commercial in vitro tests for the evaluation of FQ allergy. Determination of specific IgE (sIgE) in IR has been performed using FQ coupled to an epoxy-activated Sepharose 6B as the solid phase (Sepharose-radioimmunoassay [RIA]). This technique has shown a high specificity, although it varies between studies from 30% to 55%.[9,27] This difference may be due to the quinolone involved in each study and the severity of the reactions, with better results found when the FQs involved were mainly ciprofloxacin and the reactions were less severe, such as urticaria. On the other hand, we must take into account the time interval between the reaction and the performance of the test because significantly higher sIgE levels were found in patients evaluated within a few months after the reaction, whereas patients showing negative results were generally evaluated after a longer time period.[27]

Basophil activation tests (BATs) have shown to be useful for the in vitro evaluation of FQ hypersensitivity.[9,22,38,39] It has been reported to have a sensitivity of 71% with a higher rate of positive cases for severe reactions (69%).[9] This technique has also been shown to have a good negative predictive value, with subjects presenting negative results with both BAT and DPT,[38] making it easier for the clinician to decide whether to perform DPT in suspected FQ allergic patients. As mentioned earlier, BAT sensitivity is affected by the FQ investigated. Moreover, the use of additional FQs, as well as the suspected culprit, can affect the results. For example, in moxifloxacin allergic patients, BAT results were better when both moxifloxacin and ciprofloxacin were included in the test, with BAT sensitivity increasing from 41.7% to 79.2% compared with the results obtained using only the culprit. However, in ciprofloxacin allergic patients, the inclusion of moxifloxacin in the test did not improve the sensitivity, suggesting a previous sensitization to ciprofloxacin in moxifloxacin allergic patients because the latter was introduced to the market later.[9] In all cases, the inclusion of ciprofloxacin in the test leads to increased sensitivity. This could be due to various reasons. First, it may be due to the chemical structure and photodegradation of the molecules. Moxifloxacin has been shown to have a higher rate of photodegradation than ciprofloxacin,[40] and the performance of the test under laboratory light conditions may affect moxifloxacin BAT results, reducing

the positivity of the test from 35.7% when carried out in dark conditions to 17.9%.[40] The activation marker used in the test is also crucial. It has been observed that ciprofloxacin induces a greater upregulation of CD63, particularly for milder reactions, whereas moxifloxacin preferentially upregulates CD203c in more severe reactions (Fig. 13.1). Thus the choice of marker can have a strong bearing on the sensitivity of BAT when testing FQs, and use of both is recommended when possible.[39] Finally, as for other drugs, it is important to take into account the time interval between reaction occurrence and BAT performance. In BAT to FQ, a negative correlation has been found between the time interval and the upregulation of the activation marker, highlighting the importance of performing the test as soon as possible after the reaction.[39]

Regarding DR, most studies use the lymphocyte transformation test (LTT)[12,19,41] to demonstrate the involvement of T cells in the pathogenesis of clinical

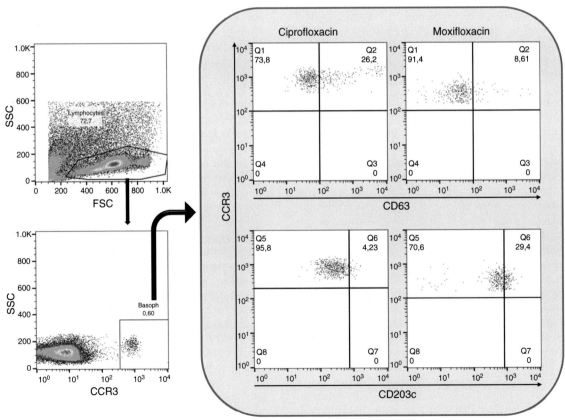

FIG. 13.1 Flow cytometry dot plots showing the classical analysis strategy of basophil activation test and an example of the differential expression of activation markers depending on the drug tested.

entities such as MPE and AGEP induced by FQs. Moreover, LTT has shown a higher sensitivity than PTs, making it potentially a promising in vitro diagnostic tool. This increased sensitivity may be due to a low capacity of FQs to penetrate the skin, or to the use of low FQ concentrations in PT.[12] Further proof of the involvement of T cells in DR can be obtained by assessing whether peripheral blood mononuclear cells photomodified with quinolones using ultraviolet A light are able to stimulate homologous cell proliferation, as has been demonstrated in photoallergy studies.[41,42]

Drug provocation test

DPT is considered the gold standard to establish or exclude the diagnosis of hypersensitivity to FQ when no other test is available. It is also useful to choose an alternative FQ if diagnosis is confirmed[28,31] and to evaluate cross-reactivity in patients who are ST or in vitro test positive.[7] DPT is not a risk-free procedure and must be performed by trained personnel in a clinical setting where rapid and adequate treatment can be administered if a reaction occurs[31] and should be considered only after balancing the risks and benefits for the individual patient.[26]

DPT should be performed in a single-blind placebo-controlled manner, although in some cases a double-blind procedure may be necessary.[31] The doses and number of steps used in DPT vary and depend on the study (Table 13.2).

The necessity of DPT for quinolone hypersensitivity evaluation is clear given that only 7%–32% of those with suspected IR and DR to FQ who underwent DPT could be confirmed as allergic.[26,28] In other words, up to 93% of patients evaluated for FQ allergy were not truly allergic, indicating that clinical history alone is often an unreliable indicator of true FQ hypersensitivity and can lead to overdiagnosis. One reason for this could be that initial symptoms first interpreted as signs of FQ hypersensitivity, such as urticaria or exanthema, are really caused by other factors such as infectious agents[26] or by other drugs taken simultaneously to quinolone, leading to difficulties in the assessment of causality. Moreover, a loss of sensitivity to drugs over time has been reported for IgE-mediated hypersensitivity reactions, as has been shown in IRs to β-lactams,[43] dypirone,[44] and neuromuscular blocking agent.[45] Therefore, the time interval between the suspected hypersensitivity reaction and the DPT can affect the outcome of the tests.

CROSS-REACTIVITY

The presence of cross-reactivity among FQ remains a controversial issue. It has been suggested to be associated with the common FQ structure, a 4-oxo-1,4-dihydroquinoleine ring core that may act as the antigenic determinant,[46] although the structure of groups bound to the C1, C5, C7, and C8 positions may also play a role.

In IR, a high degree of cross-reactivity has been reported between the first- (nalidixic acid) and second-generation (norfloxacin and ciprofloxacin) FQs.[21] Some second-generation FQs have shown cross-reactivity[29]; however, this does not always occur[10,35] and may be due to the production of different metabolites.

The same phenomena can occur with the newer FQ (moxifloxacin) and the second- (ciprofloxacin) and third-generation (levofloxacin) FQ.[3,5,24,25] Regarding levofloxacin, a low degree of cross-reactivity with ciprofloxacin has been found.[6] Using Sepharose-RIA, sIgE toward more than one quinolone was detected in 63.6%–80% of cases, although only 16% of these patients reported a reaction to several quinolones.[9,27] Regarding BAT, positive results from more than one quinolone have been found in 48.2% of cases.[9,40] This suggests that IgE can recognize the chemical structure of ciprofloxacin despite the reaction being induced by moxifloxacin.[9] Therefore, in vitro cross-reactivity may overrepresent true cross-reactivity based on DPT.

TABLE 13.2 Doses of Quinolones Used in Drug Provocation Testing					
Drug (mg)	Chang et al.[3]	Aranda et al.[9]	Lobera et al.[6] Gonzalez et al.[25] Seitz et al.[26]	Lobera et al.[6]	Seitz et al.[26]
Ciprofloxacin	250	5-50-100-150-200	50-125-250-500		
Levofloxacin		5-50-100-150-200	50-125-250-500		
Moxifloxacin	200	5-50-100-100-150	40-100-200-400	40-100-200-400	25-50-100-200
Ofloxacin					25-50-100-200

In DR, different grades of cross-reactivity between FQs from different generations have been reported for the different clinical entities.[47–49] An evaluation of the recognition of ciprofloxacin-specific T cell clones from patients who have suffered MPE[12] showed three main patterns: clones that reacted only to ciprofloxacin; others that reacted to two related quinolones, ciprofloxacin and norfloxacin; and clones that reacted to up to five quinolones.[13,16,35] A study of photoreactivity in a murine model of photoallergy showed cross-reactivity among six FQs for both in vivo and in vitro responses. This suggests that photohaptens also share a common epitope that is recognized by T cells, particularly Th1.[42] In vitro cross-reactivity studies seem to indicate that T cells recognize a common structure, whereas IgE recognizes smaller components such as side chains or small groups, although with lower affinity.[50]

In addition, cross-reactivity with other drugs has been reported in IR. Previously confirmed hypersensitivity to β-lactams is a risk factor for the development of hypersensitivity to FQ,[7] and quaternary ammonium sIgE has been detected in 53% of patients with IR to FQ, suggesting cross-reactivity with neuromuscular blocking agents[51]; however, the clinical relevance of this finding remains undefined. Quinolones can induce IR after a single use,[8,51] suggesting that sensitization was induced by another component that shares a common antigenic determinant.[8] Moreover, quinolones can induce a direct stimulation of mast-cell degranulation, mediated nonimmunologically.[52]

MANAGEMENT

Patients with a diagnosis of hypersensitivity to FQ must avoid the culprit drug. It is also important to establish an accurate diagnosis of hypersensitivity to related drugs, and to assess cross-reactivity to other quinolones. This is especially important for patients with a previous history of hypersensitivity to other antibiotics, for whom the therapeutic possibilities decrease dramatically.

When allergy to a quinolone has been proved, tolerance to another one can be assessed if necessary. Cross-reactivity between quinolones is not well known because of the small number of patients included in the scarce studies published performing DPT to several quinolones.[6,10,21,24,25,29]

When FQ is the only therapeutic option available, clinical tolerance induction may be required. There are only five reports about desensitization to FQ.[11,53–56] Three of them are patients with IR induced by ciprofloxacin[53–55] confirmed by DPT or ST. Another report[56] describes two cases of DR induced by ciprofloxacin confirmed by DPT. Although the induction is normally temporary, a case has been described in which long-term tolerance to ciprofloxacin was achieved after the desensitization of a patient with a history of FDE related to this drug.[11]

CONCLUSIONS

The number of documented cases of hypersensitivity to quinolones has increased in the last few decades, particularly for IR and for reactions induced by moxifloxacin. Diagnosis is complex, because clinical history is often unreliable and ST can induce false-positive results. Therefore, in many cases, the only way to diagnose tolerance is with DPT, a procedure that can carry some risks. FQs present a variable degree of cross-reactivity with other FQs that is difficult to predict. Importantly, hypersensitivity to FQs may be influenced by allergy to other drugs such as β-lactams and neuromuscular blocking agents, although further studies are needed to understand the underlying mechanism.

CONFLICT OF INTEREST

None of the authors has any conflict of interest, nor have they received any money for the present study.

FUNDING

The present study has been supported by the Institute of Health "Carlos III" of the Ministry of Economy and Competitiveness cofounded by European Regional Development Fund (ERDF): PI12/02529, PI15/01206, Red de Reacciones Adversas a Alergenos y Farmacos: RD12/0013/0001 and RETIC ARADYAL RD16/0006/0001. I Doña hold a Juan Rodes research contract (JR15/00036)and MI Montañez holds a Miguel Servet I research contact (CP15/00103), both by Institute of Health "Carlos III" of the Ministry of Economy and Competitiveness (grants cofunded by European Social Fund (ESF)).

REFERENCES

1. Hooper DC. Mechanisms of action of antimicrobials: focus on fluoroquinolones. *Clin Infect Dis.* 2001;32(suppl 1):S9–S15.
2. Dona I, Blanca-Lopez N, Torres MJ, et al. Drug hypersensitivity reactions: response patterns, drug involved, and temporal variations in a large series of patients. *J Invest Allergol Clin Immunol.* 2012;22(5):363–371.

3. Chang B, Knowles SR, Weber E. Immediate hypersensitivity to moxifloxacin with tolerance to ciprofloxacin: report of three cases and review of the literature. *Ann Pharmacother*. 2010;44(4):740–745.

4. Joana Sousa GA, Fortuna A, Falcao A. Third and fourth generation fluoroquinolone antibacterials: a systematic review of safety and toxicity profiles. *Curr Drug Safety*. 2014;9(2):89–105.

5. Blanca-Lopez N, Andreu I, Torres Jaen MJ. Hypersensitivity reactions to quinolones. *Curr Opin Allergy Clin Immunol*. 2011;11(4):285–291.

6. Lobera T, Audicana MT, Alarcon E, Longo N, Navarro B, Munoz D. Allergy to quinolones: low cross-reactivity to levofloxacin. *J Invest Allergol Clin Immunol*. 2010;20(7):607–611.

7. Blanca-Lopez N, et al. Hypersensitivity reactions to fluoroquinolones: analysis of the factors involved. *Clin Exp Allergy*. 2013;43(5):560–567.

8. Sachs B, Riegel S, Seebeck J, et al. Fluoroquinolone-associated anaphylaxis in spontaneous adverse drug reaction reports in Germany: differences in reporting rates between individual fluoroquinolones and occurrence after first-ever use. *Drug Safety*. 2006;29(11):1087–1100.

9. Aranda A, Mayorga C, Ariza A, et al. In vitro evaluation of IgE-mediated hypersensitivity reactions to quinolones. *Allergy*. 2011;66(2):247–254.

10. Fernandez-Rivas M. Fixed drug eruption (FDE) caused by norfloxacin. *Allergy*. 1997;52(4):477–478.

11. Garcia Rodriguez R, Galindo Bonilla PA, Feo Brito FJ, et al. Chronic desensitization to quinolones in fixed drug eruption. *J Invest Allergol Clin Immunol*. 2011;21(1):76–77.

12. Schmid DA, Depta JP, Pichler WJ. T cell-mediated hypersensitivity to quinolones: mechanisms and cross-reactivity. *Clin Exp Allergy*. 2006;36(1):59–69.

13. Davila G, Ruiz-Hornillos J, Rojas P, De Castro F, Zubeldia JM. Toxic epidermal necrolysis induced by levofloxacin. *Ann Allergy Asthma Immunol*. 2009;102(5):441–442.

14. Islam AF, Rahman MS. Levofloxacin-induced fatal toxic epidermal necrolysis. *Ann Pharmacother*. 2005;39(6):1136–1137.

15. Yoon SY, Bae YJ, Cho YS, Moon HB, Kim TB. Toxic epidermal necrolysis induced by ofloxacin. *Acta Derm Venereol*. 2010;90(5):550–551.

16. Rodriguez-Morales A, Llamazares AA, Benito RP, Cocera CM. Fixed drug eruption from quinolones with a positive lesional patch test to ciprofloxacin. *Contact Dermatitis*. 2001;44(4):255.

17. Salvo F, Polimeni G, Cutroneo PM, et al. Allergic reactions to oral drugs: a case/non-case study from an Italian spontaneous reporting database (GIF). *Pharmacol Res*. 2008;58(3–4):202–207.

18. Mockenhaupt M, Viboud C, Dunant A, et al. Stevens-Johnson syndrome and toxic epidermal necrolysis: assessment of medication risks with emphasis on recently marketed drugs. The EuroSCAR-study. *J Invest Dermatol*. 2008;128(1):35–44.

19. Scherer K, Bircher AJ. Hypersensitivity reactions to fluoroquinolones. *Curr Allergy Asthma Rep*. 2005;5(1):15–21.

20. Mayorga C, Torres MJ, Fernandez J, Canto G, Blanca M. Cutaneous symptoms in drug allergy: what have we learnt? *Curr Opin Allergy Clin Immunol*. 2009;9(5):431–436.

21. Davila I, Diez ML, Quirce S, Fraj J, De La Hoz B, Lazaro M. Cross-reactivity between quinolones. Report of three cases. *Allergy*. 1993;48(5):388–390.

22. Ben Said B, Berard F, Bienvenu J, Nicolas JF, Rozieres A. Usefulness of basophil activation tests for the diagnosis of IgE-mediated allergy to quinolones. *Allergy*. 2010;65(4):535–536.

23. Gonzalez-Mancebo E, Fernandez-Rivas M. Immediate hypersensitivity to levofloxacin diagnosed through skin prick test. *Ann Pharmacother*. 2004;38(2):354.

24. Sanchez-Morillas L, Rojas Perez-Ezquerra P, Reano-Martos M, Laguna-Martinez JJ, Gomez-Tembleque P. Systemic anaphylaxis caused by moxifloxacin. *Allergol Immunopathol*. 2010;38(4):226–227.

25. Gonzalez I, Lobera T, Blasco A, del Pozo MD. Immediate hypersensitivity to quinolones: moxifloxacin cross-reactivity. *J Invest Allergol Clin Immunol*. 2005;15(2):146–149.

26. Seitz CS, Brocker EB, Trautmann A. Diagnostic testing in suspected fluoroquinolone hypersensitivity. *Clin Exp Allergy*. 2009;39(11):1738–1745.

27. Manfredi M, Severino M, Testi S, et al. Detection of specific IgE to quinolones. *J Allergy Clin Immunol*. 2004;113(1):155–160.

28. Venturini Diaz M, Lobera Labairu T, del Pozo Gil MD, Blasco Sarramian A, Gonzalez Mahave I. In vivo diagnostic tests in adverse reactions to quinolones. *J Invest Allergol Clin Immunol*. 2007;17(6):393–398.

29. Alonso MD, Martin JA, Quirce S, Davila I, Lezaun A, Sanchez Cano M. Fixed eruption caused by ciprofloxacin with cross-sensitivity to norfloxacin. *Allergy*. 1993;48(4):296–297.

30. Brockow K, Romano A, Blanca M, Ring J, Pichler W, Demoly P. General considerations for skin test procedures in the diagnosis of drug hypersensitivity. *Allergy*. 2002;57(1):45–51.

31. Aberer W, Bircher A, Romano A, et al. Drug provocation testing in the diagnosis of drug hypersensitivity reactions: general considerations. *Allergy*. 2003;58(9):854–863.

32. Valdivieso R, Pola J, Losada E, Subiza J, Armentia A, Zapata C. Severe anaphylactoid reaction to nalidixic acid. *Allergy*. 1988;43(1):71–73.

33. Demoly P, Kropf R, Bircher A, Pichler WJ. Drug hypersensitivity: questionnaire. EAACI interest group on drug hypersensitivity. *Allergy*. 1999;54(9):999–1003.

34. Perez E, Callero A, Martinez-Tadeo JA, et al. Are skin tests useful in fluoroquinolone hypersensitivity diagnosis? *Ann Allergy Asthma Immunol*. 2013;111(5):423–425.

35. Lozano Ayllon M, Gomez Martinez M, Mosquera MR, Laguna Martinez JJ, Orta Martiartu M, Fernandez de Miguel C. Fixed eruption caused by ciprofloxacin without cross-sensitivity to norfloxacin. *Allergy*. 1995;50(7):598–599.

36. Holzle E, Neumann N, Hausen B, et al. Photopatch testing: the 5-year experience of the German, Austrian, and Swiss Photopatch Test Group. *J Am Acad Dermatol.* 1991;25(1 Pt 1):59–68.

37. Shiohara T. Fixed drug eruption: pathogenesis and diagnostic tests. *Curr Opin Allergy Clin Immunol.* 2009;9(4):316–321.

38. Rouzaire P, Nosbaum A, Denis L, et al. Negativity of the basophil activation test in quinolone hypersensitivity: a breakthrough for provocation test decision-making. *Int Arch Allergy Immunol.* 2012;157(3):299–302.

39. Fernandez TD, Ariza A, Palomares F, et al. Hypersensitivity to fluoroquinolones: The expression of basophil activation markers depends on the clinical entity and the culprit fluoroquinolone. *Medicine (Baltimore).* 2016;95(23):e3679.

40. Mayorga C, Andreu I, Aranda A, et al. Fluoroquinolone photodegradation influences specific basophil activation. *Int Arch Allergy Immunol.* 2013;160(4):377–382.

41. Campi P, Pichler WJ. Quinolone hypersensitivity. *Current Opin Allergy Clin Immunol.* 2003;3(4):275–281.

42. Tokura Y, Seo N, Ohshima A, Yagi H, Furukawa F, Takigawa M. Lymphocyte stimulation test with drug-photomodified cells in patients with quinolone photosensitivity. *J Dermatol Sci.* 1999;21(1):34–41.

43. Fernandez TD, Torres MJ, Blanca-Lopez N, et al. Negativization rates of IgE radioimmunoassay and basophil activation test in immediate reactions to penicillins. *Allergy.* 2009;64(2):242–248.

44. Gomez E, Blanca-Lopez N, Torres MJ, et al. Immunoglobulin E-mediated immediate allergic reactions to dipyrone: value of basophil activation test in the identification of patients. *Clin Exp Allergy.* 2009;39(8):1217–1224.

45. Kvedariene V, Kamey S, Ryckwaert Y, et al. Diagnosis of neuromuscular blocking agent hypersensitivity reactions using cytofluorimetric analysis of basophils. *Allergy.* 2006;61(3):311–315.

46. Nishijima S, Nakagawa M. Fixed drug eruption caused by tosufloxacin tosilate. *J Int Med Res.* 1997;25(6):359–363.

47. Kameswari PD, Selvaraj N, Adhimoolam M. Fixed drug eruptions caused by cross-reactive quinolones. *J Basic Clin Pharm.* 2014;5(2):54–55.

48. Ball P, Mandell L, Patou G, Dankner W, Tillotson G. A new respiratory fluoroquinolone, oral gemifloxacin: a safety profile in context. *Int J Antimicrob Agents.* 2004;23(5):421–429.

49. Howard-Thompson A, Cartmell B, Suda KJ. Toxic epidermal necrolysis reaction associated with the use of moxifloxacin. *Int J Antimicrob Agents.* 2014;44(2):178–179.

50. Depta JP, Altznauer F, Gamerdinger K, Burkhart C, Weltzien HU, Pichler WJ. Drug interaction with T-cell receptors: T-cell receptor density determines degree of cross-reactivity. *J Allergy clin Immunol.* 2004;113(3):519–527.

51. Rouzaire P, Nosbaum A, Mullet C, et al. Immediate allergic hypersensitivity to quinolones associates with neuromuscular blocking agent sensitization. *J Allergy Clin Immunol Prac.* 2013;1(3):273–279. e1.

52. Subramanian H, Gupta K, Ali H. Roles of Mas-related G protein-coupled receptor X2 on mast cell-mediated host defense, pseudoallergic drug reactions, and chronic inflammatory diseases. *J Allergy Clin Immunol.* 2016;138(3):700–710.

53. Erdem G, Staat MA, Connelly BL, Assa'ad A. Anaphylactic reaction to ciprofloxacin in a toddler: successful desensitization. *Pediatr Infect Dis J.* 1999;18(6):563–564.

54. Gea-Banacloche JC, Metcalfe DD. Ciprofloxacin desensitization. *J Allergy Clin Immunol.* 1996;97(6):1426–1427.

55. Lantner RR. Ciprofloxacin desensitization in a patient with cystic fibrosis. *J Allergy Clin Immunol.* 1995;96(6 Pt 1):1001–1002.

56. Bircher AJ, Rutishauser M. Oral "desensitization" of maculopapular exanthema from ciprofloxacin. *Allergy.* 1997;52(12):1246–1248.

CHAPTER 14

Sulfonamide Drug Allergy

JOSHUA M. DORN, MD • GERALD W. VOLCHECK, MD

KEY POINTS

- Sulfonamide hypersensitivity is a common clinical entity that can have multiple clinical manifestations. The mechanisms of reactions vary and objective diagnostic methods are lacking. Take multiple forms with uncertainty regarding mechanism of reactions, diagnostic methods, and cross-reactivity.
- As data have accumulated, cross-reactivity between sulfonamide antibiotics and nonantibiotics has become less of a concern.
- There is a significant experience with desensitization to sulfonamide antibiotics in the HIV population and non-HIV population.

INTRODUCTION

Sulfonamide medications, and especially antibiotics, are commonly used and frequently associated with adverse and hypersensitivity reactions. Hypersensitivity reactions to sulfonamide antibiotics occur in roughly 4%–6% of the general population and in up to 50%–60% of patients with HIV.[1,2] After β-lactam antibiotics, sulfonamide antibiotics are the most commonly implicated antibiotics in allergic reactions.[3] In both children and adults, they cause a disproportionate number of severe reactions such as erythema multiforme, Stevens-Johnson syndrome (SJS), and toxic epidermal necrolysis (TEN).[4,5] Reactions to sulfonamide medications can be especially difficult to clinically diagnose and manage because reactions are highly variable in presentation. Furthermore, unlike β-lactam antibiotics, objective diagnostic tools are lacking. There is, however, significant experience with desensitization to sulfonamide antibiotics especially with the most commonly used antibiotic, trimethoprim-sulfamethoxazole (TMP-SMX). This chapter will address sulfonamide antibiotic hypersensitivity with specific focus on cross-reactivity with other sulfonamide-containing medications and management.

TERMINOLOGY AND CLASSIFICATION

Sulfonamide

Understanding and applying proper terminology for classification of sulfonamide medications is imperative. The term "sulfa drug" can be ambiguous and contribute to both patient and clinician misunderstanding. The defining feature of all "sulfa drugs" is the sulfonamide group (Fig. 14.1). The term sulfonamide drug should be used instead as other drugs contain a sulfur molecule and are clinically distinct from the discussion of sulfonamide medication hypersensitivity. The sulfonamide functional group contains a sulfur atom bound to nitrogen, another variable functional group, and double-bonded to two oxygen molecules. Sulfonamide medications can further be categorized based on structure into sulfonamide antibiotics and nonantibiotics.

Sulfonamide Antibiotics

Sulfonamide antibiotics contain two unique structures, important to both function and pathophysiology of hypersensitivity reactions that distinguish them from nonantibiotic sulfonamides. The first is an arylamine group at the N4 position of the sulfonamide moiety (Fig. 14.2). Because of this, the sulfonamide antibiotics are sometimes referred to as "sulfonylarylamines." The second unique structure is a five- or six-membered nitrogen-containing ring attached to the N1 nitrogen of the sulfonamide.[6]

Sulfonamide Nonantibiotics

Sulfonamide nonantibiotics, in contrast, do not contain a sulfonylarylamine group. Common examples of medication classes of which certain drugs contain sulfonamide groups include loop diuretics, thiazide diuretics, sulfonylureas, COX-2 inhibitors, sulfasalazine, protease inhibitors, carbonic anhydrase inhibitors, and triptans, among others. Select sulfonamide medications and their structures can be seen in Table 14.1. Clinical cross-reactivity between sulfonamide antibiotics and nonantibiotics will be reviewed later.

MECHANISMS OF REACTIONS TO SULFONAMIDE ANTIBIOTICS

The types of reactions to sulfonamides are numerous as are the proposed mechanisms. The mechanisms are most well elucidated with TMP-SMX. Reactions mediated by both humoral and cellular mechanisms are clinically relevant, with the latter being much more frequently encountered. Table 14.2 outlines the most commonly encountered clinical reactions to TMP-SMX.

Metabolism

Metabolism of the SMX to its intermediate metabolites is important to the pathology of hypersensitivity reactions. Upon ingestion, most SMX is metabolized in the liver by *N*-acetyltransferases and *N*-glucoronyltransferase, which leads to nontoxic metabolites.[7] A small amount of SMX is also metabolized by CYP-450 to form hydroxylamine (SMX-NHOH) and then nitrososulfonamide (SMX-NO) (Fig. 14.2).[8] The SMX-NO molecule can bind to small structures such as cysteines and other serum proteins, and this combination has been shown to be highly immunogenic and is thought to be central to many hypersensitivity reactions. This molecule can then also be acetylated and excreted in urine or reduced back to hydroxylamine.[6,9]

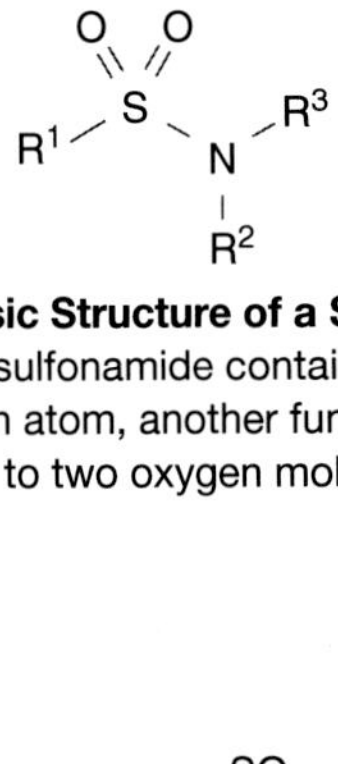

FIG. 14.1 The Basic Structure of a Sulfonamide. The basic structure of a sulfonamide contains a sulfur atom bonded to a nitrogen atom, another functional group (R^1), and double-bonded to two oxygen molecules.

Cellular Mechanisms

Cellular mechanisms are most often implicated in hypersensitivity reactions to sulfonamides. These have been shown to occur through multiple mechanisms. In the past, SMX had been thought to be too small to elicit an immune response on its own. To explain how it was so immunogenic, the hapten theory and p-i concept were employed. Drug haptenation is the process by which a drug or metabolite is bound to small proteins through covalent, stable binding before immune recognition. The immune response is generated through the innate immune system and antigen presentation with subsequent activation of B or T cells. The p-i concept of drug antigenicity, in contrast, involves exclusive T cell stimulation by binding of drug/metabolite directly to HLA or TCR proteins and direct reaction to the modified HLA/peptide complex. This is done without any innate immune response.[10]

Certain molecules on the SMX structure have been shown to be more immunogenic. The N4 position, or arylamine group, on SMX is modified during metabolism and is the epitope usually implicated in cellular reactions. In vitro models have been somewhat contradicting in that some have shown response primarily to the SMX-NO metabolite, yet others have shown direct reactivity to SMX alone. The SMX-NO metabolite has been shown to form multiple potent antigenic determinants for T cells from hypersensitive patients.[9] In contrast, other studies have shown that SMX alone may not be too small to stimulate a response because T cells have been shown to respond to noncovalently bound SMX directly and not to SMX-NO.[7] This may still be accomplished through interactions with HLA receptor and p-i mechanism and with specific variable domains of T cell receptors.[11] Direct cytotoxicity has also been proposed as a mechanism of hypersensitivity.[12]

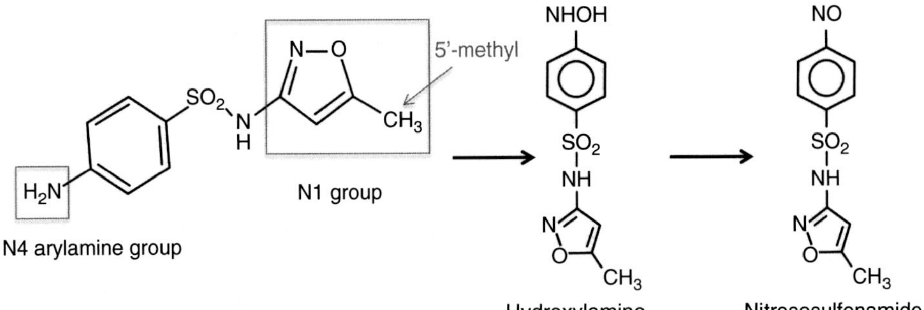

FIG. 14.2 Sulfamethoxazole and Breakdown Products. The structure of sulfamethoxazole with the substituents thought to be clinically important to hypersensitivity reactions highlighted in red. The N1 group, and specifically the 5'-methyl, has been thought to be important in IgE-mediated reactions. The N4 substituent has been implicated in delayed reactions. The CYP-450 breakdown products of sulfamethoxazole are also shown. Of them, nitrososulfonamide has been thought to be commonly implicated in hypersensitivity reactions.

Humoral Mechanisms

For immediate reactions, which are less prevalent, IgE binding to SMX and other sulfonamide antibiotics has been demonstrated.[13] The 5-methyl-3-isoxazolyl group (Fig. 14.2) on the SMX molecule was shown to be the antigenic determinant in three patients with immediate reactions to TMP-SMX.[13] Other drug-specific antibodies have been implicated as well, most notably in HIV patients. In a group of HIV patients, SMX-specific IgM and more so IgG titers were found to be significantly higher in those with previous adverse reaction to SMX compared with those who had exposure and no reaction.[14] The clinical relation of this antibody response in hypersensitivity is, however, unclear.

Reactions in HIV

Hypersensitivity reactions to sulfonamide antibiotics occur much more frequently in HIV patients. Many mechanisms have been proposed to explain this including direct cytotoxicity, reduced glutathione stores, or slow acetylator phenotypes, which result in increased exposure to reactive metabolites and possibly oxidative damage.[15] Many of these mechanisms revolve around the concept of impaired detoxification of SMX metabolites. Glutathione is partly responsible for protecting cells from damage by the SMX metabolites, and there can be reduced stores in HIV patients.[15] There have also been genetic polymorphisms described in the enzyme responsible for biosynthesis of glutathione in HIV patients.[16]

TABLE 14.1
Sulfonamide Nonantibiotics and Structures

Medication Class or Drug Name	Structure	Example Medications With Sulfonamide Structures
Loop diuretics		Furosemide Torsemide Bumetanide
Thiazide diuretics		Hydrochlorothiazide Chlorthalidone Metolazone
Sulfonylureas		Glipizide Glyburide Glimepiride
COX-2 inhibitors		Celecoxib Valdecoxib
Sulfasalazine		Sulfasalazine
Protease inhibitors		Darunavir Amprenavir Fosamprenavir Simeprevir
Sulfones*		Dapsone
Carbonic anyhydrase inhibitors		Acetazolamide Methazolamide Brinzolamide
Triptans		Sumatriptan

*Sulfones do not contain a sulfonamide group and thus are not sulfonamides. Reactions to sulfones however, are clinically similar to sulfonamides and are thus included in this discussion.

TABLE 14.2
Clinical Classification of Sulfonamide Antibiotic Reactions

Reaction Type	Clinical Manifestations	Usual Timing	Candidate for Desensitization
Immediate-type reaction	• Urticaria and/or angioedema • Wheezing, abdominal cramping or pain, nausea, vomiting • Anaphylaxis with or without shock	Often within minutes to hours of one of first 1–2 doses	Yes
Delayed cutaneous reaction	• Variable erythematous rash, often morbilliform/maculopapular, discrete lesions or confluent, flat or slightly raised, can be urticarial • With or without pruritus • Rarely photosensitivity, can progress to exfoliative dermatitis • Can be with or without fever • Does not always recur after reexposure to the drug	0–14 days after initiation of therapy; usually resolves soon after discontinuation or within 7–14 days	Yes
Organ hypersensitivity with or without cutaneous involvement	• Can have features listed above with additional variable end-organ damage including renal toxicity and hepatotoxicity, pneumonitis, myocarditis, eosinophilia. • May have very significant eosinophilia, lymphadenopathy, hepatitis (DRESS is severe form, previously "hypersensitivity syndrome")	7 days to 6 weeks after initiation of therapy	No
Severe cutaneous reaction	• Erythema multiforme: target lesions, dark centers, and lighter periphery • Stevens-Johnson syndrome/toxic epidermal necrolysis: bullous lesions, mucous membrane involvement, desquamation/skin detachment • Acute generalized exanthematous pustulosis: rare	1–3 weeks after initiation of therapy	No
Other systemic reactions	• Serum sickness–like reaction with fever, arthritis, arthralgias, pruritic rash, urticarial-type lesions • Rarely drug-induced systemic lupus erythematosus, Henoch-Schönlein purpura	7–14 days for serum sickness–like	No

Hypersensitivity to Trimethoprim

It is important to note that allergy to TMP can be the inciting factor behind hypersensitivity reaction to TMP-SMX. Clinically, this cannot be differentiated via the history of the reaction. In one series of 73 patients with HIV and history of hypersensitivity reaction to TMP-SMX, 14/73 had hypersensitivity reactions to TMP only.[17] There are several case reports of hypersensitivity reaction to TMP in the non-HIV population as well.[18] These are primarily cutaneous in nature. It is likely that TMP hypersensitivity does account for a small but significant number of hypersensitivity reactions to TMP-SMX.

APPROACH TO THE PATIENT

Types of Reactions to Sulfonamide Antibiotics

Sulfonamide hypersensitivity reactions vary greatly in their clinical presentation, severity, and timing. Reactions specifically to sulfonamide antibiotics are best described. A practical approach to reaction classification into clinically useful categories can be found in Table 14.2.

Type I, immediate hypersensitivity reactions occurring soon after ingestion of one of the first few doses are less common than more delayed reactions. Immediate reactions to sulfonamides are similar to those of other allergens and may feature urticaria, angioedema, wheezing, gastrointestinal symptoms, and less commonly shock. IgE-specific antibodies have been shown to specific parts of the SMX molecule, supporting the fact that immediate reactions can occur.[13]

Delayed reactions involving the skin are the most common hypersensitivity reaction encountered in clinical practice. Features commonly seen in cutaneous hypersensitivity reactions include a morbilliform/maculopapular eruption, urticarial rash, pruritus, and occasionally photosensitivity.[18a] In a review of 91 reactions to SMX, cutaneous reactions occurred in 38 of 91 patients and were the most common reaction to occur.[19] In another series of 72 patients selected for TMP-SMX desensitization, the most common initial reactions to TMP-SMX included rash (54%) and hives (13%).[20] Features of rashes included erythema, urticaria, and pruritus. There were no severe reactions. Half of the reactions occurred in days 0–3 after initial exposure and the other half from days 4–13. They resolved soon after drug discontinuation.[19]

Cutaneous reactions may occur with or without evidence of systemic involvement. Fever can accompany a rash or occur alone in relation to sulfonamide usage. A sulfonamide hypersensitivity syndrome was commonly described in the past and included rash and organ involvement such as hepatitis. This often included eosinophilia as well and may have been referred to in current terms as drug rash with eosinophilia and systemic symptoms (DRESS) syndrome. Many specific organ hypersensitivities may occur with or without further systemic involvement. These include hepatitis and hepatotoxicity, renal involvement in the form of acute interstitial nephritis, pneumonitis, and myocarditis.[21] Hematologic abnormalities may include eosinophilia, cytopenias, macrocytosis, and agranulocytosis. Neurologic effects have been noted with TMP-SMX; it is the most common antibiotic to cause drug-induced aseptic meningitis.[22]

Unfortunately, limited cutaneous reactions can be an early sign of a more severe reaction. Other less commonly encountered but more severe cutaneous reactions include exfoliative dermatitis, erythema multiforme, SJS, TEN, and acute generalized exanthematous pustulosis. TMP-SMX is the most common medication to cause SJS and TEN; however, other sulfonamides such as thiazide diuretics and sulfonylureas do not have elevated rates of these severe cutaneous reactions.[5]

Other severe systemic syndromes such as Henoch-Schönlein purpura and drug-induced systemic lupus erythematosis, as well as serum sickness–type reactions, have also been reported.[23]

Types of Reactions in HIV
Hypersensitivity reactions to TMP-SMX have long been known to occur at a higher rate in HIV positive patients. Cutaneous reactions are the most common and occur in 24%–50% of patients with HIV. Rashes are typically maculopapular, generalized, and pruritic.[24] Typically, a reaction will begin 8–12 days after initiation of the drug and last for 3–5 days. When fever occurs, it may also include, as with non-HIV reactions, other organ involvement such as nephrotoxicity, hepatotoxicity, and cytopenias. There is a higher rate, only 1 in 10,000–50,000 in the general population and up to 4% in the HIV population, of more severe reactions such as SJS.[15]

Adverse Effects
TMP-SMX has a long list of possible adverse effects that affect all organ systems. These are appropriate to differentiate from hypersensitivity reactions because management and consideration for future use is impacted. Some adverse effects of TMP-SMX include nausea, vomiting, *Clostridium difficile* diarrhea, agranulocytosis, aplastic anemia, hepatic necrosis, rhabdomyolysis, and creatinine elevation.[23]

CLINICAL EVALUATION
History
There are key details particularly important in the history of sulfonamide antibiotic hypersensitivity. In obtaining details of past reactions, terminology and clarification of the actual medication in question is of utmost importance.[3] There can be great misunderstanding from both patients and clinicians regarding sulfonamide terminology. The presenting complaint may be limited to "sulfa allergy" only. While this most commonly indicates sulfonamide antibiotic allergy, specific drug, timing of reaction after ingestion, all organ systems involved, and duration of reaction are important. If there was a rash, a description and the presence or absence of mucosal surface involvement and the presence or absence of blistering or lesions consistent with erythema multiforme are imperative for future decision-making. Past records from the time of the reaction should be obtained, if available, to further delineate details and physical examination findings at the time of the reaction. Other factors of the history to note are other medications used in close proximity and the underlying illness. Comorbid conditions are important to note in helping determine likelihood of future need for sulfonamide antibiotics.

Physical Examination
Ideally, physical examination can be done at the time of the reaction; however, in clinical practice this is often not the case. Vital signs including temperature should be

documented. A thorough skin examination should be performed with special attention to the mucous membranes. In particular, evidence of desquamation or target lesions classically seen in erythema multiforme should be noted. Specific classification of the reaction and features of cutaneous involvement can be found in Table 14.2.

Laboratory Testing

Careful review of all laboratory tests at the time of the reaction can be helpful in determining the type of reaction and examining for possible organ involvement. The most helpful laboratory tests include CBC with differential to examine for eosinophilia, anemia, and cytopenias. If anaphylaxis is in question, then a tryptase drawn 0.5–2 h after a reaction can be helpful to confirm.[25] An electrolyte metabolic panel including creatinine and sodium helps assess kidney involvement. Urine eosinophils may be present in acute interstitial nephritis. Liver function testing should be performed to examine for evidence of hepatotoxicity or part of a DRESS syndrome.

Diagnostic Testing

Multiple objective diagnostic tests have been explored to improve diagnosis and classification of sulfonamide antibiotic reactions. Unfortunately, there has not been specific testing shown to be consistently reliable and useful in the diagnosis and evaluation of hypersensitivity reactions. Skin testing, including skin prick, intradermal, and patch testing, has been explored in patients with history of sulfonamide antibiotic reaction. When used, they have not shown acceptable level of sensitivity.[1] The prevalence and pretest probability of immediate reactions are quite low, requiring a large number of study patients to make any definitive claims. A combination of skin prick testing and intradermal (ID) testing for immediate reactions, and delayed ID testing and patch testing for delayed reactions in a small cohort of children showed good sensitivity in a group of children with history of both immediate and delayed reactions to sulfonamides.[26] This type of combination testing would be a possible target for future diagnostic testing if shown in a larger number of patients including adults. Other tests that have been explored including lymphocyte transformation and lymphocyte toxicity assay have shown some promise, but the true clinical applicability has not been fully elucidated.

Given the complexity and diversity of sulfonamide hypersensitivity reactions as well as their underlying mechanisms, it would be difficult to imagine one specific test being clinically predictive or diagnostic of all reactions. Thus, a combination of tests would need to be used. With the currently reported testing methods, this would be tedious and expensive, and final decision-making regarding treatment would likely not be altered given the current predictive value.[1,27]

CROSS-REACTIVITY

Cross-reactivity Among Sulfonamide Antibiotics

TMP-SMX is by far the most frequently used sulfonamide antibiotic. Other sulfonamide antibiotics include sulfamerazine, sulfamethizole, sulfamoxole, sulfamethazine, sulfisoxazole, sulfapyridine, sulfadoxine, sulfadiazine, sulfaguanidine, sulfamethazine, and sulfisoxazole.[28] From mechanistic in vitro studies, over 50% of T cells responsive to SMX metabolites would also react to metabolites of other sulfonamide antibiotics.[9] This has been demonstrated to a limited extent in vivo as well.[29] Clinically, this question does not arise often; however, it is important to know that there is potential for cross-reactivity among sulfonamide antibiotics, but the cross-reactivity may be variable.[29]

Cross-reactivity Between Sulfonamide Antibiotics and Nonantibiotics

For decades there has been debate regarding cross-reactivity between sulfonamide antibiotics and nonantibiotics. A number of package inserts to sulfonamide nonantibiotics do note contraindication in those with previous reactions to sulfonamide antibiotics. As is noted in the "Mechanisms of Reactions to Sulfonamide Antibiotics" section and in Figs. 14.1 and 14.2 and Table 14.1, most immunologic mechanisms and targets on the sulfonamide antibiotic molecule are absent on nonantibiotic sulfonamides. Thus, theoretically, there should be no cross-reactivity. Numerous case reports and series of reported cross-sensitivity reactions have been fueling this debate. Two significant studies have helped more definitively answer this question.

The first study, in 2003, examined a large database of patients who had received a sulfonamide antibiotic (primarily TMP-SMX), subsequently had a likely hypersensitivity reaction, and then were given a sulfonamide nonantibiotic.[2] This was compared with a similar group who did not react to the initial sulfonamide antibiotic. Adjusted odds ratios (ORs) for a reaction to sulfonamide nonantibiotic were elevated (2.8 [95% confidence interval, 2.1 to 3.7]) in those who reacted to initial TMP-SMX compared with those who did not. However, this was similar to the ratio of those reacting to sulfonamide nonantibiotic after previously reacting to penicillin antibiotic in the same timeframe (OR 3.9 [95% confidence interval, 3.5 to 4.3]). Thus, it was concluded that the increased rate of reaction in those with previous reaction to sulfonamide antibiotics may be the result of a predisposition to hypersensitivity reactions to drugs or antibiotics in general and not necessarily a class effect of cross-reactivity.[2]

The second study in 2006 examined 94 patients admitted to the hospital with reported sulfonamide allergy (42/94 were to TMP-SMX, 42/94 could not recall the drug, and 10/94 were to other sulfonamide agents some of which were topical).[30] Forty three percent had outpatient use of at least one sulfonamide nonantibiotic. Ten percent did not receive outpatient sulfonamide nonantibiotics but received one inpatient, all without difficulty. It was concluded that previously reported sulfonamide allergy did not increase risk for reactions to other sulfonamide nonantibiotics.[30] The majority of patients had greater than one drug allergy, possibly supporting the previously discussed hypothesis that drug allergy itself puts one at higher risk to react to other drugs rather than chemical similarities of structures.

The combination of these data makes true chemical cross-reactivity unlikely. There are also likely many unreported cases of tolerance of nonantibiotics in those with previous hypersensitivity to sulfonamide antibiotics. Specific classes of medications and possible cross-reactivity are discussed below.

SULFONAMIDE–NONANTIBIOTIC HYPERSENSITIVITY

Loop Diuretics

Sulfonamide-containing loop diuretics, including furosemide, torsemide, and bumetanide, are frequently used medications that facilitate sodium and water excretion. The structure of furosemide is outlined in Table 14.1. Few case reports exist proposing possible cross-reaction of sulfonamide antibiotics with loop diuretics. One study examined reactions through oral challenge to multiple drugs including furosemide in those who previously had a sulfonamide antibiotic fixed drug eruption.[29] Cross-reactions with furosemide did not occur. Two other small series of patients with self-reported history of sulfonamide reaction (or reported "sulfa allergy"), many to antibiotics, tolerated furosemide without difficulty.[30,31] Ethacrynic acid is the only nonsulfonamide-containing loop diuretic, but its availability is variable.

Thiazide Diuretics

Thiazide diuretics are frequently used antihypertensive medications. A list of common medications in this class can be seen in Table 14.1. There are known hypersensitivity reactions to thiazides, however, not at a significantly high rate. It is unclear if there is significant cross-reactivity among thiazide diuretics. There have not been reliable reports of cross-reactivity between sulfonamide nonantibiotics and thiazide diuretics. However, the package insert for hydrochlorothiazide does note contraindication in those with previous hypersensitivity reactions to sulfonamide-containing medications. There are case reports of severe reactions to HCTZ in those with previous sulfonamide antibiotic reaction,[32] but a clear causal link is lacking. It is likely there are multiple unreported cases of tolerance of those with history of sulfonamide allergy.

Sulfonylureas

Sulfonylureas are a group of oral antidiabetic agents and were the first such agents to be introduced. The class of medications is divided into first and second generation, with second generation being primarily used. There are not significantly high rates of hypersensitivity to sulfonylureas.

There is a paucity of literature regarding cross-reactivity among sulfonylureas. Very small observational data have shown possible cross-reactivity within generations of sulfonylureas (first, not second), but not between generations.[33] Regarding cross-reactivity with other sulfonamides and especially antibiotics, this has not been consistently shown. Few case reports have proposed this occurrence; however, there have not been conclusive links.[34,35]

COX-2 Inhibitors

COX-2 selective NSAIDs can be used in those needing NSAIDs but unable to tolerate some specific side effects of COX-1 inhibitors. Celecoxib and valdecoxib contain a sulfonamide group; however, others such as rofecoxib, etoricoxib, and parecoxib do not contain a sulfonamide group. There are relatively more data on cross-reactivity with sulfonamide antibiotics and COX-2 inhibitors compared with other classes of sulfonamides. A meta-analysis of celecoxib trials showed that 135 patients had previously reported sulfonamide hypersensitivity reaction.[36] Of 135 patients 73 went on to receive celecoxib, 30/135 received an active comparator (nonsulfonamide-containing NSAID), and 32/135 received a placebo medication. The subsequent rates of hypersensitivity reaction were 11%, 3.3%, and 18.8% respectively. These differences were not statically significant. It was concluded that these data failed to show elevated risk of reaction to celecoxib in those with history of sulfonamide hypersensitivity compared with nonsulfonamide NSAIDs or placebo.[36] A number of other case reports have been published with proposed cross-reactivity but without consistent or conclusive evidence.[34] A pilot study of 28 patients with history of sulfonamide antimicrobial allergy in which patients were orally challenged with celecoxib all tolerated it.[37]

Sulfasalazine

Sulfasalazine is an antiinflammatory agent, which does have more structural similarity to sulfonamide antibiotics than other nonantibiotics. It is a prodrug split into sulfapyridine, an aromatic sulfonamide antibiotic, in the colon. It can cause severe hypersensitivity reactions that can be quite variable in presentation.[38] In vitro studies using lymphocyte transformation tests have shown cross-reactivity, with SMX and sulfapyridine.[9,38] There remains no convincing clinical evidence that there is significant cross-reactivity; however, there remains higher clinical concern of cross-reactivity compared with other sulfonamide classes. This is primarily because there may be cross-reactivity among sulfonamide antibiotics of which sulfapyridine is one. It is most prudent to manage potential cross-reactivity based on the severity of the previous reaction and availability of alternative effective agents.

Protease Inhibitors

Protease inhibitors are antiviral medications used in HIV/AIDS and more recently hepatitis C. Darunavir, amprenavir, fosamprenavir, simeprevir, and tipranavir are the protease inhibitors that contain sulfonamide moieties. There are relatively high rates of rash to both darunavir and amprenavir. Rash occurs to darunavir at a rate of around 6%.[39] In a series of 405 patients with HIV who had received both TMP-SMX and Darunavir, 79 patients had a history of allergy to TMP-SMX.[40] Darunavir hypersensitivity was seen in 5.1% of those with TMP-SMX allergy compared with 1.2% without TMP-SMX allergy. The authors concluded that there is likely increased hypersensitivity to Darunavir in those with history of sulfonamide hypersensitivity. However, the reactions were all mild, and thus they thought it may be safe to administer Darunavir in those who had previous sulfonamide hypersensitivity history.

Dapsone

Dapsone is not a sulfonamide but a sulfone. It was originally used for leprosy and also has antiinflammatory effects. It can be used in a number of conditions including dermatitis herpetiformis and as an alternative in *Pneumocystis jirovecii* pneumonia prophylaxis and treatment. Hypersensitivity reactions to dapsone are similar to that of sulfonamides; thus there is often a question of possible cross-reactivity. The most common symptoms of dapsone hypersensitivity are fever and skin symptoms (96.6% of those with hypersensitivity reaction and 92%, respectively).[41] Furthermore, when metabolized, it forms a hydroxylamine structure, as does SMX. There is an entity termed "dapsone syndrome" (or sulfone syndrome), similar to the hypersensitivity syndrome of sulfonamide antibiotics, which includes fever, lymphadenopathy, generalized rash, and hepatitis. It can be quite severe and even fatal.[41]

In one series of patients with HIV, 13 of 60 who had previously reacted to TMP-SMX and then were switched to dapsone also had a hypersensitivity reaction to dapsone.[42] The reactions were generally mild though, and 4 of 13 continued treatment with dapsone. Interestingly, individual reactions within a single patient were similar in those who reacted to both medications. In general, there are elevated rates of hypersensitivity to dapsone in those with history of sulfonamide antibiotic reaction. True rates of possible cross-reaction are low, and it is unclear if there is true chemical cross-reactivity or if HIV patients, the most commonly affected, are more likely to react to either drug individually. Unless there is severe hypersensitivity reaction to TMP-SMX, a trial of dapsone as an alternative in those with previous hypersensitivity to TMP-SMX is reasonable.[43]

Carboxy Anhydrase Inhibitors

Carboxy anhydrase inhibitors such as acetazolamide have a number of indications including altitude sickness and glaucoma. There have been few studies on cross-reactivity. One case series of 27 patients receiving acetazolamide with reported history of "sulfa allergy" (self-reported by patients) demonstrated that 2/27 had hypersensitivity reactions to acetazolamide. The authors concluded that there was no significant evidence of cross-reaction, and the drugs could be used in those with self-reported sulfa allergy if benefits outweigh the risks.[31] Another small series of three patients with a history of sulfonamide antibiotic hypersensitivity showed no evidence of cross-reactivity.[44]

5-HT Agonists

Both sumatriptan and naratriptan are used primarily as migraine medications. They have not been shown to be cross-reactive in those with sulfonamide hypersensitivity; however, there are limited data.[34]

MANAGEMENT

Management of sulfonamide allergy can be difficult given the limited diagnostic testing and still ongoing questions of cross-reactivity. Similar to other drug allergies, once features of the hypersensitivity reaction, as well as patient characteristics and likelihood of future need for sulfonamide medications, have been classified, there are three general ways to proceed. These are avoidance with use of alternatives, challenge testing either in a graded manner or full test dose, or drug desensitization. In general, avoidance of the offending agent and possibly cross-reacting drugs should be employed when there is a history of a severe reaction including SJS, TEN, DRESS, serum sickness, vasculitis, severe mucosal ulcerations, severe reactions with significant systemic involvement such as drug-induced SLE, cytopenias, or other significant systemic symptoms.[45] Graded challenge or full-dose challenge can be considered when there is a low likelihood of reaction.

Desensitization

Desensitization has long been the mainstay of treatment for those needing sulfonamide medications, primarily antibiotics that previously caused a hypersensitivity reaction. Desensitization has also been performed with several nonantibiotics. It is the process by which induction of immune tolerance is obtained with increasing doses of a medication. It is used most often to induce tolerance in those with IgE-mediated reactions; however, it is also used in patients with delayed reactions to sulfonamides of varying mechanisms. There is extensive literature on TMP-SMX desensitization in the HIV population, and less so in the HIV negative population. Desensitization should be performed only when a reasonable alternative is not available and with informed consent of the patient. There are other options for *P. jirovecii* pneumonia prophylaxis and treatment; however, TMP-SMX remains first line for both and has been shown to be more effective than other therapies when direct comparisons have been performed.[46,47] This is used both in HIV populations and other immunosuppressed populations such as organ transplant recipients.

TMP-SMX Desensitization in HIV Negative Patients

Few case series with varying protocols for desensitization have been published in HIV negative populations. In 2014, a large retrospective series of outpatient oral desensitizations of TMP-SMX in HIV negative patients was published.[20] Within this series of 72 patients, three different desensitization protocols were used. A short protocol with 6 steps (36 of 72 patients), a long 1-day protocol with 14 steps (7/72), and a >1 day protocol with 10 steps (43/72) were all utilized. These protocols can be found in Fig. 14.3. All protocols were effective; however, 98% completed the initial desensitization for 1-day protocols and only 76% completed >1-day protocols. In those who completed any protocol, long-term success when reassessed over 7 months was 95%.[20] There was also a higher long-term failure rate in those who completed the initial desensitization with the >1-day protocol versus the 1-day protocol (19% vs. 2%). Overall, the 1-day protocols appeared more efficacious; however, given the retrospective design, patients who were at higher risk to have a reaction may have been selected at a higher rate for the >1-day protocols. No one protocol has been directly compared with another in a randomized manner.

Trimethoprim-Sulfamethoxazole Desensitization in HIV Positive Patients

Adverse reactions to TMP-SMX occur more frequently in HIV positive patients. There have been multiple studies and protocols for desensitization to HIV positive individuals, many of which are over multiple days. Success may not be as high with induction of tolerance or desensitization in HIV patients. This could be related to the higher rate of hypersensitivity reactions at baseline. There have not been clearly established predictors of a successful outcome either; however, it is possible that a lower CD4 count is a positive marker for desensitization success.[48] An example of a protocol that has been used in HIV positive patients can be seen in Fig. 14.4.[49] One study did show comparable effectiveness of desensitization versus rechallenge in HIV patients.[17] However, a subsequent metaanalysis of three studies, including that study, showed improved outcomes for desensitization compared with rechallenge. Specifically, there were decreased rates of discontinuation before 6 months of follow-up (risk ratio [RR] 0.64 [95%; 0.45–0.91]; number needed to treat [NNT] to prevent one discontinuation 7.14), rate of adverse reaction (RR 0.51 [95%; 0.36–0.73]; NNT 4.55), and rate of fever (RR 0.41 [95% 0.2–0.83]).[50] No significant benefit of desensitization compared with rechallenge was seen for cutaneous reactions or hospitalizations. There were no severe hypersensitivity events. On the basis of the available evidence in HIV positive patients and for those who require sulfonamide antibiotics, desensitization is the most appropriate course.

**TMP-SMX graded administration protocols:
TMP-SMX 6 step (1 day)**

Step	Dose of TMP/SMX, mg/mg
1	0.004/0.02
2	0.04/0.2
3	0.4/2
4	4/20
5	40/200
6	Final dose: single, 80/400 PO, or double, 160/800 PO

Dosing intervals are flexible and can be 15, 30 or 60 min apart.

**TMP-SMX graded administration protocols:
TMP-SMX 14 step (1 day)**

Step	Dose of TMP/SMX, mg/mg
1	0.016/0.08
2	0.032/0.16
3	0.064/0.32
4	0.128/0.64
5	0.256/1.28
6	0.512/2.5
7	1/5
8	2/10
9	4/20
10	8/40
11	16/80
12	32/160
13	64/320
14	88/440

Dosing intervals are flexible and can be 15 min apart.

FIG. 14.3 **Sample Desensitization Protocols for Trimethoprim-Sulfamethoxazole (TMP-SMX) in HIV Negative Patients.** (Adapted with permission from Pyle RC, Butterfield JH, Volcheck GW, et al. Successful outpatient graded administration of trimethoprim-sulfamethoxazole in patients without HIV and with a history of sulfonamide adverse drug reaction. *J Allergy Clin Immunol Pract.* 2014;2(1):52–58. http://dx.doi. org/10.1016/j.jaip.2013.11.002.)

Dosing level (daily)	Dose of Trimethoprim/Sulfamethoxazole (mg/mg)
1	10/50
2	20/100
3	30/150
4	40/200
5	60/300
6	80/400

FIG. 14.4 **Sample Desensitization Protocol for Trimethoprim-Sulfamethoxazole (TMP-SMX) in HIV Positive Patients.** Induction of tolerance protocol procedure adapted with permission from Ref. 49. There was 75% success rate with this protocol compared with 57% with direct rechallenge. Each dose is a daily dose; patients must take each dose at least once. It was permitted to repeat a specific dose level once. The last dose was taken no later than day 13. Patients were permitted to withhold study drug for 2 days during the procedure. Patients were required to take an antihistamine during dose escalation once, twice, or three times daily. (Adapted with permission from Leoung GS, Stanford JF, Giordano MF, et al. Trimethoprim-sulfamethoxazole (TMP-SMZ) dose escalation versus direct rechallenge for *Pneumocystis carinii* pneumonia prophylaxis in human immunodeficiency virus-infected patients with previous adverse reaction to TMP-SMZ. *J Infect Dis.* 2001;184:992–997.)

CONCLUSION

Sulfonamide hypersensitivity is a common clinical entity that can take multiple forms with uncertainty regarding mechanism of reactions, diagnostic methods, and cross-reactivity. As data have accumulated, cross-reactivity between sulfonamide antibiotics and nonantibiotics has become less of a concern. There is significant experience with desensitization to sulfonamide antibiotics in the HIV population and non-HIV population. Further studies are needed to determine direct rechallenge against desensitization for each of the different types of reactions amenable to future use of the medication. SJS, TEN, DRESS, serum sickness, vasculitis, severe mucosal ulcerations, severe reactions with significant systemic involvement such as drug-induced SLE, cytopenias, or other significant systemic symptoms are contraindications to further use of the same sulfonamide-containing medication group.

REFERENCES

1. Gruchalla RS. Diagnosis of allergic reactions to sulfonamides. *Allergy*. 1999;54(58):28–32.
2. Strom BL, Schinnar R, Apter AJ, et al. Absence of cross-reactivity between sulfonamide antibiotics and sulfonamide nonantibiotics. *N Engl J Med*. 2003;349(17):1628–1635.
3. Dibbern DA, Montanaro A. Allergies to sulfonamide antibiotics and sulfur-containing drugs. *Ann Allergy Asthma Immunol*. 2008;100:91–101. http://dx.doi.org/10.1016/S1081-1206(10)60415-2.
4. Forman R, Koren G, Shear NH. Erythema multiforme, Stevens-Johnson syndrome and toxic epidermal necrolysis in children: a review of 10 years' experience. *Drug Saf*. 2002;25(13):965–972.
5. Roujeau J-C, Kelly J, Luigi N, Berthold R, Stern R. Medication use and the risk of Stevens–Johnson syndrome or toxic epidermal necrolysis. *N Engl J Med*. 1995;333(24):1600–1607.
6. Brackett CC, Harleen S, Block J. Likelihood and mechanisms of cross-allergenicity between sulfonamide antibiotics and other drugs containing a sulfonamide functional group. *Pharmacotherapy*. 2004;24(7):856–870.
7. Schnyder B, Burkhart C, Schnyder-Frutig K, et al. Recognition of sulfamethoxazole and its reactive metabolites by drug-specific CD4+ T cells from allergic individuals. *J Immunol*. 2000;164:6647–6654. http://dx.doi.org/10.4049/jimmunol.164.12.6647.
8. Cribb AE, Miller M, Leeder JS, Hill J, Spielberg SP. Reactions of the nitroso and hydroxylamine metabolites of sulfamethoxazole with reduced glutathione implications for idiosyncratic toxicity. *Drug Metab Dispos*. 1991;19(5):900–906.
9. Castrejon JL, Berry N, El-Ghaiesh S, et al. Stimulation of human T cells with sulfonamides and sulfonamide metabolites. *J Allergy Clin Immunol*. 2010;125(2):411–418. http://dx.doi.org/10.1016/j.jaci.2009.10.031.
10. Pichler WJ. The p-i concept: pharmacological interaction of drugs with immune receptors. *WAO J*. 2008;(June):96–102.
11. Watkins S, Pichler WJ. Sulfamethoxazole induces a switch mechanism in T cell receptors containing TCRVβ20-1, altering pHLA recognition. *PLoS One*. 2013;8(10):1–23. http://dx.doi.org/10.1371/journal.pone.0076211.
12. Naisbitt DJ, Gordon SF, Pirmohamed M, et al. Antigenicity and immunogenicity of sulphamethoxazole: demonstration of metabolism-dependent haptenation and T-cell proliferation in vivo. *Br J Pharmacol*. 2001;133:295–305. http://dx.doi.org/10.1038/sj.bjp.0704074.
13. Harle DG, Baldo BA, Wells JV. Drugs as allergens: detection and combining site specificities of IgE. *Mol Immunol*. 1988;25(12):1347–1354.
14. Pirouz Daftarian M, Filion LG, Cameron W, et al. Immune response to sulfamethoxazole in patients with AIDS. *Clin Diagn Lab Immunol*. 1995;2(2):199–204.
15. Lin D, Tucker MJ, Rieder MJ. Increased adverse drug reactions to antimicrobials and anticonvulsants in patients with HIV infection. *Ann Pharmacother*. 2006. http://dx.doi.org/10.1345/aph.1G525.
16. Wang D, Curtis A, Papp AC, Koletar SL, Para MF. Polymorphism in glutamate cysteine ligase catalytic subunit (GCLC) is associated with sulfamethoxazole-induced hypersensitivity in HIV/AIDS patients. *BMC Med Genomics*. 2012;5(32):1–9. http://dx.doi.org/10.1186/1755-8794-5-32.
17. Bonfanti P, Pusterla L, Parazzini F, et al. The effectiveness of desensitization versus rechallenge treatment in HIV-positive patients with previous hypersensitivity to TMP-SMX: a randomized multicentric study. *Biomed Pharmacother*. 2000;54:45–49. http://dx.doi.org/10.1016/S0753-3322(00)88640-0.
18. Moreno Escobosa M, Granados SC, Quesada MM, Lopez JA. Enanthema and fixed drug eruption caused by trimethoprim. *J Investig Allergol Clin Immunol*. 2009;19(3):237–252.
18a. Cribb AE, Lee BL, Trepanier LA, Spielberg SP. Adverse reactions to sulphonamide and sulphonamide-trimethoprim antimicrobials: clinical syndromes and pathogenesis. *Advers Drug React Toxicol Rev*. 1996;15(1):9–50.
19. Jick H. Adverse reactions to trimethoprim-sulfamethoxazole in hospitalized patients. *Rev Infect Dis*. 2016;4(2):426–428.
20. Pyle RC, Butterfield JH, Volcheck GW, et al. Successful outpatient graded administration of trimethoprim-sulfamethoxazole in patients without HIV and with a history of sulfonamide adverse drug reaction. *J Allergy Clin Immunol Pract*. 2014;2(1):52–58. http://dx.doi.org/10.1016/j.jaip.2013.11.002.
21. Cribb AE, Lee BL, Trepanier LA, Spielberg SP. Documents to U (MNU/MNUG). *Advers Drug React Toxicol Rev*. 1996;15(1):9–50.
22. Bruner KE, Coop CA, White KM. Trimethoprim-sulfamethoxazole-induced aseptic meningitis – not just another sulfa allergy. *Ann Allergy Asthma Immunol*. 2014;113:520–526. http://dx.doi.org/10.1016/j.anai.2014.08.006.
23. AR Scientific. *Bactrim DS, Bactrim Product Information*. DailyMed National Libr Med (US); 2009. https://dailymed.nlm.nih.gov/dailymed/archives/fda.

24. Jung AC, Paauw DS. Management of adverse reactions to trimethoprim-sulfamethoxazole in human immunodeficiency virus-infected patients. *Arch Intern Med.* 1994;154:2402–2406.

25. Solensky R, Khan DA, Leonard B, Bloomberg G. Drug allergy: an updated practice parameter. *Ann Allergy Asthma Immunol.* 2010;105:1–78. http://dx.doi.org/10.1016/j.anai.2010.08.002.

26. Atanaskovic-Markovic M, Medjo B, Radovic P, Petrovic M. Immediate and non-immediate allergic reaction to sulfonamides in children. *Allergy Eur J Allergy Clin Immunol.* 2015;70:224.

27. Neuman MG, Malkiewicz IM, Shear NH. A novel lymphocyte toxicity assay to assess drug hypersensitivity syndromes. *Clin Biochem.* 2000;33(7):517–524.

28. Slatore CG, Tilles SA. Sulfonamide hypersensitivity. *Immunol Allergy Clin North Am.* 2004;24:477–490.

29. Tornero P, De Barrio M, Baeza ML, Herrero T. Cross-reactivity among p-amino group compounds in sulfonamide fixed drug eruption: diagnostic value of patch testing. *Contact Dermatitis.* 2004;51:57–62. http://dx.doi.org/10.1111/j.0105-1873.2004.00274.x.

30. Hemstreet BA, Page RL. Sulfonamide allergies and outcomes related to use of potentially cross-reactive drugs in hospitalized patients. *Pharmacotherapy.* 2006;26(4):551–557. http://dx.doi.org/10.1592/phco.26.4.551.

31. Lee AG, Anderson R, Kardon RH, Wall M. Presumed "sulfa allergy" in patients with intracranial hypertension treated with acetazolamide or furosemide: cross-reactivity, myth or reality? *Am J Ophthalmol.* 2004;138(1):114–118. http://dx.doi.org/10.1016/j.ajo.2004.02.019.

32. Mineo MC, Pharm D, Cheng EY. Severe allergic reaction to hydrochlorothiazide mimicking septic shock. *Pharmacotherapy.* 2009;29:357–361.

33. Chichmanian RM, Papasseudi G, Hieronimus S, et al. Allergies aux sulfonylurees hypoglycemiantes: les reactions croisees existent-elles? [Hypersensitivity to hypoglycemic sulfonylurea compounds: are there cross-reactions?]. *Therapie.* 1991;46:163–167.

34. Johnson KK, Green DL, Rife JP, Limon L. Sulfonamide cross-reactivity: fact or fiction? *Ann Pharmacother.* 2005;39:290–301. http://dx.doi.org/10.1345/aph.1E350.

35. Wulf NR, Matuszewski KA. Sulfonamide cross-reactivity: is there evidence to support broad cross-allergenicity? *Am J Heal Pharm.* 2013;70:1483–1494. http://dx.doi.org/10.2146/ajhp120291.

36. Patterson R, Bello AE, Lefkowith J. Immunologic tolerability profile of celecoxib. *Clin Ther.* 1999;21(12):2065–2079. http://dx.doi.org/10.1016/S0149-2918(00)87238-0.

37. Shapiro LE, Knowles SR, Weber E, Neuman MG, Shear NH. Safety of celecoxib in individuals allergic to sulfonamide: a pilot study. *Drug Saf.* 2003;26(3):187–195. http://dx.doi.org/10.2165/00002018-200326030-00004.

38. Zawodniak A, Lochmatter P, Beeler A, Pichler WJ. Cross-reactivity in drug hypersensitivity reactions to sulfasalazine and sulfamethoxazole. *Int Arch Allergy Immunol.* 2010;153:152–156. http://dx.doi.org/10.1159/000312632.

39. Tibotec Therapeutics. *PREZISTA – darunavir ethanolate tablet.* DailyMed National Libr Med (US); 2010. https://dailymed.nlm.nih.gov/dailymed/drugInfo.cfm.

40. Buijs BS, Van Den Berk GE, Boateng CP, Hoepelman AI, Van Maarseveen EM, Arends JE. Cross-reactivity between darunavir and trimethoprim- sulfamethoxazole in HIV-infected patients. *AIDS.* 2015;29:785–791. http://dx.doi.org/10.1097/QAD.0000000000000612.

41. Lorenz M, Wozel G, Schmit J. Hypersensitivity reactions to dapsone: a systematic review. *Acta Derm Venereol.* 2012;92:194–199. http://dx.doi.org/10.2340/00015555-1268.

42. Holtzer CD, Flaherty JFJ, Coleman RL. Cross-reactivity in HIV-infected patients switched from trimethoprim-sulfamethoxazole to dapsone. *Pharmacotherapy.* 1998;18(4):831–835.

43. Beumont MG, Graziani A, Ubel PA, MacGregor RR. Safety of dapsone as *Pneumocystis carinii* pneumonia prophylaxis in human immunodeficiency virus-infected patients with allergy to trimethoprim/sulfamethoxazole. *Am J Med.* 1996;100(6):611–616. http://dx.doi.org/10.1016/S0002-9343(96)00008-3.

44. Platt D, Griggs RC. Use of acetazolamide in sulfonamide-allergic patients with neurologic channelopathies. *Arch Neurol.* 2012;69(4):527–529. http://dx.doi.org/10.1001/archneurol.2011.2723.

45. Scherer K, Brockow K, Aberer W, et al. Desensitization in delayed drug hypersensitivity reactions – an EAACI position paper of the Drug Allergy Interest Group. *Allergy Eur J Allergy Clin Immunol.* 2013;68:844–852. http://dx.doi.org/10.1111/all.12161.

46. Sattler FR, Cowan R, Nielsen DM, Ruskin J. Trimethoprim-sulfamethoxazole compared with pentamidine for treatment of *Pneumocystis carinii* pneumonia in the acquired immunodeficiency syndrome. A prospective, noncrossover study. *Ann Intern Med.* 1988;109(4):280–287.

47. Stern A, Green H, Paul M, Vidal L, Leibovici L. Prophylaxis for Pneumocystis pneumonia (PCP) in non-HIV immunocompromised patients (review). *Cochrane Database Syst Rev.* 2014;10:1–67. http://dx.doi.org/10.1002/14651858.CD005590.pub3. www.cochranelibrary.com.

48. Caumes E, Guermonprez G, Lecomte C, Katlama C, Bricaire F. Efficacy and safety of desensitization with sulfamethoxazole and trimethoprim in 48 previously hypersensitive patients infected with human immunodeficiency virus. *Arch Dermatol.* 1997;133:465–469.

49. Leoung GS, Stanford JF, Giordano MF, et al. Trimethoprim-sulfamethoxazole (TMP-SMZ) dose escalation versus direct rechallenge for *Pneumocystis carinii* pneumonia prophylaxis in human immunodeficiency virus–infected patients with previous adverse reaction to TMP-SMZ. *J Infect Dis.* 2001;184:992–997.

50. Lin D, Li W, Reider M. Cotrimoxazole for prophylaxis or treatment of opportunistic infections of HIV/AIDS in patients with previous history of hypersensitivity to cotrimoxazole. *Cochrane Database Syst Rev.* 2007;(2):1–16.

CHAPTER 15

Other Antibiotic Allergy

JAMES M. FERNANDEZ, MD, PHD • ANTHONY P. FERNANDEZ, MD, PHD •
DAVID M. LANG, MD

KEY POINTS

- Adverse reactions occur to antibiotics other than the more frequently prescribed β-lactams.
- Other antibiotics that cause adverse reactions to be discussed in this chapter include vancomycin, metronidazole, tetracyclines, dapsone, clindamycin, and aminoglycosides.
- Although these adverse reactions are less commonly encountered, clinicians should also be aware of the appropriate management of patients with adverse reactions to these antibiotics.

INTRODUCTION

Adverse reactions occur to antibiotics other than the more frequently prescribed β-lactams, sulfonamide-containing antibiotics and fluoroquinolones, including vancomycin, metronidazole, tetracyclines, dapsone, clindamycin, and aminoglycosides.

Although these adverse reactions are less commonly encountered, clinicians should also be aware of the appropriate management of patients with adverse reactions to these agents.

VANCOMYCIN

Vancomycin is a tricyclic glycopeptide antibiotic, first introduced in the 1950s.[1] Based on its risk for adverse reactions, including nephrotoxicity, ototoxicity, and thrombophlebitis, vancomycin was supplanted by semisynthetic penicillins.[1] However, with the emergence of methicillin-resistant *Staphylococcus aureus* (MRSA) and *Clostridium difficile* (antibiotic-associated) pseudomembranous colitis, vancomycin has been commonly used in the past four decades for the treatment of septicemia, pneumonia, endocarditis, meningitis, and other infections, particularly those caused by MRSA and also in patients who relate a history of allergy to penicillins.[2]

Vancomycin has been associated with a number of adverse reactions.

Red Man Syndrome

The most commonly observed adverse reaction to vancomycin is termed red man syndrome (RMS), also known as "red neck syndrome" or "red person syndrome."[2] RMS typically occurs with parenteral infusion of vancomycin, although RMS has also been observed after oral administration.[3] RMS may occur promptly during or after vancomycin administration and typically entails flushing, warmth, erythema, pruritus, and urticaria, affecting the face, neck, and upper torso. The reaction is usually self-limited; however, back pain, chest pain, dyspnea, and more serious reactions with life-threatening hypotension and cardiovascular depression may also occur.[4] RMS results from nonimmunologic mast cell and basophil histamine release and may be accompanied by an elevated level of serum tryptase.[5] Patients with mast cell disorders, or who are receiving agents that are also associated with nonimmunologic histamine release (e.g., opiates or contrast media), may be more prone to experience RMS.[2] The frequency of RMS is related to the vancomycin dose and infusion rate: in normal volunteers who received 1 g of vancomycin as a 60-min infusion, the rate of RMS was 80% to 90%[6]; a reduction in the dose or infusion rate, or administration of premedication with H1 and H2 antihistamines, can successfully prevent RMS in most patients.[6,7]

It may be difficult in some cases to distinguish RMS from an IgE-mediated (allergic/anaphylactic) reaction. In contrast to RMS, anaphylaxis requires prior exposure to vancomycin and may entail other symptoms such as angioedema and respiratory distress, which are uncommon manifestations of RMS.[2] Immediate hypersensitivity skin testing has not been validated in terms of its positive or negative predictive value, either for predicting RMS or for determining whether IgE-mediated potential to vancomycin is present.[8] When vancomycin is clearly indicated, without an equally effective alternative, desensitization can be performed successfully in cases of severe, recurrent RMS or suspected anaphylaxis,[9] even for cases in which life-threatening reactions have occurred.[10]

Linear IgA Bullous Dermatosis

Linear IgA bullous dermatosis (LABD) is an autoimmune, vesiculobullous disorder[11] characterized by the linear deposition of IgA at the dermoepidermal junction of the basement membrane zone on direct immunofluorescence of perilesional skin (shown in Fig. 15.1). The first case of vancomycin-induced LABD was reported in 1988.[12] LABD has become a more commonly identified adverse reaction in association with vancomycin.[13] This acute blistering dermatosis may be difficult to distinguish from erythema multiforme, dermatitis herpetiformis, or bullous pemphigoid. LABD generally resolves after discontinuation of vancomycin.

Other Adverse Reactions

Vancomycin administration also may be associated with drug rash with eosinophilia and systemic symptoms (DRESS) syndrome, Stevens-Johnson syndrome (SJS), toxic epidermal necrolysis (TEN), leukocytoclastic vasculitis, fixed drug eruptions, neutropenia, drug-induced fever, nephrotoxicity, ototoxicity, and other adverse reactions.[2] As with LABD, management of the above-mentioned reactions entails discontinuation

of vancomycin. Desensitization is not recommended for adverse reactions to vancomycin other than severe recurrent RMS or a suspected IgE-mediated reaction.

METRONIDAZOLE

Metronidazole is an imidazole that is used for the treatment of antibacterial and antiprotozoal infections, including bacterial vaginosis and antibiotic-associated colitis. Metronidazole is the first drug of choice for the treatment of *Trichomonas vaginalis*. IgE-mediated and non-IgE-mediated reactions, including SJS, TEN, serum sickness, and fixed drug eruptions, have been described in association with metronidazole.[14]

The negative predictive value of skin testing to metronidazole has not been established.[15] For this reason, even if skin testing is negative, it is prudent to avoid not only metronidazole but also other imidazoles to which metronidazole is structurally similar, including ketoconazole, miconazole, and clotrimazole.

For patients whose history is consistent with an IgE-mediated reaction and who require metronidazole for an indication (e.g., trichomonas vaginalis) for which there is no equally efficacious alternative, desensitization can be performed to permit its safe administration. Successful metronidazole desensitization was initially reported in 1991[16]; a modified desensitization protocol that offers a more gradual dose escalation was published in 2014.[17]

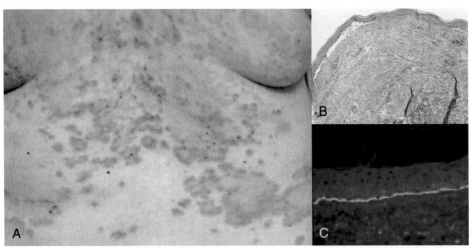

FIG. 15.1 Vancomycin-Induced Linear IgA Dermatosis. **(A)** An urticarial and annular-to-polycyclic eruption on the trunk of a 64-year-old woman occurring after 5 days of intravenous vancomycin treatment. **(B)** Lesional biopsy for hematoxylin and eosin staining reveals a subepidermal blister with a superficial dermal inflammatory infiltrate. **(C)** Perilesional biopsy for direct immunofluorescence reveals linear deposition of IgA at the basement membrane zone.

TETRACYCLINES

Tetracyclines are antibiotics with activity against bacteria, mycoplasmas, chlamydia, rickettsia, spirochetes, and some parasites. In addition, they have antiinflammatory properties that have resulted in broad clinical application for chronic inflammatory and autoimmune diseases. Tetracycline medications are numerous and can be categorized based on whether they are short acting or long acting. Doxycycline and minocycline (both long acting) are by far the most commonly prescribed and will be the focus of this section.

Minocycline causes significantly more serious adverse effects than doxycycline.[18,19] The reason for this is unclear, but it is hypothesized that minocycline's metabolism plays a role.[18] Minocycline shares the basic four-ring structure of the other common tetracyclines but uniquely has a substitution of a dimethylamino group in the seven position. This is thought to result in the generation of reactive minocycline metabolites that bind to tissue macromolecules and act as haptens, eliciting secondary immune responses.[18]

Immune-mediated adverse reactions to tetracyclines can be categorized into two groups—early and late. Early reactions typically occur within 2 months of treatment onset. Both doxycycline and minocycline have been reported to cause such reactions, including urticaria,[18] serum sickness—like reactions,[18] DRESS,[18] fixed drug eruption,[20,21] Sweet syndrome,[22,23] and SJS/TEN.[24-26] Both medications can also cause photosensitivity, with doxycycline being more photosensitizing than minocycline. The mechanism of photosensitivity is thought to be immunologic at least in part, because complement seems to be required.[27] Eosinophilic pneumonitis and interstitial nephritis have been reported secondary to minocycline.[20,28,29] Isolated single organ dysfunction reportedly caused by doxycycline is most commonly severe cutaneous reactions, whereas with minocycline it is most commonly pneumonitis.[18]

Late reactions consist of autoimmune disorders, which can occasionally be fatal, including drug-induced lupus erythematosus (DIL), polyarteritis nodosum (PAN), and autoimmune hepatitis (AH).[18,26,30] These reactions are almost exclusively associated with minocycline, although rare reports associated with doxycycline may exist. Most cases occur in young women treated for acne.[19,31,32] Minocycline-induced autoimmune syndromes are characterized by polyarthralgia, fever, frequent skin involvement, and occasional chronic hepatitis.[33] Most cases present with positive antinuclear antibody (ANA) and perinuclear neutrophil antibodies

(pANCA.), although some may have negative ANA with pANCA being the only positive autoimmune marker.[34]

Numerous cases of systemic PAN with positive serology (+ANA, +pANCA) have been described.[34] Skin lesions often have a livedoid pattern, and onset occurs after ≥6 months of minocycline use.[34] pANCA antibodies associated with minocycline use typically have reactivity against various antigens, including myeloperoxidase, elastase, bactericidal permeability increasing protein, lactoferrin, or cathepsin G.[34]

Minocycline-induced AH can be associated with hypersensitivity reactions (including DRESS) or occur as AH.[33] In a review of AH cases, the mean daily dosage of minocycline was 127 mg (range 10–500 mg).[33] Cases associated with a hypersensitivity reaction tend to have a more rapid onset (within 10 weeks), whereas AH generally occurs after >1 year of therapy.[33]

DIL begins on average 19 months after initiation of therapy.[31] A study involving 27,588 patients with acne revealed that taking minocycline is associated with an 8.5-fold risk of developing DIL compared with controls.[35] The median daily minocycline dose at DIL onset has been found to be 100 mg (range, 50–200 mg). Patients with minocycline-induced DIL tend to be ANA positive, but antihistone antibodies, the classic marker of DIL in 95% of cases, are rarely detected.[32] Elevated C-reactive protein is a typical feature of minocycline-induced DIL but is unusual in idiopathic lupus unless there is superimposed infection, serositis, macrophage activation syndrome, or vasculitis.

The treatment of minocycline autoimmune events includes glucocorticoid administration and discontinuation of minocycline. Autoimmune diseases will typically resolve 3 days to 12 months after minocycline is discontinued.[32] Doxycycline can be given in place of minocycline without concern that the autoimmune disease will recur. Rarely, autoimmune sequelae can persist after minocycline discontinuation.[36] Secondary to these significant adverse effects, it has been recommended that minocycline be reserved for patients who do not show improvement with other tetracyclines.[37] It has also been found that minocycline is more often prescribed as a long-term therapy compared with other tetracyclines.[18] Thus, avoiding long-term minocycline use may also help minimize autoimmune adverse events. Although some clinicians suggest baseline liver function tests, ANA, and ANCAs be ordered in patients expected to require therapy >1 year, others argue these tests do not help predict or prevent reactions and it is best to simply make a diagnosis once the reaction has begun.[26,38]

DAPSONE

Dapsone is a sulfone medication with important antibiotic activity against *Mycobacterium tuberculosis* and *Mycobacterium leprae*. However, its ability to inhibit neutrophil myeloperoxidase and eosinophil myeloperoxidase makes it effective in treating numerous diseases characterized by inflammatory infiltrates with neutrophils and eosinophils. Importantly, general cross-reactivity between dapsone and other sulfonamide-derived drugs is not observed.[39]

The main immunologic adverse event noted with dapsone is "dapsone hypersensitivity syndrome (DHS)," or DRESS syndrome. DHS typically presents with fever, cutaneous eruption, and often systemic organ involvement. Cutaneous lesions can display variable morphologies, ranging from a maculopapular rash to bullous lesions reminiscent of TEN.[40-43] The most common extracutaneous organs involved include the hematopoietic system (peripheral eosinophilia) and liver (hepatitis). Hepatitis can be fulminant and life-threatening.[43] Based on the published epidemiologic studies, the prevalence of DHS is 1.4% and the fatality rate is 9.9%.[44] Latency between dapsone initiation and occurrence of the first DHS symptoms is about 28 days.[44]

Dapsone has also been reported to cause various other immune-mediated skin eruptions.[41,44] Although rarely seen, dapsone photosensitivity occurs via a photoallergic mechanism, supported by photopatch testing.[45] Other rare immune-mediated adverse effects include eosinophilic pneumonitis and agranulocytosis.[46] Dapsone-induced agranulocytosis has been proposed to be mediated by dapsone metabolites that function as haptens and trigger a hypersensitivity-like immune reaction.[47]

CLINDAMYCIN

Clindamycin is a 7(S)-chloro-7-deoxy derivative of semisynthetic lincomycin, a natural antibiotic produced by the actinobacterium *Streptomyces lincolnensis*. It inhibits bacterial protein synthesis by binding to bacterial 50S ribosomal subunits and may be bacteriostatic but is primarily bactericidal. Clindamycin is used primarily to treat anaerobic infections of the oral cavity, respiratory tract, skin, and soft tissue. It is frequently used as an alternative treatment to penicillin in penicillin-allergic individuals.

Although side effects are not uncommon, true hypersensitivity reactions to clindamycin are rare. Common adverse reactions consist mainly of diarrhea, pseudomembranous colitis, elevated liver enzymes, and thrombocytopenia. Of note, clindamycin is one of the more common causes of *Clostridium difficile* colitis, although this is also considered a nonimmunologic reaction.

Of the rare immunologic reactions to clindamycin, delayed maculopapular eruptions are the most frequent. In a retrospective review, immunologic reactions were reported in 0.4% (14 of 3896) courses of clindamycin. Most commonly, the maculopapular eruption occurred approximately 7 to 10 days after initiation of the drug.[48] Other cutaneous reactions caused by clindamycin have included some severe and potentially life-threatening cases of SJS, TEN, and DRESS, as well as a few reports of acute generalized exanthematous pustulosis (AGEP).[2,49-51] Although rare, suspected IgE-mediated reactions including anaphylactic shock, urticaria, and angioedema have been reported.[52,53]

As with any type of drug reaction, evaluation begins with a thorough history and review of medications with timing of ingestion. In one case series of patients with a maculopapular rash caused by clindamycin, one-half reported an onset of symptoms on days 1 to 6 of the treatment course and the other half on day 6 or later. Skin prick testing was performed in all patients and was negative at 20 min in all patients (intradermal testing was not performed).[54] In another study of 31 patients with delayed reactions suspected to be caused by clindamycin, all patients underwent skin prick and intradermal testing with readings at 20 min and 48 to 72 h.[55] None of the patients had positive skin tests at 20 min, but two were positive at 48 h. All patients were challenged with a single dose of 150 mg of oral clindamycin. Of 31 patients, 10 (32%) experienced reactions. In eight patients, the reaction occurred 2 to 6 h after the challenge, and in two it occurred 1 to 2 days after challenge. The reactions consisted of eight pruritic maculopapular rashes, one urticaria, and one angioedema.[55]

Patch testing has been evaluated as a diagnostic tool for non-IgE-mediated hypersensitivity to clindamycin. A study of patients with a history suggestive of clindamycin skin reactions found that 5 of 33 patients (15%) had positive clindamycin patch tests using solubilized 150-mg tablets.[54] False-negative patch tests were seen in 6 of 26 patients (24%). Oral challenges using hourly dosing of 75, 150, 300, and 450 mg of clindamycin were performed and 6 of 26 subjects had positive challenges, all with only cutaneous reactions. Another study of 30 patients with delayed cutaneous reactions associated with clindamycin found positive patch tests in 30% of patients using clindamycin 10% in petrolatum.[56] Therefore, because of the poor sensitivity and specificity of diagnostic testing to clindamycin, a graded oral challenge or drug desensitization is typically pursued if a patient specifically requires treatment with clindamycin.

AMINOGLYCOSIDES

Aminoglycosides are classified into two groups: (1) desoxystreptamine group, including kanamycin, amikacin, gentamicin, tobramycin, and neomycin, and (2) streptidine group, including streptomycin. Aminoglycosides inhibit bacterial protein synthesis and are particularly active against gram-negative bacteria but are used in combination with penicillin or vancomycin to produce synergistic bactericidal effects against enterococcus, streptococcus, and staphylococcus. Aminoglycosides are frequently used in systemic, topical, and ophthalmic forms. The rates of drug reactions differ based on the route of administration.

The most common nonimmunologic side effects of the aminoglycosides are nephrotoxicity and ototoxicity, occurring in up to 20% of patients. Immunologic hypersensitivity reactions are much rarer, with the most frequent being a Type IV contact dermatitis to topical aminoglycosides. The prevalence of allergic contact reactions to topical neomycin has been estimated between 1 and 29 of 10,000, occurring in 30% of persons who have stasis ulcers, 15% of patients who have chronic otitis externa, and 5% of those who have chronic eczematous plaques.[51] Other topical aminoglycosides appear to be less allergenic than neomycin. Other more serious cutaneous manifestations to aminoglycosides such as TEN and DRESS have also been reported.[51]

Type IV hypersensitivity may be evaluated with patch testing with readings most commonly at 72 and 96 h. In fact, contact reactions to neomycin are so prevalent that neomycin is included in the T.R.U.E. TEST panel and other commercial diagnostic products. It is usually used at a concentration of 20% in petroleum.[2] A 20% concentration is also recommended for gentamicin and tobramycin, whereas a much lower 1% concentration is recommended for streptomycin.[2] The percentage of positive patch tests with neomycin in patients with contact dermatitis is 2.5% to 3.6%, and in patients with leg ulcers it varies from 9% to 15%. Based on patch testing data in patients with contact dermatitis, cross-reactivity among aminoglycosides is high.[57] Cross-reactivity is close to 50% or more among those from the desoxystreptamine group, but not surprisingly cross-reactivity to streptomycin is less common (1%–5%).[58]

IgE-mediated hypersensitivity, including anaphylactic reactions to gentamicin, streptomycin, and framycetin, has been reported.[59-62] Inhaled tobramycin has been linked to eosinophilia with severe bronchospasm and cutaneous rash.[51] Unfortunately, as with many antibiotics, there is no validated skin test for the diagnosis of IgE-mediated hypersensitivity to aminoglycosides. However, positive skin prick or intradermal skin tests have been observed with tobramycin, gentamicin, framycetin, and streptomycin, with one prick test to streptomycin resulting in a systemic reaction.[63] The starting concentrations suggested for prick tests range from 0.1 to 1 ng/mL, with a suggested increase in strength reaching the concentration of 20 mg/mL. Studies evaluating intradermal testing are less robust, but nonirritating concentrations for intradermal testing have been established for gentamicin and tobramycin at 4 mg/mL.[63] There is no evidence of positive serum-specific IgE to aminoglycosides. If the patient has positive skin testing or oral challenge or a particularly concerning history (even with negative skin testing), a rapid drug desensitization could be considered. Successful desensitizations with intravenous streptomycin and both intravenous and inhaled tobramycin for urticaria have been reported.[64]

REFERENCES

1. Levy M, Koren G, Dupuis L, Read SE. Vancomycin-induced red man syndrome. *Pediatrics*. 1990;86:572–580.
2. Sanchez-Borges M, Thong B, Blanca M, et al. Hypersensitivity reactions to non beta-lactam antimicrobial agents, a statement of the WHO special committee on drug allergy. *World Allergy Organ J*. 2013;6:18.
3. Killian AD, Sahai JV, Memish ZA. Red man syndrome after oral vancomycin. *Ann Intern Med*. 1991;115:410–411.
4. Newfield P, Roizen MF. Hazards of rapid administration of vancomycin. *Ann Intern Med*. 1979;91:581.
5. Fisher MM, Baldo BA. Mast cell tryptase in anaesthetic anaphylactoid reactions. *Br J Anaesth*. 1998;80:26–29.
6. Polk RE. Anaphylactoid reactions to glycopeptide antibiotics. *J Antimicrob Chemother*. 1991;27:17–29.
7. Renz CL, Thurn JD, Finn HA, et al. Antihistamine prophylaxis permits rapid vancomycin infusion. *Crit Care Med*. 1999;27:1732–1737.
8. Polk RE, Israel D, Wang J, Venitz J, Miller J, Stotka J. Vancomycin skin tests and prediction of "red man syndrome" in healthy volunteers. *Antimicrob Agents Chemother*. 1993;37:2139–2143.
9. Lin RY. Desensitization in the management of vancomycin hypersensitivity. *Arch Intern Med*. 1990;150:2197–2198.
10. Villavicencio AT, Hey LA, Patel D, Bressler P. Acute cardiac and pulmonary arrest after infusion of vancomycin with subsequent desensitization. *J Allergy Clin Immunol*. 1997;100:853–854.

11. Carpenter S, Berg D, Sidhu-Malik N, Hall RP, Rico MJ. Vancomycin-associated linear IgA dermatosis. *J Am Acad Dermatol*. 1992;26:45–48.

12. Baden LA, Apovian C, Imber MJ, et al. Vancomycin induced linear IgA bullous dermatosis (LABD). *Arch Dermatol*. 1988;124:1186–1188.

13. Minhas JS, Wickner PG, Long AA, Banerji A, Blumenthal KG. Immune mediated reactions to vancomycin: a systematic review and analysis. *Ann Allergy Asthma Immunol*. 2016;116:544–553.

14. Knowles S, Choudhury T, Shear NH. Metronidazole hypersensitivity. *Ann Pharmacother*. 1994;28:325.

15. Garcia-Rubio I, Martínez-Cócera C, Santos Magadán S, et al. Hypersensitivity reactions to metronidazole. *Allergol Immunopathol (Madr)*. 2006;34:70–72.

16. Kurohara ML, Kwong FK, Lebherz TB, Klaustermeyer WB. Metronidazole hypersensitivity and oral desensitization. *J Allergy Clin Immunol*. 1991;88:279–280.

17. Gendelman S, Pien L, Gutta R, Abouhassan S. Modified oral metronidazole desensitization protocol. *Allergy Rhinol (Providence)*. 2014;5:66–69.

18. Shapiro LE, Knowles SR, Shear NH. Comparative safety of tetracycline, minocycline, and doxycycline. *Arch Dermatol*. 1997;133(10):1224–1230.

19. Lebrun-Vignes B, Kreft-Jais C, Castot A, Chosidow O. French network of regional centers of pharmacovigilance. Comparative analysis of adverse drug reactions to tetracyclines: results of a French national survey and review of the literature. *Br J Dermatol*. 2012;166(6):1333–1341.

20. Gul U, Gonul M, Soylu S, Kaya I. Doxycycline-induced fixed drug eruption. *J Dermatolog Treat*. 2008;19(2):126–127.

21. Shimizu Y, Shimao S. A case of minocycline-induced fixed drug eruption. *J Dermatol*. 1977;4(2):73–76.

22. Khan Durani B, Jappe U. Drug-induced Sweet's syndrome in acne caused by different tetracyclines: case report and review of the literature. *Br J Dermatol*. 2002;147(3):558–562.

23. Kalai C, Brand R, Yu L. Minocycline-induced Sweet syndrome (acute febrile neutrophilic dermatosis). *J Am Acad Dermatol*. 2012;67(6):e289–e291.

24. Shoji A, Someda Y, Hamada T. Stevens-Johnson syndrome due to minocycline therapy. *Arch Dermatol*. 1987;123(1):18–20.

25. Lau B, Mutyala D, Dhaliwal D. A case report of doxycycline-induced Stevens-Johnson syndrome. *Cornea*. 2011;30(5):595–597.

26. Knowles SR, Shapiro L, Shear NH. Serious adverse reactions induced by minocycline. Report of 13 patients and review of the literature. *Arch Dermatol*. 1996;132(8):934–939.

27. Hasan T, Kochevar IE, McAuliffe DJ, Cooperman BS, Abdulah D. Mechanism of tetracycline phototoxicity. *J Invest Dermatol*. 1984;83(3):179–183.

28. Hung SW. Minocycline-induced acute eosinophilic pneumonia: a case report and review of the literature. *Respir Med Case Rep*. 2015;15:110–114.

29. Walker RG, Thomson NM, Dowling JP, Ogg CS. Minocycline-induced acute interstitial nephritis. *Br Med J*. 1979;1(6162):524.

30. Gough A, Chapman S, Wagstaff K, Emery P, Elias E. Minocycline induced autoimmune hepatitis and systemic lupus erythematosus-like syndrome. *BMJ*. 1996;312:169–172.

31. Schlienger RG, Bircher AJ, Meier CR. Minocycline-induced lupus. A systematic review. *Dermatology*. 2000;200(3):223–231.

32. Elkayam O, Levartovsky D, Brautbar C, et al. Clinical and immunological study of 7 patients with minocycline-induced autoimmune phenomena. *Am J Med*. 1998;105(6):484–487.

33. Lawrenson RA, Seaman HE, Sundström A, Williams TJ, Farmer RD. Liver damage associated with minocycline use in acne: a systematic review of the published literature and pharmacovigilance data. *Drug Saf*. 2000;23(4):333–349.

34. Lenert P, Icardi M, Dahmoush L. ANA (+) ANCA (+) systemic vasculitis associated with the use of minocycline: case-based review. *Clin Rheumatol*. 2013;32(7):1099–1106.

35. Sturkenboom MC, Meier CR, Jick H, Stricker BH. Minocycline and lupus-like syndrome in acne patients. *Arch Intern Med*. 1999;159:493–497.

36. El-Hallak M, Giani T, Yeniay BS, et al. Chronic minocycline-induced autoimmunity in children. *J Pediatr*. 2008;153(3):314–319.

37. Somech R, Arav-Boger R, Assia A, Spirer Z, Jurgenson U. Complications of minocycline therapy for acne vulgaris: case reports and review of the literature. *Pediatr Dermatol*. 1999;16(6):469–472.

38. Driscoll MS, Rothe MJ, Abrahamian L, Grant-Kels JM. Long term oral antibiotics for acne: is laboratory monitoring necessary? *J Am Acad Dermatol*. 1993;28:595–602.

39. Strom BL, Schinnar R, Apter AJ, et al. Absence of cross-reactivity between sulfonamide antibiotics and sulfonamide nonantibiotics. *N Engl J Med*. 2003;349:1628–1635.

40. Prussick R, Shear NH. Dapsone hypersensitivity syndrome. *J Am Acad Dermatol*. 1996;35:346–349.

41. Frey HM, Gershon AA, Borkowsky W, et al. Fatal reaction to dapsone during treatment of leprosy. *Ann Intern Med*. 1981;94:777–779.

42. Lawrence WA, Olsen HW, Nickles DJ. Dapsone hepatitis. *Arch Intern Med*. 1987;147:175.

43. Coleman MD. Dapsone: modes of action, toxicity and possible strategies for increasing patient tolerance. *Br J Dermatol*. 1993;129:507–513.

44. Lorenz M, Wozel G, Schmitt J. Hypersensitivity reactions to dapsone: a systematic review. *Acta Derm Venereol*. 2012;92(2):194–199.

45. Kar BR. Dapsone-induced photosensitivity: a rare clinical presentation. *Photodermatol Photoimmunol Photomed*. 2008;24(5):270–271.

46. Jaffuel D, Lebel B, Hillaire-Buys D, et al. Eosinophilic pneumonia induced by dapsone. *BMJ*. 1998;317(7152):181.

47. Besser M, Vera J, Clark J, Chitnavis D, Beatty C, Vassiliou G. Preservation of basophils in dapsone-induced agranulocytosis suggests a possible pathogenetic role for leucocyte peroxidases. *Int J Lab Hematol*. 2009;31(2):245–247.

48. Mazur N, Greenberger PA, Regalado J. Clindamycin hypersensitivity appears to be rare. *Ann Allergy Asthma Immunol.* May 1999;82(5):443–445.

49. Sulewski Jr RJ, Blyumin M, Kerdel FA. Acute generalized exanthematous pustulosis due to clindamycin. *Dermatol Online J.* 2008;14:14.

50. Kapoor R, Flynn C, Heald PW, Kapoor JR. Acute generalized exanthematous pustulosis induced by clindamycin. *Arch Dermatol.* 2006;142:1080–1081.

51. Chiou CS, Lin SM, Lin SP, Chang WG, Chan KH, Ting CK. Clindamycin-induced anaphylactic shock during general anesthesia. *J Chin Med Assoc.* November 2006;69(11):549–551.

52. Lochmann O, Kohout P, Vymola F. Anaphylactic shock following the administration of clindamycin. *J Hyg Epidemiol Micrbiol Immunol.* 1977;21:441–447.

53. Seitz CS, Bröcker EB, Trautmann A. Allergy diagnostic testing in clindamycin-induced skin reactions. *Int Arch Allergy Immunol.* 2009;149(3):246–250.

54. Notman MJ, Phillips EJ, Knowles SR, Weber EA, Shear NH. Clindamycin skin testing has limited diagnostic potential. *Contact Dermatitis.* December 2005;53(6):335–338.

55. Pereira N, Canelas MM, Santiago F, Brites MM, Goncalo M. Value of patch tests in clindamycin-related drug eruptions. *Contact Dermatitis.* 2011;65:202–207.

56. Gehrig KA, Warshaw EM. Allergic contact dermatitis to topical antibiotics: epidemiology, responsible allergens, and management. *J Am Acad Dermatol.* 2008;58(1):1.

57. Menéndez Ramos F, Llamas Martín R, Zarco Olivo C, Dorado Bris JM, Merino Luque MV. Allergic contact dermatitis from tobramycin. *Contact Dermatitis.* 1990;22:305–306.

58. Schulze S, Wollina U. Gentamicin-induced anaphylaxis. *Allergy.* January 2003;58(1):88–89.

59. Proebstle TM, Jugert FK, Merk HF, Gall H. Severe anaphylactic reaction to topical administration of framycetin. *J Allergy Clin Immunol.* September 1995;96(3):429–430.

60. Romano A, Viola M, Di Fonso M, Rosaria Perrone M, Gaeta F, Andriolo M. Anaphylaxis to streptomycin. *Allergy.* November 2002;57(11):108.

61. Bensaid B, Rozieres A, Nosbaum A, Nicolas J, Berard F. Amikacin-induced drug reaction with eosinophilia and systemic symptoms syndrome: delayed skin test and ELISPOT assay results allow the identification of the culprit drug. *J Allergy Clin Immunol.* 2012;130:1413–1414.

62. Yoo JY, Al Naami M, Markowitz O, Hadi SM. Allergic contact dermatitis: patch testing results at Mount Sinai Medical Center. *Skinmed.* 2010;8:257–260.

63. Empedrad R, Darter AL, Earl HS, Gruchalla RS. Nonirritating intradermal skin test concentration for commonly prescribed antibiotics. *J Allergy Clin Immunol.* 2003;112:629–630.

64. Earl H, Sullivan TJ. Acute desensitization of a patient with CF to both beta-lactam and aminoglycoside antibiotics. *J Allergy Clin Immunol.* 1987;79:477–483.

CHAPTER 16

Multiple Drug Intolerance Syndrome

ERIC MACY, MS, MD

KEY POINTS

- Multiple drug intolerance syndrome is more common in elderly females with relatively high levels of healthcare and medication utilization.
- Immunologically-mediated multiple drug hypersensitivity is extremely uncommon in individuals with multiple drug intolerance syndrome.
- Avoidance of unnecessary drugs, substitution of alternative drugs, and rechallenges are the mainstays of multiple drug intolerance syndrome management.

INTRODUCTION

Multiple drug intolerance syndrome (MDIS) is typically defined as three or more unrelated medication intolerances reported in the medical record.[1] Adverse reactions are associated with and reported after a certain fraction of all medication use.[2] The most common drug intolerances reported, not unexpectedly, are to antibiotics, nonsteroidal antiinflammatory drugs, opiates, antihypertension medications, and cholesterol-lowering medications.[3] Drug intolerance reports accumulate with age. Reported drug intolerances are rarely confirmed with rechallenge. Drug intolerances are more commonly reported by females. Most individuals with MDIS are elderly females and actively using multiple medications. The terminology used to describe each specific drug intolerance in the electronic health record (EHR) is critical to subsequent management.[4] Desensitization is only possible with IgE-mediated allergy, drugs that are direct mast cell activators, or drugs that induce antigen-specific IgG, which can activate complement. Desensitization is not possible with T cell—mediated benign or serious cutaneous adverse drug reactions (SCARs). Fortunately, IgE-mediated drug allergy or serious T cell—mediated delayed-type hypersensitivity to multiple unrelated medications is rarely a significant factor in MDIS.[5] Desensitization is also not possible with nonimmunologically mediated or most pharmacologically mediated reactions such as coughing or angioedema with angiotensin converting enzyme inhibitors, myalgias with HMG-CoA reductase inhibitors, or tendonitis with fluoroquinolones. Most individuals with MDIS can be effectively managed by a combination of drug avoidance, substitution, and rechallenge when needed.

EPIDEMIOLOGY

The two largest population-based studies on the prevalence of MDIS to date were published in 2012 and 2014.[1,6] The 2012 report reviewed the drug intolerances reported by 2,375,424 Kaiser Permanente Southern California health plan members, who had at least 11 months of health plan coverage and at least one health-care visit during 2009.[1] We identified 49,582 (2.1% of the population) patients who use healthcare with three or more unrelated drug intolerances reported in their EHR. There were 537 patients in this cohort with severe MDIS (defined as 4 or more unrelated drug class intolerances and 10 or more individual drug intolerance entries) and 49,045 patients with moderate MDIS (all other MDIS that was not severe MDIS). These groups were then compared with the 478,283 patients without MDIS but with two or fewer drug intolerances and the 1,897,141 patients with no reported drug intolerances. There were significant increases in the percent of females, the elderly, patients with higher body mass indexes, patients seen in psychiatry or allergy, and patients with any urticaria diagnosis between the four groups as one went from the no drug intolerance group to those with any drug intolerance, moderate MDIS, and finally to severe MDIS. There were also significant increases in the current number of different medications chronically used, total annual prescriptions filled, total courses of antibiotics used, total dispensing of narcotics, rates at which new drug intolerances were reported, outpatient visits, emergency department visits, hospital days, and total radiology procedures as one went from the no drug intolerance group to those with any drug intolerance, moderate MDIS, and finally severe MDIS.

There was only one case of confirmed Steven-Johnson syndrome, associated with fluconazole use, and only two confirmed cases of anaphylaxis, one attributed to lidocaine and one attributed to cephalexin, in the entire cohort of 49,582 MDIS patients in 2009.

The 2014 study reported on hospitalized individuals in Birmingham, England, admitted between January 1, 2009, and July 31, 2013.[6] Omar and coworkers identified 1250 (4.9%) hospitalized individuals with three or more unrelated drug intolerances. Multivariable analysis showed that MDIS was significantly correlated with having two or more comorbidities, female gender, and previous hospital admissions. Age was not an independent cofactor because the hospitalized population tended to be older.

TRUE IMMUNOLOGICALLY MEDIATED MULTIPLE DRUG INTOLERANCE

There are rare reports of documented IgE-mediated allergy or T cell—mediated delayed-type hypersensitivity to multiple unrelated medications.[4,5] The best studied are those rare individuals who mount clinically significant IgE-mediated reactions against side chains shared between penicillins and cephalosporins.[7] When looking at populations, there is very little clinically significant IgE-mediated immunologic cross-reactivity between penicillins and cephalosporins.[8–12] There have also been rare individuals documented to develop T cell—mediated reactions to multiple unrelated medications.[13–15] What is known about the genetics of serious T cell—mediated adverse drug reactions and IgE-mediated skin test positivity to penicillins and cephalosporins supports the observed rarity of true immunologically mediated multiple drug intolerance. There are very specific, often population-restricted, and relatively unique HLA associations with a number of serious T cell—mediated adverse drug reactions.[16] The HLA-DRA variants that are associated with positive IgE-mediated allergy test results to penicillins are not associated with positive IgE-mediated allergy test results to cephalosporins.[17]

RISK FACTORS FOR MULTIPLE DRUG INTOLERANCE

There are many medical conditions that will predispose individuals to report multiple drug intolerances. These include AIDS, autoimmunity, congestive heart failure, chronic spontaneous urticaria, cystic fibrosis, G6PD deficiency, immune deficiencies, liver disease, renal dysfunction, and serious mental illness. The underlying infections can increase the probability of reporting MDIS. Individuals who are HIV positive are more likely to report multiple drug intolerances to antituberculosis medications.[18] Untreated or just newly treated HIV-positive individuals report sulfonamide antibiotic—associated intolerance at very high rates and then often tolerate sulfonamide antibiotics when HIV is treated. Individuals with any underlying urticarial syndrome are more likely to report multiple drug intolerances.[19] Individuals with urticaria associated with multiple drug exposures are more likely to have positive autologous serum skin tests and have increased basophil histamine—releasing activity in their sera.[20,21] There are several small basic peptides and cationic medications, including icatibant, tubocurarine, atracurium, and fluoroquinolones, that can directly activate mast cells through the G protein—coupled receptor MrgprX2.[22]

CLINICAL MANAGEMENT OF TYPICAL CASES

When confronted with a patient with multiple drug intolerances listed in his/her EHR, first look for duplicates.[2,23] If multiple penicillins, narcotics, HMG-CoA reductase inhibitors, or nonsteroidal antiinflammatory medications are listed, group these into drug class intolerances and enter only one listing in the drug intolerance field. Determine the date of the index adverse reaction, the nature of the adverse reaction, and the time after the start of the last exposure that the adverse reaction occurred.[2,23] See Table 16.1 for the seven essential elements of a drug intolerance evaluation. If an individual has subsequently tolerated the medication listed, remove the listing from his/her EHR. Determine possible pathologic mechanisms for each adverse reaction based on the clinical symptoms and the time to onset. Determine if the medication implicated can function as a hapten or is large enough to be a directly immunogenic. Allergy testing or rechallenge should be contemplated only in individuals with a history of anaphylaxis, hives, other benign rashes, gastrointestinal (GI) symptoms, headaches, other benign symptoms, or unknown reactions associated with the previous use of an implicated drug. The underlying mechanisms associated with potentially safe testing or rechallenge include possible IgE-mediated reactions, direct mast cell activation, IgG- and complement-mediated reactions, and many of those adverse drug reactions with no potential immunologic etiology, such as GI upset or headaches. Do not test for allergy or rechallenge any individual with any SCARs, including anyone with drug reaction with eosinophilia and systemic symptoms (DRESS), toxic epidermal necrolysis (TEN), and Stevens-Johnson syndrome (SJS), serious hepatitis, hemolytic anemia, or

TABLE 16.1
Seven Essential Elements of a Drug Intolerance Evaluation

1	Date of the index adverse reaction
2	Time to initial symptoms after start of last exposure ($<1\,h$, $1-6\,h$, $7-48\,h$, $>48\,h$)
3	Symptoms noted with adverse reaction (hives, other benign rashes, GI upset, headaches, SCARs, and others)
4	Treatments given for adverse drug reaction symptoms (none, antihistamines, steroids, adrenaline, and others)
5	Time to symptom resolution ($<1\,day$, $1-7\,days$, $>7\,days$)
6	Suspected mechanism of adverse drug reaction (IgE-mediated, T cell—mediated, pharmacologically mediated, and others)
7	Management plan (avoidance, alternatives, rechallenge, desensitization, and others)

GI, gastrointestinal; *SCARs*, serious cutaneous adverse drug reactions.

interstitial nephritis, given our current state of knowledge, outside of a clinical trial.

DRUG CHALLENGES

The mainstay of MDIS management is rechallenging with acutely needed medications when there is no reasonable alternative.[2,23–25] Give oral challenges whenever possible. Allow adequate time after the drug reexposure for previously noted symptoms to recur. Mild delayed onset symptoms can be noted by the patient at home. A single therapeutic dose is typically adequate to document acute tolerance and the lack of any clinically significant T cell—mediated reaction occurring over the next 2–5 days. Multistep challenges, using three or more steps, are generally no safer than using only one or two steps in appropriately selected subjects.[26] It is essential to use 10-fold dosing increments in challenges to avoid the potential for desensitization that can occur when using only 2-fold dosing increments.

If there had been a reaction that started within 1 h of a previous exposure, give 10% of a therapeutic dose, observe for at least 30 min, give the remaining 90% of the dose, and observe for at least one additional hour. For NSAIDs, observe for at least 2 h after a therapeutic dose. If the reaction started more than 6 h after the index exposure, just give the whole dose. Expect

subjective reactions, such as itching without any rashes, headaches, anxiety, or GI upset, with all challenges, but treat only objective reactions. Be observant for objective reactions, such as hypotension, hives, changes in spirometry, or pulse oximetry. Individuals with more severe underlying anxiety are more likely to have more subjective rechallenge reactions.

Consider using placebo-controlled blinded challenges if needed.[27,28] With agents expected to induce an acute reaction, placebo challenges and active agent challenges can be done on the same day, but it is necessary to allot enough time to observe the patient for objective reactions after each dose. Immatteo and coworkers noted a 7%–8% rate of subjective reactions with placebo challenges, all in women, 20 out of 183 females versus 0 out of 46 males ($P = .02$), but only 4.4% of the 229 total patients challenged had objective reactions with active drugs.[29] Placebo-controlled challenges for delayed onset reactions may need to be done over a several-day period, with several days of follow-up after each challenge.

If a delayed onset rash appears, with lesions lasting more than 24 h, arrange to have it biopsied to help determine ethology. If only hives occur, it is enough to just treat with antihistamines. Drug challenges can cause significant anxiety, and even a negative result is sometimes not convincing to the patient.[30] It is very important to address the patients' needs and concerns before and after the rechallenge.[31] Try to reduce overall drug exposure; use all medications at the lowest possible effective dose and the shortest possible duration.

CONCLUSIONS

MDIS can be managed effectively in most individuals by initially determining as accurately as possible the mechanisms of the medication-associated adverse reactions. Then it is important to fully explain multiple drug intolerances to the patient. By using challenges when needed, it is usually possible to demonstrate to the affected individuals that they can, when needed, tolerate many medications they have been previously associated with intolerance. Avoidance of unneeded medications, using the lowest-effective dose, shortest possible duration, and stopping chronic medication use whenever possible should also be the goals of MDIS management to help prevent future reactions. Clear directions should be placed in the drug *allergy* field of the EHR. Each patient should be given a "Drug Allergy Passport" including a list of medications that should continue to be avoided, medications they could tolerate if needed, and a management plan to address future reactions to new medications.[32]

REFERENCES

1. Macy E, Ho NJ. Multiple drug intolerance syndrome: prevalence, clinical characteristics, and management. *Ann Allergy Asthma Immunol.* 2012;108:88–93.
2. Macy E, Poon KWT. Self-reported antibiotic allergy incidence and prevalence: age and sex effects. *Am J Med.* 2009;122:778e1–778e7.
3. Blumenthal KG, Park MA, Macy EM. Redesigning the allergy module of the electronic health record. *Ann Allergy Asthma Immunol.* June 14, 2016. pii:S1081–1206(16)30267-8.
4. Chiriac AM, Demoly P. Multiple drug hypersensitivity syndrome. *Curr Opin Allergy Clin Immunol.* 2013;13:323–329.
5. Macy E. Multiple antibiotic allergy syndrome. *Immunol Allergy Clin North Am.* 2004;24:533–543.
6. Omar HMRB, Hodson J, Thomas SK, Coleman JJ. Multiple drug intolerance syndrome: a large-scale retrospective study. *Drug Saf.* 2014;37:1037–1045.
7. Romano A, Gaeta F, Arribas Poves MF, Valluzzi RL. Cross-reactivity among beta-lactams. *Curr Allergy Asthma Rep.* 2016:24. http://dx.doi.org/10.1007/s11882-016-0594-9.
8. Khoury L, Warrington R. The multiple drug allergy syndrome: a matched-control retrospective study in patients allergic to penicillin. *J Allergy Clin Immunol.* 1996;98:462–464.
9. Warrington R. Multiple drug allergy syndrome. *Can J Clin Pharmacol.* 2000;7:18–19.
10. Park J, Matsui D, Rieder MJ. Multiple antibiotic sensitivity syndrome in children. *Can J Clin Pharmacol.* 2000;7:38–41.
11. Macy E. Penicillin and beta-lactam allergy: epidemiology and diagnosis. *Curr Allergy Asthma Rep.* 2014;14:476. http://dx.doi.org/10.1007/s11882-014-0476-y.
12. Macy E, Contreras R. Adverse reactions associated with oral and parenteral cephalosporin use: a retrospective population-based analysis. *J Allergy Clin Immunol.* 2015;135:745–752.e5.
13. Nagayama H, Nakamura Y, Shinkai H. A case of drug eruption due to simultaneous sensitization with three different kinds of drugs. *J Dermatol.* 1996;23:899–901.
14. Voltolini S, Bignardi D, Minale P, Pellegrini S, Troise C. Phenobarbital-induced DiHS and ceftriaxone hypersensitivity reaction: a case of multiple drug allergy. *Eur Ann Allergy Clin Immunol.* 2009;41:62–63.
15. Özkaya E, Yazganoğlu KD. Sequential development of eczematous type "multiple drug allergy" to unrelated drugs. *J Am Acad Dermatol.* 2011;65:e26–e29.
16. Chung WJH, Wang CW, Dao RL. Severe cutaneous adverse drug reactions. *J Dermatol.* 2016;43:758–766.
17. Guéant JL, Romano A, Cornejo-Garcia JA, et al. HLA-DRA variants predict penicillin allergy in genome-wide fine-mapping genotyping. *J Allergy Clin Immunol.* January 2015;135(1):253–259.
18. Pozniak AL, MacLeod GA, Mahari M, Legg W, Weinberg J. The influence of HIV status on single and multiple drug reactins to antituberculosis therapy in Africa. *AIDS.* 1992;6:809–814.
19. Asero R. Intolerance to nonsteroidal anti-inflammatory drugs might precede by years the onset of chronic urticaria. *J Allergy Clin Immunol.* 2003;111:1095–1098.
20. Asero R, Tedeschi A, Lorini M, Caldironi G, Barocci F. Sera from patients with multiple drug allergy syndrome contain circulating histamine-releasing factors. *Int Arch Allergy Immunol.* 2003;131:195–200.
21. Asero R, Tedeschi A, Riboldi P, et al. Coagulation cascade and fibrinolysis in patients with multiple-drug allergy syndrome. *Ann Allergy Asthma Immunol.* 2008;100:44–48.
22. McNeil BD, Pundir P, Meeker S, et al. Identification of a mast cell specific receptor crucial for pseudo-allergic drug reactions. *Nature.* 2015;519:237–241.
23. Blumenthal KG, Saff RR, Banerji A. Evaluation and management of a patient with multiple drug allergies. *Allergy Asthma Proc.* 2014;35:197–203.
24. Asero R. Detection of patients with multiple drug allergy syndrome by elective tolerance tests. *Ann Allergy Asthma Immunol.* 1998;80:185–188.
25. Schiavino D, Nucera E, Roncallo C, et al. Multiple-drug intolerance syndrome: clinical findings and usefulness of challenge tests. *Ann Allergy Asthma Immunol.* 2007;99:136–142.
26. Iammatteo M, Blumenthal KG, Saff R, Long AA, Banerji A. Safety and outcomes of test doses for the evaluation of adverse drug reactions: a 5-year retrospective review. *J Allergy Clin Immunol Pract.* 2014;2:768–774.
27. Aun MV, Bisaccioni C, Garro LS, et al. Outcomes and safety of drug provocation tests. *Allergy Asthma Proc.* 2011;32:301–306.
28. Kao L, Rajan J, Roy L, Kavosh E, Khan DA. Adverse reactions during drug challenges: a single US institution's experience. *Ann Allergy Asthma Immunol.* 2013;110:86–91.e1.
29. Iammatteo M, Ferastraoaru D, Koransky R, et al. *J Allergy Clin Immunol Pract.* November 22, 2016. http://dx.doi.org/10.1016/j.jaip.2016.09.041. pii: S2213–2198(16)30495-0.
30. Gomes ER, Kvedariene V, Demoly P, Bousquet PJ. Patients' satisfaction with diagnostic drug provocation tests and perception of its usefulness. *Int Arch Allergy Immunol.* 2011;156:333–338.
31. Davies SJC, Jackson PR, Ramsey LE, Ghahramani P. Drug intolerance due to non-specific adverse effects related to psychiatric morbidity in hypertensive patients. *Arch Intern Med.* 2003;163:592–600.
32. Brockow K, Aberer W, Atanaskovic-Markovic M, et al. Drug allergy passport and other documentation for patients with drug hypersensitivity-an ENDA/EAACI drug allergy interest group position paper. *Allergy.* 2016;71:1533–1539.

CHAPTER 17

Aspirin-Exacerbated Respiratory Disease

TANYA M. LAIDLAW, MD

KEY POINTS

- Oral aspirin challenge has remained the gold standard for the diagnosis of AERD.
- There are no clinically available in vitro tests or diagnostic biomarkers that are recommended for the routine diagnosis of AERD.
- The diagnosis of AERD can be reliably made based on history alone if patients provide a clear clinical history of adult-onset asthma, recurrent nasal polyposis, and respiratory reactions to COX-1 inhibitors. Patients for whom the history is less clear should be offered a provocative aspirin challenge.
- AERD is underdiagnosed by clinicians, and also patients may underreport their symptoms.

INTRODUCTION

Definition and Classification

Aspirin-exacerbated respiratory disease (AERD) is an acquired inflammatory syndrome of the upper and lower airways that is classically characterized by the triad of recurrent eosinophilic nasal polyps, asthma, and respiratory reactions induced by aspirin and all medications that inhibit cyclooxygenase 1 (COX-1). The onset of the disease is usually in young adulthood, beginning with nasal congestion and persistent rhinitis, sinus disease, and nasal polyposis, followed by the development of asthma, and then hypersensitivity to COX-1 inhibitors.[1] Once the syndrome has fully progressed, reactions will be induced within 30–120 min of ingestion of any medication that inhibits COX-1, including aspirin and all nonselective nonsteroidal antiinflammatory drugs (NSAIDs). These reactions typically involve respiratory symptoms in the upper and/or lower airways, including increased rhinorrhea, acute nasal congestion, ocular erythema, chest tightness, and bronchoconstriction as measured by a fall in FEV1. In addition to the respiratory symptoms, up to 30% of patients also note that their reactions are accompanied by extrapulmonary findings, including skin changes such as pruritic rash and flushing, or gastrointestinal symptoms such as abdominal pain, vomiting, or diarrhea.[1–3]

The association of aspirin-induced reactions, nasal polyps, and asthma was first published in 1922 by Widal and colleagues who described this constellation of symptoms in a 37-year-old woman.[4] In 1968, Samter and Beers expanded considerably on the available literature and described the clinical features of 182 aspirin-sensitive patients, and for many years following, the syndrome was referred to as "Samter's triad."[3] Then in 2001, Drs. Stevenson, Sanchez-Borges, and Szczeklik proposed an updated classification of hypersensitivity reactions to COX inhibitors and introduced the term AERD to best describe the underlying disease in this subset of patients.[5] This term has been helpful because it stresses that for patients with AERD, exposure to and reactions caused by COX-1 inhibitors are neither the root cause of their disease nor even usually their main medical issue. Instead, the chronic underlying inflammatory respiratory disease, which persists and progresses even when all COX inhibitors are carefully avoided, is exacerbated during reactions to NSAIDs.[6] These hypersensitivity reactions in AERD are universally cross-reactive among all medications that inhibit COX-1 and are not considered to be true "allergic" reactions, as they are not IgE mediated. The cross-reactivity is an important point of clinical education that should be provided to patients, as even an NSAID that is new to the patient will induce a reaction on the first exposure, and therefore a careful understanding of all medications that fall within this class is a key to patient safety.

Prevalence

The published prevalence rates of AERD have varied based on the population studied and the diagnostic methods and clinical criteria used. Prevalence has been suggested to be as low as 4.3% of adult asthmatics when self-reported and assessed by questionnaire alone[7] or as high as 21% of asthmatics if assessed by direct oral provocation,[8] and the true rates must fall somewhere in between. To better clarify the prevalence of AERD, a metaanalysis of studies among asthmatic adults was performed and published in 2015, and it was found that the prevalence of AERD in typical adult asthmatics is 7.2% and rises to 14.9% among patients with severe asthma.[9] Of note, studies that were performed in a tertiary referral center for AERD and therefore had known referral bias were excluded from the analysis, further confirming that these rates likely reflect the true prevalence in the general asthmatic population. Therefore, according to asthma prevalence rates in adults as listed in the 2014 National Health Interview Survey Data, approximately 1.2 million adults in the United States are estimated to have AERD.

DIAGNOSIS BASED ON CLINICAL HISTORY

Timely and accurate diagnosis of AERD is both crucial for patient safety and allows patients to pursue disease-tailored therapies, including aspirin desensitization and high-dose daily aspirin, which provides long-term therapeutic benefit for the majority of patients with AERD.[10-14] Unfortunately, delay to diagnosis is common, and for many patients there is a lag time of over 10 years between the onset of symptoms and correct diagnosis.[15] Furthermore, of 638 patients who had been electronically identified as having all three features of the clinical triad (nasal polyps, asthma, and NSAID-induced reactions), listed within their medical record, and then classified as having clinical AERD through complete chart review, 12.4% had no diagnosis or mention of AERD or a similar term by any treating caregiver.[16] This suggests that even for patients who are aware of their symptoms and properly report them to treating physicians, the diagnosis of AERD is often missed.

The identification of AERD requires a careful medical history, and in some cases the clinical history alone may be sufficient for diagnosis. The current literature suggests that up to 17% of patients with a history consistent with clinical criteria for AERD may have a negative oral aspirin challenge.[17,18] However, the clinical experience from our institution, involving more than 200 aspirin challenges, is that less than 5% of patients with asthma, recurrent nasal polyposis, and a recent respiratory reaction to an NSAID go on to have a negative oral aspirin challenge. At our center, for patients who present with the complete triad of adult-onset asthma, recurrent nasal polyps, and a reliable history of at least two prior NSAID-induced respiratory reactions, at least one of which was within the last 5 years, we are comfortable making the diagnosis of AERD based on clinical history alone and do not require a provocative challenge.

Additional findings that are often present and help to further substantiate the diagnosis of AERD include mild-to-moderate peripheral blood eosinophilia[19] and a rapid rate of nasal polyp recurrence following surgical polypectomy. A history of alcohol-induced respiratory reactions can provide another clue, as 77%–83% of patients with AERD report the onset of upper (nasal congestion and rhinorrhea) and/or lower (wheezing, shortness of breath) respiratory symptoms on consumption of alcoholic beverages.[20-22]

However, diagnosis based solely on patient-reported history of NSAID allergy can be insufficient. Specifically, the presence of NSAID hypersensitivity can be difficult to establish based on patient-report alone. As far back as 1968 with Samter's initial case series, it has been noted that up to 15% of patients with AERD are seemingly unaware that they are intolerant to aspirin or maintain that they can take NSAIDs without ill effects—these patients do not become aware of their hypersensitivity until a reaction is induced during a physician-observed provocation test.[1,3] Therefore, it is unreliable to simply ask patients "are you allergic to aspirin or NSAIDs?". We have identified many patients with AERD who had a delay in diagnosis because they had answered "no" to this question during previous evaluations.

These patients usually fall into one of the four categories, and a provocative challenge is required to determine proper diagnosis:

1. Patients with no recent use of NSAIDs.

   Patients who have not used aspirin or NSAIDs recently or since the development of their respiratory disease may not recall any NSAID-induced reactions. However, in the absence of recent NSAID exposure, they may not know whether they are currently hypersensitive. A physician-observed provocative challenge is required for diagnosis.

2. Patients whose reaction symptoms may be pharmacologically blocked.

   The use of leukotriene-modifying agents, such as the leukotriene receptor antagonist montelukast or the 5-lipoxygenase inhibitor zileuton, can completely block or blunt the symptomatic manifestations of NSAID-induced reactions enough that the reactions go unnoticed by the patient.[23,24]

Therefore, for patients on a leukotriene-modifying drug, we recommend these medications are stopped at least 7 days before a physician-observed provocative challenge.

3. Patients who do not perceive their reactions.

There is a subset of patients with AERD who present with both asthma and recurrent nasal polyps but maintain that they can use aspirin or NSAIDs and do not note adverse effects. This general insensitivity to reaction symptoms seems to occur in patients with the most severe chronic sinus polyposis, who simply do not notice the acutely worsening symptoms that followed NSAID ingestion. For patients who live with complete nasal obstruction, intermittent episodes of worsened nasal congestion may go unnoticed. Therefore a physician-observed provocative challenge can be helpful.

4. Patients on daily low-dose aspirin.

A recent study highlighted the finding that some patients with AERD who are already taking 81 mg aspirin for cardiac protection at the time of initial clinical evaluation may not report symptoms of NSAID-induced hypersensitivity. These patients, who tended to have very mild asthma symptoms, historically tolerated low-dose aspirin, but after stopping low-dose aspirin for at least 10 days, did develop aspirin-induced respiratory symptoms during a provocative oral aspirin challenge.[15] This apparent tolerance of low-dose aspirin may have been because the aspirin-induced symptoms on initiation of low-dose aspirin were mild enough that they went unnoticed by the patient, or because their initiation of low-dose aspirin had been before the development of their respiratory disease.

DIAGNOSTIC TESTING WITH PROVOCATION CHALLENGES

Safety Requirements and Circumstances for Performing Provocation Challenges

A provocation challenge using aspirin, or occasionally another COX-1 inhibitor, is the gold standard to confirm the diagnosis of AERD. There are no validated or reliable clinically available in vitro diagnostics. Oral aspirin challenge is the most commonly available challenge method in the United States. Intranasally administered ketorolac challenges can also be performed at some centers in the United States. Both inhalational and intravenous testing procedures are performed at several European and Asian centers, but these modalities require the administration of lysine-aspirin, which is not approved for use in the United States.[25–27]

Provocative challenges should be performed at a facility equipped with emergency resuscitation equipment and under the direct supervision of a physician and a medical team who are experienced in provocation testing. An outpatient setting is appropriate for most patients with AERD, provided they meet the following safety criteria:

1. Stable clinical condition and without any underlying medical condition that would make management of severe reaction symptoms more difficult
2. Relatively well-controlled asthma
3. Baseline FEV1 of at least 60% of predicted
4. Not currently using a β-receptor blocker (for patients on β-blockers, the outpatient setting is still appropriate if the medication can be safely held for at least two half-lives before a challenge)

The availability of albuterol for treatment of reaction-induced bronchoconstriction is an important safety requirement. It is also recommended to have oral zileuton available for treatment of possible extrapulmonary reaction symptoms, which can be administered for patient comfort. For patients not meeting the above safety criteria, an inpatient challenge may be warranted. Early guidelines had recommended that a peripheral IV be placed before aspirin challenges.[27,28] However, recent additional safety data have been reassuring enough that aspirin challenges are now done without a peripheral IV in place at most major academic centers in the United States that routinely perform these tests.

It is recommended that patients temporarily discontinue all oral antihistamines and leukotriene modifiers at least 1 week before any diagnostic provocative challenge for AERD, to decrease the likelihood of a false-negative challenge. Patients in the United States are generally allowed to continue their usual dose of daily inhaled and/or oral corticosteroids and long-acting bronchodilators, although European centers will often recommend that long-acting bronchodilators are withdrawn 24 h before a challenge. Higher doses of systemic steroids (>15 mg/day oral prednisone) may blunt the aspirin-induced bronchospasm and nasal symptoms, so ideally patients should be reduced to the lowest achievable steroid dose.[29] If it is safe to do so from a cardiac perspective, patients on daily low-dose aspirin (81 mg/day) for cardioprotection[15] should stop aspirin for at least 10 days before a provocative challenge.

Oral Aspirin Challenge

Oral aspirin provocation testing is considered the gold standard for the diagnosis of AERD. The benefits and risks of the procedure should be discussed thoroughly

TABLE 17.1
Procedure for Oral Aspirin Challenge

1 week before the challenge	Confirm that patient (A) will stop all oral antihistamines, leukotriene-modifying drugs, and/or daily low-dose aspirin; patient (B) is able to avoid all β-blockers for the day of challenge; and patient (C) has not had a recent exacerbation of his/her underlying asthma
Morning of the challenge	Before administering the first dose of aspirin, measure baseline vital signs, FEV1, and the patient-recorded total AERD symptom score (Table 17.2)
Throughout the challenge procedure	Measure vital signs, FEV1, and patient-recorded total AERD symptom score (Table 17.2) just before each dose, and again if there is any change in symptoms noted by the patient

Time	Dose[a] of Aspirin Administered per Step	Tablets[b] Used for Oral Aspirin Dosing
0	40.5 mg	Half of a 81 mg tablet
90 min	81 mg	One 81 mg tablet
3 h	162 mg	Two 81 mg tablets
4.5 h	325 mg	One 325 mg tablet

[a]The doses recommended here are based on the common over-the-counter aspirin dosages available in the United States.
[b]Nonenteric-coated aspirin tablets are recommended for oral challenges, as they are more quickly absorbed and enteric-coated tablets could delay the onset of symptoms.
AERD, aspirin-exacerbated respiratory disease.

with each patient, and written informed consent should be obtained. There are several distinct protocols available,[27,28] which differ in the exact doses of aspirin administered and the length of time between doses. At the Brigham and Women's Hospital AERD Center, we generally use a four-dose challenge protocol with 90-min intervals between doses, based on commercially available 81-mg and 325-mg aspirin tablets with the aid of a pill cutter to obtain the lower doses.[28] Starting early in the morning (Table 17.1), we measure vital signs and FEV1, record the patient's baseline symptoms, and then administer 40.5 mg aspirin, followed by 81, 162, and 325 mg. Lung function and vital signs are again measured every 90 min before proceeding with dose escalation and also at the onset of any symptom. A challenge is confirmed as "positive" with a lower respiratory tract reaction if there is a ≥15% decrease in the FEV1 from baseline FEV1, and/or with a nasoocular reaction if there is an acute and physician-observable increase in at least two of the following: nasal congestion, rhinorrhea, sneezing, nasal or eye itching, or eye redness or tearing. The development of extrapulmonary symptoms, including gastrointestinal discomfort, skin flushing or rash, and headache, is recorded, but in the absence of any respiratory symptoms, this is not sufficient to confirm a diagnosis of AERD.

To improve quantification methods for the measurement of these aspirin-induced symptoms, we have developed a 12-symptom questionnaire as a patient-recorded total AERD symptom score (Table 17.2). Using this scoring system, patients are asked to fill out the questionnaire multiple times throughout the day of the aspirin challenge procedure. They are confirmed to have an aspirin-induced reaction if the total score increases from baseline by at least three points, reflecting increased symptoms in at least two separate symptom categories, at least one of which is in the first nine categories, which are more specific to the respiratory and nasoocular system.

Following the onset of aspirin-induced symptoms, patients are monitored closely in the clinic and observed for at least a 3-h period. The symptoms tend to peak within 60 min of the onset of reaction, although some patients do continue to worsen for up to 2 h, and are generally resolving by the end of the 3-h observation period. Lower respiratory reactions and acute bronchoconstriction are treated with nebulized albuterol, and a single dose of zileuton can be administered to quickly improve any aspirin-induced gastrointestinal pain and skin rash.[23] Many patients will report a globus sensation or tickling sensation in their throat during the reaction, which is usually mild and self-limiting. For the very rare cases of significant laryngeal edema or hypotension, intramuscular epinephrine is used.

Interestingly, for patients who are challenged more than once, there can be quite a bit of variability in the spectrum and severity of aspirin-induced symptoms during repeated challenges. In fact, 14% of the patients

TABLE 17.2
Total Aspirin-Exacerbated Respiratory Disease Symptom Score

		None	A Little	Moderate	Quite a Bit	Severe	Very Severe
1	Nasal congestion	0	1	2	3	4	5
2	Runny nose	0	1	2	3	4	5
3	Itchy nose	0	1	2	3	4	5
4	Sneezing	0	1	2	3	4	5
5	Itchy eyes	0	1	2	3	4	5
6	Eye tearing	0	1	2	3	4	5
7	Itchy ears or throat	0	1	2	3	4	5
8	Eye redness	0	1	2	3	4	5
9	Cough, wheezing, chest tightness, shortness of breath	0	1	2	3	4	5
10	Abdominal cramps, nausea, vomiting, or diarrhea	0	1	2	3	4	5
11	Skin rash, flushing, or itching	0	1	2	3	4	5
12	Headache	0	1	2	3	4	5
Totals							
Grand total							

with confirmed AERD who had multiple oral aspirin challenges over a period of several years had a negative oral aspirin challenge at least once, and therefore a single negative challenge does not necessarily rule out AERD in a patient whose clinical history otherwise suggests it.[18]

Intranasal Challenge With Ketorolac

Intranasal provocation testing can be done using the parenteral form of ketorolac, which is a potent nonselective COX inhibitor used for moderate and severe pain in the United States. The reaction symptoms induced by intranasal ketorolac tend to be less severe than those induced during oral aspirin challenges. Compared with oral aspirin challenge, intranasal ketorolac is less likely to cause severe bronchoconstriction or to cause extrapulmonary gastrointestinal or skin symptoms.[30,31] However, the sensitivity of intranasal ketorolac challenges is only 78%.[30] Therefore, lack of response to intranasal ketorolac is not sufficient to rule out AERD and may need to be followed by an oral aspirin challenge to make a definitive diagnosis.

The procedure for intranasal challenge with ketorolac requires the preparation and dilution of the injectable form of ketorolac tromethamine (Table 17.3) for use in a nasal spray bottle. Increasing doses of ketorolac are given every 30–60 min until reaction symptoms are noted. If no symptoms develop within 1 h after the highest dose of ketorolac, the challenge procedure can be converted into an oral aspirin challenge and would proceed with administering 40.5 mg of aspirin, to continue as in Table 17.1.

IN VITRO DIAGNOSIS

As the mechanism of AERD is known to involve abnormal arachidonic acid metabolism with overproduction of cysteinyl leukotrienes,[32] several studies have explored the diagnostic value of urinary leukotriene E4 (LTE_4) in AERD. LTE_4 is the stable metabolite of LTC_4 and LTD_4, and urinary LTE_4 level is a biomarker of increased systemic cysteinyl leukotriene production. The diagnostic utility of both single "spot" urine[33] and 24-h urinary excretion[34] levels of LTE_4 have been investigated in small numbers of patients. Although these rely on arbitrary study-specific LTE_4 cutoff values, the results have been encouraging, suggesting sensitivity and specificity of over 85% for identifying aspirin sensitivity in patients with respiratory disease. Further research will be needed to validate the diagnostic reliability of

TABLE 17.3
Procedure for Intranasal Ketorolac Challenge

1. Mix ketorolac tromethamine (60 mg/2 mL) and preservative-free normal saline (2.75 mL) into any empty nasal spray bottle, for which each spray actuates 0.1 mL, equivalent to 1.26 mg of ketorolac per spray.
2. Prime with 5 sprays before use.
3. Instruct patient to tilt head down while spraying and sniff gently to avoid swallowing solution.
4. Incremental doses of ketorolac sprays are given every 30 min with accompanying PNIF measurement and spirometry is repeated before each dose.

Time	Sprays Administered per Step	Dose of Ketorolac Administered per Step
0	1 spray (1 in 1 nostril)	1.26 mg
30 min	2 sprays (1 in each nostril)	2.52 mg
60 min	4 sprays (2 in each nostril)	5.04 mg
90 min	6 sprays (3 in each nostril)	7.56 mg

PNIF, peak nasal inspiratory flow.
Adapted from Lee RU, White AA, Ding D, et al. Use of intranasal ketorolac and modified oral aspirin challenge for desensitization of aspirin-exacerbated respiratory disease. *Ann Allergy Asthma Immunol.* 2010;105(2):130–135.

urinary LTE_4. Currently, there are no clinically available in vitro tests that can be recommended for the routine diagnosis of AERD, and there are no diagnostic biomarkers that have been identified as exclusive to AERD.

SUMMARY

In the absence of reliable biomarkers or noninvasive testing methodologies, oral aspirin challenges have remained the gold standard for the diagnosis of AERD. However, for many patients, the diagnosis of AERD can be confidently made based on a clear clinical history. For those patients in whom the history is unclear, or for whom the status of their sensitivity to COX-1 inhibitors is unknown, a provocative challenge with aspirin is warranted and can safely be performed in an outpatient setting for nearly all patients.

REFERENCES

1. Szczeklik A, Nizankowska E, Duplaga M. Natural history of aspirin-induced asthma. AIANE investigators. European network on aspirin-induced asthma. *Eur Respir J.* 2000;16(3):432–436.
2. Cahill KN, Bensko JC, Boyce JA, Laidlaw TM. Prostaglandin D(2): a dominant mediator of aspirin-exacerbated respiratory disease. *J Allergy Clin Immunol.* 2015;135(1): 245–252.
3. Samter M, Beers Jr RF. Intolerance to aspirin. Clinical studies and consideration of its pathogenesis. *Ann Intern Med.* 1968;68(5):975–983.
4. Widal F, Abrami P, Lermoyez J. Anaphylaxie et idiosyncrasie. *Presse Med.* 1922;30:189–192.
5. Stevenson DD, Sanchez-Borges M, Szczeklik A. Classification of allergic and pseudoallergic reactions to drugs that inhibit cyclooxygenase enzymes. *Ann Allergy Asthma Immunol.* 2001;87(3):177–180.
6. Berges-Gimeno MP, Simon RA, Stevenson DD. The natural history and clinical characteristics of aspirin-exacerbated respiratory disease. *Ann Allergy Asthma Immunol.* 2002;89(5):474–478.
7. Kasper L, Sladek K, Duplaga M, et al. Prevalence of asthma with aspirin hypersensitivity in the adult population of Poland. *Allergy.* 2003;58(10):1064–1066.
8. Jenkins C, Costello J, Hodge L. Systematic review of prevalence of aspirin induced asthma and its implications for clinical practice. *BMJ.* 2004;328(7437):434.
9. Rajan JP, Wineinger NE, Stevenson DD, White AA. Prevalence of aspirin-exacerbated respiratory disease among asthmatic patients: a meta-analysis of the literature. *J Allergy Clin Immunol.* 2015;135(3):676–681 e671.
10. Stevenson DD, Pleskow WW, Simon RA, et al. Aspirin-sensitive rhinosinusitis asthma: a double-blind crossover study of treatment with aspirin. *J Allergy Clin Immunol.* 1984;73(4):500–507.
11. McMains KC, Kountakis SE. Medical and surgical considerations in patients with Samter's triad. *Am J Rhinol.* 2006;20(6):573–576.
12. Berges-Gimeno MP, Simon RA, Stevenson DD. Early effects of aspirin desensitization treatment in asthmatic patients with aspirin-exacerbated respiratory disease. *Ann Allergy Asthma Immunol.* 2003;90(3):338–341.
13. Stevenson DD, Hankammer MA, Mathison DA, Christiansen SC, Simon RA. Aspirin desensitization treatment of aspirin-sensitive patients with rhinosinusitis-asthma: long-term outcomes. *J Allergy Clin Immunol.* 1996;98(4): 751–758.

14. Świerczyńska-Krępa M, Sanak M, Bochenek G, et al. Aspirin desensitization in patients with aspirin-induced and aspirin-tolerant asthma: a double-blind study. *J Allergy Clin Immunol*. 2014;134(4):883–890.

15. Lee-Sarwar K, Johns C, Laidlaw TM, Cahill KN. Tolerance of daily low-dose aspirin does not preclude aspirin-exacerbated respiratory disease. *J Allergy Clin Immunol Pract*. 2015;3(3):449–451.

16. Cahill KN, Johns CB, Cui J, et al. Automated identification of an aspirin-exacerbated respiratory disease cohort. *J Allergy Clin Immunol*. 2016.

17. White AA, Stevenson DD, Simon RA. The blocking effect of essential controller medications during aspirin challenges in patients with aspirin-exacerbated respiratory disease. *Ann Allergy Asthma Immunol*. 2005;95(4):330–335.

18. Pleskow WW, Stevenson DD, Mathison DA, Simon RA, Schatz M, Zeiger RS. Aspirin-sensitive rhinosinusitis/asthma: spectrum of adverse reactions to aspirin. *J Allergy Clin Immunol*. 1983;71(6):574–579.

19. Fountain CR, Mudd PA, Ramakrishnan VR, Sillau SH, Kingdom TT, Katial RK. Characterization and treatment of patients with chronic rhinosinusitis and nasal polyps. *Ann Allergy Asthma Immunol*. 2013;111(5):337–341.

20. Cardet JC, White AA, Barrett NA, et al. Alcohol-induced respiratory symptoms are common in patients with aspirin exacerbated respiratory disease. *J Allergy Clin Immunol Pract*. 2014;2(2):208–213.

21. White A, Ta V. Survey-defined patient experiences with aspirin exacerbated respiratory disease (AERD). *J Allergy Clin Immunol Pract*. 2015;3(5):711–718.

22. De Schryver E, Derycke L, Campo P, et al. Alcohol hyperresponsiveness in chronic rhinosinusitis with nasal polyps. *Clin Exp Allergy*. 2017;47:245–253.

23. Israel E, Fischer AR, Rosenberg MA, et al. The pivotal role of 5-lipoxygenase products in the reaction of aspirin-sensitive asthmatics to aspirin. *Am Rev Respir Dis*. 1993;148 (6 Pt 1):1447–1451.

24. Stevenson DD, Simon RA, Mathison DA, Christiansen SC. Montelukast is only partially effective in inhibiting aspirin responses in aspirin-sensitive asthmatics. *Ann Allergy Asthma Immunol*. 2000;85(6 Pt 1):477–482.

25. Melillo G, Balzano G, Bianco S, et al. Report of the INTERASMA working group on standardization of inhalation provocation tests in aspirin-induced asthma. Oral and inhalation provocation tests for the diagnosis of aspirin-induced asthma. *Allergy*. 2001;56(9):899–911.

26. Mita H, Higashi N, Taniguchi M, Higashi A, Akiyama K. Increase in urinary leukotriene B4 glucuronide concentration in patients with aspirin-intolerant asthma after intravenous aspirin challenge. *Clin Exp Allergy*. 2004;34(8):1262–1269.

27. Nizankowska-Mogilnicka E, Bochenek G, Mastalerz L, et al. EAACI/GA2LEN guideline: aspirin provocation tests for diagnosis of aspirin hypersensitivity. *Allergy*. 2007;62(10):1111–1118.

28. Macy E, Bernstein JA, Castells MC, et al. Aspirin challenge and desensitization for aspirin-exacerbated respiratory disease: a practice paper. *Ann Allergy Asthma Immunol*. 2007;98(2):172–174.

29. Nizankowska E, Szczeklik A. Glucocorticosteroids attenuate aspirin-precipitated adverse reactions in aspirin-intolerant patients with asthma. *Ann Allergy*. 1989;63(2):159–162.

30. White A, Bigby T, Stevenson D. Intranasal ketorolac challenge for the diagnosis of aspirin-exacerbated respiratory disease. *Ann Allergy Asthma Immunol*. 2006;97(2):190–195.

31. Lee RU, White AA, Ding D, et al. Use of intranasal ketorolac and modified oral aspirin challenge for desensitization of aspirin-exacerbated respiratory disease. *Ann Allergy Asthma Immunol*. 2010;105(2):130–135.

32. Christie PE, Tagari P, Ford-Hutchinson AW, et al. Urinary leukotriene E4 concentrations increase after aspirin challenge in aspirin-sensitive asthmatic subjects. *Am Rev Respir Dis*. 1991;143(5 Pt 1):1025–1029.

33. Celejewska-Wojcik N, Mastalerz L, Wojcik K, et al. Incidence of aspirin hypersensitivity in patients with chronic rhinosinusitis and diagnostic value of urinary leukotriene E4. *Pol Arch Med Wewn*. 2012;122(9):422–427.

34. Divekar R, Hagan J, Rank M, et al. Diagnostic utility of urinary LTE4 in asthma, allergic rhinitis, chronic rhinosinusitis, nasal polyps, and aspirin sensitivity. *J Allergy Clin Immunol Pract*. 2016;4(4):665–670.

CHAPTER 18

Other NSAIDs Reactions

NATALIA BLANCA-LOPEZ, MD, PHD • MARIA GABRIELA CANTO, MD, PHD • MIGUEL BLANCA, MD, PHD

KEY POINTS

- Nonsteroidal antiinflammatory drugs (NSAIDs), are the most commonly prescribed drugs all over the world.
- Five major groups of entities are presently considered: respiratory manifestations, now recognized as NSAID-exacerbated respiratory disease (NERD); chronic spontaneous urticaria that is aggravated after the intake of an NSAID, designated as NSAID-exacerbated cutaneous disease (NECD); and urticaria and angioedema that appears in the absence of chronic urticaria, recognized as NSAID-induced urticaria and angioedema (NIUA), are among them.
- Desensitization to NSAIDs is successful in specific cases including NERD.
- It is known that in cases of selective responders to one single COX-2 inhibitor, alternative drugs from the same group can be safely administered.

INTRODUCTION

Nonsteroidal antiinflammatory drugs (NSAIDs) are the most commonly prescribed drugs all over the world[1] and are responsible for a wide spectrum of adverse events.[2] In this chapter we, focus specifically on hypersensitivity reactions to NSAIDs.[3] Although several classifications have been provided,[4–7] we will follow the latest, proposed in 2012 by the Expert Committee of the European Academy of Allergy and Clinical Immunology. This classification unifies those previously used and terms such as anaphylactoid reactions and pseudoallergic reactions, and others that are rather imprecise have been included within this new classification.[8,9]

A new nomenclature for hypersensitivity reactions is provided in this chapter that includes reactions produced by specific immunologic mechanisms and reactions where no immunologic recognition of the drug occurs.[10] The former category includes allergic reactions and the latter includes reactions that are currently defined as nonallergic drug hypersensitivity to NSAIDs (Fig. 18.1).[9]

A growing interest in NSAID hypersensitivity has emerged over recent years because new data indicate that the skin is the organ most frequently involved,[11] with others emphasizing this finding.[12,13] Importantly, this interest has extended to children, in whom allergic and nonallergic hypersensitivity reactions to NSAIDs are also occurring with increasing frequency[14,15]

The category of NSAIDs includes a large group of nonchemically related drugs that belong to different classes shown in Table 18.1.[16] Not all these drugs are prescribed in all countries, and those commonly used in all countries have different patterns of consumption although there is a common denominator, with paracetamol (acetaminophen) and ibuprofen being greatly utilized everywhere. In fact, paracetamol and ibuprofen (and in some countries ASA) can be obtained over the counter.[17,18] Ibuprofen and diclofenac are strong COX-1 inhibitors and therefore more liable to induce hypersensitivity reactions than ASA.

Paracetamol, a relatively safe drug, is a very common ingredient in US medications, appearing in more than 600 pharmaceutical products.[18,19] Although paracetamol is not a classical antiinflammatory drug but rather an analgesic and antipyretic, in allergy textbooks and reviews, it is usually included within the category of NSAIDs when dealing with hypersensitivity reactions to NSAIDs.[3,4] Paracetamol is implicated in both nonallergic hypersensitivity reactions to NSAIDs[13] and in selective reactions.[16] In addition, paracetamol has also been implicated (although with a very low frequency) in selective nonimmediate allergic reactions, such as Stevens-Johnson syndrome, toxic epidermal necrolysis, and acute generalized exanthematous pustulosis, as well as organ-specific reactions considered to have serious

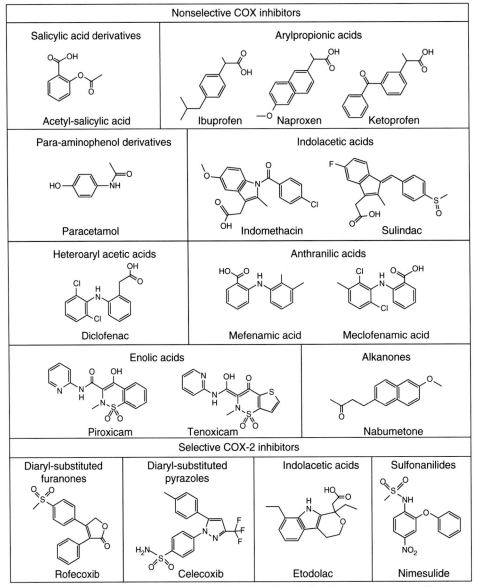

FIG. 18.1 Nonsteroidal antiinflammatory drugs involved in drug hypersensitivity reactions.

adverse effects that can often be fatal or produce serious sequelae.[19]

This chapter deals with hypersensitivity reactions to NSAIDs, focusing on those with skin involvement.[8,9] We will also consider those reactions of the skin accompanied by other manifestations, whether systemic or organ-specific. Skin manifestations include those that occur in patients who experience chronic spontaneous urticaria (CSU) and those where cutaneous manifestations occur in the absence of CSU. Much emphasis is now being given to the latter because patients present with these symptoms frequently.[1,20] Other important entities such as anaphylaxis, which involves not just the skin but other organs also, will be considered. As anaphylaxis may occur in patients who are cross-intolerant, suggestions have been made to reevaluate the classification we use in this chapter.[21–23]

TABLE 18.1
Classification of Nonsteroidal Antiinflammatory Drug (NSAID) Hypersensitivity Reactions

Type of Reaction	Clinical Manifestation	Timing	Underlying Disease	Cross-reactivity		PUTATIVE MECHANISM
NSAID-exacerbated respiratory disease (NERD)	Rhinitis/asthma	Acute	Asthma/rhinosinusitis	Yes	Nonallergic	Cox-1 inhibition
NSAID-exacerbated cutaneous disease (NECD)	Urticaria/angioedema		Chronic urticaria			Cox-1 inhibition
NSAID-induced urticaria/angioedema (NIUA)	Urticaria/angioedema		No underlying chronic diseases			Unknown, probably COX-1 inhibition
Single NSAID-induced urticaria/angioedema/anaphylaxis (SNIUAA)	Urticaria/angioedema/anaphylaxis		No underlying chronic diseases	No	Allergic	IgE mediated
Single NSAID-induced delayed reactions (SNIDRs)	Various symptoms and organs involved	Delayed	No underlying chronic diseases			T cell mediated

CLASSIFICATION AND MECHANISMS

As mentioned above, we will follow the classification proposed by the ENDA group within the European Academy of Allergy.[9] This classification has been adopted by many groups. Although it is subject to further updates, as analyzed later in this chapter, it is currently the most appropriate for classifying the different clinical entities occurring in patients.[21]

The recently proposed concept of nonallergic drug hypersensitivity[10] includes reactions involving nonimmunologic mechanisms. Drugs involved include radiocontrast media, vancomycin, quinolones, muscle relaxants, opioids, chemotherapeutic agents, and others,[24] although NSAIDs are by far the most common.[25,26] This latter group includes strong COX-1 inhibitors such as ASA and propionic acid derivatives, weak COX-1 inhibitors such as paracetamol and meloxicam, and selective COX-2 inhibitors such as the coxib group of drugs.[25] In addition, there is a second category comprising those reactions involving specific immunologic mechanisms. In this category, immediate reactions, usually occurring within 1 h after drug intake,[16] are the second most frequent of the whole group, with T cell–mediated reactions being rather infrequent, particularly the more severe reactions.[27,28]

Following the classification of Kowalski, five types of reactions to NSAIDs are recognized (see Table 18.1). These are NSAID-exacerbated respiratory disease (*NERD*); NSAID-exacerbated cutaneous disease (*NECD*); NSAID-induced urticaria angioedema in the absence of chronic urticaria (*NIUA*); single

NSAID-induced urticaria, angioedema, and anaphylaxis (*SNIUAA*); and single NSAID-induced delayed hypersensitivity reaction (*SNDR*). The first three are considered nonallergic hypersensitivity reactions, and the last two are allergic reactions and comprise a larger number of entities in which IgE or T cell mechanisms participate.

Those reactions with respiratory airway involvement, formerly considered aspirin-exacerbated respiratory disease (AERD) and now identified within the NERD group, will be presented in another chapter. In fact, *NERD* seems more appropriate than AERD because ASA is not the most frequent drug involved, at present, because it has been progressively replaced by other NSAIDs, the most important of which are the arylpropionic derivatives, with ibuprofen being the main culprit.[11,25] In any case, skin reactions may or may not be accompanied by systemic involvement and/or participation of the respiratory airways. Whether this represents a unique phenotype or concerns well-differentiated entities will be considered in this chapter. Indeed, the first reported reaction, by Widal, was anaphylaxis with skin involvement.[29]

Instances exist where cutaneous reactions are imputed to NSAIDs, but after completing the allergological work-up, good tolerance is observed. These cases may occur in combination with the intake of certain food allergens, combined or not with exercise. In these circumstances the NSAIDs act more as a cofactor triggering the symptoms than a true causative agent. In patients with anaphylaxis induced by gliadin plus exercise, it has been proposed that ASA increases gastrointestinal absorption, enabling a higher amount of the protein to be absorbed, inducing mast cell and basophil activation. It has been shown that blood gliadin levels correlate with clinical symptoms induced by exercise and ASA.[30] A pharmacological effect of NSAIDs favoring histamine release in these circumstances has also been proposed.[31]

EPIDEMIOLOGY

Studies on the prevalence of hypersensitivity reactions to NSAIDs are variable and include those generally dealing with adverse side effects,[32,33] with fewer studies focusing on the hypersensitivity reaction. Information concerning the prevalence of the different entities according to the more recent classification is scarce.[11]

Data based on spontaneous reports in large population surveys show cutaneous reactions to NSAIDs to be the most frequently reported after antimicrobials.[34] In this study, dipyrone and ASA were the NSAIDs most frequently involved, with a female to male ratio of 1.58. For self-reporting cutaneous manifestations, NSAIDS were the most frequently reported after β-lactam antibiotics.[35] Although allergy-based surveys indicate NSAIDs after antibiotics,[36] recent studies suggest that NSAIDs are, in fact, the most frequent drugs involved in hypersensitivity drug reactions.[11,26] When the different entities are considered, cutaneous manifestations are the most common.[25,26,36] NSAIDs also follow antibiotics as the most frequent cause of anaphylaxis in patients attending emergency departments,[37] although other studies have shown NSAIDs as the leading cause.[38,39] Data based on spontaneous reporting have shown that compared with other drugs, NSAIDs have the highest relative risk for inducing anaphylaxis, with diclofenac, ibuprofen, and naproxen being among the most common.[40]

Concerning severe reactions, the SCAR study plus a population-based study carried out in Germany and the US Food and Drug Administration (FDA) spontaneous reporting system shows that the prevalence of these reactions is low, with the absolute risk of SJS and TEN being higher for oxicams, although these findings were not observed by others.[41]

Although NSAID hypersensitivity reactions are less frequent in children, these drugs have been implicated since the early days.[4] NSAIDs follow β-lactam antibiotics as the most frequent cause of reactions.[42]

Two large studies have summarized the epidemiologic data on the type of reactions induced. Our group reported a large series of cases between 2005 and 2010.

From a total of 4994 patients evaluated by clinical history, 37% of the episodes were attributed to NSAIDs and 29.4% to β-lactam antibiotics. Of this 37%, 47% were confirmed to be hypersensitivity reactions to NSAIDs and 18% to β-lactam antibiotics.[11] The NSAID reactions included both allergic and nonallergic hypersensitivity. These data support previous studies also undertaken in a large population that included children and adolescents.[26]

TYPES OF NSAIDS IN SPECIFIC NSAID HYPERSENSITIVITY PHENOTYPES

We will consider the clinical entities involved in cutaneous manifestations following the ENDA classification. Concerning *NECD*, in addition to ASA, all drugs that are strong COX-1 inhibitors can induce symptoms in patients with CSU. This includes ibuprofen and the other arylpropionic derivatives.[43] Piroxicam, indomethacin, pyrazolone derivatives such as metamizol and paracetamol, and in a few cases selective COX-2 inhibitors have all been implicated.[44-46] Although CSU is less frequent in children than in adults, figures for positive responses to ASA are similar to those in adults.[22] Because symptoms in CSU may fluctuate,[47] the response may be related with the course of the disease.[48,49]

One characteristic of patients with *NIUA* is that the same drugs involved in *NERD* and *NECD* are also common triggers for this entity.[1,20] When weak COX-1 inhibitors such as paracetamol are administered, up to 25% of cases have been shown to have skin symptoms, and even subjects tolerating paracetamol may respond to selective COX-2 inhibitors such as etoricoxib.[46] A study carried out by Asero et al. found that pyrazolone derivatives were implicated in 64% of the cases.[50] Isolated angioedema is also an entity that can be included within NIUA, although cases with idiopathic angioedema aggravated by the intake of NSAIDs may also occur. The prevalence of drug-induced angioedema in the absence of urticaria has been estimated at 2.3%, with a mean age of the patients being 47 years; of these, NSAIDs were the responsible agent in more than 50% of cases.[51] As in the case of urticaria, the drugs involved were ASA, ibuprofen, dipyrone, and acetaminophen, followed at lower percentages by diclofenac, nimesulide, ketoprofen, and naproxen.[52]

Although the classic drugs contributing to *SNIUA* for many years were pyrazolone derivatives such as metamizol and propyphenazone,[44,45,53] the progressive use of arylpropionic derivatives, particularly ibuprofen, has seen an increase in these drugs. A study published in 2010 evaluating a large series of patients over a period of 30 years between 1980 and 2010 found a decrease in pyrazolones and an increase in propionic acid derivatives, although the predominance was still significant for pyrazolones, which contributed to 44% of the selective responders in contrast to 25% for propionic acid derivatives.[25] More recently this predominance has been shown in a large series of cases with immediate reactions to arylpropionic derivatives, where 17% were considered. Within this group, selectivity to ibuprofen or naproxen was observed with cross-reactivity between the different arylpropionics, although there were also selective responses to ibuprofen with good tolerance to naproxen and dexketoprofen and vice versa.[54]

Concerning single NSAID-induced delayed hypersensitivity reaction (*SNIDHR*), although the classic drugs involved in T cell–mediated reactions are anticonvulsants, such as carbamazepine and hidantoins or allopurinol, plus a few others,[55,56] some studies have shown that NSAIDs are also involved.[1,20] Maculopapular exanthema and contact eczema are the most frequent manifestations.[11] The relative contribution of the different NSAIDs to SNIDHR can vary according to the clinical entity. For example, in fixed drug eruptions (FDEs), pyrazolone derivatives, paracetamol, nabumetone, and COX-2 inhibitors have been reported more frequently than the other NSAIDs.[57,58]

Although the risk of severe reactions to NSAIDs is extremely low, healthcare providers and patients should be aware of the possibility.[58] The incidence for SJS-TEN ranges from 0.9 to 7.1 cases per million.[59,60] Of particular relevance for severe reactions are COX-2 inhibitors, although the incidence of SJS-TEN and DRESS is very low.[61–63] Although NSAIDs are not among the main drugs involved, they may also contribute to severe reactions.[55]

NSAIDs are frequently involved in photoallergic and phototoxic reactions,[64] also included within the group of SNIDHR. Among the arylpropionic derivatives, the most frequently involved is ketoprofen, a drug widely used as a topical agent.[64] Piketoprofen has also been implicated, although with a lower photosensitizing capacity.[65] Other NSAIDS involved are etofenamate,[66,67] diclofenac,[68] and oxicams.[69]

PHENOTYPES OF NSAID HYPERSENSITIVITY

As stated above, although in the past most basic and clinical research has been devoted to the respiratory entities now included within the NERD group,[3] the more frequently occurring reactions involve the skin, with or without systemic symptoms.[1,20] Although urticaria and angioedema were initially included within

the syndrome of ASA idiosyncrasy,[4] this was not usually considered, and most studies focused on the respiratory involvement.[1,20]

NSAID-Exacerbated Cutaneous Disease

In the early 70´s the association between NSAID intolerance and CSU was reported.[70] Up to 30%–40% of patients with CSU may experience an exacerbation after the intake of strong COX-1 inhibitors, such as ASA, ibuprofen, diclofenac, piroxicam, and others.[70–72] The symptoms not only worsen in cases with active disease, but there may also be an exacerbation of CSU. Exposure may not only worsen the clinical entity, but the patient may also develop anaphylaxis. *NECD* can be unveiled after a clinical evaluation because the patient has not taken these drugs during the course of the active disease.[50] Reactions may appear within an interval of minutes to hours after drug administration, although in most subjects the reaction occurs within 2 h.[49,73] In general, this phenomenon is dose-dependent, but the ingestion of doses as low as 100 mg can cause the symptoms.[74] NSAID intolerance may precede the appearance of CSU.[72] Although the route of administration is usually oral or parenteral, reactions can also been triggered by topical application.[74]

Although NECD is more frequent in the adult population, this reaction has also been reported in children.[75] In some cases the only manifestation may be eyelid angioedema.[76,77]

Concerning the pathophysiologic mechanisms, a common basis with NERD has been proposed because nonchemically related strong COX-1 inhibitors can precipitate or aggravate CSU. Masterlanz et al. reported that patients with CSU showed eicosanoid alterations similar to those present in NERD.[71] However, only a few studies have been carried out on the mechanisms involved, which can be complex.[78] Because of its pharmacological effect, ASA can enhance the release of mediators of allergic reactions, such as histamine, by several mechanisms, including being triggered by allergens.[79] The analysis of biopsies from patients with *NECD* shows the presence of dermal edema and lymphatic dilatation with a perivascular mononuclear cell infiltrate that may include eosinophils and neutrophils. No evidence of leukocytoclastic vasculitis with fibrin deposits has been found.[80] The finding can also be observed in CSU. Isolated angioedema induced by NSAIDs was also reported very early on.[4]

NSAID-Induced Urticaria and Angioedema

The *NIUA* groups include those cases with urticaria and/or angioedema triggered by the intake of NSAIDs in the absence of CSU. Recent studies suggest that this is the most common clinical entity within hypersensitivity reactions to NSAIDs. The clinical history and drug provocation testing show that NIUA accounts for at least 60% of cases.[25] After the intake of ASA or any NSAID, patients may develop symptoms within just 1 h or even sooner in 46% of cases, with 21% developing symptoms after 1–6 h. In the remaining cases symptoms may appear after 24–48 h or even later. In general, there is a good correlation between the symptoms after challenge and the clinical history.[14] In those cases with isolated angioedema, symptoms may also appear a long time after the drug intake. Although initially it was thought that patients with urticaria could be selective responders to a number of NSAIDs, several studies have shown that this must be classified within the category of cross-intolerance (CI).[50]

Although the ENDA classification included urticaria, urticaria with angioedema, and isolated angioedema within the *NIUA* group, it has been shown that cases with anaphylaxis must be included.[78] In our experience, within the category of cross-intolerance, 7% of cases develop an anaphylactic response with the involvement of more than two organs.[25] In children, anaphylactic reactions to multiple NSAIDs have also been reported.[22] Although it is claimed that this may constitute a different phenotype, as is the case in adults, these must be included within the *NIUA* category.[78]

An important question is whether *NIUA* can evolve to NECD or whether it is a well-defined entity. Although Asero et al. have reported that in the course of NIUA, patients sooner or later develop CSU,[3] a study by our group showed that in a large series of subjects with *NIUA* followed during a period of 12 years, the number of cases developing NECD was low and no different from the control group.[81] Another question concerning natural evolution relates to the disappearance of *NIUA* over time. In cases with NERD, some evidence indicates that this may occur,[82,83] but no studies are currently available concerning this entity. This is a matter of investigation for the coming years.

Single NSAID-Induced Urticaria, Angioedema, and Anaphylaxis

SNIUAA patients can develop urticaria and/or angioedema and anaphylaxis in response to a single drug, even if it is a weak or selective COX-2 inhibitor.[16] Studies by Perlmutter showed cases that were skin-test positive to ASA-polylisine who also had urticaria, angioedema, and anaphylaxis.[84] Other studies have shown that aspirin anhydride, a reactive compound as a contaminant of ASA, is able to bind proteins and

induce specific IgE antibodies.[85] However, neither this contaminant nor others exist in current drug formulations. Selective immediate reactions have been reported to all NSAIDs prescribed,[16] with the two main drugs currently being pyrazolones and arylpropionic acid derivatives.[11] The contribution of different NSAIDS can vary according to country,[86] and a tendency for these drugs to vary over time has also been reported.[11,25] The number of selective (SNIUAA) versus CI (NIUA) varies according to different studies. Most studies have been carried out in adult populations or in both adults and adolescents.[25,26,36,86–88] In a large series of over 600 cases, including adults and adolescents, it was shown that 76% were CI and 24 selective responders,[11] but these figures may vary according to country. Over a period of about 5 years, the proportion of CI remains almost constant, with figures of around 50%, but there was a slight but significant decrease later for selective responders, varying from 11% of the drug hypersensitivity reactions reported to 4.96% ($P<.0001$).[11] The most severe clinical entity within this group was anaphylaxis, occurring in 42% of cases with SNIUAA compared with 7% of cases with NIUA ($P<.0001$). A high frequency of anaphylaxis may also appear in children.[39] In some instances, coronary spasm may occur because of histamine release.[88] Although aged persons with cardiovascular risks are more prone, this has also been reported in younger patients.[89]

In some countries, diclofenac is another NSAID involved in immediate selective reactions, and it has been responsible for severe or fatal anaphylaxis.[90] This drug is metabolized to acyl glucuronide that binds to proteins and is able to induce an immune response.[91–93] It has been proposed that gastric acid suppression facilitates the production of diclofenac protein conjugates in the stomach because of the high pH conditions, and these can be a causative mechanism for the induction of diclofenac-specific IgE antibodies.[94] Harrier et al. have covalently coupled phase I and phase II diclofenac metabolites to a protein carrier in a search for specific IgE by immunoassay and basophil activation. Although this group was able to detect specific IgG antibodies, no IgE antibodies were found. Other studies have found support for the presence of IgE antibodies to propyphenazone,[53] pyrazolones,[95] paracetamol,[96] and ibuprofen.[97] With another pyrazolone, metamizol, there is indirect evidence that this drug and some of its metabolites can induce basophil activation in cases with selective immediate responses that are skin-test positive,[98] but direct proof of the presence of specific IgE antibodies has not yet been found. The list of drugs to which an IgE mechanism is attributed has been reviewed by Canto et al.[16]

Concerning children aged under 14 years, immediate selective responses can also occur. In a study carried out by Cavkaytar, 41% were selective,[99] but figures have varied from 30% to 75%.[22,100–103] These variations can be explained by the different protocols used for the diagnosis (the diagnosis was not confirmed by challenge in all cases) and by patterns of drug consumption, among other factors.[78]

It is assumed that in most instances we are dealing with an IgE mechanism, and the natural history follows the same tendency as that observed in cases with immediate reactions to β-lactams.[104] Studies based on basophil activation in patients with SNIUAA to metamizol indicate that over time there is a tendency for basophil activation tests to become negative.[98]

Single NSAID-Induced Delayed Reactions

The single NSAID-induced delayed reaction (SNIDR) group includes reactions involving a T cell–mediated response. Although much less frequent in number of reactions, they are the most heterogeneous among the clinical entities induced (see Table 18.2). The Type IV reactions in the classification by Gell and Coombs include four major pathophysiologic mechanisms, corresponding to different entities.[28] These are as follows:

Type IVa, such as contact eczema, is considered a Th1 reaction with the production of IFN-γ. Drugs typically involved in contact eczema are arylpropionic acid derivatives, fenamates, oxicams, and diclofenac.[105–108]

Type IVb is maculopapular exanthema, often followed by bullae formation. The pathology consists of a perivascular mononuclear infiltrate, often accompanied by eosinophilia, with the presence of CD3+ T cells and predominance of CD4+. A Th2 mechanism is proposed, with the involvement of IL-5 and IL-4.[109–111] Drugs typically eliciting this kind of reaction are pyrazolones, paracetamol, and propionic acid derivatives.[25,32,112,113]

Type IVc comprises lesions consisting of maculopapular exanthema with bullous lesions. Activated T cells release perforin and Granzyme B, which are able to kill keratinocytes. The CD8+ T cells are responsible for the bullae formation by killing the keratinocytes. In the case of TEN, there is a predominance of CD8+ T cells with natural killer cells, which together with monocytes are responsible for the massive apoptosis of keratinocytes.[114,115] NSAIDs involved include arylpropionic acid derivatives, such as ibuprofen,[116] paracetamol,[117] pyrazolone derivatives,[118] and selective COX-2 inhibitors.[119–121]

Type IVd is formed by pustular exanthema with disseminated small aseptic pustules. Skin biopsy reveals intraepidermal pustules with the presence of CD4+ and CD8+ T cells and neutrophils.[28] Typical drugs include ibuprofen[122] and selective COX-2 inhibitors.[123]

Although this classification has proved to be of value, not all lesions can be easily categorized within these four subgroups. In the case of DRESS, for example, there is systemic involvement with liver injury and the presence of activated CD8+ T cells in the circulation and eosinophilia.[124,125] Typical drugs involved are arylpropionic acid derivatives[126] and COX-2 inhibitors.[127]

Of relevance within the SNIDR group are the photosensitivity reactions.[128] NSAIDs, particularly some propionic acid derivatives, etofenamate, and oxicams are important contributors. These drugs can be administered through parenteral, oral, or topical routes. NSAIDs are photoactivated after exposure to light, generating a photoallergen[129] by binding to proteins forming adducts that interact with the immune system.[130] In experimental models, it has been shown that CD4

TABLE 18.2
Clinical Entities Induced by a T Cell Response (Single NSAID-Induced Delayed Reactions, SNIDRs)

Maculopapular exanthema (MPE)
Nonimmediate urticaria (NIU)
Fixed drug eruption (FDE)
Acute generalized exanthematous pustulosis (AGEP)
Drug rash with eosinophilia and systemic symptoms (DRESS)
Stevens-Johnson syndrome/toxic epidermal necrolysis (SJS-TEN)
Contact dermatitis (CD)
Photocontact dermatitis (PCD)
Organ-specific reactions (e.g., hepatitis, pneumonitis, pancreatitis)

TABLE 18.3
Escalating Doses of NSAIDs for Cross-intolerance (CI) and Selective Responders (SRs)

	DOSES OF NSAIDS USED IN CHALLENGES	
Drug	**(A) Doses Used in Challenges in Suspected or Confirmed CI. The Doses Were Administered at 90-min Intervals (Total Accumulated Dose)**	**(B) Doses Used in Challenges in Suspected or Confirmed SR. The Doses Were Administered at 90-min Intervals (Total Accumulated Dose)**
Paracetamol	50, 100, 350, 500 mg (1000 mg)	5, 50, 100, 350 mg (500 mg)
Piroxicam	5, 15 mg (20 mg)	5, 5, 10 mg (20 mg)
Diclofenac	12.5, 12.5, 25 mg (50 mg)	5, 15, 30 mg (50 mg)
Dipyrone	50, 100, 150, 300 mg (575 mg)	1st day: 5, 10, 50 mg 2nd day: 50, 150, 300 mg (575 mg)
Ibuprofen	150, 150, 300 mg (600 mg)	5, 50, 100, 200, 250 mg (600 mg)
Indomethacin	10, 20, 20 mg (50 mg)	5, 5, 15, 25 mg (50 mg)
ASA	50, 100, 150, 250 mg (500 mg)	1st day: 5, 30, 100 mg 2nd day: 150, 300 mg (500 mg)

ASA, ASA-sensitive asthma; *NSAIDs*, nonsteroidal antiinflammatory drugs.

T cells participate as effector cells with a Th2 cytokine pattern.[131,132]

Although this group of hypersensitivity reactions to NSAIDs contributes fewer cases, it nevertheless includes the largest number of clinical entities (see Table 18.3).

Maculopapular exanthema

This is the most common clinical entity induced in this category.[133] Although NSAIDs are not the most common drug involved, they may still contribute.[20] This reaction consists of macules and/or papules disseminated over the skin, usually pruritic with a predominance on the chest and abdomen, although the arms and legs can also be affected. The lesions usually subside over several days.[28,133] Often the lesions can show a more severe maculopapular eruption followed by angioedema, including on the face, and followed by desquamation.[28]

Fixed drug eruption

This consists of one or several lesions usually pigmented, sometimes forming bullae, that persist for several days or longer leaving a pigmented region. Repeated exposure to the drug induces the lesion again and sometimes a nonchemically related drug may precipitate it. Often the affected skin can be very extensive, and it may be confused with SJS.[134]

Acute generalized exanthematous pustulosis

This consists of many small, aseptic pustules, located in the epidermis, that are confluent. Lesions resolve once the drug is withdrawn.[28,123]

Drug rash with eosinophilia and systemic symptoms

This is a clinical entity that results from the combination of cutaneous plus systemic symptoms with liver involvement. The cutaneous lesions, which may be maculopapular with generalized erythema, are accompanied by fever, with lymphadenopathy, hepatitis, and pneumonitis; kidney involvement may also occur. An increase in the eosinophil number with atopic lymphocytes appears in peripheral blood.[28]

Stevens-Johnson syndrome/toxic epidermal necrolysis

These two entities form part of a spectrum with variable detachment of the skin. SJS is considered <10%, SJS-TEN an overlap (10%–30%), and TEN (>30%). Symptoms appear from 1 to 8 weeks after drug intake and initiate with a cutaneous eruption that is often mistaken for classic maculopapular exanthema. In a very short time, they evolve to mucosal involvement with conjunctivitis, ulcers in the mouth and esophagus, and genital involvement. Systemic symptoms and liver or kidney involvement may also occur in the most severe cases.

Contact dermatitis and photoallergic dermatitis

Several NSAIDs applied to the skin have been implicated in contact dermatitis (CD). At the sites of skin application, small papules appear followed by vesicles, with the presence of a cutaneous infiltrate. Sometimes the lesions can extend beyond the areas of direct skin contact. In the case of photoallergic dermatitis, the lesions can appear after the topical administration of an NSAID or after its oral or parenteral intake. The areas affected are those exposed to the light, and the usual appearance is red erythematous and/or maculopapular lesions that can evolve to more severe reactions.[64]

MIXED REACTIONS

The concept of respiratory plus skin involvement was originally designated as a blended reaction.[3,4] In a study on the prevalence of ASA-induced asthma in a Polish population, 50% of those considered as AIA had skin reactions.[135] In patients with NERD, a challenge with ASA may trigger, in addition to respiratory symptoms, extrapulmonary manifestations such as generalized urticaria, facial angioedema, conjunctival hyperemia, stomach pain, and other gastrointestinal manifestations.[135] This is due to mast cell activation with the release of inflammatory mediators that leak to the circulation and further involve different organs.[136–138] Cases that, after drug administration, experience systemic and/or upper and lower airway manifestations, in addition to skin symptoms, have also been reported. It has been suggested that several phenotypes may exist within this category.[78]

Currently, we consider most of these reactions as anaphylaxis. In a study carried out by our group, a mixed reaction appeared in 7.1% of cases in the CI group, and in 18.2% of cases, the patients reported symptoms of the skin and airway that could be considered anaphylaxis.[25] Subjects with systemic symptoms may also appear in cases with CU after the intake of NSAIDs.[139] Of particular relevance is the role of mixed reactions in children.[140] Development of wheezing in a subject who reported angioedema and generalized urticaria has also occurred after diclofenac intake.[141] A case has also been reported of a severe respiratory reaction after a low dose of ibuprofen, consisting of nasal obstruction and chest tightening, followed by facial angioedema with erythema.[142]

Although rather uncommon, combined immediate and delayed allergy to metamizol has been reported. The patient developed an episode of eyelid angioedema, followed by generalized angioedema and difficulty breathing 6 h after taking metamizol. Intradermal reading was positive at 5 mm after 20 min but negative after 24 h, and patch testing was positive at 72 h.[143]

COFACTORS, RISK FACTORS, AND ATOPY

Instances exist where a preexisting condition may precipitate a reaction after the intake of an NSAID,

particularly in the case of those that are strong COX-1 inhibitors.[1,20] Experimental evidence suggests that the intake of ASA can amplify the allergic response.[144,145] The mechanism proposed is an increase in gastrointestinal permeability, with the passage of allergens into the systemic circulation.[146,147] In some instances, the administration of ASA can be soon before or after the intake of the offending food allergen, and the cause can be attributed to the NSAID.[147] In other instances, the intake of NSAIDs induces respiratory and cutaneous symptoms, including anaphylaxis after performing exercise.[148] The mechanism involved is not known, although the administration of leukotriene antagonists has prevented cases of bronchospasm, suggesting an activation of the leukotriene pathway.[138] To further complicate the situation, cases also exist where the combination of an NSAID plus food intake precedes the exercise inducing the reaction.[149,150] The mechanism proposed here is that exercise facilitates histamine release because of the interaction of food with specific IgEs.[151,152] The threshold of mast cell histamine release may be lowered by exercise and NSAIDs. Weak COX-1 or selective COX-2 inhibitors do not produce this effect.[151]

When atopy is referred as a risk factor for hypersensitivity to NSAIDs, different criteria must be considered: skin testing to common environmental inhalant or food allergens, total serum IgE levels, and the clinical entity. Through the years, data on the prevalence of atopy have been contradictory. Initially, in cases with respiratory involvement, a low prevalence of atopy was found, around 10%–15%.[4] Within the group with *NERD*, most patients with nasal polyposis have negative immediate skin tests although others have found a higher prevalence of atopy.[4] Bochenek et al. undertook a study comparing AIA with cases of selective responses to pyrazolones and found differences only in the prevalence of atopy with the control group, but not in the results between the entities.[153] Vervloet et al. have suggested that atopy was not a risk factor for ASA intolerance or hypersensitivity to pyrazolones.[154] In a study carried out by Doña et al., three parameters were considered for atopic status: the implementation of a clinical questionnaire for the diagnosis of the atopic disease, prick testing with a panel of prevalent allergens, and total serum IgE levels. Significant differences were observed comparing CI with the control group in the skin test results and the total IgE levels when patients with *NIUA* were compared with negative controls. The allergens most significantly associated were housedust mite and dog epithelia. When two criteria were used, higher differences were found. When the clinical entities were compared, strong significant associations with rhinitis and asthma ($P=.004$ and $P<.0001$) and a lower significance with food allergy were found ($P<.04$).[11] Differences have also been observed in children. In one study carried out in children, atopy, defined by skin testing, was 72% in NIUA versus 27% in SNUAA ($P<.0045$), and a significant difference was also observed when a combination of prick testing to inhalant allergens, total IgE, and clinical symptoms were compared. The most relevant allergens contributing to these differences were house-dust mite, Olea europaea pollen, and alternaria.[99] Similar results for the association between atopy and NAIAD hypersensitivity have been found by others,[22,103] although some studies have failed to find these differences.[100,155]

NATURAL HISTORY OF NSAID HYPERSENSITIVITY

When we consider the natural history in NSAID hypersensitivity, it is rational to consider this topic in the different entities now recognized.[9] Because the number of clinical entities is large and several mechanisms can take place, the natural course and evolution can differ for many of these entities.

In NERD the classic view is that the natural history indicates that patients worsen over time.[3,4] However, in a series of three cases with intrinsic asthma, nasal polyposis, and ASA intolerance evaluated >10 years later, the patients had a negative challenge with L-ASA and good tolerance with the oral route of up to 1000 mg.[83] In another study evaluating patients with CI to NSAIDs with angioedema, anaphylaxis, or respiratory symptoms, 78% tolerated ASA.[156] Concerning NECD, strong COX-1 inhibitors can not only aggravate preexisting urticaria but also elicit the disease.[47] It is reasonable to assume that as soon as the CSU is resolved, NSAIDs can be tolerated. No information is available so far on the natural course of NIUA.

In SNIUAA, as is the case with other drugs such as β-lactams that elicit immediate allergic IgE reactions, subjects may become skin-test negative over time.[104] In fact, a follow-up study of patients with SNIUAA to metamizol and a positive basophil activation test found that positivity decreased over time, with an important number of subjects becoming negative.[98] However, the opposite may occur and a study has shown that patients with SNIUAA to a single drug may develop additional selective responses to other drugs if further exposure occurs.[157]

Concerning T cell responses to NSAIDs, no information is available at present to show that these reactions will persist for a long time or resolve. As there are several clinical entities in this group, the natural evolution in each group probably differs.[28]

DIAGNOSIS

As no reliable diagnostic tests exist in many hypersensitivity reactions to NSAIDs (with some exceptions such as CD), the history has become essential in the diagnosis of NSAID hypersensitivity.[158] Major problems arise distinguishing patients with NECD and NIUA and discriminating between anaphylaxis and mixed reactions.[78]

Because the most frequent clinical entity within the CI group is NIUA, no specific immunologic mechanism is involved, and therefore neither skin tests nor in vitro tests areavailable for the diagnosis, with the only alternative being the DPT.[1] However, in many instances patients have experienced repeated episodes with two or more NSAIDs that are strong COX-1 inhibitors and in some instances with weak COX-1 or even selective COX-2 inhibitors, and diagnosis can be established based on the clinical history.[20,25] Although some studies have indicated that the value of the clinical history is not reliable and that 75% of the patients with this entity have a negative challenge with ASA,[159] our view differs. A study carried out by Blanca-Lopez et al. showed that 63% of the cases with two episodes to two different drugs could be diagnosed based on the clinical history, and this increased to 92% when there were three or more drugs involved.[158] This implies that in cases with many episodes and a consistent history most of the patients will have a reaction in the event that an NSAID is administered again.

In Vivo Tests

As stated above, in vivo tests are not indicated in those clinical entities belonging to the cross-intolerant group.[20] The DPT is the only alternative (described in another section below), although there are cases where several episodes have occurred, and in these circumstances the clinical history can be valid. This is particularly relevant in cases of SNUIUA, where in the event of two or more severe anaphylactic episodes it is not advisable to perform any confirmatory tests but rather to provide an alternative drug.[16] With this entity the only drug that has been validated is metamizol, and concentrations of 0.1 mg/mL have been used for intradermal administration; in those cases with severe reactions, this concentration must be first assayed by prick and diluted 10-fold or lower. Because severe reactions after intradermal testing have been reported,[95,159,160] it is advisable not to use intradermal skin testing in high-risk patients. The basophil activation test is an in vitro assay that can be used as an alternative.[98] Case studies and small series have been reported with diclofenac, paracetamol, nimesulide, and others,[16] but no validation has been undertaken in larger series and it is not advised in routine practice.

The two common approaches for evaluating in vivo SNIDHR are patch and intradermal testing.[161,162] As is the case with immediate reactions, any drug belonging to the NSAID category can induce any of the nonimmediate reactions outlined in Table 18.2.

Intradermal testing. Delayed reading intradermal testing has been used for the diagnosis of nonimmediate reactions to drugs.[162] The negative predictive value for both intradermal and patch testing is low, in general, for all drugs including NSAIDs.[163,164] The positive predictive value for an intradermal test is high.[162]

Patch testing. This procedure has also been used in SNIDHR such as CD, FDE, SJS-TEN, exanthematic reactions, and photoallergic reactions. Although patch testing can be performed with soluble drugs, the advantage is that insoluble NSAIDs can also be used. The drug can be smashed and mixed with vaseline. In this case, in addition to testing the active drug, the additive(s) should also be tested to avoid false positives.[161] A positive patch test is also highly predictive.[162]

For photoallergic reactions such as those produced by arylpropionic derivatives, fenamates, and oxicams, a modification consisting of the photopatch is used. The NSAID is fixed on the back of the patient and after 1 day the patch is removed and the skin is irradiated with ultraviolet light, 5 or 10 J/cm^2 UVA (Hozle). This test is read after 2, 3, and 4 days. Further details can be consulted in Refs. 130,162.

In Vitro Tests

For quantitation of IgE antibodies, experimental prototypes have been published with series of cases or single cases reported for propyfenazone,[53] ASA,[85] and paracetamol,[96] but no additional studies of series validated by other groups exist.[16] An alternative for indirect quantitation of IgE antibodies is the basophil activation assay. This technique has proved to be valid for methamizol.[98] In a series of cases with SNIUAA, the sensitivity was 54.9% with good specificity.

In the case of NERD and NIUA, both in the CI category, there is no place for immunoassays seeking specific antibodies, but histamine and leukotriene release assays have been used. The quantitation by enzyme immunoassay of cysteinyl leukotriene C_4, D_4, and E_4 release by peripheral blood cells after being stimulated

by ASA has been used,[165,166] and in some studies the combination of in vitro stimulation of ASA + C5a is recommended for increasing the sensitivity of the assay.[165] In fact, in one study the sensitivity was 61% with a specificity of 91%, and the positive predictive value was 92%.[167] However, these data have not been confirmed by other groups,[168,169] and further studies are required for the improvement of this methodology.[170] Although other in vitro assays have been proposed, these are beyond the scope of this chapter.

Drug Provocation Tests

Although DPTs have been mainly used for the diagnosis of *NERD*, over the years[135] this technique has been progressively used for the diagnosis of the other entities, mainly *NIUA*.[1,11]

In *NIUA* in many instances, patients are evaluated years after the episode occurs, and many subjects report having had multiple episodes to several NSAIDs.[11] The more episodes that have occurred in the past (providing they are consistent and reproducible in the clinical response), the more accurate can be the diagnosis based solely on the clinical history. This situation does not occur if the patient has only had one episode, even if it is recent and shortly before the evaluation.

There is general agreement within the ENDA group that ASA must be administered to assess CI.[9,135] Escalating doses administered by the oral route must be given until a full therapeutic dose is achieved. Placebo can be administered one day before[171] or on the same day, thus saving time in the performance of the tests. The doses and time intervals that we used for NIUA are shown in Table 18.3, column A. In this we include paracetamol in addition to strong COX-1 inhibitors. After giving the placebo and waiting for a period of 90 min, the drug is given at intervals of 90 min until a full therapeutic dose is reached. In cases where ASA was the culprit drug and no reactions occurred to other NSAIDs, the alternative should be to start with indomethacin.[25] After receiving a full therapeutic dose, the patient waits for 48 h and a full therapeutic dose is then repeated twice a day for 2 days.

The use of an alternative strong COX-1 inhibitor different from ASA to challenge, for example, ibuprofen in the case of diclofenac or vice versa, although used in the past,[25,87] is not currently recommended because cases with a positive response to both but good tolerance to ASA have been reported.[157] Although this possibility seems to be low, it must nevertheless be considered.

In patients with NECD, ASA challenge should be made when urticaria is in remission and a minimum interval of 1–2 weeks has elapsed with no symptoms.[171]

Medications such as antihistamines must be withdrawn, and the test must be single blind placebo-controlled. Procedures for challenge are similar to those shown above for NIUA.

A case of SNIUA must be suspected when the subject refers having had one or several episodes of urticaria and/or angioedema to one or more NSAIDs with good tolerance to ASA. If this has occurred, the first approach in these patients is to verify tolerance to ASA. If any positive response occurs, the case must be diagnosed as CI. If good tolerance occurs, we must consider the possible existence of a selective response. In cases of SNIUA, anaphylaxis is the most frequent clinical entity, and figures are of the order of 42% compared with those of CI, with just 7%.[25] This may also occur in children.[14,15] This is particularly relevant for those countries where pyrazolones are highly prescribed,[1] although drugs such as diclofenac and ibuprofen have been progressively involved in NSAID-induced anaphylaxis.[54] Because of the severity of anaphylaxis, caution must be taken in these cases. In these circumstances in the event a DPT is required to establish the diagnosis, starting doses must be low and often cases need to be studied over 2 days to reach the therapeutic dose (see Table 18.3, column B).

Cross-intolerant reactions to NSAIDs, although less known, also occur in children.[14] In some studies CI are more than 50% in those under 14 years of age.[22,99,102,103] A clear suspicion currently under evaluation is that the younger the child, in the event a CI reaction appears, the more likely it is to belong to this group.

Less experience exists in DPT with NSAIDs in children than in adults, and at present, an expert group of the ENDA is drawing up a consensus document providing relevant recommendations. In the mean time we provide a list of articles by several authors with the dose recommended for challenge in Table 18.4.

CHALLENGE WITH ALTERNATIVE DRUGS

Some patients refuse to undertake a study to confirm the diagnosis, but alternative NSAIDs must be recommended even if no diagnosis can be made. If tolerance to weak COX-1 or selective COX-2 inhibitors is not known after the occurrence of the episode, this must be verified. In fact, some studies recommend avoiding all NSAIDs, including weak COX-1 or even selective COX-2 inhibitors, while tolerance remains unverified.[172] The choice of an alternative drug is paracetamol, the most widely used at all ages.[46] However, other drugs can also be considered.

Tolerance to paracetamol has been studied by various groups. Asero et al. reported that 19% of subjects with NIUA and 23% of subjects with NECD have symptoms after being challenged with paracetamol or nimesulide, but no specific information for the individual drugs was provided.[45]

In a series of patients with NSAID hypersensitivity, tolerance to paracetamol was verified in those who had not taken this drug, with the response being positive in 2.7% of the cases.[172] In this study, although most cases had urticaria and/or angioedema, some cases with respiratory and anaphylactic reactions were also included. Furthermore, whether patients with urticaria and/or angioedema belonged to the NIUA or NECD groups was not detailed.

Another study concerning meloxicam showed that 10 of 116 patients (8.6%) developed mild UR/AE or only erythema and pruritus at a one-quarter or cumulative dose of 7.5 mg of meloxicam. The remaining subjects (91.4%) tolerated meloxicam. In this study, 7.5 mg meloxicam was a safe alternative for ASA/NSAID-intolerant UR/AE patients. The reactions in those subjects who developed them were mild.[173] Another study carried out by Ispano et al. showed that 7.8% of the cases challenged responded to paracetamol and 4.9% to nimesulide.[171] Similar data with nimesulide have been reported by other authors. Benzydamine is also a weak COX-1 inhibitor used in some countries. Nettis et al. challenged a group of patients with urticaria, with good tolerance in 98% of cases.[173] Nevertheless, it must be noted that in most of these studies, and others carried out when patients with urticaria and angioedema to NSAID hypersensitivity are considered, particularly in those with CI, no clear specification was given as to whether they were dealing with NIUA or NECD.

In a study carried out by Doña et al. in patients with NIUA, tolerance to etoricoxib was tested in two groups. In those already positive after challenge to paracetamol, 25% responded to etoricoxib, but even in those with good tolerance to paracetamol, 6% developed skin manifestations after being challenged with paracetamol.[46]

Concerning tolerance to selective COX-2 inhibitors, a study carried out by Asero et al. in subjects with NIUA or NECD found a similar response to rofecoxib in both groups, with 18% and 17% of cases responding, respectively.[174] However, in a later study the same authors reported that in a group of 17 patients with CSU, etoricoxib was well tolerated.[175] Another study undertaken with rofecoxib in patients with urticaria and/or angioedema showed that all cases tolerated rofecoxib, although in this study challenge with ASA was not

TABLE 18.4
Proposed Protocols for Challenging in Children

Author	Age	Challenge Protocol	Duration
Zambonino[99]	6–13	Ibuprofen ¼, ¼, and ½ of TCD (10 mg/kg), ASA 1st day 1/4, ¼, and ½ of TCD, second day ½ and ½ of TCD (20 mg/kg), methamizol ¼, ¼, and ½ of TCD, (20 mg/kg), paracetamol one dose 15 mg/kg TBW	
Cavkaytar[22]	5–12	Four to five doses at 90 min intervals until a cumulative dose equal to the therapeutic dose adjusted for weight and age	1 day follow 48 h
Alves[155]	5–14	Incremental doses starting at 1/10 therapeutic dose adjusted for weight and age	1 day
Calvo-Campoverde[101]	0.2–16	First day placebo three capsules at 90 min intervals; second day four doses of 27, 44, 117 and 312; or a cumulative dose of 10 mg/kg of ASA	2 days
Guvenir[100]	0.2–16	Ibuprofen 10 mg/kg, ASA 20 mg/kg, methamizol 20 mg/kg, paracetamol 10–15 mg/kg, meloxicam 15 mg, Natumetone 500 mg (1/100 to 1/10, FTD)	1 day
Yilmaz[102]	0.3–17	Ibuprofen 10, 20, 80, 150, 300: ASA 10, 20, 50, 100, 200; methamizol 62, 125, 250; paracetamol 10, 50, 250, 500, dose adjusted for weight and age	
Hassani[103]	7–17	1/10 mg of NSAID according to severity, increasing gradually every 20 min until achieving FTD adjusted for weight and age. Second and third days half of the therapeutic dose and supervise 17–18 h followed by on-call supervision	24 h IR48-73 NIR
Kidon[42,140,141]		Ibuprofen 5 mg/kg divided in four doses 1 h interval each. Paracetamol 10 mg/kg divided in 4 doses 1 h interval each	1 day

TCD: total cumulative dose

performed in all patients, with some cases diagnosed only by clinical history.[176] Tolerance to both rofecoxib and celecoxib has also been determined. Celik et al. reported that in a large series of 309 patients, 95% of the cases tolerated rofecoxib and 94.9% celecoxib.[177] However, because these drugs have been documented to have cardiac toxicity, both medications were removed from the market in 2003.

Etoricoxib is a COX-2 inhibitor becoming increasingly used, and several studies have assessed tolerance in patients with NSAID hypersensitivity. Nettis et al. evaluated 141 subjects with a history of cutaneous hypersensitivity to NSAIDs and found a positive response in 1.4% of cases. In this study, some cases had CSU, but no further details of the clinical entities according to the modern classification were provided.[173] In another study, etoricoxib was tolerated in 97% of the cases, but no detailed information was provided.

As far as we know two studies have attempted to evaluate tolerance to selective COX-2 inhibitors according to the ENDA classification. Doña et al. reported that after challenging with etoricoxib, 25% of those patients who were positive to paracetamol had a positive challenge to etoricoxib, but this decreased to 6% if the subjects had good tolerance to 1 g of paracetamol.[46] The other study evaluated tolerance to celecoxib and found that in patients with NECD the response was 17.4%, and in NIUA less than 10% of cases responded.[178]

DESENSITIZATION

Although aspirin desensitization has been mainly carried out in subjects with NERD[3,179] and the indications are not so well established in cases with cutaneous manifestations, some studies have nevertheless been carried out in this context. It is generally accepted that patients with cutaneous reactions to aspirin and NSAIDs form a heterogeneous group, and they may require different desensitization protocols.[179]

A study in 22 subjects with urticaria and angioedema found good tolerance to 600 mg of ASA after giving increasing doses of ASA. More than half of these cases also had tolerance to indomethacin. The protocol for desensitization was rather long, varying from 2 to 14 days. In the course of desensitization not only did cutaneous symptoms appear, but in some patients upper and/or lower respiratory symptoms also appeared. Details on the protocol for desensitization are provided.[180] Another study evaluated 11 patients with urticaria and/or angioedema with one patient also having respiratory symptoms, carrying out a rapid protocol for desensitization. Desensitization was successful in all patients except two who had previously had urticaria and angioedema in the absence of NSAID intake. To reduce the desensitization time, the intravenous route was used.[181] In this study the criteria for including patients was based on the clinical history, so there may have been cases with NIUA or SNIUA.

In another study desensitization was carried out in a case with CSU. The regimen started with a dose of 40 mg, followed by incremental doses up to the final dose. During the course of desensitization, the patient showed mild adverse effects until reaching a dose of 325 mg. In spite of tolerating the drug, the subject needed daily cetirizine treatment for symptom control.[182]

Desensitization to other NSAIDs can also be undertaken in cases of special indications. For example, celecoxib, a COX-2 inhibitor, is indicated in addition to an antiinflammatory drug as an inhibitor of angiogenesis.[183] Desensitization to this drug was attempted in a patient with cutaneous reactions.[184] However, in this case we do not know whether the patient had CI or he/she was a selective responder. It is known that in cases of selective responders to one single COX-2 inhibitor, alternative drugs from the same group can be safely administered.[185]

REFERENCES

1. Cornejo-Garcia JA, Blanca-Lopez N, Doña I, et al. Hypersensitivity reactions to non-steroidal anti-inflammatory drugs. *Curr Drug Metab.* 2009;10:971–980.
2. Hunziker T, Bruppacher R, Kuenzi UP, et al. Classification of ADRs: a proposal for harmonization and differentiation based on the experience of the Comprehensive Hospital Drug Monitoring Bern/St. Gallen, 1974-1993. *Pharmacoepidemiol Drug Saf.* 2002;11:159–163.
3. Szczeklik A, Nizankowska-Mogilnicka E, Sanak M. Hypersensitivity to aspirin and nonsteroidal anti-inflammatory drugs. In: Adkinson N, Busse WW, Bochner BS, Holgate ST, Simons ER, Lemanske RF, eds. *Middleton's Allergy.* 7th ed. 2009.
4. Harnet JC, Spector SL, Farr RS. Aspirin idiosyncrasy: asthma and urticaria. In: Middleton Jr E, Reed CE, Ellis EF, eds. *Allergy Principles and Practice.* Philadelphia, USA: Mosby C; 1978:1002–1022.
5. Quiralte J, Blanca C, Delgado J, et al. Challenge-based clinical patterns of 223 spanish patients with nonsteroidal anti-inflammatory –drug induced reactions. *J Investig Allergol Clin Immunol.* 2007;17:182–188.
6. Stevenson DD, Sanchez-Borges M, Szczeklik A. Classification of allergic and pseudoallergic reactions to drugs that inhibit cyclooxygenase enzymes. *Ann Allergy Asthma Immunol.* 2001;87:177–180.
7. Kowalski ML, Stevenson DD. Classification of reactions to non steroidal anti-inflammatory drugs. *Immunol Allergy Clin North Am.* 2013;33:135–145.
8. Kowalski ML, Makowska JS, Blanca M, et al. Hypersensitivity to nonsteroidal anti-inflammatory drugs (NSAIDs) – classification, diagnosis and management: review of the EAACI/ENDA(#) and GA2LEN/HANNA. *Allergy.* 2011;66:818–829.
9. Kowalski ML, Asero R, Bavbek S, et al. Classification and practical approach to the diagnosis and management of hypersensitivity to nonsteroidal anti-inflammatory drugs. *Allergy.* 2013;68:1219–1232.
10. Johanson SG, Bieber T, Dahl R, et al. Revised nomenclature for allergy for global use: report of the Nomenclature Review Committee of the World Allergy Organization. *J Alllergy Clin Immunol.* 2004;113:832–836.
11. Doña I, Blanca-López N, Torres MJ, et al. Drug hypersensitivity reactions: response patterns, drug involved, and temporal variations in a large series of patients. *J Investig Allergol Clin Immunol.* 2012;22:363–371.
12. Brockow K. Time for more clinical research on non-steroidal anti-inflammatory drug-induced urticaria/angioedema and anaphylaxis. *Clin Exp Allergy.* 2013;43:5–7.
13. Quiralte J, Avila-Castellano R, Cimbollek S. A phenotype-based classification of NSAIDs hypersensitivity: new patients, new challenges. *Allergy.* 2014;69:814–815.
14. Blanca-Lopez N, Cornejo-Garcia JA, Plaza-Seron MC, et al. Hypersensitivity to non steroidal anti-inflammatory drugs in children and adolescents: cross-intolerance reactions. *J Investig Allergol Clin Immunol.* 2015;25:259–269.
15. Blanca-López N, Cornejo-García JA, Pérez-Alzate D, et al. Hypersensitivity reactions to nonsteroidal anti-inflammatory drugs in children and adolescents: selective reactions. *J Investig Allergol Clin Immunol.* 2015;25:385–395.
16. Canto MG, Andreu I, Fernandez J, et al. Selective immediate hypersensitivity reactions to NSAIDs. *Curr Opin Allergy Clin Immunol.* 2009;9:293–297.
17. Arencibia ZB, Choonara I. Balancing the risks and benefits of the use of over-the-counter pain medications in children. *Drug Saf.* 2012;35:1119–1125.
18. Kogan MD, Pappas G, Yu SM, et al. Over-the-counter medication use among US preschool-age children. *JAMA.* 1994;272:1025–1030.
19. Kuehn BM. FDA: acetaminophen may trigger serious skin problems. *JAMA.* 2013;310:785.
20. Torres MJ, Barrionuevo E, Kowalski M, Blanca M. Hypersensitivity reactions to non steroidal antiinflammatory drugs. *Immunol Allergy Clin North Am.* 2014;34:507–524.

21. Blanca-López N, Bogas G, Doña I, et al. ASA must be given to classify multiple NSAID-hypersensitivity patients as selective or cross-intolerant. *Allergy.* 2016;71:576–578.

22. Cavkaytar O, Yilmaz EA, Karaatmaca B, et al. Different phenotypes of non-steroidal anti-inflammatory drug hypersensitivity during childhood. *Int Arch Allergy Immunol.* 2015;167:211–221.

23. Arikoglu T, Aslan G, Yildirim DD, et al. Discrepancies in the diagnosis and classification of non steroidal anti-inflammatory drug hypersensitivity reactions in children. *Allergol Int.* November 16, 2016. pii: S1323-8930(16)30158-7.

24. Farnam FK, Chang C, Teuber S, et al. Nonallergic drug hypersensitivity reactions. *Int Arch Allergy Immunol.* 2012;159:327–345.

25. Doña I, Blanca-López N, Cornejo-García JA, et al. Characteristics of subjects experiencing hypersensitivity to non-steroidal anti-inflammatory drugs: patterns of response. *Clin Exp Allergy.* 2011;41:86–95.

26. Messaad D, Sahla H, Benahmed S, et al. Drug provocation tests in patients with a history suggesting an immediate drug hypersensitivity reaction. *Ann Intern Med.* 2004;140:1001–1006.

27. Coombs PR, Gell PG. Classification of allergic reactions responsible for clinical hypersensitivity and disease. In: Gell RR, ed. *Clinical Aspects of Immunology.* Oxford: Oxford Univ Pr; 1968:575–596.

28. Pichler WJ. Delayed drug hypersensitivity reactions. *Ann Intern Med.* 2003;139:683–693.

29. Settipanne GA. Landmark commentary: history of aspirin intolerance. *Allergy Proc.* 1990;11:251–253.

30. Matsuo H, Morimotow K, Akaki T, et al. Exercise and aspirin increase levels of circulating gliadin peptides in patients with wheat-dependent exercise-induced anaphylaxis. *Clin Exp Allergy.* 2005;35:461–466.

31. Shirai T, Matsui T, Uto T, et al. Ninsteroidal antiinflammatory drugs enhance allergic reactions in a patient with wheat-induced anaphylaxis. *Allergy.* 2003;58:1071–1081.

32. Drago F, Cogorno L, Agnoletti AF, et al. A retrospective study on cutaneous drug reactions in an outpatient population. *Int J Clin Pharm.* 2015;37:739–743.

33. Parretta E, Rafaniello C, Magro L, et al. Improvement of patient adverse drug reaction reporting through a community pharmacist-based intervention in the Campania region of Italy. *Expert Opin Drug Saf.* 2014;13:S21–S29.

34. Gomes E, Cardoso MF, Praça F, et al. Self-reported drug allergy in a general adult Portuguese population. *Clin Exp Allergy.* 2004;34:1597–1601.

35. Naldi L, Conforti A, Venegoni M, et al. Cutaneous reactions to drugs. An analysis of spontaneous reports in four Italian regions. *Br J Clin Pharmacol.* 1999;48:839–846.

36. Chalabianloo F, Berstad A, Schjott J, et al. Clinical characteristics of patients with drug hypersensitivity in Norway: a single-centre study. *Pharmacoepidemiol Drug Saf.* 2011;20:506–513.

37. Cianferoni A, Novembre E, Mugnaini L, et al. Clinical features of acute anaphylaxis in patients admitted to a university hospital: an 11-year retrospective review (1985–1996). *Ann Allergy Asthma Immunol.* 2001;87:27–32.

38. Faria E, Rodrigues-Cernadas J, Gaspar A, et al. Drug-induced anaphylaxis survey in Portuguese allergy departments. *J Investig Allergol Clin Immunol.* 2014;24:40–48.

39. Jares EJ, Baena-Cagnani CE, Sánchez-Borges M, et al. Drug-induced anaphylaxis in Latin American countries. *J Allergy Clin Immunol Pract.* 2015;3:780–788.

40. van Puijenbroek EP, Egberts ACG, Meyboom RHB, et al. Different risks for NSAID-induced anaphylaxis. *Ann Pharmacother.* 2002;36:24–29.

41. Mockenhaupt M, Kelly JP, Kaufman D, et al. The risk of Stevens-Johnson syndrome and toxic epidermal necrolysis associated with nonsteroidal antiinflammatory drugs: a multinational perspective. *J Rheumatol.* 2003;30:2234–2240.

42. Kidon MI, See Y. Adverse drug reactions in Singaporean children. *Singapore Med J.* 2004;45:574.

43. Fukunaga A, Shimizu H, Tanaka M, et al. Limited influence of aspirin intake on mast cell activation in patients with food-dependent exercise-induced anaphylaxis: comparison using skin prick and histamine release tests. *Acta Derm Venereol.* 2012;92:480–483.

44. Carmona MJ, Blanca M, Garcia A, et al. Intolerance to piroxicam in patients with adverse reactions to non-steroidal anti-inflammatory drugs. *J Allergy Clin Immunol.* 1992;90:873–879.

45. Asero R. Detection of aspirin reactivity in patients with pirazolones-induced skin disorders. *Allergy.* 1998;53:214–215.

46. Doña I, Blanca-López N, Jagemann LR, et al. Response to a selective COX-2 inhibitor in patients with urticaria/angioedema induced by nonsteroidal anti-inflammatory drugs. *Allergy.* 2011;66:1428–1433.

47. Zuberbier T, Bindslev-Jensen C, Canonica W, et al. EAACI/GA2LEN/EDF guideline: management of urticaria. *Allergy.* 2006;61:321–331.

48. Szczeklik A, Gryglewski RJ, Czerniawska-Mysik G. Clinical patterns of hypersensitivity to NSAIDs and pathogenesis. *J Allergy Clin Immunol.* 1977;60:276–284.

49. Grattan CE. Aspirin sensitivity and urticaria. *Clin Exp Dermatol.* 2003;28:123–127.

50. Asero R. Multiple sensitivity to NSAID. *Allergy.* 2000;55:893–894.

51. Leeyaphan C, Kulthanan K, Jongjarearnprasert K, et al. Drug-induced angioedema without urticaria: prevalence and clinical features. *J Eur Acad Dermatol Venereol.* 2010;24:685–691.

52. Sánchez-Borges M, Capriles-Behrens E, Caballero-Fonseca F. Hypersensitivity to non-steroidal anti-inflammatory drugs in childhood. *Pediatr Allergy Immunol.* 2004;15:376–380.

53. Himly M, Jahn-Schmid B, Pittertschatscher K, et al. IgE-mediated immediate-type hypersensitivity to the pyrazolone drug propyphenazone. *J Allergy Clin Immunol.* 2003;111:882–888.

54. Blanca-López N, Pérez-Alzate D, Andreu I, et al. Immediate hypersensitivity reactions to ibuprofen and other arylpropionic acid derivatives. *Allergy.* 2016;71:1048–1056.

55. Houwerzijl J, De Gast GC, Nater JP, et al. Lymphocyte-stimulation tests and patch tests to carbamazepine hypersensitivity. *Clin Exp Immunol.* 1977;29:272–277.

56. Pichler WJ, Yawalkar N, Britschgi M, et al. Cellular and molecular pathophysiology of cutaneous drug reactions. *Am J Clin Dermatol.* 2002;3:229–238.

57. Ponce V, Muñoz-Bellido F, Moreno E, et al. Fixed drug eruption caused by etoricoxib with tolerance to celecoxib and parecoxib. *Contact Dermatitis.* 2012;66:106–112.

58. Ward KE, Archambault R, Mersfelder TL. Severe adverse skin reactions to nonsteroidal antiinflammatory drugs: a review of the literature. *Am J Health-Syst Pharm.* 2010;67:206–213.

59. Strom BL, Carson JL, Halpern AC, et al. A population-based study of Stevens-Johnson syndrome: incidence and antecedent drug exposures. *Arch Dermatol.* 1991;127:831–838.

60. Schopf E, Stuhmer A, Rzany B, et al. Toxic epidermal necrolysis and Stevens-Johnson syndrome: an epidemiologic study from West Germany. *Arch Dermatol.* 1991;127:839–842.

61. Layton D, Marshall V, Boshier A, et al. Serious skin reactions and selective COX-2 inhibitors. *Drug Saf.* 2006;29:687–696.

62. Marques S, Milpied B, Foulc P, et al. Severe cutaneous reaction to celebrex. *Clin Rheumatol.* 2006;25:S22–S29.

63. Atzori L, Pinna AL, Aste N, et al. Adverse cutaneous reactions to selective cyclooxygenase 2 inhibitors: experience of an Italian drug-surveillance center. *J Cutan Med Surg.* 2006;10:31–35.

64. Andreu I, Mayorga C, Miranda MA. Generation of reactive intermediates in photoallergic dermatitis. *Curr Opin Allergy Clin Immunol.* 2010;10:303–308.

65. Miralles JC, Negro JM, Sanchez-Gascon F, Garcia M. Ketoprofen contact dermatitis with good piketoprofen tolerance. *Allergol Immunol Clin.* 2001;16:105–108.

66. Consuegra-Romero G, Castro-Gutierrez B, Gonzalez-Lopez MA. Photoallergic contact dermatitis. *Eur J Intern Med.* pii: S0953-6205(16)30253-9 (Epub ahead of print). http://dx.doi.org/10.1016/j.ejim.2016.08.013.

67. Kerr A, Becher G, Ibbostson S, et al. Action spectrum for etofenamate photoallergic contact dermatitis. *Contact Dermatitis.* 2011;65:117–118.

68. Fernandez-Jorge B, Goday-Bujan JJ, Murga M, et al. Photoallergic contact dermatitis due to diclofenac with cross-reaction to aceclofenac: two casereports. *Contact Dermatitis.* 2009;61:236–247.

69. Stingeni L, Foti C, Cassano N, et al. Photocontact allergy to arylpropionic acid non-steroidal anti-inflammatory drugs in patients sensitized to fragrance mix I. *Contact Dermatitis.* 2010;63:108–110.

70. Sánchez-Borges M, Caballero-Fonseca F, Capriles-Hulett A, et al. Aspirin-exacerbated cutaneous disease (AECD) is a distinct subphenotype of chronic spontaneous urticaria. *J Eur Acad Dermatol Venereol.* 2015;29:698–701.

71. Mastalerz L, Setkowicz M, Sanak M, et al. Hypersensitivity to aspirin: common eicosanoid alterations in urticaria and asthma. *J Allergy Clin Immunol.* 2004;113:771–775.

72. Asero R. Intolerance to nonsteroidal antiinflammatory drugs might precede by years the onset of chronic urticaria. *J Allergy Clin Immunol.* 2003;111:1095–1098.

73. Setkowicz M, Mastalerz L, Podolec-Rubis M, et al. Clinical course and urinary eicosanoids inpatients with aspirin-induced urticaria followed up for 4 years. *J Allergy Clin Immunol.* 2009;123:174–178.

74. Fukunaga A, Hatakeyama M, Taguchi K, et al. Aspirin-intolerant chronic urticaria exacerbated by cutaneous application of a ketoprofen poultice. *Acta Derm Venereol.* 2010;90:413–415.

75. Kang LW, Kison MI, Chin CW, et al. Severe anaphylactic reaction in a child with recurrent urticaria. *Pediatrics.* 2007;120:e742.

76. Sánchez-Borges M, Caballero-Fonseca F, Capriles-Hulett A. Aspirin-exacerbated cutaneous disease. *Immunol Allergy Clin North Am.* 2012.

77. Quiralte J, Blanco C, Castillo R, et al. Intolerance to nonsteroidal anti-inflammatory drugs: results of controlled drug challenges in 98 patients. *J Allergy Clin Immunol.* 1996;98:678–685.

78. Ayuso P, Blanca-López N, Roña I, et al. Advanced phenotyping in hypersensitivity drug reactions to NSAIDs. *Clin Exp Allergy.* 2013;43:1097–2009.

79. Wojnar RJ, Hearn T, Starkweather S. Augmentation of allergic histamine release from human leukocytes by nonsteroidal anti-inflammatory-analgesic agents. *J Allergy Clin Immunol.* 1980;66:37–45.

80. Zembowicz A, Mastalerz L, Setkowicz M, et al. Safety of cyclooxygenase 2 inhibitors and increased leukotriene synthesis in chronic iiopathic uricaia with sensitivity to nonsteroidal anti-inflammatory drugs. *Arch Dermatol.* 2003;139:1577–1582.

81. Doña I, Blanca Lopez N, Torres MJ, et al. NSAID-induced urticaria/angioedema does not evolve into chronic urticaria: a 12-year follow-up study. *Allergy.* 2014;69:438–444.

82. Choi IS. Disappearance of aspirin intolerance with anti-asthma treatment. *J Allergy Clin Immunol.* 2002;110:665–666.

83. Rosado A, Vives R, Gonzalez R, et al. Can NSAIDs intolerance disappear? A study of three cases. *Allergy.* 2003;58:689–690.

84. Philis JA, Perlmutter L. IgE mediated and non IgE mediated allergic type reactions to aspirin. *Acta Allergol.* 1974;29:474–490.

85. Blanca M, Perez E, Garcia JJ, et al. Angioedema and IgE antibodies to aspirin: a case report. *Ann Allergy.* 1989;62:295–298.

86. Harrer A, Lang R, Grims R, et al. Diclofenac hypersensitivity: antibody responses to the parent drug and relevant metabolites. *PLoS One.* 2010;5:e13707.

87. Caiado J, Ravasqueira A, Rodrigues Alves R, et al. Diclofenac hypersensitivity as cause of hospitalization in an immunoallergology department. *Allergy.* 2007;62:21–22.

88. Woessner KM, Castells M. NSAID single-drug-induced reactions. *Immunol Allergy Clin North Am.* 2013;33:237–249.

89. Kumar A, Berko NS, Gothwal R, et al. Kounis syndrome secondary to ibuprofen use. Kounis syndrome secondary to ibuprofen use. *Int J Cardiol.* 2009;137:79–80.

90. Sen I, Mitra S, Gombar KK. Fatal anaphylactic reaction to oral diclofenac sodium. *Eur J Anaesthesiol.* 2001;18:763–765.

91. Riley RJ, Leeder JS. In vitro analysis of metabolic predisposition to drug hypersensitivity reactions. *Clin Exp Immunol.* 1995;99:1–6.

92. Ware JA, Graf ML, Martin BM, et al. Immunochemical detection and identification of protein adducts of diclofenac in the small intestine of rats: possible role in allergic reactions. *Chem Res Toxicol.* 1998;11:164–171.

93. Naisbitt DJ, Sanderson LS, Meng X, et al. Investigation of the immunogenicity of diclofenac and diclofenac metabolites. *Toxicol Lett.* 2007;168:45–50.

94. Riemer AB, Gruber S, Pali-Scholl I, et al. Suppression of gastric acid increases the risk of developing immunoglobulin E-mediated drug hypersensitivity: human diclofenac sensitization and a murine sensitization model. *Clin Exp Allergy.* 2010;40:486–493.

95. Kowalski ML, Bienkiewicz B, Woszczek G. Diagnosis of pyrazolone drug sensitivity: clinical history versus skin testing and in vitro testing. *Allergy Asthma Proc.* 1999;20:347–352.

96.

97. Bluth MH, Beleza P, Hajee F, et al. IgE-mediated hypersensitivity after ibuprofen administration. *Ann Clin Lab Sci.* 2007;37:362–365.

98. Gómez Martinez M, Fernandez de Miguel C, Domínguez Lázaro A, et al. Fixed exanthema due to paracetamol. *J Investig Allergol Clin Immunol.* 1996;6:131–132.

99. Zambonino MA, Torres MJ, Muñoz C, et al. Drug provocation tests in the diagnosis of hypersensitivity reactions to non-steroidal anti-inflammatory drugs in children. *Pediatr Allergy Immunol.* 2013;24:151–159.

100. Guvenir H, Misirlioglu ED, Vezir E, et al. Nonsteroidal anti-inflammatory drug hypersensitivity among children. *Allergy Asthma Proc.* 2015;36:386–393.

101. Calvo Campoverde K, Giner-Muñoz MT, Martínez Valdez L, et al. Hypersensitivity reactions to non-steroidal anti-inflammatory drugs and tolerance to alternative drugs. *An Pediatr (Barc).* 2016;84:148–153.

102. Yilmaz O, Ertoy Karagol IH, Bakirtas A, et al. Challenge-proven nonsteroidal anti-inflammatory drug hypersensitivity in children. *Allergy.* 2013;10:1111.

103. Hassani A, Ponvert C, Karila C, et al. Hypersensitivity to cyclooxygenase inhibitory drugs in children: a study of 164 cases. *Eur J Dermatol.* 2008;18:561–565.

104. Blanca M, Torres MJ, Garcia JJ, et al. Natural evolution of skin test sensitivity in patients allergic to beta-lactam antibiotics. *J Allergy Clin Immunol.* 1999;103:918–924.

105. Pigatto PD, Mozzanica N, Bigardi AS, et al. Topical NSAID allergic contact dermatitis. Italian experience. *Contact Dermatitis.* 1993;29:39–41.

106. Goday Buján JJ, Pérez Varela L, et al. Allergic and photoallergic contact dermatitis from etofenamate: study of 14 cases. *Contact Dermatitis.* 2009;61:118–120.

107. Gonçalo M, Figuerireido A, Tavares P, et al. Photosensitivity to piroxicam: absence of cross-reaction with tenoxicam. *Contact Dermatitis.* 1992;27:287–290.

108. Gulin SJ, Chirac A. Diclofenac-induced allergic contact dermatitis: a series of four patients. *Drug Saf Case Rep.* 2016;3:15.

109. Yawalkar N, Egli F, Hari Y, et al. Infiltration of cytotoxic T cells in drug-induced cutaneous eruptions. *Clin Exp Allergy.* 2000;30:847–855.

110. Britschgi M, Steiner UC, Schmid S, et al. T-cell involvement in drug-induced acute generalized exanthematous pustulosis. *J Clin Invest.* 2001;107:1433–1441.

111. Barbaud AM, Bene MC, Schmutz J, et al. Role of delayed cellular hypersensitivity and adhesion molecules in amoxicillin induced morbilliform rashes. *Arch Dermatol.* 1997;133:481–486.

112. Tian XY, Liu B, Shi H, et al. Incidence of cutaneous reactions in 22.866 Chinese inpatients: a prospective study. *Arch Dermatol Res.* 2015;307:829–834.

113. Jurakić Tončić R, Marinović B, Lipozencić J. Nonallergic hypersensitivity to nonsteroidal antiinflammatory drugs, angiotensin-converting enzyme inhibitors, radio contrast media, local anesthetics, volume substitutes and medications used in general anesthesia. *Acta Dermatocenerol Croat.* 2009;17:54–69.

114. Viard I, Wehrli P, Bullani R, et al. Inhibition of toxic epidermal necrolysis by blockade of CD95 with human intravenous immunoglobulin. *Science.* 1998;282:490–493. Acta Dermatovenerol Croat. 2009;17:54–69.

115. Sharma K, Wang RX, Zhang LY, et al. Death the Fas way: regulation and pathophysiology of CD95 and its ligand. *Pharmacol Ther.* 2000;88:333–347.

116. Angadi SS, Kam A. Ibuprofen induced Stevens-Johnson syndrome – toxic epidermal necrolysis in Nepal. *Asia Pac Allergy.* 2016;6:70–73.

117. Pena MA, Perez S, Zazo MC, et al. Case of toxic epidermal necrolysis secondary to acetaminophen in a child. *Curr Drug Saf.* 2016;11:90–101.

118. Vas CJ. An unusual complication of phenylbutazone therapy–toxic epidermal necrolysis. *Postgrad Med J.* 1963;39:94–95.

119. Layton D, Marshall V, Friedman P, et al. Serious skin reactions and selective COX-2 inhibitors: a case series from prescription-event monitoring in England. *Drug Saf.* 2006;29:687–696.

120. Berger P, Dwyer D, Corallo CE. Toxic epidermal necrolysis after celecoxib therapy. *Pharmacotherapy.* 2002;22:1193–1195.

121. Layton RJ, Wilton LV, et al. Safety profile of rofecoxib as used in general practice in England: results of a prescription-event monitoring study. *Br J Clin Pharmacol.* 2003;55:166–174.

122. Arochena L, Zafra MP, Fariña MC, et al. Acute generalized exanthematic pustulosis due to ibuprofen. *Ann Allergy Asthma Immunol.* 2013;110:386–387.

123. Goeschke B, Braathen LR. Acute generalized exanthematic pustulosis: a case and an overview of side effects affecting the skin caused by celecoxib and other COX-2 inhibitors reported so far. *Dermatology.* 2004;209:53–56.

124. Knowles SR, Shapiro LE, Shear NH. Anticonvulsant hypersensitivity syndrome: incidence, prevention and management. *Drug Saf.* 1999;21:489–501.

125. Carroll MC, Yueng-Yue KA, Esterly NB, et al. Drug-induced hypersensitivity syndrome in pediatric patients. *Pediatrics.* 2001;108:485–492.

126. Rosales-Gomez V, Molero AI, Perez-Amarilla I, et al. DRESS syndrome secondary to ibuprofen as a cause of hyperacute liver failure. *Rev Esp Enferm Dig.* 2014;106:482–486.

127. Lee JH, Park HK, Heo J, et al. Drug rash with eosinophilia and systemic symptoms (DRESS) syndrome induced by celecoxib and anti-tuberculosis drugs. *J Korean Med Sci.* 2008;23:521–525.

128. Andrew N, Gabb G, Del Fante M. ACEI associated angioedema: a case study and review. *Aust Fam Physician.* 2011;40:985–988.

129. Tokura Y. Immune responses to photohaptens: implications for the mechanisms of photosensitivity to exogenous agents. *J Dermatol Sci.* 2000;23:S6–S9.

130. Holzle E, Lehmann P, Neumann N. Phototoxic and photoallergic reactions. *J Dtsch Dermatol Ges.* 2009;7:643–649.

131. Imai S, Atarashi K, Ikesue K, et al. Establishment of murine model of allergic photocontact dermatitis to ketoprofen and characterization of pathogenic T cells. *J Dermatol Sci.* 2006;41:127–136.

132. Karlberg AT, Bergstrom MA, Borje A, et al. Allergic contact dermatitis–formation, structural requirements, and reactivity of skin sensitizers. *Chem Res Toxicol.* 2008;21:53–69.

133. Torres MJ, Mayorga C, Blanca M. Nonimmediate allergic reactions induced by drugs: pathogenesis and diagnostic tests. *J Investig Allergol Clin Immunol.* 2009;19:80–90.

134. Shiohara T. Fixed drug eruption: pathogenesis and diagnostic tests. *Curr Opin Allergy Clin Immunol.* 2009;9:316–321.

135. Makowska JS, Grzegorczyk YJ, Bienkiewicz B, et al. Systemic responses after bronchial aspirin challenge in sensitive patients with asthma. *J Allergy Clin Immunol.* 2008;121:348–354.

136. Bochenek G, Nizankowska E, Gielicz A, et al. Plasma 9a, 11b-PGF2, a PGD2 metabolite, as a sensitive marker of mast cell activation by allergen in bronchial asthma. *Thorax.* 2004;59:459–464.

137. Nasser S, Christie PE, Pfister R, et al. Effect of endobronchial aspirin challenge on inflammatory cells in bronchial biopsy samples from aspirin-sensitive asthmatic subjects. *Thorax.* 1996;51:64–70.

138. Kowalski ML, Grzegorczyk J, Wojciechowska B, et al. Intranasal challenge with aspirin induces cell influx and activation of eosinophils and mast cells in nasal secretions of ASA-sensitive patients. *Clin Exp Allergy.* 1996;26:807–814.

139. Karakaya G, Celebioglu E, Kalyoncu FA. Non-steroidal anti-inflammatory drug hypersensitivity in adults and the factors associated with asthma. *Respir Med.* 2013;107:967–974.

140. Kidon MI, Kang LW, Chin CW, et al. Non-steroidal anti-inflammatory drug hypersensitivity in preschool children. *Allergy Asthma Clin Immunol.* 2007;3:114–122.

141. Kidon MI, Liew WK, Chiang WC, et al. Hypersensitivity to paracetamol in Asian children with early onset of nonsteroidal antiinflammatory drug allergy. *Int Arch Allergy Immunol.* 2007;144:51–56.

142. King G, Byrne A, Fleming P. A case of severe NSAID exacerbated respiratory disease (NERD) following a dental procedure in a child. *Eur Arch Paediatr Dent.* 2016;17:277–281.

143. Bellegrandi S, Rosso R, Mattiacci G, et al. Combined immediate and delayed-type hypersensitivity to metamizole. *Allergy.* 1999;54:78–92.

144. Yamashita M. Aspirin intolerance: experimental models for bed-to-bench. *Curr Drug Targets.* 2016;17:1963–1970.

145. Flemstrom G, Marsden NVB, Richter W. Passive cutaneous anaphylaxis in guinea pigs elicited by gastric absorption of dextran induced by acetylsalicylic acid. *Int Arch Allergy Appl Immunol.* 1976;51:627–636.

146. Bjarnason I, Williams P, Smwthurst P, et al. Effect of nonsteroidal anti-inflammatory drugs and prostaglandins on the permeability of the human small intestine. *Gut.* 1986;27:1292–1297.

147. Cant AJ, Gibson P. Food hypersensitivity made life threatening by ingestion of aspirin. *Br Med J (Clin Res Ed).* 1984;288:755–756.

148. Van Wijk RG, de Groot H, Bogaard JM. Drug-dependent exercise-induced anaphylaxis. *Allergy.* 1995;50:992–994.

149. Dohi M, Suko M, SuGiYAMA H, et al. Food-dependent, exercise-induced anaphylaxis: a study on 11 Japanese cases. *J Allergy Clin Immunol.* 1991;87:34–40.

150. Kohno K, Matsuo H, Takahashi H, et al. Serum gliadin monitoring extracts patients with false negative results in challenge tests for the diagnosis of wheat-dependent exercise-induced anaphylaxis. *Allergol Int.* 2013;62:229–238.

151. Aihara M, Miyazawa M, Osuna H, et al. Food-dependent exercise-induced anaphylaxis: influence of concurrent aspirin administration on skin testing and provocation. *Br J Dermatol.* 2002;146:466–472.

152. Sheffer AL, Tong AKF, Murphy GF, et al. Exercise-induced anaphylaxis: a serious form of physical allergy associated with mast cell degranulation. *J Allergy Clin Immunol.* 1985;74:479–484.

153. Vervloet D, Pradal M. *Drug allergy.* Sweden, Sundbyerg: S-M Ewert; 1992.

154. Bochenek G, Nizankowska E, Szczeklik A. The atopy trait in hypersensitivity to nonsteroidal anti-inflammatory drugs. *Allergy.* 1996;51:16–23.

155. Alves C, Romeira AM, Abreu C, et al. Non-steroidal anti-inflammatory drug hypersensitivity in children. *Allergol Immunopathol.* July 27, 2016. pii: S0301-0546(16)30066-0. http://dx.doi.org/10.1016/j.aller.2016.04.004.

156. Malskat WSJ, van der Tas C, Knulst AC, et al. Aspirin tolerance in patients with NSAID-hypersensitivity. *Allergy.* 2010;10:1197–1198.

157. Pérez-Alzate D, Cornejo-García JA, Pérez-Sánchez N, et al. Immediate reactions to more than one NSAID must not be considered as cross-hypersensitivity unless as a tolerance is verified. *J Investig Allergol Clin Immunol.* May 18, 2016. http://dx.doi.org/10.18176/jiaci.0080.

158. Blanca-Lopez N, J. Torres M, Doña I, et al. Value of the clinical history in the diagnosis of urticaria/angioedema induced by NSAIDs with cross-intolerance. *Clin Exp Allergy.* 2013;43:85–91.

159. Viola M, Rumi G, Valluzzi LR, et al. Assessing potential determinants of positive provocation tests in subjects with NSAID hypersensitivity. *Clin Exp Allergy.* 2011;41:96–103.

160. de Paramo BJ, Gancedo SQ, Cuevas M, et al. Paracetamol (acetaminophen) hypersensitivity. *Ann Allergy Asthma Immunol.* 2000;85:508–511.

161. Barbaud A. Skin testing and patch testing in non-IgE-mediated drug allergy. *Curr Allergy Asthma Rep.* 2014;14:442.

162. Bruynzeel DP, Ferguson J, Andersen K, et al. Photopatch testing: a consensus methodology for Europe. *J Eur Acad Dermatol Venereol.* 2004;18:679–682.

163. Blanca-López N, Zapatero L, Alonso E, et al. Skin testing and drug provocation in the diagnosis of nonimmediate reactions to aminopenicillins in children. *Allergy.* 2009;64:229–233.

164. Padial A, Antunez C, Blanca-Lopez N, et al. Non-immediate reactions to beta-lactams: diagnostic value of skin testing and drug provocation test. *Clin Exp Allergy.* 2008;38:822–828.

165. May A, Weber A, Gall H, et al. Means of increasing sensitivity of an in vitro diagnostic test for aspirin intolerance. *Clin Exp Allergy.* 1999;29:1402–1411.

166. Koroseca P, Tislerb U, Bajrovica N, et al. Acetylsalicylic acid-triggered 15-HETE generation by peripheral leukocytes for identifying ASA sensitivity. *Respir Med.* 2011;105:81–83.

167. Kim MS, Cho YJ. Flow-cytometry assisted basophil activation test as a safe diagnostic tool for aspirin/NSAID hypersensitivity. *Allergy Asthma Immunol Res.* 2012;4:137–142.

168. Pierzchalska M, Mastalerz L, Sanak M, et al. A moderate and unspecific release of cysteinyl leukotrienes by aspirin from peripheral blood leucocytes precludes its value for aspirin sensitivity testing in asthma. *Clin Exp Allergy.* 2000;30:1785–1791.

169. Sanz ML, Gamboa P, de Weck AL. A new combined test with flowcytometric basophil activation and determination of sulfidoleukotrienes is useful for in vitro diagnosis of hypersensitivity to aspirin and other nonsteroidal anti-inflammatory drugs. *Int Arch Allergy Immunol.* 2005;136:58–72.

170. Çelik GE, Schroeder JT, Hamilton RH, et al. Effect of in vitro aspirin stimulation on basophils in patients with aspirin exacerbated respiratory disease. *Clin Exp Allergy.* 2009;39:1522–1531.

171. Niankowska-Mogilnicka E, Bochenek G, Mastalerz L, et al. EAACI/GA2LEN guideline: aspirin provocation tests for diagnosis of aspirin hypersensitivity. *Allergy.* 2007;62:1111–1118.

172. Ispano M, Fontana A, Scibilia J, et al. Oral challenge with alternative nonsteropdal anti-inflamatory drugs (NSAIDs) and paracetamol in patients intolerant to these agents. *Drugs.* 1993;46:253–256.

173. Nettis E, Di Paola R, Napoli G, et al. Benzydamine: an alternative nonsteroidal anti-inflammatory drug in patients with nimesulide-induced urticaria. *Allergy.* 2002;57:442–445.

174. Asero R. Tolerability of rofecoxib. *Allergy.* 2001;56:916–917.

175. Asero R. Etoricoxib challenge in patients with chronic urticaria with NSAID.

176. Nettis E, Colanardi MC, Ferrannini A, et al. Short-term tolerability of etoricoxib in patients with cutaneous hypersensitivity reactions to nonsteroidal anti-inflammatory drugs. *Ann Allergy Asthma Immunol.* 2005;95:438–442.

177. Çelik G, Bavbeck S, Misirligil Z, et al. Release of cysteinyl leukotrienes with aspirin stimulation and the effect of prostaglandin E2 on this release from peripheral blood leucocytes in aspirin-induced asthmatic patients. *Clin Exp Allergy.* 2001;31:1615–1622.

178. Kim KH, Lim KH, Kim MY, et al. Cross-reactivity to acetaminophen and celecoxib according to the type of nonsteroidal anti-inflammatory drug hypersensitivity. *Allergy Asthma Immunol Res.* 2014;6:156–162.

179. Macy E, Bernstein JA, Castells MC, et al. Aspirin challenge and desensitization for aspirin exacerbated respiratory disease: a practice paper. *Ann Allergy Asthma Immunol.* 2007;98:172–174.

180. Grzelewska-Rzymowska I, Roznlecki J, Szmidt M. Aspirin desensitization in patients with aspirin-induced urticaria and angioedema. *Allergol Immunopathol.* 1988;16:305–308.

181. Wong JT, Sagy CS, Krinzman SJ, et al. Rapid oral challenge-desensitization for patients with aspirin-related urticaria-angioedema. *J Allergy Clin Immunol.* 2000;106:997–1001.

182. Slowik SM, Slavin RG. Aspirin desensitization in a patient with aspirin sensitivity and chronic idiopathic urticaria. *Ann Allergy Asthma Immunol.* 2009;102:171–172.

183. Stockhammer F, Misch M, Koch A, et al. Continuous low-dose temozolomide and celecoxib in recurrent glioblastoma. *J Neurooncol.* 2010;100:407–415.

184. Burbach GJ, Vajkoczy P, Zuberbier T. Celecoxib desensitization: continued temozolomide/celecoxib chemotherapy after a celecoxib-induced hypersensitivity reaction. *Anti-Cancer.* 2012;23:1118–1120.

185. Cimbollek S, Quiralte J, Avila R. COX-2 inhibitors in patients with sensitivity to nonselective NSAIDs. *N Engl J Med.* 2009;361:2197–2198.

FURTHER READING

1. Kulthanan K, Jiamton S, Boochangkool K, Jongjarearnprasert K. Angioedema: clinical and etiological aspects. *Clin Dev immunol.* 2007:26438.
2. Stevenson DD. Diagnosis, prevention, and treatment of adverse reactions to aspirin and nonsteroidal anti-inflammatory drugs. *J Allergy Clin Immunol.* 1984;74:617–622.
3. Terrados S, Blanca M, Garcia J, et al. Allergy. Nonimmediate reactions to betalactams: prevalence and role of the different penicillins. *Allergy.* 1994;49:317–322.
4. Romano A, Blanca M, Torres MJ, et al. Diagnosis of non-immediate reactions to beta-lactam antibiotics. *Allergy.* 2004;59:1153–1160.
5. Romano A, Caubet JC. Antibiotic allergies in children and adults: from clinical symptoms to skin testing diagnosis. *J Allergy Clin Immunol Pract.* 2014;2:3–12.

CHAPTER 19

Chemotherapy Allergy

MARIANA CASTELLS, MD, PHD • MARLENE GARCIA-NEUER, MS • KATHLEEN MARQUIS, PHARM D, PH D • DONNA LYNCH, MSN, FNP-BC

KEY POINTS

- The evaluation of patients with hypersensitivity reactions to chemotherapy has become a key function of allergy specialists in the 21st century.
- A thorough and personalized diagnostic evaluation and risk stratification, including a detailed history, physical examination, and skin testing (if appropriate and available), are required.
- Rapid drug desensitization is a safe and groundbreaking procedure for the management of immediate drug hypersensitivity reactions, to protect patients against anaphylaxis.
- To be successful in providing patients with first-line therapies through desensitization, a tight collaboration between allergy, nursing, pharmacy, and other specialists is required.

INTRODUCTION

The increased use of chemotherapies in the 21st century has led to an increase in hypersensitivity reactions (HSRs) worldwide. This has prevented the use of first-line therapies, which has affected patients' survival and quality of life.[1] Reactions to medications can be immediate/acute or delayed, with different clinical patterns and presentations. Acute or immediate reactions include type I HSRs with IgE and/or mast cell/basophil involvement and occur immediately or within 24 h after the drug administration.[2] Use of premedication in patients before their treatment may mask and delay the onset of HSRs.[3,4] These reactions range from mild cutaneous reactions to life-threatening anaphylaxis and result from the release of histamine, leukotrienes, prostaglandins, and other mediators from basophils and/or mast cells, whose actions are implicated in cutaneous, respiratory, gastrointestinal, and cardiovascular symptoms (Table 19.1).[5] Atypical symptoms such as pain have been associated with taxanes and oxaliplatin.[10] Other systemic symptoms seen with some platins, such as oxaliplatin, include general malaise, chills, and fever.[5,6,11] The etiology appears to be non-IgE mediated and one explanation would be a *cytokine storm–like* reaction caused by the release of proinflammatory cytokines tumor necrosis factor α, interleukin-1, and interleukin-6 from activated macrophages and other immune cells with FcγR receptors.[5–7,11,12] These symptoms can also present as a combination reaction with cytokine storm–like symptoms and typical type I HSRs, such as flushing, urticaria, shortness of breath, and hypotension.[4,13,14] Deaths have been reported when reexposing patients who have presented with immediate HSRs.[3,15,16]

Delayed reactions occurring more than 24 h after the infusion of chemotherapy have been shown to be type IV reactions with T cells as effector cells and typically with maculopapular rashes. In addition to these rashes, other symptoms, such as flushing, urticaria, or shortness of breath, can present as mast cell/basophil mediators-related symptoms.[5,8] Delayed anaphylactic reactions have been rarely reported.[17,18]

Through drug desensitization, patients with immediate and delayed HSRs to chemotherapy have been safely reexposed despite their allergic or HSR history.[5,19,20] Protocols for drug desensitization utilize small incremental doses of the culprit allergic medication that are reintroduced to an allergic patient through multiple steps, achieving the target dose over several hours most commonly.[5,21] The technique takes advantage of inhibitory mast cell/basophil mechanisms, protecting the patients against anaphylaxis and inducing a state of temporary tolerization, which can be maintained as long as the drug is continuously administered (Fig. 19.1).[12,22] The inherent toxicity of chemotherapy medications makes continuous dosing not always possible, and patients typically need to be desensitized with each administration.[14,23] Most patients with immediate and delayed reactions can benefit from drug desensitization. Patients with severe cutaneous and systemic reactions,

TABLE 19.1
Immediate Hypersensitivity Reactions to Platinum- and Taxane-Based Chemotherapy

Drugs	Reaction Timing	Reaction Percentage	Characteristics of Reaction
PLATINUM AGENTS			
Carboplatin	Within the first 30 min of infusion, generally after 7 exposures, BRACAI/II at a higher risk	1–44	Urticaria, itching, erythema (palms and soles), cutaneous (face swelling, diffuse erythema), gastrointestinal, (abdominal cramps, diarrhea), respiratory (dyspnea, desaturation, bronchospasm), cardiovascular (chest pain, tachycardia, hypertension, hypotension), seizure, laryngeal edema
Oxaliplatin	Within minutes from infusion, generally after 6 exposures	10–19	Itching, erythema (palms and soles), urticaria, angioedema, bronchospasm, and atypical symptoms such as fever, chills, pain, and generalized malaise
Cisplatin	Within minutes of infusion start, between 4th and 8th exposure, generally after 6	5–20	Rash, pruritus, dyspnea, bronchospasm, hypotension. Increase with concomitant radiation. Variable reactions sometimes lethal
TAXANES			
Paclitaxel	Within first minutes of infusion, during 1st or 2nd exposure (rarely subsequent)	8–45	Dyspnea (with or without bronchospasm), urticaria, erythema, hypotension (or sometimes hypertension), back pain, chest pain, or pelvic pain. Minor reactions in 40% of patients, 1.3% with severe reactions
Docetaxel	Within first minutes of infusion, during 1st or 2nd exposure	25–50	Dyspnea (with or without bronchospasm) urticaria, hypotension (or sometimes hypertension), erythema, fluid retention syndrome. Severe anaphylactic reactions in 2% of patients

Data from Castells MC, Tennant NM, Sloane DE, et al. Hypersensitivity reactions to chemotherapy: outcomes and safety of rapid desensitization in 413 cases. *J Allergy Clin Immunol*. 2008;122(3):574–580; Gamarra RM, McGraw SD, Drelichman VS, Maas LC. Serum sickness-like reactions in patients receiving intravenous infliximab. *J Emerg Med*. 2006;30(1):41–44; Caiado J, Castells M. Presentation and diagnosis of hypersensitivity to platinum drugs. *Curr Allergy Asthma Rep*. 2015;15(4):15; Brennan PJ, Rodriguez Bouza T, Hsu FI, Sloane DE, Castells MC. Hypersensitivity reactions to mAbs: 105 desensitizations in 23 patients, from evaluation to treatment. *J Allergy Clin Immunol*. 2009;124(6):1259–1266 and Galvão VR, Castells MC. Hypersensitivity to biological agents—updated diagnosis, management, and treatment. *J Allergy Clin Immunol Pract*. 2015;3(2):175–185.

such as Steven-Johnson syndrome (SJS), toxic epidermal necrolysis (TEN), drug reactions with eosinophilia and systemic symptoms (DRESS), and acute generalized exanthematous pustulosis (AGEP), for which the pathogenesis is poorly understood, and some cases under viral and/or specific human leukocyte antigen haplotype control would not qualify (Table 19.2).[23–26]

Drug desensitization is not recommended for patients with type II HSR, such as immune thrombocytopenia, or type III serum sickness–like reactions, because of the risk of bleeding and immune complex deposition in skin, kidney, and other organs (Table 19.2).[13,27,28]

For patients with type I and type IV HSRs, desensitization protocols are available with demonstrated efficacy

and safety.[5,29,30] The success of drug desensitization relies on personalized protocols based on the nature and severity of the initial reaction, tryptase levels, skin testing, and risk stratification based on associated comorbidities such as decreased lung function and cardiovascular diseases (Table 19.1).[19,20,31–34] Common chemotherapy drugs for which desensitization protocols exist include platins (carboplatin, cisplatin, and oxaliplatin) and taxanes (paclitaxel, docetaxel, and cabazitaxel).[5,8,30]

PLATIN HYPERSENSITIVITY

Platinum compounds are used to treat ovarian, colorectal, endometrial, glioblastoma, and pancreatic

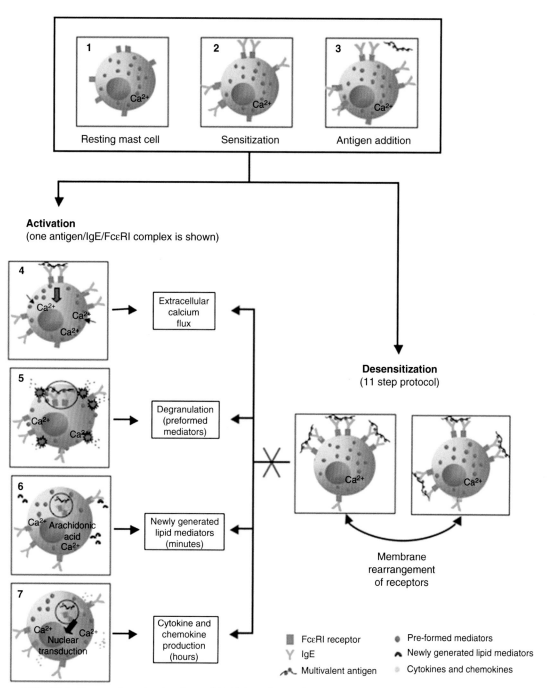

FIG. 19.1 Proposed mechanism for rapid IgE drug desensitization. (From Castells MC, Sancho-Serra MC, Simarro M. Hypersensitivity to antineoplastic agents: mechanisms and treatment with rapid desensitization. *Cancer Immunol Immunother*. May 2012;61:1575–1584; with permission.)

TABLE 19.2
Indications and Contraindications for Rapid Drug Desensitizations

Indications	High-Risk Patients	Contraindications
Type I reactions (IgE and/or mast cell/basophil) Reaction type IV	Severe anaphylaxis (intubation)	Severe cutaneous adverse reactions (SJS/TEN, DIHS/DRESS, AGEP)
No alternative drug	Decreased FEV_1 <1 L	Immunocytotoxic reactions (type II reactions)
Drug is more effective and/or associated with less side effects	Cardiac disease	Vasculitis
Drug has a unique mechanism of action	Use of β-blockers, ACE inhibitors Pregnancy	Serum sickness–like (type III reactions)

ACE, angiotensin converting enzyme; *AGEP*, acute generalized exanthematous pustulosis; *DIHS*, drug-induced hypersensitivity syndrome; *DRESS*, drug reaction (rash) with eosinophilia and systemic symptoms; *FEV₁*, forced expiration volume in the first second of expiration; *SJS*, Stevens-Johnson syndrome; *TEN*, toxic epidermal necrolysis.
Data from Castells MC, Tennant NM, Sloane DE, et al. Hypersensitivity reactions to chemotherapy: outcomes and safety of rapid desensitization in 413 cases. *J Allergy Clin Immunol*. 2008;122(3):574–580 and Sloane D, Govindarajulu U, Harrow-Mortelliti J, et al. Safety, costs, and efficacy of rapid drug desensitizations to chemotherapy and monoclonal antibodies. *J Allergy Clin Immunol Pract*. 2016;4(3):497–504.

cancer as initial chemotherapy and in second-line or salvage settings.[7,35] Carboplatin is more commonly used because of its relative lack of nephrotoxicity and neurotoxicity and lower incidence of severe emesis, in comparison with its parent compound, cisplatin.[4] Most allergic reactions to platins are IgE mediated and sensitization occurs through multiple exposures of the drug.[12,36,37] The incidence of carboplatin allergy is upward to 27% after seven lifetime exposures and as high as 46% in patients with 15 lifetime doses.[3,4] Sensitized patients present with HSRs, including flushing, pruritus, and shortness of breath, which can progress to anaphylaxis with hypotension and oxygen desaturation (Table 19.1).[36] In a study by Galvão et al., patients bearing BRCA 1 and 2 mutations have an increased risk for carboplatin reactions, which can occur with fewer exposures than in patients not bearing BRCA mutations (Fig. 19.2).[38,39] Most reactions to platins occur during drug infusion with consistent symptoms of typical type I HSRs.[1,40] In a report of 413 desensitizations by Castells et al., the distribution of symptoms in the 60 carboplatin-sensitized patients were 100% cutaneous, 60% pulmonary, 40% respiratory, and 42% gastrointestinal.[5]

Immediate reactions to oxaliplatin include typical IgE-mediated symptoms and atypical symptoms such as back and pelvic pain, as well as cytokine-mediated reactions with fever and chills.[6,11] Rare HSRs include antibody-mediated thrombocytopenia and immune complex–mediated syndromes with urticaria and proteinuria.[41,42] Idiosyncratic reactions to oxaliplatin

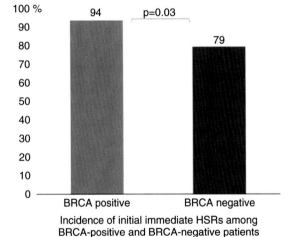

Incidence of initial immediate HSRs among BRCA-positive and BRCA-negative patients

FIG. 19.2 Incidence of initial immediate hypersensitivity reactions among BRCA-positive and BRCA-negative patients. (From Galvão VR, Phillips E, Giavina-Bianchi P, Castells MC. Carboplatin-allergic patients undergoing desensitization: prevalence and impact of the BRCA 1/2 mutation. *J Allergy Clin Immunol Pract*. October 2016. http://dx.doi.org/10.1016/j.jaip.2016.08.012; with permission.)

include pulmonary fibrosis, with no clinical or serologic markers to predict patients at risk (Table 19.1).[36,41–43]

Skin testing to platins has been safely done and is used to identify IgE/mast-cell mechanism in platin-sensitized patients.[44–46] For patients with six or more exposures of carboplatin or cisplatin, the positive predictive value of skin testing is up to 86% in patients with recent exposure (less than 6 months).[3,46] However, 50% of patients presenting with type I reactions to oxaliplatin may have negative skin test, indicating that skin test reagents may not reflect in vivo allergenic determinants or non-IgE mechanisms.[13,46,47]

A study of the potential cross-reactivity among platins by analyzing serum-specific IgE demonstrated that some patients sensitized to oxaliplatin and never exposed to cisplatin or carboplatin had developed cross-reactive antibodies against carboplatin and cisplatin. Conversely, patients exposed and reacting to carboplatin and cisplatin had specific IgE to the offending agent but not to oxaliplatin. Oxaliplatin seems more immunogenic than carboplatin or cisplatin and patients exposed to oxaliplatin may be at potential risk for hypersensitive reactions when exposed to carboplatin and cisplatin.[37] A study by Hesterberg et al. reported that skin test (ST)-negative patients with a remote history of HSR to carboplatin were at a higher risk for conversion to positive ST through reexposure to carboplatin during desensitization, as well as presenting with more severe HSRs.[19] In the study of 38 women with a history of carboplatin HSR, 11 women had negative ST and 27 had positive ST to carboplatin. All of these patients had preemptive carboplatin desensitization. Of the patients with negative ST, three tolerated the infusions without any HSRs and remained negative on ST. The other eight patients converted to positive ST and six (75%) developed HSRs during drug desensitization, with severe reactions and elevated tryptase level.[19] The authors hypothesize that a risk-stratification protocol using three repeat skin tests can lead to fewer desensitizations for patients who remain negative ST. Converters have an increased risk for HSRs during subsequent carboplatin treatments.[19] In the Wang study, 142 patients with HSRs to carboplatin and oxaliplatin were analyzed through 574 desensitizations; 54 (38%) had positive ST, 63 (44%) had negative ST, and 25 (17.6%) had conversions from negative to positive ST.[47] Of the patients with negative ST, 33 (17 carboplatin and 16 oxaliplatin reactors) safely completed 154 outpatient infusions, without desensitizations.[47] For carboplatin and oxaliplatin, negative ST was associated with an interval of greater than 6 months from the HSR to the ST.[47] Other studies indicate that increasing the skin test concentration for carboplatin to 10 mg/mL can identify some of those patients but may induce some skin irritant effect (413 castells)[5] (Table 19.3).

In patients with platin-induced HSRs, slow infusions or increased premedications have not provided protection against anaphylaxis and/or switching to another platin also carries a cross-reactivity risk.[16,37] Patients

TABLE 19.3
Nonirritant Skin Testing Concentrations for Common Chemotherapy Drugs

Medication	Prick (mg/mL)	Intradermal (mg/mL)
Carboplatin[a]	10	1, 5 (10 for patients exposed more than 6 months ago)
Cisplatin	1	0.1 and 1
Oxaliplatin	5	0.5 and 5
Cyclophosphamide	10	0.1, 1, and 10
Methotrexate	25	0.25 and 2.5
Paclitaxel	1–6	0.001 and 0.01

[a]10 mg/mL of carboplatin can cause local and reversible skin necrosis.
[b]Cannot be diluted per manufacturer.

with severe cutaneous adverse reactions to drugs are currently not candidates because of the possibility of inducing a severe reaction with minimal amount of medication delivered.[23,26]

TAXANES HYPERSENSITIVITY

Taxanes are used for the treatment of lung, breast, and prostate cancers and include paclitaxel, docetaxel, cabacitaxel, and albumin bound paclitaxel (Abraxene).[35,48,49] Cremophor is the solubilizing agent for paclitaxel, and docetaxel is solubilized by polysorbate 80.[4,49,50] These lipid solvents have been shown to activate complement, leading to the generation of anaphylatoxins and mast-cell activation.[51-55] Early studies leading to the US Food and Drug Administration approval of paclitaxel showed HSRs were associated to Cremophor, which responded to antihistamines and corticosteroids.[14,56] Despite these standardized premedications, HSRs are present in 1%–10% of patients treated with paclitaxel and can be severe enough to necessitate the discontinuation of the medication.[51,52,54,55] Reactions occur typically during the first or second lifetime drug exposure, and typical symptoms can include throat tightening, skin flushing, cardiovascular changes such as hypo/hypertension, and respiratory symptoms such as dyspnea (Table 19.1).[20,30] Atypical symptoms include severe chest pain with normal chest X-ray and electrocardiogram and back and/or pelvic pain.[20]

IgE-mediated HSRs to taxanes are rare but have been documented, generating interest in a standardized skin test to evaluate patients.[20,49,57] In one study,

164 patients were treated for taxane-related HSR; 145 patients received skin testing, of which 103 (71%) were positive.[49] A total of 138 patients received a taxane desensitization, with 49 reported reactions: 29 (21%) had mild immediate HSRs and 20 (14%) had mild delayed HSRs. Patients with negative skin test were challenged, and two patients developed mild immediate HSRs and one delayed HSR.[49] Risk factors for reactions during challenge included the diagnosis of ovarian, fallopian, or peritoneal cancer and the presence of atopy for immediate reactions, and older age for delayed reactions.[49] No patients had severe immediate HSRs with desensitization or challenge. Of the desensitized patients, 36 (22%) eventually resumed regular infusions; most of them had delayed or mild immediate initial HSRs.[49] This study demonstrates that patients with taxanes HSRs can be stratified for risk of HSR during reexposure using skin test and the severity of the initial HSR.[20,49]

EVALUATION OF PATIENTS WITH HYPERSENSITIVITY REACTIONS TO CHEMOTHERAPY

Patients presenting symptoms consistent with type I or type IV reactions can be evaluated with skin testing. Recent data indicate that serum-specific IgE and basophil activation test (BAT) may also be of utility to evaluate platin-sensitized patients (Fig. 19.3, Table 19.4).[58,59] Patch testing has not been recommended because of the local toxicity of chemotherapy agents.[60] During the initial reaction, serum tryptase levels can help determine the mechanism and extent of the reaction. Tryptase, the major mast cell protease, is released during anaphylactic reactions and peaks at 30–60 min of the onset of symptoms compatible with basophil/mast-cell activation and declines with a half-life of about 2 h.[32–34] Acute serum tryptase level above normal range (11.4 ng/mL) or increased by 20% plus 2 ng/mL over the baseline level is indicative of mast-cell activation.[32–34] Skin testing is not available for all chemotherapeutic agents because some are vesicants, such as doxorubicin.[61] Table 19.4 includes common skin tests available with nonirritating concentrations. Carboplatin has a positive predictive value of 87%. Patients reactive on prick testing are at a higher risk for anaphylaxis when reexposed to the drug.[21] In patients with negative skin tests and normal tryptase levels, if a reaction occurs during the challenge, desensitization is recommended. Patients who do not react during a challenge can be treated with regular administration of the medication without the need for desensitization.[20,60]

The indications for desensitization include type I and IV reactions, the absence of an alternative medication, and/or a medication without equal efficacy.[21,62] Patients at risk during desensitization include pregnant women, patients with previous near-fatal anaphylaxis, patients with severe systemic, respiratory, or cardiac-associated diseases, and patients given β-blockers or angiotensin converting enzyme inhibitors who cannot tolerate discontinuation of these medications.[1,20,21,62] Contraindications for desensitization include severe cutaneous reactions, such as SJS, TEN, AGEP, DRESS, and type III reactions or vasculitis (Table 19.2).[22,23,26,60]

PREMEDICATIONS AND PROTOCOLS FOR RAPID DRUG DESENSITIZATION FOR CHEMOTHERAPY

Premedications for desensitizations are personalized to protect the patient against the symptoms presented during the initial reaction or to breakthrough reactions, which might still occur during desensitization. Antihistamines for blockage of H1 and H2 receptors can address cutaneous symptoms of pruritus, urticaria, angioedema, and flushing.[1] Anxiolytics, such as lorazepam, are used to address fear and anxiety. Nonsteroidal antiinflammatory drugs, such as aspirin and ibuprofen, address cytokine storm–like symptoms, such as malaise, chills, fever, and pain.[63] Antileukotriene therapy, such as montelukast and zileuton (5LO (Arachidonate 5-lipoxygenase inhibitor) inhibitor), are used for respiratory symptoms and cutaneous symptoms, such as angioedema.[64] Steroids are not typically used during chemotherapy desensitization but are part of standard premedications for patients receiving taxanes.[60]

A flexible 12- to 20-step protocol that delivers ×2 to ×2.5 incremental doses of drug antigens at fixed time intervals starting at 1/1000 to 1/100 dilutions of the final concentration is the most widely used intravenous protocol. Patients categorized as moderate risk are desensitized with 12 steps and patients at high risk are desensitized with 16 to 20 steps (Fig. 19.4A and B). The aim of the protocol is to gradually increase the dose of medication without reaching a threshold concentration that would trigger anaphylaxis (Fig. 19.5).[5,8]

Immediate and delayed type IV injection-site reactions elicited by subcutaneous agents (such as adalimumab and etanercept) have been addressed with desensitization protocols administered subcutaneously (Table 19.4).[65] The starting dose is typically 1/100 to 1/10 of the target doses, and the doses are doubled until the target dose is reached in seven or more steps with an interval of 30 min per step.[65]

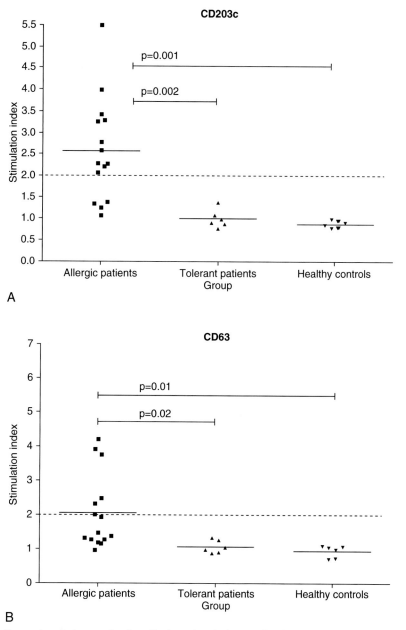

FIG. 19.3 Comparison between allergic patients and controls regarding basophil activation tests measured by expressions of CD203c **(A)** and CD63 **(B)**. Stimulation index of two or more is considered significant (*dashed line*, twofold increase over saline stimulation). (From Giavina-Bianchi P, Galvão VR, Picard M, Caiado J, Castells MC. Basophil activation test is a relevant biomarker of the outcome of rapid desensitization in platinum compounds-allergy. *J Allergy Clin Immunol Pract.* http://dx.doi.org/10.1016/j.jaip.2016.11.006.)

TABLE 19.4
Subcutaneous Desensitization to Adalimumab

Step	Time (min)	Concentration (mg/mL)	Volume Administered per Step (mL)	Dose Administered With This Step (mg)	Cumulative Dose (mg)
1	0	0.5	1	0.5	0.5
2	30	5	0.15	0.75	1.25
3	60	5	0.25	1.25	2.5
4	90	5	0.5	2.5	5
5	120	50	0.1	5	10
6	150	50	0.2	10	20
7	180	50	0.4	20	40

Time per step, 30 min; number of steps, seven; total dose, 40 mg.
From Bavbek S, Ataman Ş, Akinci A, Castells M. Rapid subcutaneous desensitization for the management of local and systemic hypersensitivity reactions to etanercept and adalimumab in 12 patients. *J Allergy Clin Immunol Pract*. July–August 2015;3(4):629–632.

Successful desensitization protocols are available for rituximab, ofatumumab, obinutuzumab, trastuzumab, cetuximab, tocilizumab, infliximab, etanercept, adalimumab, golimumab, certolizumab, brentuximab, bevacizumab, and omalizumab.[5,8,30,62]

OUTCOMES OF RAPID DRUG DESENSITIZATION FOR CHEMOTHERAPY AND MONOCLONAL ANTIBODIES

The largest study of desensitization on patients with chemotherapy allergy that provided data on outcomes and safety was published.[30] The patient population included 370 patients who presented 402 HSRs and received 2177 successful desensitization to 15 drugs. In 93% of these desensitization procedures, there were no HSRs or mild HSRs, whereas 7% had moderate to severe reactions, which did not preclude the completion of the treatment, and there were no deaths (Fig. 19.6).[30]

The study also provided the first cost-effectiveness analysis of desensitized patients and indicated that the overall health costs were not increased over the standard treatment (Table 19.5).[30] Most importantly, a group of women with ovarian cancer sensitized to carboplatin had a nonstatistically significant lifespan advantage over nonallergic controls, indicating that the efficacy of carboplatin through rapid drug desensitization protocols was at least as effective as regular infusions (Fig. 19.7). This raised the intriguing possibility that patients with ovarian cancer desensitized to carboplatin may be better armed to fight cancer.[30]

CONCLUSION

The evaluation of patients with HSRs to chemotherapy has become a key function of the allergy specialists in the 21st century. A thorough and personalized diagnostic evaluation and risk stratification, including a detailed history, physical examination, and skin testing (if appropriate and available), are required (Fig. 19.8). Specific serum IgE and BATs are future tools with demonstrated ability to identify reactors and to predict severity of reactions during desensitization. Immediate and delayed IgE- and non-IgE-mediated chemotherapy HSRs can be managed by desensitization with appropriate premedications, enabling the sensitized patient to receive the full treatment safely, and represents an important advancement in the patient's treatment and overall prognosis. Most patients with HSRs are candidates for desensitization, except for patients with severe cutaneous adverse reactions.

Rapid drug desensitization is a safe and groundbreaking procedure for the management of immediate drug hypersensitivity reactions, protecting patients against anaphylaxis. To be successful in providing patients with first-line therapies through desensitization, a tight collaboration between allergy, nursing, pharmacy, and other specialists is required. Future advances in drug desensitizations will include the role of biological treatments directed against Th2 cytokines or IgE, such as omalizumab. It is important to further understand the mechanism of non-IgE-mediated reactions, the role of excipients, and the presence of preexisting cross-reactivity. Identifying potential reactors through improved skin testing and in vitro testing, including genetic testing, will lead to increased safety in the administration of drug desensitization protocols.

Name of medication:			Rituximab			
Target dose(mg):			500			
Standard volume per bag (mL):			250			
Final rate of infusion (mL/hour):			80			
Calculated target concentration (mg/mL):			2			

	Volume		Concentration (mg/mL)		Total mg per bag	Amount infused (mL)
Solution 1	250	mL of	0.020	mg/mL	5.000	9.25
Solution 2	250	mL of	0.200	mg/mL	50.000	18.75
Solution 3	250	mL of	1.984	mg/mL	496.065	250.00

PLEASE NOTE The total volume and dose dispensed are more than the final dose given to patient because many of the solutions are not completely infused.

Step	Solution	Rate (mL/hour)	Time (minutes)	Volume infused per step (mL)	Dose administered with this step (mg)	Cumulative dose (mg)
1	1	2.0	15	0.50	0.0100	0.0100
2	1	5.0	15	1.25	0.0250	0.0350
3	1	10.0	15	2.50	0.0500	0.0850
4	1	20.0	15	5.00	0.1000	0.1850
5	2	5.0	15	1.25	0.2500	0.4350
6	2	10.0	15	2.50	0.5000	0.9350
7	2	20.0	15	5.00	1.0000	1.9350
8	2	40.0	15	10.00	2.0000	3.9350
9	3	10.0	15	2.50	4.9607	8.8957
10	3	20.0	15	5.00	9.9213	18.8170
11	3	40.0	15	10.00	19.8426	38.6596
12	3	80.0	174.375	232.50	461.3405	500.0000

Total time: 5.66 hours

A

Name of medication:			Paclitaxel			
Target dose(mg):			200			
Standard volume per bag (mL):			250			
Final rate of infusion (mL/hour):			80			
Calculated target concentration (mg/mL):			0.8			

	Volume		Concentration (mg/mL)		Total mg per bag	Amount infused (mL)
Solution 1	250	mL of	0.000	mg/mL	0.100	9.38
Solution 2	250	mL of	0.008	mg/mL	2.000	9.38
Solution 3	250	mL of	0.080	mg/mL	20.000	18.75
Solution 4	250	mL of	0.794	mg/mL	198.421	250.00

PLEASE NOTE The total volume and dose dispensed are more than the final dose given to patient because many of the solutions are not completely infused.

Step	Solution	Rate (mL/hour)	Time (minutes)	Volume infused per step (mL)	Dose administered with this step (mg)	Cumulative dose (mg)
1	1	2.5	15	0.625	0.0003	0.0003
2	1	5	15	1.25	0.0005	0.001
3	1	10	15	2.5	0.0010	0.002
4	1	20	15	5	0.0020	0.004
5	2	2.5	15	0.625	0.005	0.009
6	2	5	15	1.25	0.010	0.019
7	2	10	15	2.5	0.020	0.039
8	2	20	15	5	0.040	0.079
9	3	5	15	1.25	0.100	0.179
10	3	10	15	2.5	0.200	0.379
11	3	20	15	5	0.400	0.779
12	3	40	15	10	0.800	1.579
13	4	10	15	2.5	1.984	3.563
14	4	20	15	5	3.968	7.531
15	4	40	15	10	7.937	15.468
16	4	80	174.375	232.5	184.532	200.000

Total time: 6.66 hours

B

FIG. 19.4 **(A)** BWH 3 (Brigham and Women's Hospital's 3 bag 12 step protocol) bags 12 steps desensitization protocol for 500 mg of rituximab. **(B)** BWH 4 (Brigham and Women's Hospital's 4 bag 16 step protocol) bags 16 steps desensitization protocol for 200 mg of paclitaxel. (From Mezzano V, Giavina-Bianchi P, Picard M, Caiado J, Castells M. Drug desensitization in the management of hypersensitivity reactions to monoclonal antibodies and chemotherapy. *BioDrugs.* April 2014;28(2):133–144.)

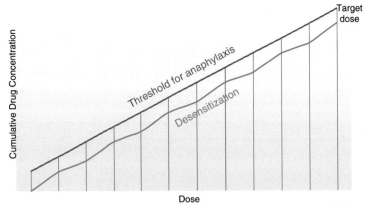

FIG. 19.5 Putative mechanism of clinical rapid drug desensitization. (From Bonamichi-Santos R, Castells M. Diagnoses and management of drug hypersensitivity and anaphylaxis in cancer and chronic inflammatory diseases: reactions to taxanes and monoclonal antibodies. *Clin Rev Allergy Immunol*. June 2016. http://dx.doi.org/10.1007/s12016-016-8556-5.)

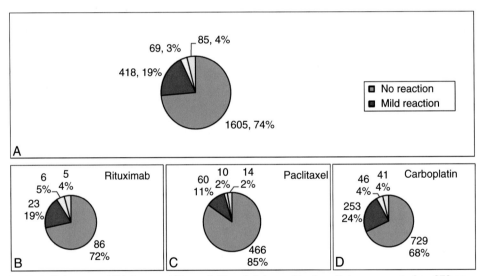

FIG. 19.6 Outcomes of Brigham and Women's Hospital desensitization. Data are reported on 370 patients for 2177 desensitizations and 15 medications (carboplatin, cisplatin, oxaliplatin, paclitaxel, docetaxel, doxorubicin, cyclophosphamide, methotrexate, rituximab, infliximab, trastuzumab, bevacizumab, tocilizumab, cetuximab, and gemcitabine). Overall outcomes in **(A)** and specific outcomes for rituximab **(B)** paclitaxel **(C)** and carboplatin **(D)**. (From Sloane D, Govindarajulu U, Harrow-Mortelliti J, et al. Safety, costs, and efficacy of rapid drug desensitizations to chemotherapy and monoclonal antibodies. *J Allergy Clin Immunol Pract*. 2016;4(3):497–504; with permission.)

TABLE 19.5

Overall Health Costs of Drug Desensitizations for Carboplatin Allergic Patients With Ovarian Cancer and Nonallergic Controls

Patients and Cost Data	Patients/ Encounters	Age	Total Encounters	Average (Range) Encounters/Patients	Average Cost[a]	Total Costs
Desensitized	171/146	62 (36–95)	532	3.1 (1–16)	$6796	$26,605
Control	186/170	57(18–88)	592	3.2 (1–16)	$9256	$29,825

[a]Significantly different between groups by t-test at $P < .0001$.

From Sloane D, Govindarajulu U, Harrow-Mortelliti J, et al. Safety, costs, and efficacy of rapid drug desensitizations to chemotherapy and monoclonal antibodies. *J Allergy Clin Immunol Pract.* 2016;4(3):497–504.

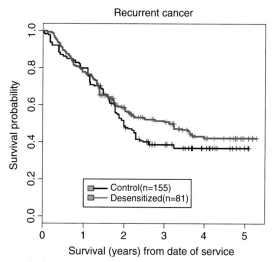

Plot of Kaplan-Meier survival curves from propensity-weighted data on carboplatin-treated recurrent cancer patients

FIG. 19.7 Kaplan-Meyer survival curves for patients with ovarian cancer with carboplatin allergy and desensitized to carboplatin and for ovarian cancer carboplatin treated controls without allergy to carboplatin. (From Sloane D, Govindarajulu U, Harrow-Mortelliti J, et al. Safety, costs, and efficacy of rapid drug desensitizations to chemotherapy and monoclonal antibodies. *J Allergy Clin Immunol Pract.* 2016;4(3):497–504.)

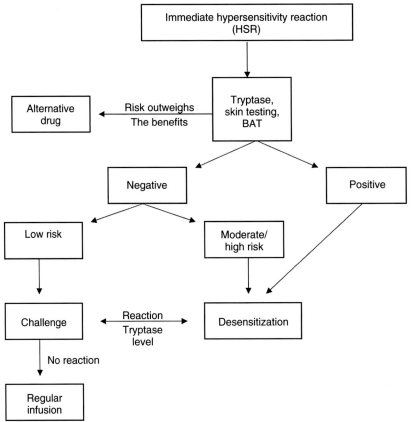

FIG. 19.8 Proposed algorithm for the evaluation of chemotherapy drugs hypersensitivity and indications for rapid drug desensitization. *BAT*, basophil activation test. (From Bonamichi-Santos R, Castells M. Diagnoses and management of drug hypersensitivity and anaphylaxis in cancer and chronic inflammatory diseases: reactions to taxanes and monoclonal antibodies. *Clin Rev Allergy Immunol.* June 2016. http://dx. doi.org/10.1007/s12016-016-8556-5.)

REFERENCES

1. Castells Guitart MC. Rapid drug desensitization for hypersensitivity reactions to chemotherapy and monoclonal antibodies in the 21st century. *J Investig Allergol Clin Immunol.* 2014;24(2):72–79. quiz 2 p following 79.
2. Gruchalla RS. 10. Drug allergy. *J Allergy Clin Immunol.* 2003;111(2 Suppl.):S548–S559.
3. Markman M. Toxicities of the platinum antineoplastic agents. *Expert Opin Drug Saf.* 2003;2(6):597–607.
4. Sakaeda T, Kadoyama K, Yabuuchi H, et al. Platinum agent-induced hypersensitivity reactions: data mining of the public version of the FDA adverse event reporting system, AERS. *Int J Med Sci.* 2011;8(4):332–338.
5. Castells MC, Tennant NM, Sloane DE, et al. Hypersensitivity reactions to chemotherapy: outcomes and safety of rapid desensitization in 413 cases. *J Allergy Clin Immunol.* 2008;122(3):574–580.
6. Gamarra RM, McGraw SD, Drelichman VS, Maas LC. Serum sickness-like reactions in patients receiving intravenous infliximab. *J Emerg Med.* 2006;30(1):41–44.
7. Caiado J, Castells M. Presentation and diagnosis of hypersensitivity to platinum drugs. *Curr Allergy Asthma Rep.* 2015;15(4):15.
8. Brennan PJ, Rodriguez Bouza T, Hsu FI, Sloane DE, Castells MC. Hypersensitivity reactions to mAbs: 105 desensitizations in 23 patients, from evaluation to treatment. *J Allergy Clin Immunol.* 2009;124(6):1259–1266.
9. Galvão VR, Castells MC. Hypersensitivity to biological agents—updated diagnosis, management, and treatment. *J Allergy Clin Immunol Pract.* 2015;3;3(2):175–185.
10. Feldweg AM, Lee C-W, Matulonis UA, Castells M. Rapid desensitization for hypersensitivity reactions to paclitaxel and docetaxel: a new standard protocol used in 77 successful treatments. *Gynecol Oncol.* 2005;96(3):824–829.

11. Luheshi GN. Cytokines and fever. Mechanisms and sites of action. *Ann N Y Acad Sci.* 1998;856:83–89.

12. Sancho-Serra MC, Simarro M, Castells M. Rapid IgE desensitization is antigen specific and impairs early and late mast cell responses targeting FcεRI internalization. *Eur J Immunol.* 2011;41(4):1004–1013.

13. Wong JT, Ling M, Patil S, Banerji A, Long A. Oxaliplatin hypersensitivity: evaluation, implications of skin testing, and desensitization. *J Allergy Clin Immunol Pract.* 2014;2(1):40–45.

14. Kadoyama K, Kuwahara A, Yamamori M, Brown JB, Sakaeda T, Okuno Y. Hypersensitivity reactions to anticancer agents: data mining of the public version of the FDA adverse event reporting system, AERS. *J Exp Clin Cancer Res.* 2011;30:93.

15. A fatal anaphylactic reaction to paclitaxel is described, which was preceded by a possible delayed reaction to the initial infusion. *Allergy Asthma Proc.* 2011;32(1):79.

16. Zweizig S, Roman LD, Muderspach LI. Death from anaphylaxis to cisplatin: a case report. *Gynecol Oncol.* 1994;53(1):121–122.

17. Cheifetz A, Mayer L. Monoclonal antibodies, immunogenicity, and associated infusion reactions. *Mt Sinai J Med.* 2005;72(4):250–256.

18. Nucera E, Schiavino D, Hohaus S, et al. Desensitization to thalidomide in a patient with multiple myeloma. *Clin Lymphoma Myeloma.* 2008;8(3):176–178.

19. Hesterberg PE, Banerji A, Oren E, et al. Risk stratification for desensitization of patients with carboplatin hypersensitivity: clinical presentation and management. *J Allergy Clin Immunol.* 2009;123(6):1262–1267.e1.

20. Picard M, Pur L, Caiado J, et al. Risk stratification and skin testing to guide re-exposure in taxane-induced hypersensitivity reactions. *J Allergy Clin Immunol.* 2016;137(4). 1154–1164.e1–e12.

21. Cernadas JR, Brockow K, Romano A, et al. General considerations on rapid desensitization for drug hypersensitivity–a consensus statement. *Allergy.* 2010;65(11):1357–1366.

22. Bonamichi-Santos R, Castells M. Diagnoses and management of drug hypersensitivity and anaphylaxis in cancer and chronic inflammatory diseases: reactions to taxanes and monoclonal antibodies. *Clin Rev Allergy Immunol.* June 2016. http://dx.doi.org/10.1007/s12016-016-8556-5.

23. Phillips EJ, Chung W-H, Mockenhaupt M, Roujeau J-C, Mallal SA. Drug hypersensitivity: pharmacogenetics and clinical syndromes. *J Allergy Clin Immunol.* 2011;127(3 Suppl.):S60–S66.

24. Bachot N, Roujeau J-C. Differential diagnosis of severe cutaneous drug eruptions. *Am J Clin Dermatol.* 2003;4(8):561–572.

25. Zaraa I, Jones M, Trojjet S, et al. Severe adverse cutaneous drug eruptions: epidemiological and clinical features. *Int J Dermatol.* 2011;50(7):877–880.

26. Pirmohamed M, Friedmann PS, Molokhia M, et al. Phenotype standardization for immune-mediated drug-induced skin injury. *Clin Pharmacol Ther.* 2011;89(6):896–901.

27. Arnold DM, Kukaswadia S, Nazi I, et al. A systematic evaluation of laboratory testing for drug-induced immune thrombocytopenia. *J Thromb Haemost.* 2013;11(1):169–176.

28. Aster RH. Drug-induced immune thrombocytopenia: an overview of pathogenesis. *Semin Hematol.* 1999;36(1 Suppl. 1):2–6.

29. Giavina-Bianchi P, Caiado J, Picard M, Pur Ozyigit L, Mezzano V, Castells M. Rapid desensitization to chemotherapy and monoclonal antibodies is effective and safe. *Allergy.* 2013;68(11):1482–1483.

30. Sloane D, Govindarajulu U, Harrow-Mortelliti J, et al. Safety, costs, and efficacy of rapid drug desensitizations to chemotherapy and monoclonal antibodies. *J Allergy Clin Immunol Pract.* 2016;4(3):497–504.

31. Patil SU, Long AA, Ling M, et al. A protocol for risk stratification of patients with carboplatin-induced hypersensitivity reactions. *J Allergy Clin Immunol.* 2012;129(2):443–447.

32. Ruëff F, Przybilla B, Biló MB, et al. Predictors of severe systemic anaphylactic reactions in patients with *Hymenoptera venom* allergy: importance of baseline serum tryptase—a study of the European Academy of Allergology and Clinical Immunology Interest Group on Insect Venom Hypersensitivity. *J Allergy Clin Immunol.* 2009;124(5):1047–1054.

33. Laroche D, Vergnaud MC, Sillard B, Soufarapis H, Bricard H. Biochemical markers of anaphylactoid reactions to drugs. Comparison of plasma histamine and tryptase. *Anesthesiology.* 1991;75(6):945–949.

34. Sala-Cunill A, Cardona V, Labrador-Horrillo M, et al. Usefulness and limitations of sequential serum tryptase for the diagnosis of anaphylaxis in 102 patients. *Int Arch Allergy Immunol.* 2013;160(2):192–199.

35. Morgan Jr RJ, Alvarez RD, Armstrong DK, et al. Ovarian cancer, version 3.2012. *J Natl Compr Canc Netw.* 2012;10(11):1339–1349.

36. Nektaria M, Ekaterini S, Ioannis K, Leonidas M, Muhammad Wasif S. Hypersensitivity reactions associated with platinum antineoplastic agents: a systematic review. *Met Based Drugs.* 2010;2010. http://downloads.hindawi.com/journals/mbd/2010/207084.pdf.

37. Caiado J, Venemalm L, Pereira-Santos MC, Costa L, Barbosa MP, Castells M. Carboplatin-, oxaliplatin-, and cisplatin-specific IgE: cross-reactivity and value in the diagnosis of carboplatin and oxaliplatin allergy. *J Allergy Clin Immunol Pract.* 2013;1(5):494–500.

38. Moon DH, Lee J-M, Noonan AM, et al. Deleterious BRCA1/2 mutation is an independent risk factor for carboplatin hypersensitivity reactions. *Br J Cancer.* 2013;109(4):1072–1078.

39. Galvão VR, Phillips E, Giavina-Bianchi P, Castells MC. Carboplatin-allergic patients undergoing desensitization: prevalence and impact of the BRCA 1/2 mutation. *J Allergy Clin Immunol Pract.* October 2016. http://dx.doi.org/10.1016/j.jaip.2016.08.012.

40. Callahan MB, Lachance JA, Stone RL, Kelsey J, Rice LW, Jazaeri AA. Use of cisplatin without desensitization after carboplatin hypersensitivity reaction in epithelial ovarian and primary peritoneal cancer. *Am J Obstet Gynecol.* 2007;197(2). 199.e1–e4; discussion 199.e4-e5.

41. Thomas RR, Quinn MG, Schuler B, Grem JL. Hypersensitivity and idiosyncratic reactions to oxaliplatin. *Cancer.* 2003;97(9):2301–2307.

42. Maindrault-Goebel F, André T, Tournigand C, et al. Allergic-type reactions to oxaliplatin: retrospective analysis of 42 patients. *Eur J Cancer*. 2005;41(15):2262–2267.

43. Bhargava P, Gammon D, McCormick MJ. Hypersensitivity and idiosyncratic reactions to oxaliplatin. *Cancer*. 2004;100(1):211–212.

44. Leguy-Seguin V, Jolimoy G, Coudert B, et al. Diagnostic and predictive value of skin testing in platinum salt hypersensitivity. *J Allergy Clin Immunol*. 2007;119(3):726–730.

45. Garufi C, Cristaudo A, Vanni B, et al. Skin testing and hypersensitivity reactions to oxaliplatin. *Ann Oncol*. 2003;14(3):497–498.

46. Zanotti KM, Rybicki LA, Kennedy AW, et al. Carboplatin skin testing: a skin-testing protocol for predicting hypersensitivity to carboplatin chemotherapy. *J Clin Oncol*. 2001;19(12):3126–3129.

47. Wang AL, Patil SU, Long AA, Banerji A. Risk-stratification protocol for carboplatin and oxaliplatin hypersensitivity: repeat skin testing to identify drug allergy. *Ann Allergy Asthma Immunol*. 2015;115(5):422–428.

48. Hennenfent KL, Govindan R. Novel formulations of taxanes: a review. Old wine in a new bottle? *Ann Oncol*. 2006;17(5):735–749.

49. Picard M, Castells MC. Re-visiting hypersensitivity reactions to taxanes: a comprehensive review. *Clin Rev Allergy Immunol*. 2015;49(2):177–191.

50. Banerji A, Lax T, Guyer A, Hurwitz S, Camargo Jr CA, Long AA. Management of hypersensitivity reactions to carboplatin and paclitaxel in an outpatient oncology infusion center: a 5-year review. *J Allergy Clin Immunol Pract*. 2014;2(4):428–433.

51. Weiss RB, Donehower RC, Wiernik PH, et al. Hypersensitivity reactions from taxol. *J Clin Oncol*. 1990;8(7):1263–1268.

52. Kwon JS, Elit L, Finn M, et al. A comparison of two prophylactic regimens for hypersensitivity reactions to paclitaxel. *Gynecol Oncol*. 2002;84(3):420–425.

53. Markman M, Kennedy A, Webster K, Kulp B, Peterson G, Belinson J. Paclitaxel-associated hypersensitivity reactions: experience of the gynecologic oncology program of the Cleveland Clinic Cancer Center. *J Clin Oncol*. 2000;18(1):102–105.

54. Squibb B-M. *TAXOL®(Paclitaxel) Injection Prescribing Information*; 2012.

55. Sanofi-Aventis US. *Taxotere Prescribing Information*; 2008.

56. Vasey PA, Jayson GC, Gordon A, et al. Phase III randomized trial of docetaxel–carboplatin versus paclitaxel–carboplatin as first-line chemotherapy for ovarian carcinoma. *J Natl Cancer Inst*. 2004;96(22):1682–1691.

57. Madrigal-Burgaleta R, Berges-Gimeno MP, Angel-Pereira D, et al. Hypersensitivity and desensitization to antineoplastic agents: outcomes of 189 procedures with a new short protocol and novel diagnostic tools assessment. *Allergy*. 2013;68(7):853–861.

58. Piva E, Chieco-Bianchi F, Krajcar V, Aversa S, Plebani M. Adverse reactions in patients with B-cell lymphomas during combined treatment with rituximab: in vitro evaluation of rituximab hypersensitivity by basophil activation test. *Am J Hematol*. 2012;87(11):E130–E131.

59. Giavina-Bianchi P, Galvão VR, Picard M, Caiado J, Castells MC. Basophil activation test is a relevant biomarker of the outcome of rapid desensitization in platinum compounds-allergy. *J Allergy Clin Immunol Pract*. 2016. http://dx.doi.org/10.1016/j.jaip.2016.11.006.

60. Hsu Blatman KS, Castells MC. Desensitizations for chemotherapy and monoclonal antibodies: indications and outcomes. *Curr Allergy Asthma Rep*. 2014;14(8):453.

61. Brockow K, Romano A, Blanca M, Ring J, Pichler W, Demoly P. General considerations for skin test procedures in the diagnosis of drug hypersensitivity. *Allergy*. 2002;57(1):45–51.

62. Liu A, Fanning L, Chong H, et al. Desensitization regimens for drug allergy: state of the art in the 21st century. *Clin Exp Allergy*. 2011;41(12):1679–1689.

63. Vultaggio A, Maggi E, Matucci A. Immediate adverse reactions to biologicals: from pathogenic mechanisms to prophylactic management. *Curr Opin Allergy Clin Immunol*. 2011;11(3):262–268.

64. Breslow RG, Caiado J, Castells MC. Acetylsalicylic acid and montelukast block mast cell mediator–related symptoms during rapid desensitization. *Ann Allergy Asthma Immunol*. 2009;102(2):155–160.

65. Bavbek S, Ataman Ş., Akinci A, Castells M. Rapid subcutaneous desensitization for the management of local and systemic hypersensitivity reactions to etanercept and adalimumab in 12 patients. *J Allergy Clin Immunol Pract*. 2015 Jul-Aug;3(4):629–632.

FURTHER READING

1. Ow TJ, Sandulache VC, Skinner HD, Myers JN. Integration of cancer genomics with treatment selection: from the genome to predictive biomarkers. *Cancer*. 2013;119(22):3914–3928.

2. O'Neil BH, Allen R, Spigel DR, et al. High incidence of cetuximab-related infusion reactions in Tennessee and North Carolina and the association with atopic history. *J Clin Oncol*. 2007;25(24):3644–3648.

3. Chung CH, Mirakhur B, Chan E, et al. Cetuximab-induced anaphylaxis and IgE specific for galactose-alpha-1,3-galactose. *N Engl J Med*. 2008;358(11):1109–1117.

4. Yoshiki R, Nakamura M, Tokura Y. Drug eruption induced by IL-6 receptor inhibitor tocilizumab. *J Eur Acad Dermatol Venereol*. 2010;24(4):495–496.

5. Boulanger J, Boursiquot JN, Cournoyer G, et al. Management of hypersensitivity to platinum- and taxane-based chemotherapy: CEPO review and clinical recommendations. *Curr Oncol*. 2014;21(4):e630–e641.

6. Mezzano V, Giavina-Bianchi P, Picard M, Caiado J, Castells M. Drug desensitization in the management of hypersensitivity reactions to monoclonal antibodies and chemotherapy. *BioDrugs*. April 2014;28(2):133–144.

7. Castells MC, Sancho-Serra MC, Simarro M. Hypersensitivity to antineoplastic agents: mechanisms and treatment with rapid desensitization. *Cancer Immunol Immunother*. May 2012;61:1575–1584.

CHAPTER 20

Hypersensitivity Reactions to Monoclonal Antibodies

ANNE Y. LIU, MD

Therapeutic monoclonal antibodies (mAbs) are produced by harnessing the immunologic machinery, and they are a departure from synthesized small molecule drugs. This field has risen out of a greater understanding of the mechanistic pathways of diseases and a desire for narrowly targeted therapeutics. Improvements in recombinant antibody (Ab) technology have made production for clinical use in patients feasible. As large-molecular-weight proteins, their immunogenic potential has created a rapidly growing branch within the field of drug allergy.

At the time of this writing, there are over 60 US Food and Drug Administration (FDA)-approved mAbs and many more investigational agents. The proliferation of these drugs makes a comprehensive cataloging of reported adverse effects and hypersensitivity reactions (HSRs) impractical. The goals of this chapter are:

- to provide a background on mAb production relevant to their immunogenicity;
- to describe ways in which mAbs may differ in their immunogenicity from small molecules;
- to review a classification scheme of immunologically mediated reactions based on possible mechanisms, with a focus on HSRs and on adverse reactions that mimic HSRs;
- to discuss in greater detail several mAbs that illustrate and highlight considerations important to allergists;
- to review diagnostic and management options, including skin testing and desensitization.

The scope of this discussion focuses on FDA-approved therapies and excludes non-mAb biologics, such as insulin, cytokines, and fusion proteins.

BASICS OF MAB PRODUCTION

mAb production was first described by Köhler and Milstein in 1975, and early mAb production harnessed the hybridoma technology, which allows unlimited production of Abs of selected specificity.[1] Mice immunized against an antigen produce B cells, which are then fused with immortalized myeloma cells to produce hybridomas, from which a clone is selected based on epitope specificity for continued production of mAbs.[2] Limitations in this system, including the immunogenicity of xenogenic proteins, have led to the development of other mAb production methods that utilize transgenic mice, mammalian milk glands, human plasmablasts, and phage display technologies. Phage display is an in vitro technique for the production of fully human mAbs, in which human DNA sequences are inserted into filamentous phage genes, allowing for display of recombinant human proteins on phages and consistent production upon infection of *Escherichia coli*.[3,4]

IMMUNOGENICITY

A number of factors that determine the immunogenicity of mAbs are distinct from those of small molecule drugs. Early mAbs revealed that the risk of HSRs depends in large part on the proportion of murine and human sequences, with murine components increasing immunogenicity and provoking human anti-mouse Ab development. The importance of the source species is reflected in the nomenclature of mAbs: murine mAbs end in *–omab*, chimeric mAbs in *–ximab*, humanized mAbs in *–zumab*, and fully human mAbs in *–umab*.[5,6]

Isotype selection, posttranslational and cotranslational modifications, and protein aggregate formation are among other factors that determine the likelihood of HSRs, infusion reactions, and complement activation.[7-9] The primary amino acid sequence does not completely predict the structure of a mAb, which is subject to posttranslational and cotranslational modifications, such as glycosylation, phosphorylation, sulfation, deamidation, and more; for a given IgG molecule, these modifications can produce 10^8 isoforms. For example, the glycosylation pattern of cetuximab is largely responsible for its immunogenicity, which is discussed further in this chapter.

Excipients such as polysorbate and polyethylene glycol may act as unintended adjuvants or as immunogenic substances. Polysorbate is a nonionic surfactant included in many mAb preparations to prevent aggregate formation but can itself cause clinically significant sensitization.[10,11] Cases of delayed-onset omalizumab HSRs have been rarely attributed to polysorbate 80.[12]

CLASSIFICATION OF ADVERSE REACTIONS TO MABS

Classification of adverse drug reactions and HSRs is traditionally based on small molecule therapeutics, which are usually synthesized chemicals. Ab-based therapies should be considered differently as they are large, complex molecules designed to mimic human proteins. For example, small molecules can elicit an immunologic response when they act as haptens or prohaptens; in these interactions, a drug or its metabolite becomes antigenic and subject to recognition by T cells only when bound to an endogenous or exogenous protein.[13] In contrast, mAbs can act as complete antigens.

Pichler proposed a classification of adverse reactions to biologics based on putative mechanisms.[14,15] This classification structure differentiates the target-related effects from the effects specific to the structure of the agent. As a mechanistically driven classification, it may not clarify reactions whose clinical symptoms straddle more than one mechanistic category and for which we lack proper diagnostic tests with sufficient predictive value. Although this chapter focuses on HSRs, non-HSR adverse reactions that mimic hypersensitivities are also highlighted.

Type α reactions arise from high circulating cytokine concentrations, from Ab-mediated immune cell lysis and/or activation resulting in cytokine release syndrome (CRS). Examples include some reactions observed with rituximab, muromonab, and TGN1412:

1. TGN1412, a fully humanized mAb targeting the costimulatory molecule CD28 on T cells, was thought to preferentially activate T-regulatory cells, but its activity as a superagonistic Ab to trigger T cell proliferation and cytokine release had catastrophic consequences.[16] In a Phase I study, infusion into six healthy volunteers unexpectedly and rapidly precipitated overwhelming T cell activation and cytokine storm. Subjects experienced multiorgan failure and necrotic vasculitis with subsequent digital gangrene.
2. Muromonab (OKT3), an early murine mAb directed against the T cell receptor CD3, has been used for the prevention of allograft rejection. In some patients, it triggered T cell activation and pre-

cipitous cytokine release, resulting in arthralgias, aseptic meningitis, capillary leak syndrome with pulmonary edema, encephalopathy, fever, and gastrointestinal distress.[17]

3. Rituximab, an anti-CD20 mAb, can trigger B cell destruction and release of contents, manifesting as fever, rigors, hypotension, and dyspnea. This is further detailed later in the discussion.

CRS may involve a wide variety of immune cells, releasing cytokines, such as tumor necrosis factor (TNF)-α, interferon (IFN)-γ, interleukin (IL)-8, and IL-6.[18] In situations without a direct mechanism of T cell or B cell activation, it has been suggested that CRS can be triggered by the interaction of the mAb with the FcγR on immune cells and/or via complement activation.[19]

Type β reactions are immunologically mediated HSRs. This group parallels those seen with low-molecular-weight compounds (chemicals/drugs), conventionally classified as Gell-Coombs types I through IV. When elicited by mAbs, there are some notable departures from traditional patterns of drug allergy.

- Type I: IgE-mediated reactions are usually characterized by a rapid onset of symptoms, with some combination of urticaria, angioedema, bronchospasm, laryngospasm, diarrhea, vomiting, and anaphylaxis within an hour of administration; with mAbs, the time to onset of these symptoms can be delayed for days. The presence of anti-drug IgE Abs has been demonstrated by skin testing and/or specific IgE detection for a number of mAbs, including infliximab, tocilizumab, cetuximab (see later discussion), rituximab, trastuzumab, natalizumab, and muromonab.[20–24] As with IgE-type reactions to other drugs, long intervals between doses of a mAb could potentiate a clinical HSR.

- Types II and III: Production of anti-drug IgG Abs against mAbs can precipitate the formation of immune complexes and activation of Fc-IgG receptors, resulting in serum sickness, vasculitis, nephritis, and cytopenias that are usually delayed in onset.[25–27] More frequently, anti-drug IgG Abs result in mAb inaction without other clinically apparent symptoms. These reactions generally occur in a delayed fashion as with small molecule agents. An instructive example came from 125 patients with Crohn disease, in whom the development of anti-infliximab Abs correlated with infusion reactions and reduced infliximab concentrations.[28] Patients concurrently treated with a nonsteroidal immunosuppressive regimen (azathioprine, mercaptopurine, or methotrexate) were significantly less likely to develop anti-infliximab Abs. This phenomenon appears to generalize to patients with a variety of rheumatologic disorders.[29]

- Type IV: T cell–mediated delayed-type HSRs that manifest as drug exanthems, including maculopapular rashes, Stevens-Johnson syndrome, drug rash eosinophilia and systemic symptoms (DRESS)/drug-induced hypersensitivity syndrome, acute generalized exanthematous pustulosis, and fixed drug eruptions, are relatively rare with mAbs, as compared with small molecule drugs. Delayed rashes that are not HSRs, however, are very common with some mAbs, as discussed in the following text.[30]

Type γ reactions in the Pichler classification scheme arise from immune/cytokine imbalances. These are immunologically mediated by virtue of the intended effect of the mAb, rather than from a hypersensitivity response against the mAb. Either impairment of normal immune function or overactivity leading to a proinflammatory state may be observed in type γ reactions. Examples include:

- TNF-α inhibitors, such as infliximab and adalimumab, have not only been successfully used in a variety of autoinflammatory conditions, such as rheumatoid arthritis and inflammatory bowel disease, but also expose patients to significant risks from impaired inflammation, including malignancies, tuberculosis, endemic mycoses, and more. Many other mAbs also increase the infection risk, the discussion of which is beyond the scope of this chapter.
- Immunostimulating mAbs produce immune balance–mediated side effects that may mimic HSRs. Checkpoint inhibitors in this group target molecules that serve as brakes on effector T cells; these drugs thus nonspecifically reduce tolerance to self-antigens.[31] Ipilimumab inhibits cytotoxic T-lymphocyte-associated protein 4 (CTLA-4). Nivolumab and pembrolizumab target programmed cell death 1 (PD-1).

Half of patients who receive ipilimumab develop cutaneous complications, ranging from reticular erythema and maculopapular rashes to neutrophilic and eosinophilic dermatoses, usually several weeks after the initiation of therapy.[32–34] Although most ipilimumab-related cutaneous findings are not HSRs, rare cases of Stevens-Johnson syndrome and DRESS have been reported.[35,36] About 30%–40% of patients who receive nivolumab and pembrolizumab will have dermatologic findings similar to those associated with ipilimumab. Other complications of these mAbs that may mimic HSRs include hepatitis, pneumonitis, and cytopenias.

Many more immune-activating therapeutics are in development at the time of this writing. As cancer immunotherapy plays an expanding role in oncologic treatments, allergists may be called upon to help distinguish inflammatory sequelae of their use from HSRs against these drugs.

Type δ reactions result from cross-reactivity when antigens similar or identical to the target antigen are expressed on different tissues. An example of this phenomenon is an acneiform rash that commonly appears during treatment with cetuximab and panitumumab. Their target is epidermal growth factor receptor (EGFR) expressed on various types of carcinoma, but EGFR is also expressed in the epidermis. The rash occurs in two-thirds of recipients and may predict oncologic response.[37]

Type ε reactions include a wide variety of nonimmunologic side effects, such as depression and thrombosis.

INFUSION REACTIONS

Infusion reactions can be difficult to categorize when using mechanistic classification schemes. Strictly speaking, infusion reactions may be type α CRS, type β immediate-type IgE-mediated HSRs, or neither. CRS and HSRs constitute only a fraction of all mAb infusion reactions. More common, "typical" infusion reactions (TIRs) range from mild to severe, with occasional fatal reactions. TIRs may exhibit a combination of fever and/or rigors, flushing, hemodynamic changes (including hypertension, hypotension, or tachycardia), shortness of breath, chest pressure and tightness, gastrointestinal distress including nausea, vomiting, and/or diarrhea, and back pain. These reactions do not usually include nasal congestion, urticaria, angioedema, hoarseness, or wheezing, which are more characteristic of HSRs. Conversely, HSRs usually do not exhibit fever, rigors, or myalgias.

TIRs and CRS typically occur with the first or second infusion, whereas IgE-mediated HSRs require an initial exposure for sensitization. However, the discovery of patients who are presensitized (e.g., to cetuximab via α-gal) and can have anaphylaxis on the first exposure to a mAb has made this point of distinction less useful in specific cases. HSRs can become more severe with each exposure, whereas TIRs usually become successively milder. The severity of CRS may depend on the burden of disease (e.g., lymphocyte count).[38] In clinical practice, aside from a few characteristic features, mechanistically distinct reactions can be clinically indistinguishable. The overlapping presentations may account for some variability in terminology found in the literature. Although immediate treatment of these reactions can be similar, categorization should be attempted to determine how to readminister in the future.

Infusion reactions may utilize uncategorized pathways to complement activation, mast cell degranulation, and pyrogen release. Anti-drug Abs of IgG or IgM isotype have only occasionally been correlated with infusion reactions.[23,39] Although mAb skin testing and/or anti-drug Ab assays can be sought, routine diagnostic testing is generally not standardized or widely available for most mAbs.

Subcutaneously administered mAbs commonly induce local injection-site erythema and induration that is usually not correlated with the development of systemic reactions. Rarely these have been reported to represent delayed T cell–mediated responses.[40]

RITUXIMAB

Rituximab is a mouse-human chimeric mAb directed against CD20 used in several rheumatologic diseases and hematologic malignancies. Reactions to rituximab illustrate that mechanistically distinct adverse reactions may have overlapping manifestations, a phenomenon common to many mAbs.

The majority of recipients experience infusion reactions, most of which are TIRs as described earlier, but CRS and HSRs can also occur. Infusion reactions are more common in patients with hematologic malignancies than in those with rheumatologic disease, approximately 50%–80% and 12%–30%, respectively,[41] on initial infusion and decline with successive administration, possibly related to the decreasing burden of disease. HSRs represent a small subset of all infusion reactions. Most reactions are mild and subside with the interruption of the infusion, but severe reactions have resulted in pulmonary edema, acute respiratory distress syndrome, cardiogenic shock, myocardial infarction, cardiac arrhythmias, and death.[42,43] This spectrum, from mild TIRs to severe CRS, is thought to represent varying degrees of complement-dependent and Ab-dependent cytotoxicity triggered by the binding of rituximab to CD20 on B cells. CRS to rituximab is associated with the release of IL-2, IL-6, and TNF-α, carries a higher mortality, and is more likely to occur in the presence of very high lymphocyte counts in B cell chronic lymphocytic leukemia.[38] Dose fractionation is recommended by the manufacturer for all recipients with additional rate modifications on subsequent infusions for patients with risk factors for CRS (high lymphocyte count, malignancy type). Other management options are discussed later in this chapter.

Rituximab can cause cytopenias apart from the expected B cell depletion. Both early and late rituximab-associated neutropenia are commonly observed, with multiple possible mechanisms including type β HSR with autoantibody formation, autoimmune myelopathy, Fas-dependent neutrophil apoptosis, and hematopoietic lineage competition from reconstituting B cells.[44–48] Rituximab-associated anemia has occasionally been attributed to autoimmune hemolytic anemia, even as it is often used off-label for the treatment of this entity.[49,50] Thrombocytopenia has been associated with TNF-α elevation and complement activation, even in the absence of rituximab-dependent Abs.[51]

Immune complex–mediated reactions, including serum sickness and small-vessel vasculitis, may occur with rituximab treatment.[52–54] Many pulmonary adverse events have been attributed to rituximab, including cases of hypersensitivity pneumonitis.[55]

CETUXIMAB

A particularly curious story emerged from investigations into cetuximab anaphylaxis, revealing connections to delayed mammalian meat anaphylaxis and possibly to tick bite exposures. Cetuximab is a chimeric anti-EGFR mAb used in colorectal cancer and squamous cell cancers of the head and neck. HSRs to cetuximab were noted during clinical trials, occurring during or within 20 min of the first infusion, and were occasionally fatal.[56,57] Pretreatment sera that were prospectively collected from cetuximab-treated subjects revealed anti-cetuximab IgE Abs in 68% of patients who experienced HSRs and 2% of patients who did not.[57] The preexisting anti-cetuximab IgE was found to have specificity against a carbohydrate moiety called galactose-α-1,3-galactose, or "α-gal," located primarily on both heavy chain portions of the Fab fragment of cetuximab.

α-Gal is a blood group substance of nonprimate mammals. Its synthesis requires an enzyme that is nonfunctional in higher primates but active in other mammals, whose erythrocytes and other tissues display α-gal.[58] Some murine cell lines, including that used to produce cetuximab, employ α-gal in posttranslational glycosylation of proteins. Humans and primates normally synthesize IgG and IgM molecules against α-gal, which is a limiting factor in xenotransplantation. α-Gal-specific IgE appears to be responsible for many cetuximab HSRs.

These findings opened up the possibility that α-gal IgE might have broader implications for reactions to glycoproteins from nonprimate mammals. Indeed, a group of patients presenting with anaphylaxis 2–6 h after ingestion of mammalian meat and positive meat skin tests were found to have α-gal IgE.[59] Other patients presenting with idiopathic anaphylaxis, angioedema, or urticaria were found to have α-gal IgE and retrospectively confirmed delayed anaphylaxis to mammalian meat. These patients had all previously tolerated meat without reaction.

The sensitizing event to α-gal has been hypothesized to be a lone star tick bite. An Australian report had previously linked meat allergy to tick bites.[60] Cetuximab reactions, delayed meat allergy in the United States, and α-gal IgE disproportionately occur in the southeastern states, in a distribution pattern matching that of the lone star tick.[56,57] Pre–tick bite and post–tick bite sera have revealed significant increases in α-gal IgE. Commins et al. noted a correlation between lone star tick IgE and α-gal IgE.[61] Many patients with both meat allergy and α-gal IgE report recent tick bites.[62] At the time of this writing, the mechanism of α-gal sensitization has not yet been described.

Panitumumab is a fully human anti-EGFR mAb. It lacks murine sequences and lacks α-gal, and has a much lower rate of TIRs and HSRs than cetuximab. It has been used successfully in patients who have had reactions to cetuximab,[63,64] including a patient with α-gal IgE who had positive skin testing to cetuximab and gelatin.[65] Desensitization to cetuximab can also be an option after an HSR.[64,66,67]

Whether α-gal IgE will generalize to adverse reactions against other α-gal containing substances, including bioprosthetic heart valves, is being explored. The cetuximab story highlights the complexity of mAbs as whole antigens and variables introduced by posttranslational modification to recombinant drugs.

OMALIZUMAB

Omalizumab is a subcutaneously administered humanized anti-IgE mAb and primarily binds free IgE, indirectly reducing the concentrations of high-affinity IgE receptors. It is approved for the treatment of allergic asthma and chronic idiopathic/spontaneous urticaria and has been used in a variety of other allergic disorders and to facilitate allergen desensitization.[68,69] Injection-site reactions were no more common than with placebo.[70] Rarely serum sickness reactions have been reported.[71,72]

Of great concern have been the apparent omalizumab-associated HSRs with anaphylaxis, particularly of a delayed type. Although the rate of anaphylaxis to omalizumab is low (0.1%–0.2%), caution is warranted because approximately 25% of anaphylactic reactions have occurred outside the recommended

observation period (2 h after the first three injections, and 30 min after subsequent injections).[70,73,74] One-third of anaphylactic reactions occurred more than 6 h, with 5% more than 24 h, after injection. Anaphylaxis may occur up to several days after injection, with some reactions occurring a year or more into the omalizumab therapy. About 90% had respiratory compromise, and 15%–30% were considered life-threatening and/or resulted in hospitalization.[75] Moreover, the FDA noted in a subset of patients (8%) an unusually protracted progression of symptoms not resembling biphasic reactions, with some patients needing multiple doses of epinephrine. No specific risk factors for delayed onset or protracted progression of anaphylaxis were identified among the demographic and comorbidity information analyzed, but a subsequent retrospective case-control study found that a self-reported history of anaphylaxis from other causes was more common in patients with omalizumab anaphylaxis than in controls (odds ratio 8.1).[76]

A substantial proportion of reactions (39%) occurred with the first injection, suggesting a preexisting sensitization or a non-IgE-mediated mechanism. The mechanism of omalizumab hypersensitivity remains unknown, and convincing evidence of anti-omalizumab Abs has not yet been published.[70,77] A nonirritating concentration for intradermal skin testing was found to be 1:100,000 (1.25 μg/mL), but this is unusually dilute even for mAb skin testing and the predictive value is unknown.[78] Excipients may play a role in some cases of anaphylaxis, as illustrated in a report of two patients who developed anaphylaxis to omalizumab after more than a year of successful administration and were found to be sensitized to polysorbate.[12] Of patients who experienced anaphylaxis to omalizumab in the previously mentioned case-control study, none of those who underwent skin testing (to omalizumab and excipient alone) and/or anti-omalizumab IgG and IgE testing had positive results.[76] Thus, without reliable confirmatory testing, diagnosis of omalizumab hypersensitivity is based on history alone.

Because of concerns for delayed omalizumab anaphylaxis, it is standard practice in the U.S. that patients who receive omalizumab give informed consent; receive education regarding signs, symptoms, and treatment of anaphylaxis; carry epinephrine autoinjector for 24 h after omalizumab injections; have a health assessment before each injection, including vital signs and measure of lung function; and remain under observation for 2 h after the first three injections and 30 min after subsequent injections.[73,79]

Successful desensitization to omalizumab after an HSR has only been described once, in three patients who had experienced mild to moderate omalizumab reactions, two of whom also had vocal cord dysfunction.[80] Their protocol started with 0.0625 mg, doubling doses every 30 min up to a 40- to 55-mg dose, with mild to moderate reactions but subsequent tolerance occurring in all three patients. Reports of other omalizumab desensitization are sparse, and include an instructive failed desensitization in which a patient with a negative skin prick test developed severe bronchospasm during desensitization, followed by recrudescent reaction symptoms several hours later.[81]

Delayed anaphylaxis to other mAbs is extremely rare. Omalizumab may blunt or block some forms of anaphylaxis (food, venom, idiopathic)[82]; whether omalizumab itself can alter the clinical manifestations of omalizumab hypersensitivity is unknown.

Use of other mAbs for atopic and asthmatic populations may provide some insight into whether this patient population is at a greater risk for such reactions. Mepolizumab and reslizumab are both anti-IL-5 mAbs approved in 2015 and 2016, respectively, for use in eosinophilic asthma. Anaphylaxis was reported in 0% of mepolizumab recipients and 0.3% of reslizumab recipients in clinical trials.[83-86] The three cases of reslizumab-related anaphylaxis occurred shortly after the infusions. More postmarketing data will be needed to draw any conclusions.

MANAGEMENT

Most mAbs should be administered in settings where rescue medications and equipment are immediately available, with trained staff to provide resuscitation. Intravenous fluids, epinephrine, inhaled bronchodilators, antihistamines, corticosteroids, oxygen, airway equipment, and a defibrillator should be on hand. When any reaction occurs, the infusion should be slowed or stopped, assessment and treatment should be provided, and symptoms and treatments should be documented. Observation time after uneventful administration should follow the guidelines standardized for each specific mAb. For mAbs known to cause delayed anaphylaxis, such as omalizumab, patients should carry an epinephrine autoinjector and receive instruction on its use.

If the reaction is mild, then the clinician could try to differentiate between a TIR and an HSR. If it is mild and clearly a TIR, and if the patient is in a setting staffed by personnel well trained in the recognition and treatment of HSRs, then treatment and slowed rechallenge could be attempted: the infusion is paused and the reaction symptomatically treated, often with antihistamines and/or meperidine; when the symptoms have subsided, the infusion can be resumed at a reduced rate. The premedication regimen and infusion rate can be adjusted for subsequent infusions, although TIRs tend to decline in severity with successive administrations. Patients with reactions more suggestive of an HSR, even if mild, can be referred to an allergist to consider skin testing and/or desensitization. In a same-day rechallenge study of patients who received rituximab, most patients who initially had a grade one to two reaction during rituximab infusion were successfully rechallenged at a 50% rate, whereas higher-grade reactions resulted in rechallenge reactions.[87] Such a rechallenge protocol based on the reaction grade likely applies best to mAbs that commonly cause TIRs and only rarely cause HSRs.

If the reaction is moderate to severe, then the clinician should immediately stop the infusion and rapidly treat for anaphylaxis, including placing the patient in a supine position; administering intravenous fluids, intramuscular epinephrine, supplemental oxygen, bronchodilators, and antihistamines; and summoning additional assistance as needed. The role of corticosteroids is adjunctive. Multiple doses of epinephrine may be needed. If further treatment is needed, these patients should either be switched to an alternative agent or referred to an allergist. An acceptable alternative agent should be equally efficacious and tolerable. An allergy evaluation should include risk stratification, with consideration of skin testing and/or desensitization. Even severe TIRs without hypersensitivity may be ameliorated with the use of rapid desensitization regimens.[21]

For other types of delayed HSRs, patients should be treated according to the type and severity of their reactions. Serum sickness–type reactions may benefit from corticosteroid therapy. The risk of developing anti-drug IgG Abs may be reduced by concurrent immunosuppressive agents, and their presence does not appear to be cross-reactive within a class (e.g., patients with anti-infliximab IgG may be treated with adalimumab).[28]

DIAGNOSTIC TESTING

Epicutaneous and intradermal skin testing concentrations have been published for several mAbs and are shown in Table 20.1, but in some cases nonirritating concentrations were not established and none have been validated in large studies.

Tryptase should be drawn if immediate-type hypersensitivity is suspected, 30–120 min after the onset of symptoms.[102] Elevation of tryptase, produced by mast

TABLE 20.1
Published Skin Testing and Desensitization Protocols for mAbs

Monoclonal Antibody	Skin Testing	Desensitization
Adalimumab	Bavbek et al.[88] • SPT: 40 mg/mL • IDT: 0.04, 0.4, 4 mg/mL	Rodriguez-Jimenez et al.[89] Bavbek et al.[90]
Brentuximab		DeVita et al.[91] Story et al.[92]
Cetuximab	Michel et al.[93] • SPT: 1:1 • IDT: 1:100 Madrigal-Burgaleta et al.[94] • SPT: 5 mg/mL • IDT: 0.5, 5 mg/mL	Jerath et al.[66] Saif et al.[64] Hong et al.[67]
Infliximab	Brennan et al.[21] • SPT: 10 mg/mL • IDT: 0.1, 1 mg/mL Madrigal-Burgaleta et al.[94] • SPT: 10 mg/mL • IDT: 1, 10 mg/mL	Brennan et al.[21] Puchner et al.[95] Duburque et al.[96]
Omalizumab	Lieberman et al.[78] • SPT: 125 mg/mL undiluted, 1:10, 1:100, 1:1000 • IDT: 1.25 μg/mL (1:100,000)	Owens et al.[80]
Rituximab	Brennan et al.[21] • SPT: 10 mg/mL • IDT: 0.1, 1 mg/mL Madrigal-Burgaleta et al.[94] • SPT: 10 mg/mL • IDT: 1, 10 mg/mL	Brennan et al.[21] Castells et al.[97]
Tocilizumab	Rocchi et al.[98] • SPT: 0.2, 2, 20 mg/mL • IDT: 0.002, 0.02, 2, 20 mg/mL	Ye et al.[99] Justet et al.[100]
Trastuzumab	Brennan et al.[21] • SPT: 21 mg/mL • IDT: 0.21, 2.1 mg/mL	Brennan et al.[21] Melamed et al.[101]

IDT, intradermal test; *SPT*, skin prick test.

cells, can confirm mast cell–mediated anaphylaxis, although a normal tryptase level does not rule out drug-induced anaphylaxis. Basophil activation tests have been investigated as in vitro assays for mAb anaphylaxis but are not validated for clinical use. Drug-specific IgG and IgE assays are available for some agents and have been subjected to varying degrees of validation.

DESENSITIZATION

Rapid desensitization can be considered for anaphylaxis-type HSRs (immediate or delayed) and severe TIRs. Many desensitization protocols have been published,

some of which are listed in Table 20.1; the largest report of mAb desensitizations employed a three-bag, 12-step protocol that started the infusion at 1/4000 of the final concentration, doubling every 15 min, until achieving a final rate at which the infusion was continued until completion.[21,97] Reactions that occurred during desensitization were mostly mild and generally responsive to antihistamines. Montelukast and aspirin were employed for flushing, and epinephrine and other rescue medications for more severe reactions when indicated. Desensitization protocols have been published for some subcutaneously administered mAbs, including adalimumab.[88–90] Although there are many reports of successful desensitization protocols, the choice of protocol must be tailored to each patient based on reaction history, individual risk of anaphylaxis, and potential benefit.

Desensitization is generally not considered helpful for other types of delayed HSRs, or for other non-HSRs. A history of life-threatening nonanaphylactic HSRs, such as Stevens-Johnson syndrome and DRESS, is a contraindication to rechallenge and desensitization in any form. A patient's candidacy for desensitization should incorporate the baseline health status and comorbidities that could complicate treatment of an HSR. Patients should be cautioned that desensitization produces only a temporary state of tolerance. Although mAbs typically remain in circulation much longer than most small molecule drugs, their variable clearance times do not reliably predict when the mAb can be safely readministered without repeat desensitization in a sensitized patient.

CONCLUSIONS

The scope of therapeutic mAbs will continue to expand, and in the absence of predictive diagnostic testing we will continue to be challenged to understand novel reaction patterns. Although these drugs are intricately engineered and precisely targeted, the associated infusion reactions and HSRs leave much to be discovered. Continued improvements in Ab production methods hold promise for reducing immunogenicity beyond humanization.

ABBREVIATIONS

Ab   Antibody
mAb   Monoclonal antibody
HSR   Hypersensitivity reaction
CRS   Cytokine release syndrome
TIR   Typical infusion reaction

REFERENCES

1. Köhler G, Milstein C. Continuous cultures of fused cells secreting antibody of predefined specificity. *Nature*. 1975;256(5517):495–497.
2. Little M, Kipriyanov S, Le Gall F, Moldenhauer G. Of mice and men: hybridoma and recombinant antibodies. *Immunol Today*. 2000;21(8):364–370.
3. Smith G. Filamentous fusion phage: novel expression vectors that display cloned antigens on the virion surface. *Science*. 1985;228(4705).
4. Bradbury ARM, Sidhu S, Dübel S, McCafferty J. Beyond natural antibodies: the power of in vitro display technologies. *Nat Biotechnol*. 2011;29(3):245–254.
5. World Health Organization. General policies for monoclonal antibodies. In: INN Work Doc 09251. 2009.
6. Niederhuber JE, Armitage JO, Doroshow JH, et al. *Abeloff's Clinical Oncology*. 5th ed. Churchill Livingstone; 2014.
7. Salfeld JG. Isotype selection in antibody engineering. *Nat Biotechnol*. 2007;25(12):1369–1372.
8. Jefferis R. Isotype and glycoform selection for antibody therapeutics. *Arch Biochem Biophys*. 2012;526(2):159–166.
9. Jefferis R. Posttranslational modifications and the immunogenicity of biotherapeutics. *J Immunol Res*. 2016;2016:1–15.
10. Shelley WB, Talanin N, Shelley ED. Polysorbate 80 hypersensitivity. *Lancet*. 1995;345(8960):1312–1313.
11. Steele RH, Limaye S, Cleland B, Chow J, Suranyi MG. Hypersensitivity reactions to the polysorbate contained in recombinant erythropoietin and darbepoietin. *Nephrology*. 2005;10(3):317–320.
12. Price KS, Hamilton RG. Anaphylactoid reactions in two patients after omalizumab administration after successful long-term therapy. *Allergy Asthma Proc*. 2007;28(3):313–319.
13. Park BK, Sanderson JP, Naisbitt DJ. Drugs as haptens, antigens, and immunogens. In: *Drug Hypersensitivity*. Basel: KARGER; 2007:55–65.
14. Pichler WJ, Campi P. Adverse side effects to biological agents. In: *Drug Hypersensitivity*. Basel: Karger; 2007:151–165.
15. Pichler WJ. Adverse side-effects to biological agents. *Allergy*. 2006;61(8):912–920.
16. Suntharalingam G, Perry MR, Ward S, et al. Cytokine storm in a phase 1 trial of the anti-CD28 monoclonal antibody TGN1412. *N Engl J Med*. 2006;355(10):1018–1028.
17. Vasquez EM, Fabrega AJ, Pollak R. OKT3-induced cytokine-release syndrome: occurrence beyond the second dose and association with rejection severity. *Transplant Proc*. 1995;27(1):873–874.
18. Wing M. Monoclonal antibody first dose cytokine release syndromes - mechanisms and prediction. *J Immunotoxicol*. 2008;5(1):11–15.
19. Bugelski PJ, Achuthanandam R, Capocasale RJ, Treacy G, Bouman-Thio E. Monoclonal antibody-induced cytokine-release syndrome. *Expert Rev Clin Immunol*. 2009;5(5):499–521.
20. Stubenrauch K, Wessels U, Birnboeck H, Ramirez F, Jahreis A, Schleypen J. Subset analysis of patients experiencing clinical events of a potentially immunogenic nature in the pivotal clinical trials of tocilizumab for rheumatoid arthritis: Evaluation of an antidrug antibody ELISA using clinical adverse event-driven immunogenicity testing. *Clin Ther*. 2010;32(9):1597–1609.
21. Brennan PJ, Rodriguez Bouza T, Hsu FI, Sloane DE, Castells MC. Hypersensitivity reactions to mAbs: 105 desensitizations in 23 patients, from evaluation to treatment. *J Allergy Clin Immunol*. 2009;124(6):1259–1266.

22. Muñoz-Cano R, Carnés J, Sanchez-Lopez J, et al. Biological agents: new drugs, old problems. *J Allergy Clin Immunol.* 2010;126(2):394–395.

23. Vultaggio A, Matucci A, Nencini F, et al. Anti-infliximab IgE and non-IgE antibodies and induction of infusion-related severe anaphylactic reactions. *Allergy.* 2010;65(5):657–661.

24. Georgitis JW, Browning MC, Steiner D, Lorentz WB. Anaphylaxis and desensitization to the murine monoclonal antibody used for renal graft rejection. *Ann Allergy.* 1991;66(4):343–347.

25. Proctor L, Renzulli B, Warren S, Brecher ME. Transfusion medicine illustrated. Monoclonal antibody-stimulated serum sickness. *Transfusion.* 2004;44(7):955.

26. Krishna M, Nadler SG. Immunogenicity to biotherapeutics – the role of anti-drug immune complexes. *Front Immunol.* 2016;7:21.

27. Han PD, Cohen RD. Managing immunogenic responses to infliximab: treatment implications for patients with Crohn's disease. *Drugs.* 2004;64(16):1767–1777.

28. Baert F, Noman M, Vermeire S, et al. Influence of immunogenicity on the long-term efficacy of infliximab in Crohn's disease. *N Engl J Med.* 2003;348(7):601–608.

29. Thomas SS, Borazan N, Barroso N, et al. Comparative immunogenicity of TNF inhibitors: impact on clinical efficacy and tolerability in the management of autoimmune diseases. A systematic review and meta-analysis. *BioDrugs.* 2015;29(4):241–258.

30. Abdullah SE, Haigentz M, Piperdi B. Dermatologic toxicities from monoclonal antibodies and tyrosine kinase inhibitors against EGFR: pathophysiology and management. *Chemother Res Pract.* 2012;2012:1–10.

31. González N, Ratner D. Novel melanoma therapies and their side effects. *Cutis.* 2016;97(6):426–428.

32. Naidoo J, Page DB, Li BT, et al. Toxicities of the anti-PD-1 and anti-PD-L1 immune checkpoint antibodies. *Ann Oncol.* September 2015:mdv383.

33. Kyllo RL, Parker MK, Rosman I, Musiek AC. Ipilimumab-associated Sweet syndrome in a patient with high-risk melanoma. *J Am Acad Dermatol.* 2014;70(4):e85–e86.

34. Phan GQ, Yang JC, Sherry RM, et al. Cancer regression and autoimmunity induced by cytotoxic T lymphocyte-associated antigen 4 blockade in patients with metastatic melanoma. *Proc Natl Acad Sci USA.* 2003;100(14):8372–8377.

35. Voskens CJ, Goldinger SM, Loquai C, et al. The price of tumor control: an analysis of rare side effects of anti-CTLA-4 therapy in metastatic melanoma from the ipilimumab network. In: Soyer HP, ed. *PLoS One.* 2013;8(1):e53745.

36. Pathria M, Mundi J, Trufant J. A case of Stevens–Johnson syndrome in a patient on ipilimumab. *Int J Case Rep Images.* 2016;7(5):300.

37. Peréz-Soler R, Saltz L. Cutaneous adverse effects with HER1/EGFR-targeted agents: is there a silver lining? *J Clin Oncol.* 2005;23(22):5235–5246.

38. Winkler U, Jensen M, Manzke O, Schulz H, Diehl V, Engert A. Cytokine-release syndrome in patients with B-cell chronic lymphocytic leukemia and high lymphocyte counts after treatment with an anti-CD20 monoclonal antibody (rituximab, IDEC-C2B8). *Blood.* 1999;94(7):2217–2224.

39. van Schie KA, Wolbink G-J, Rispens T. Cross-reactive and pre-existing antibodies to therapeutic antibodies—effects on treatment and immunogenicity. *mAbs.* 2015;7(4):662–671.

40. Torres MJ, Chaves P, Doña I, et al. T-cell involvement in delayed-type hypersensitivity reactions to infliximab. *J Allergy Clin Immunol.* 2011;128(6):1365–1367.e1.

41. *Rituxan (Rituximab) Package Insert.* ; 2011. Biogen Idec Inc., MA, USA, and Genentech Inc., CA, USA.

42. Maloney DG, Grillo-López AJ, White CA, et al. IDEC-C2B8 (Rituximab) anti-CD20 monoclonal antibody therapy in patients with relapsed low-grade non-Hodgkin's lymphoma. *Blood.* 1997;90(6):2188–2195.

43. Grillo-López AJ, White CA, Varns C, et al. Overview of the clinical development of rituximab: first monoclonal antibody approved for the treatment of lymphoma. *Semin Oncol.* 1999;26(5 Suppl. 14):66–73.

44. Voog E, Morschhauser F, Solal-Céligny P. Neutropenia in patients treated with rituximab. *N Engl J Med.* 2003;348(26). 2691–2694.4.

45. Dunleavy K, Tay K, Wilson WH. Rituximab-associated neutropenia. *Semin Hematol.* 2010;47(2):180–186.

46. Liu JH, Wei S, Lamy T, et al. Chronic neutropenia mediated by fas ligand. *Blood.* 2000;95(10):3219–3222.

47. Terrier B, Ittah M, Tourneur L, et al. Late-onset neutropenia following rituximab results from a hematopoietic lineage competition due to an excessive BAFF-induced B-cell recovery. *Haematologica.* 2007;92(2):e20–e23.

48. Papadaki T, Stamatopoulos K, Anagnostopoulos A, Fassas A. Rituximab-associated immune myelopathy. *Blood.* 2003;102(4).

49. Cattaneo C, Spedini P, Casari S, et al. Delayed-onset peripheral blood cytopenia after rituximab: frequency and risk factor assessment in a consecutive series of 77 treatments. *Leuk Lymphoma.* 2006;47(6):1013–1017.

50. Jourdan E, Topart D, Richard B, Jourdan J, Sotto A. Severe autoimmune hemolytic anemia following rituximab therapy in a patient with a lymphoproliferative disorder. *Leuk Lymphoma.* 2003;44(5):889–890.

51. Ram R, Bonstein L, Gafter-Gvili A, Ben-Bassat I, Shpilberg O, Raanani P. Rituximab-associated acute thrombocytopenia: an under-diagnosed phenomenon. *Am J Hematol.* 2009;84(4):247–250.

52. Karmacharya P, Poudel DR, Pathak R, et al. Rituximab-induced serum sickness: a systematic review. *Semin Arthritis Rheum.* 2015;45(3):334–340.

53. Dereure O, Navarro R, Rossi JF, Guilhou JJ. Rituximab-induced vasculitis. *Dermatology.* 2001;203(1):83–84.

54. Kim MJ, Kim HO, Kim HY, Park YM. Rituximab-induced vasculitis: a case report and review of the medical published work. *J Dermatol.* 2009;36(5):284–287.

55. Lioté H, Lioté F, Séroussi B, Mayaud C, Cadranel J. Rituximab-induced lung disease: a systematic literature review. *Eur Respir J.* 2010;35(3):681–687.

56. O'Neil BH, Allen R, Spigel DR, et al. High incidence of cetuximab-related infusion reactions in Tennessee and North Carolina and the association with atopic history. *J Clin Oncol.* 2007;25(24):3644–3648.

57. Chung CH, Mirakhur B, Chan E, et al. Cetuximab-induced anaphylaxis and IgE specific for galactose-α-1,3-galactose. *N Engl J Med.* 2008;358(11):1109–1117.

58. Macher BA, Galili U. The Galalpha1,3Galbeta1,4GlcNAc-R (alpha-Gal) epitope: a carbohydrate of unique evolution and clinical relevance. *Biochim Biophys Acta.* 2008;1780(2):75–88.

59. Commins SP, Satinover SM, Hosen J, et al. Delayed anaphylaxis, angioedema, or urticaria after consumption of red meat in patients with IgE antibodies specific for galactose-α-1,3-galactose. *J Allergy Clin Immunol.* 2009;123(2):426–433.e2.

60. Van Nunen SA, O'Connor KS, Clarke LR, Boyle RX, Fernando SL. An association between tick bite reactions and red meat allergy in humans. *Med J Aust.* 2009;190(9):510–511.

61. Commins SP, James HR, Kelly LA, et al. The relevance of tick bites to the production of IgE antibodies to the mammalian oligosaccharide galactose-α-1,3-galactose. *J Allergy Clin Immunol.* 2011;127(5):1286–1293.e6.

62. Kennedy JL, Stallings AP, Platts-Mills TAE, et al. Galactose-α-1,3-galactose and delayed anaphylaxis, angioedema, and urticaria in children. *Pediatrics.* 2013;131(5):e1545–e1552.

63. Langerak A, River G, Mitchell E, Cheema P, Shing M. Panitumumab monotherapy in patients with metastatic colorectal cancer and cetuximab infusion reactions: a series of four case reports. *Clin Colorectal Cancer.* 2009;8(1):49–54.

64. Saif MW, Peccerillo J, Potter V. Successful re-challenge with panitumumab in patients who developed hypersensitivity reactions to cetuximab: report of three cases and review of literature. *Cancer Chemother Pharmacol.* 2009;63(6):1017–1022.

65. Caponetto P, Biedermann T, Yazdi AS, Fischer J. Panitumumab: a safe option for oncologic patients sensitized to galactose-α-1,3-galactose. *J Allergy Clin Immunol Pract.* 2015;3(6):982–983.

66. Jerath MR, Kwan M, Kannarkat M, et al. A desensitization protocol for the mAb cetuximab. *J Allergy Clin Immunol.* 2009;123(1):260–262.

67. Hong DI, Bankova L, Cahill KN, Kyin T, Castells MC. Allergy to monoclonal antibodies: cutting-edge desensitization methods for cutting-edge therapies. *Expert Rev Clin Immunol.* 2012;8(1):43–54.

68. Wood RA, Kim JS, Lindblad R, et al. A randomized, double-blind, placebo-controlled study of omalizumab combined with oral immunotherapy for the treatment of cow's milk allergy. *J Allergy Clin Immunol.* 2016;137(4). 1103–1110.e11.

69. Massanari M, Nelson H, Casale T, et al. Effect of pretreatment with omalizumab on the tolerability of specific immunotherapy in allergic asthma. *J Allergy Clin Immunol.* 2010;125(2):383–389.

70. Corren J, Casale TB, Lanier B, Buhl R, Holgate S, Jimenez P. Safety and tolerability of omalizumab. *Clin Exp Allergy.* 2009;39(6):788–797.

71. Dreyfus DH, Randolph CC. Characterization of an anaphylactoid reaction to omalizumab. *Ann Allergy Asthma Immunol.* 2006;96(4):624–627.

72. Pilette C, Coppens N, Houssiau FA, Rodenstein DO. Severe serum sickness-like syndrome after omalizumab therapy for asthma. *J Allergy Clin Immunol.* 2007;120(4):972–973.

73. Cox L, Platts-Mills TAE, Finegold I, et al. American Academy of Allergy, Asthma & Immunology/American College of Allergy, Asthma and Immunology Joint Task Force Report on omalizumab-associated anaphylaxis. *J Allergy Clin Immunol.* 2007;120(6):1373–1377.

74. Lin RY, Rodriguez-Baez G, Bhargave GA. Omalizumab-associated anaphylactic reactions reported between January 2007 and June 2008. *Ann Allergy Asthma Immunol.* 2009;103(5):442–445.

75. Limb SL, Starke PR, Lee CE, Chowdhury BA. Delayed onset and protracted progression of anaphylaxis after omalizumab administration in patients with asthma. *J Allergy Clin Immunol.* 2007;120(6):1378–1381.

76. Lieberman PL, Umetsu DT, Carrigan GJ, Rahmaoui A. Anaphylactic reactions associated with omalizumab administration: analysis of a case-control study. *J Allergy Clin Immunol.* 2016;138(3):913–915.e2.

77. Baker DL, Nakamura GR, Lowman HB, Fischer SK. Evaluation of IgE antibodies to omalizumab (Xolair®) and their potential correlation to anaphylaxis. *AAPS J.* 2016;18(1):115–123.

78. Lieberman P, Rahmaoui A, Wong DA. The safety and interpretability of skin tests with omalizumab. *Ann Allergy Asthma Immunol.* 2010;105(6):493–495.

79. Cox L, Lieberman P, Wallace D, et al. American Academy of Allergy, Asthma & Immunology/American College of Allergy, Asthma & Immunology Omalizumab-Associated Anaphylaxis Joint Task Force follow-up report. *J Allergy Clin Immunol.* 2011;128(1):210–212.

80. Owens G, Petrov A. Successful desensitization of three patients with hypersensitivity reactions to omalizumab. *Curr Drug Saf.* 2011;6(5):339–342.

81. Paranjpe P, Hilton K, Khan D. Failure of omalizumab desensitization resulting in anaphylaxis in a patient with severe asthma. *Ann Allergy Asthma Immunol.* 2009. Conference(103): A124[abstract].

82. Lieberman JA, Chehade M. Use of omalizumab in the treatment of food allergy and anaphylaxis. *Curr Allergy Asthma Rep.* 2013;13(1):78–84.

83. Pavord ID, Korn S, Howarth P, et al. Mepolizumab for severe eosinophilic asthma (DREAM): a multicentre, double-blind, placebo-controlled trial. *Lancet.* 2012;380(9842):651–659.

84. Ortega HG, Liu MC, Pavord ID, et al. Mepolizumab treatment in patients with severe eosinophilic asthma. *N Engl J Med.* 2014;371(13):1198–1207.

85. Castro M, Mathur S, Hargreave F, et al. Reslizumab for poorly controlled, eosinophilic asthma: a randomized, placebo-controlled study. *Am J Respir Crit Care Med.* 2011;184(10):1125–1132.

86. Castro M, Zangrilli J, Wechsler ME, et al. Reslizumab for inadequately controlled asthma with elevated blood eosinophil counts: results from two multicentre, parallel, double-blind, randomised, placebo-controlled, phase 3 trials. *Lancet Respir Med.* 2015;3(5):355–366.

87. Levin AS, Otani IM, Lax T, Hochberg E, Banerji A. Reactions to rituximab in an outpatient infusion center: a 5-year review. *J Allergy Clin Immunol Pract.* 2016;5(1):107–113.

88. Bavbek S, Ataman Ş., Akıncı A, Castells M. Rapid subcutaneous desensitization for the management of local and systemic hypersensitivity reactions to etanercept and adalimumab in 12 patients. *J Allergy Clin Immunol Pract.* 2015;3(4):629–632.

89. Rodríguez-Jiménez B, Domínguez-Ortega J, González-Herrada C, Kindelan-Recarte C, Loribo-Bueno P, Garrido-Peño N. Successful adalimumab desensitization after generalized urticaria and rhinitis. *J Investig Allergol Clin Immunol.* 2009;19(3):246–247.

90. Bavbek S, Ataman Ş., Bankova L, Castells M. Injection site reaction to adalimumab: positive skin test and successful rapid desensitisation. *Allergol Immunopathol (Madr).* 2013;41(3):204–206.

91. DeVita MD, Evens AM, Rosen ST, Greenberger PA, Petrich AM. Multiple successful desensitizations to brentuximab vedotin: a case report and literature review. *J Natl Compr Canc Netw.* 2014;12(4):465–471.

92. Story SK, Petrov AA, Geskin LJ. Successful desensitization to brentuximab vedotin after hypersensitivity reaction. *J Drugs Dermatol.* 2014;13(6):749–751.

93. Michel S, Scherer K, Heijnen IAFM, Bircher AJ. Skin prick test and basophil reactivity to cetuximab in patients with IgE to alpha-gal and allergy to red meat. *Allergy.* 2014;69(3):403–405.

94. Madrigal-Burgaleta R, Berges-Gimeno MP, Angel-Pereira D, et al. Hypersensitivity and desensitization to antineoplastic agents: outcomes of 189 procedures with a new short protocol and novel diagnostic tools assessment. *Allergy.* 2013;68(7):853–861.

95. Puchner TC, Kugathasan S, Kelly KJ, Binion DG. Successful desensitization and therapeutic use of infliximab in adult and pediatric Crohn's disease patients with prior anaphylactic reaction. *Inflamm Bowel Dis.* 2001;7(1):34–37.

96. Duburque C, Lelong J, Iacob R, et al. Successful induction of tolerance to infliximab in patients with Crohn's disease and prior severe infusion reactions. *Aliment Pharmacol Ther.* 2006;24(5):851–858.

97. Castells MC, Tennant NM, Sloane DE, et al. Hypersensitivity reactions to chemotherapy: outcomes and safety of rapid desensitization in 413 cases. *J Allergy Clin Immunol.* 2008;122(3):574–580.

98. Rocchi V, Puxeddu I, Cataldo G, et al. Hypersensitivity reactions to tocilizumab: role of skin tests in diagnosis. *Rheumatology.* 2014;53(8):1527–1529.

99. Ye W, Fifield M, Mayhew A, Nasser S, Östör A. Successful tocilizumab desensitization in an adult with juvenile idiopathic arthritis. *Scand J Rheumatol.* 2016;45(1):75–76.

100. Justet A, Neukirch C, Poubeau P, et al. Successful rapid tocilizumab desensitization in a patient with Still disease. *J Allergy Clin Immunol Pract.* 2014;2(5):631–632.

101. Melamed J, Stahlman JE. Rapid desensitization and rush immunotherapy to trastuzumab (Herceptin). *J Allergy Clin Immunol.* 2002;110(5):813–814.

102. Schwartz LB. Diagnostic value of tryptase in anaphylaxis and mastocytosis. *Immunol Allergy Clin North Am.* 2006;26(3):451–463.

CHAPTER 21

Perioperative Allergy

LENE H. GARVEY, MD, PHD

INTRODUCTION

Allergic reactions occurring in the perioperative setting pose a great challenge for both allergists, who were given the task of subsequent allergy investigations, and for attending anesthetists. Reactions are rare, but presentation is often very dramatic with life-threatening symptoms. Investigation of these reactions is thus very complicated and not always embarked on if the specialized knowledge is not available.[1] In such cases the patient may be put at great risk of developing another, and perhaps more severe, allergic reaction on reexposure to the culprit during subsequent anesthesia and surgery.

In the perioperative setting, there are numerous nonallergic causes of symptoms mimicking allergic reactions, because of the effects of potent drugs, airway instrumentation, and the surgical procedure itself.[2] Also, multiple simultaneous drug administrations and other exposures, some of which are not even recorded on the charts, make identifying the culprit difficult.[3] Subsequent allergy investigations should aim at establishing the likely mechanism behind the reaction, and in cases of an allergic mechanism, the culprit should be identified. Patients with suspected perioperative allergic reactions are probably the most complex ones in the field of drug allergy, and a successful outcome of investigations is, in most cases, dependent on close collaboration between allergists and anesthesiologists.

INCIDENCE

The exact incidence of perioperative allergic reactions is difficult to determine because of the relative rarity of events and differences in definitions and investigations used in different centers.[3,4] From retrospective surveys, the incidence is quoted to range between 1:1250 and 1:18,600 anesthetic procedures.[4] However, a much higher incidence seems to be quoted in prospective studies with 1:3180 from France,[5] 1:1480 from Spain,[6] and 1:353 in a two-week "snapshot survey" from the United Kingdom (UK).[7]

Mortality from perioperative anaphylaxis was quoted to be 4% in a study of fatalities from neuromuscular blocking agents (NMBAs) in France.[8] This is in contrast to findings in an Australian study of all causes of perioperative allergic reactions reporting fatality rates to be very low and in the range of 0%–1.4%.[9] Because of the rare occurrence of these reactions and differences in reporting, the exact mortality is difficult to determine.

DEFINITION OF TERMS AND CLASSIFICATION

Many different terms such as allergic, anaphylactic, anaphylactoid, pseudoallergic, and histaminoid have been used in the literature, reflecting differences in the definition and the underlying mechanisms.

In an attempt to standardize definitions within the field of allergy, a proposal was made by the World Allergy Organization (WAO) that the overall term "hypersensitivity reaction" should be used about all suspected reactions. According to the suggested classification, hypersensitivity reactions are divided into allergic and nonallergic, and the allergic hypersensitivity reactions are further divided into IgE mediated and non-IgE mediated. Anaphylaxis is to be used as an overall term for severe, generalized, and life-threatening reactions, which also subdivides into IgE mediated and non-IgE mediated.[10] These suggestions were recently endorsed in an international consensus (ICON) on drug allergy,[11] where it was also suggested that reactions were classified into immediate and nonimmediate related to the timing of symptom onset. For the purpose of this review, only immediate-type reactions will be discussed, and as the majority of reactions discussed will have an underlying allergic mechanism, the term "allergic reaction" will be used as an overall term, and "anaphylaxis" will be used when discussing cases of severe life-threatening reactions.

The severity of perioperative allergic reactions varies from mild reactions with only skin symptoms to severe life-threatening reactions fulfilling the criteria for anaphylaxis with multiorgan involvement and ultimately cardiac arrest. In the literature, several different systems are used to classify severity. Most guidelines use a system based on the original classification system first suggested by Ring and Messmer for classifying reactions to colloids in 1977.[12–14]

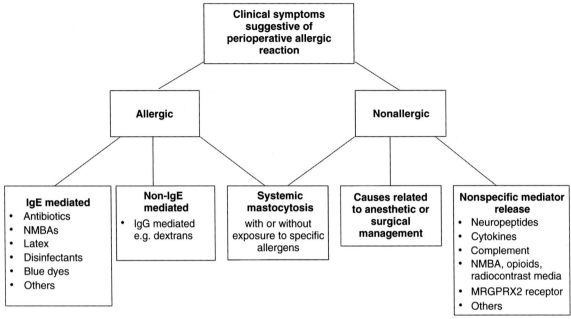

FIG. 21.1 Overview of possible mechanisms behind suspected perioperative allergic reactions.

MECHANISMS AND DIFFERENTIAL DIAGNOSES

While the above classification of drug hypersensitivity reactions proposed by WAO and ICON is useful when investigating cases of suspected allergy to single drugs, it needs modification before it can be applied to the very complex perioperative setting of multiple drug administrations and exposures (see Fig. 21.1). Clinically, it is not usually possible to distinguish between the underlying mechanisms because the symptomatology is similar.

The most important aim of allergy investigation of suspected perioperative allergic reactions is to confirm or rule out an IgE-mediated mechanism. Reexposure to the culprit allergen could cause a life-threatening reaction because of the recognition by the immune system of preformed specific IgE antibodies and the resulting mast cell degranulation with the release of mediators accounting for the clinical symptoms. Rates of confirmed IgE-mediated reactions reported from centers that carry out these specialized investigations vary considerably. The majority of centers report confirming an IgE-mediated mechanism in 40%–70% of investigated patients, while a few centers report very low rates of 10%–20%, and some report very high rates of >80% of investigated patients.[4] There is a tendency to higher rates of confirmed IgE-mediated reactions in countries with high rates of reactions to NMBAs.[2] However, these

differences are likely to be multifactorial and related to differences in drug use, sensitization patterns, referral patterns, and performance and interpretation of tests used in the investigations.[2–4]

The allergic, but non-IgE-mediated reactions are not so common but include reactions to dextrans, which have been confirmed to have an IgG-mediated mechanism.[15]

There are multiple nonallergic mechanisms causing reactions to drugs in the perioperative setting, most of which may be related to direct activation of mast cells, leading to mediator release and clinical symptoms. Different mechanisms have been suggested to cause non-IgE-mediated activation of the mast cell such as activation via the complement system or direct activation via neuropeptides and cytokines[16] or by certain drugs groups with a propensity for direct histamine release such as opioids,[17] radiocontrast media, and NMBAs. Recently, it has been suggested that certain drugs, e.g., NMBAs and ciprofloxacin, may activate mast cells via the human G protein–coupled receptor because a similar receptor in mice can be activated in this manner.[16,18]

A proportion of suspected perioperative allergic reactions may be concluded to be due to nonallergic differential diagnoses related to effects of anesthetic or surgical management and not to specific drugs. When investigations do not lead to a conclusion about a

TABLE 21.1
Nonallergic Causes of Symptoms Mimicking Perioperative Allergic Reactions

ISOLATED ANGIOEDEMA OR LARYNGEAL/PHARYNGEAL EDEMA AND NORMAL SERUM TRYPTASE

Edema due to handling of difficult airway

Contact allergy to perioperative exposures (delayed onset 8–12 h postoperative)

ACE inhibitor–elicited angioedema (onset 1–8 h after surgery)

Subcutanous emphysema

Hereditary angioedema

ISOLATED BRONCHOSPASM AND NORMAL SERUM TRYPTASE

Undiagnosed, untreated, or insufficiently treated asthma

Irritation from misplaced endotracheal tube, superficial/light anesthesia

Hyperreactive airways due to, e.g., Viral infections, smoking

ISOLATED HYPOTENSION AND NORMAL SERUM TRYPTASE

Major bleeding

Relative overdose of anesthetic agents

Vasodilatory effect of neuroaxial blockade (spinal/epidural)

Treatment with tricyclic antidepressants

Amniotic fluid embolism/pulmonary embolism

Bone cement implantation syndrome

Other types of shock

ISOLATED SKIN SYMPTOMS AND NORMAL SERUM TRYPTASE

Uriticaria or angioedema in patients with existing chronic urticaria or angioedema

Nonspecific histamine release causing transient rash, flushing, itching

COMBINATION OF TACHYCARDIA, FLUSHING, HYPOTENSION, AND NORMAL SERUM TRYPTASE

Nonspecific histamine release

Relative overdose of oxytocin

Mesenteric traction syndrome

specific allergy, the involvement of an anesthesiologist is valuable for a rereview of the charts and suggestions of possible alternatives to an allergic mechanism.[2,3] Often symptoms from a single organ system only, without elevation in serum tryptase at the time of reaction, may have an alternative explanation, e.g., isolated pharyngeal/laryngeal edema resulting from the handling of a difficult airway; isolated bronchospasm due to intubation in patients with undiagnosed or poorly treated asthma, or isolated hypotension due to bleeding, relative hypovolemia, or effects of neuroaxial blockade. Other rarer causes of nonallergic reactions have been described, such as profound isolated hypotension due to treatment with tricyclic antidepressants or bone cement implantation syndrome. A combination of tachycardia, flushing, and hypotension may be seen in

cases of relative overdose of oxytocin and mesenteric traction syndrome.[2] A list of nonallergic differential diagnoses can be seen in Table 21.1.

Lastly, systemic mastocytosis is a very rare, but probably underdiagnosed explanation for some cases of suspected perioperative allergic reactions. This should be suspected in patients who present with perioperative anaphylaxis, with or without elevated tryptase at the time of reaction, where subsequent investigation reveals no specific allergen.[3,19] An elevated baseline serum tryptase may be found, but systemic mastocytosis has been described with normal baseline tryptase values.[20] It should be remembered that mastocytosis patients can also have specific allergies, and thus allergy investigations should be performed in patients with known mastocytosis who present with perioperative allergy.[21]

CLINICAL PRESENTATION AND MANAGEMENT IN THE OPERATING ROOM

In large surveys, skin symptoms have been reported to be present in 80% of cases,[22] but in practice sterile drapes cause skin symptoms to be overlooked in many cases. Also, in cases of very profound hypotension, the skin symptoms may only appear once adequate treatment has resulted in a restored circulation.[23]

In patients with isolated skin symptoms, the nature of the symptoms may help determine whether further investigation is indicated. Widespread or generalized urticaria may be a relevant symptom of an allergic reaction, and investigation should be considered.[24,25]

On the other hand, isolated itch and localized or very transient (few minutes) rashes related to injection of known histamine-releasing substances such as NMBAs and opioids do not require further investigation.[13] Repeated mild reactions of this type occur in some patients, most likely related to nonspecific histamine release. Usually, pretreatment with oral antihistamines for a few days before subsequent surgery is effective in preventing or minimizing such symptoms.[2,26]

Respiratory symptoms can be related to both upper and lower airways. Angioedema is rarely an allergic symptom when presenting with no associated symptoms.[27] However, there are several important differential diagnoses to perioperative allergy in patients with isolated angioedema (see Table 21.1). One cause that must not be overlooked is angioedema triggered by ACE inhibitor drugs. These patients may develop very severe and life-threatening angioedema in the perioperative setting or several hours later.[28] As the mechanism is related to alterations in bradykinin metabolism, treatments for allergy are largely ineffective,[29,30] and specific bradykinin receptor antagonists may be required.[31]

Symptoms from the lower airways present with increased peak airway pressures, decreased oxygen saturation, and wheeze on auscultation. Patients with hyperreactive airways due to asthma, chronic obstructive airways disease, smoking, or concurrent viral infections are more likely to develop lower airway symptoms during an allergic reaction. Isolated lower airway symptoms have been shown to be more likely to be caused by an allergic reaction if they are severe, long-lasting, and occurring before airway instrumentation.[32]

Cardiovascular symptoms are usually changes in heart rate, most commonly tachycardia, and hypotension, which may evolve very rapidly. Hypotension can be very profound and resistant to the usual methods to increase blood pressure such as ephedrine, phenylephrine, and other vasopressors.[26] Perioperative allergic reactions may present with symptoms from one or more organ systems, and the rate of reactions with circulatory compromise is relatively high, quoted to be 45% of investigated reactions in one Danish reference center.[33] However, even if several organ systems are involved, the diagnosis can be difficult to make for the attending anesthetists. Anesthetic drugs and procedures in themselves may induce most of the mentioned symptoms, and skin symptoms are rarely visible to aid the diagnosis. In addition, because of the rare occurrence of perioperative allergic reactions, anesthetists may not consider the diagnosis or be updated on the correct management. This has led to a suggestion that cases of perioperative circulatory compromise, not responding to the usual management, should be treated with epinephrine in small intravenous bolus doses of 5–10 μg titrated to effect.[33] This will ensure that adequate circulation is restored while the diagnostic process is undertaken. The perioperative setting is ideal for this management as patients are continually monitored and observed. In addition, anesthetic personnel should have the necessary training in administering intravenous epinephrine. In contrast to most guidelines for anaphylaxis where intramuscular epinephrine is the treatment of choice, current guidelines for the treatment of perioperative anaphylaxis recommend intravenous epinephrine in small bolus doses of 10–50 μg titrated to effect.[13,26,34] First-line treatment with epinephrine should be supplemented with adequate volume expansion, and once the patient is stabilized, secondary treatment with antihistamines and steroids can be administered.[13,26]

ALLERGY EVALUATION

Because of the complexity of suspected perioperative allergic reactions, investigations should ideally be carried out in specialist centers with relevant expertise from both allergy and anesthesiology. Before evaluation, it is imperative to gather as much relevant information as possible. Ideally, direct discussions with the anesthetic personnel present during the reaction will give the most correct information on timing of administered drugs and other exposures, some of which may not be documented.[3] Information on symptoms, treatment and treatment response, and a serum tryptase value from the time of reaction may help decide if further investigations are needed. In some cases the anesthesiologist may offer alternative explanations, which, together with a correctly timed normal serum tryptase sample, may be enough evidence to conclude that the mechanism was nonallergic. However, such decisions need to be made by specialists with suitable experience in the field.

During planning of investigations, all drugs and other exposures administered before the reaction should be considered.[2] This includes all exposures that are not given intravenously such as latex, disinfectants, sterilizing agents, dyes, hemostatic agents, gels and sprays, as reactions to excipients in these substances have been described.[3,35,36] There is no evidence-based guideline with recommendations on which drugs should be tested, based on timing alone, and the criteria for selection of drugs for testing vary between centers. Some centers test all patients with common exposures such as latex, disinfectants (e.g. chlorhexidine), and sterilizing agents (e.g. ethylene oxide),[37–39] in addition to specific drugs suspected in individual cases. This is done on the presumption that perioperative exposure to these substances is highly likely, even if it is not documented on the charts.[3,39] Other centers test suspected drugs and, in addition, certain drug groups commonly implicated, such as NMBAs, to rule out cross-reactivity within these specific groups.[14,22]

The timing of a reaction to a certain allergen is dependent on the route of administration as shown in a study of fatal anaphylaxis.[40] The study showed that reactions to IV exposures occurred within few minutes, subcutaneous exposure led to reactions within 15 min, and oral exposures within 30 min. In the perioperative setting, there are multiple exposures via different routes occurring simultaneously. In this setting the timing of administration of specific drugs can help determine which drugs are more likely but cannot be used to positively confirm the culprit without investigation.[41,42]

Once the list of possible culprits has been decided, the investigations of suspected perioperative allergic reactions follow the same principles as drug allergy investigations in general. The main aim of investigations is to confirm or rule out an IgE-mediated allergy to one or more specific culprit drugs.

The commonly used tests comprise in vitro tests: serum tryptase (at the time of reaction and a later baseline sample), specific IgE tests, and in some centers additional tests such as histamine release tests or basophil activation tests (BATs). The in vivo tests are skin tests (skin prick tests [SPTs] and intradermal tests [IDTs]) considered the reference standard in perioperative allergy investigation in the literature. Provocation tests, which are usually considered the reference standard in allergy, have traditionally not been used in perioperative allergy because of the potent effect (e.g., paralysis) of several of the drug groups involved.

For many of the drugs used in the perioperative setting, experience with testing is limited and no single test has a 100% sensitivity or specificity. False-negative testing is potentially hazardous for the patients because of the risk of reexposure, whereas false-positive testing limits the choice for future anesthesia, which may seem acceptable in comparison. However, if false-positive testing leads to the wrong conclusions being made, and the real allergen not being tested, the patient is still at the risk of reexposure.

To avoid these pitfalls, systematic testing of all potential culprits should be carried out, and routine testing of drugs the patient was not exposed to should be avoided.[43] In the absence of drug provocation, the risk of false-positive testing is reduced if several different test modalities are used. It has been suggested that a positive result in two or more test modalities is one way of achieving a high sensitivity in perioperative allergy testing.[39,44]

Serum Tryptase

The baseline level of serum tryptase consists of pro-α-tryptase and pro-β-tryptase, continuously secreted from resting mast cells.[45] Mature β-tryptase is present inside granules in mast cells and only released during mast cell activation (e.g., during IgE-mediated anaphylaxis). A serum sample taken at the time of a suspected allergic reaction therefore consists of the sum of baseline tryptase and β-tryptase released during the reaction. As baseline levels have been shown to exhibit very little variation in individual subjects, a relevant increase in tryptase may occur within the normal reference range.[46,47] Therefore, a comparison should always be made with a baseline level measured at a later date (e.g., at the time of allergy investigation).[13] An algorithm for this has been proposed recently suggesting that a clinically relevant increase in serum tryptase at the time of reaction exceeds $2 + 1.2 \times$ baseline tryptase level.[48] Anaphylaxis does not always lead to an increase in serum tryptase, and allergy investigations should still be considered if the clinical reaction is suggestive of anaphylaxis. As serum tryptase peaks at 1–2 h after an allergic reaction, correct interpretation of the measured values is dependent on information about timing of blood sampling in relation to the time of reaction. The optimum sampling time is 30 min to 3 h after the reaction according to the manufacturer (ThermoFisher Scientific, Uppsala, Sweden).

In practice the blood test should be taken once the patient is stabilized. Serum tryptase is very stable in both serum and plasma, can be sent untreated at room temperature, and can be analyzed several days after sampling if needed, which is useful in the setting of a busy anesthetic department. Because of the many differential diagnoses in perioperative allergy, a serum tryptase value from the time of reaction compared with a baseline sample is a very useful tool in the diagnostic process. In some countries the distribution of an "anaphylaxis pack," (see Fig. 21.2) containing a treatment algorithm, blood collection equipment, and information about local referral procedures for allergy investigation, has increased the number of referrals where serum tryptase has been taken.[13,49]

Even in cases where no serum tryptase is available from the time of reaction, the baseline serum tryptase may provide useful information. In rare cases, an elevated baseline sample may indicate that the patient has systemic mastocytosis, and an algorithm for when this should be suspected has recently been suggested.[50] The diagnosis can be made by identifying the KIT-816 mutation in either peripheral blood or bone marrow, and in rare cases this mutation can even be seen in patients with baseline tryptase within the normal range.[20]

Presently, tryptase is the only mediator used in perioperative allergy in most centers. Only few highly specialized centers have access to measuring histamine, which has a shorter half-life and needs special handling before being processed in the laboratory, limiting its use in clinical practice.[13,14]

Specific IgE

Measurement of specific IgE antibodies in serum is available for a limited number of drugs used in the perioperative setting. The UniCAP system (Thermo-Fisher Scientific, Uppsala, Sweden) is widely used worldwide, but sensitivity and specificity vary greatly between allergens, and in practice in the perioperative setting the highest sensitivity and specificity is found for specific IgE to chlorhexidine.[39]

Specific IgE may already be elevated at the time of reaction, and this has been shown for chlorhexidine,[39,51] NMBAs,[52] and ethylene oxide.[53] Therefore, specific IgE can be measured on the sample taken for serum tryptase at the time of reaction. If levels of specific IgE are negative at the time of reaction, they should be repeated after a few weeks, as increases in specific IgE have been reported in the weeks after exposure to penicillins,[54] ethylene oxide,[53] and chlorhexidine.[55] In a follow-up study of chlorhexidine allergic patients, it has recently been shown that specific IgE levels decrease over time and may decrease below the usual cutoff limit of 0.35 KUa/L, in as little as 4 months on lack of exposure.[55] A specific IgE level below 0.35 KUa/L does not rule out a clinical allergy, regardless of the timing of the sample.

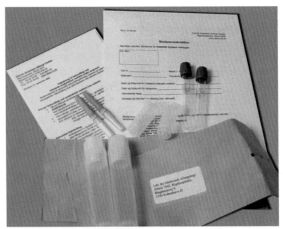

FIG. 21.2 "Anaphylaxis pack" for anesthesiologists containing anaphylaxis treatment algorithm, referral papers, and blood collection equipment for sample for serum tryptase analysis.

Basophil Histamine Release and Basophil Activation Tests

The basophil histamine release test is based on measuring histamine release in response to a suspected allergen. All drugs and substances can be tested, even catheters or solid substances that divide small enough to enter a test tube to be incubated with the patient's blood. Histamine release can be performed with passive sensitization (incubation of donor basophils with patient serum before exposure to suspected allergen), and this method detects IgE-mediated reactions.[51] While specificity is usually high, the sensitivity is low for most of the drug allergens, and therefore, in clinical practice, the histamine release test is used to supplement diagnostics in cases where other tests are not possible to perform or give doubtful results.[13]

BATs are based on using flow cytometry to analyze upregulation of activation and degranulation surface markers, primarily CD63 and CD203c, in response to stimulation with a suspected allergen.[56] Sensitivity and specificity vary with the allergen, but the BAT has especially been useful in suspected NMBA anaphylaxis because it may also be used to assess cross-reactivity within the drug group.[57,58]

Both methods are demanding on resources in the laboratory and rely on the use of freshly drawn blood samples (<24 h old). This means that their use is mostly restricted to highly specialized clinics.

Skin Testing

Skin testing has been considered the reference standard in the investigation of perioperative allergic reactions.[14,59]

For immediate-type allergy, SPTs and IDTs are most commonly used, but there is no international consensus on the method, performance, or interpretation of these tests. This leads to great variation in the way skin testing is used and interpreted between centers and countries.[60,61] The sensitivity and specificity of skin testing vary with different drugs, and with factors such as device and method used, the tester, and the skin reactivity of the patient.[62] A recent initiative to standardize skin test concentrations in perioperative allergy has come from Europe and the European Drug Allergy Network.[43] The concentrations recommended in this paper are based on a thorough literature review and the recommendations from the French Network of Anesthesia Allergy Center's GERAP[14] combined with a study in healthy volunteers of nonirritant concentrations for NMBAs.[63]

To ensure adequate reactivity in the skin, ideally skin testing should be performed at 4–6 weeks after the reaction.[64]

Skin prick testing is performed by pricking into the epidermis, which is devoid of blood vessels, through a drop of the drug to be tested. It can usually be performed up to undiluted concentrations of drugs except for direct histamine-releasing drugs such as morphine.[43] A negative control with normal saline and a positive control with histamine should be performed to confirm an adequate response in the skin and exclude an exaggerated skin response (dermographism), respectively. A SPT is considered positive when a wheal >3 mm appears at 15–20 min usually associated with flare and a degree of itching.[43,62] The risk of a systemic reaction to skin prick testing is considered very low.

Intradermal testing is performed by injecting a small volume of dilute drug into the vascularized dermis, and although intradermal testing is considered a safe procedure in experienced hands, it does carry a very small risk of inducing anaphylaxis. The safest approach, especially when testing unfamiliar drugs, is to start at low dilutions, e.g. 1/10,000 or 1/1000, and proceed to higher concentrations if tests are negative. As many drugs are irritant on intradermal injection, the maximum concentration used is usually 1/10 dilution, or lower, to avoid nonspecific reactions that could be misinterpreted as positive.[43] There are many sources of variation in both skin prick testing and, especially, intradermal testing, and standardization has been called for regarding performance and interpretation of the IDT.[43,60] Several different injection techniques have been described, but most guidelines have recommended injecting a volume creating a bleb of 3–5 mm in diameter. As the injected volume might vary greatly using this approach, it has recently been suggested to inject a fixed volume of 0.02 mL to avoid injecting large volumes, which may increase the risk of anaphylaxis.[39,65] The bleb induced by the intradermal injection is observed for 20 min, and a positive test is determined by a wheal forming, which increases the diameter of the induced bleb, usually associated with flare and a degree of itching. Several different criteria have been used for positivity of the IDT, and there is no international consensus on this at the present time. In France the GERAP and French Society of Anesthesiologists recommend that a positive IDT can be concluded when the diameter of the induced bleb doubles in size.[14,66] The European Network for Drug Allergy (ENDA) recommend an increase in wheal diameter of at least 3 mm associated with a flare after 15–20 min.[61] A third commonly used positive criterion is a wheal diameter of minimum 8 mm independent of negative control.[67] A recent study comparing these three diagnostic criteria in patients with perioperative allergic reactions to chlorhexidine concluded that the sensitivity was surprisingly low using the criteria of doubling in diameter of the induced bleb but the other two criteria had an acceptable sensitivity and specificity.[39]

Drug Provocation

While drug provocation is considered the "reference standard" in drug allergy investigation for single drugs,[11] it has not been standard practice to include provocation in the investigation of suspected perioperative allergic reactions. Some guidelines have even considered provocation contraindicated for drugs such as narcotics, opioids, and NMBAs because of their potent effects.[14]

Some highly specialized centers perform provocation for most of the drugs used in the perioperative setting,[41,68] and even cases of provocation with NMBAs have been reported recently from Australia.[69] However, because of the large number of drugs implicated and the high risk of inducing anaphylaxis, provocation with drugs used in the perioperative setting is very demanding on resources and is not likely to ever become standard practice in most centers. Provocation does, however, provide obvious benefits in the perioperative setting where there are numerous drugs showing great variation in sensitivity and specificity for both skin tests and in vitro tests. In addition, while skin tests and specific IgE testing are designed to detect IgE-mediated allergy only, provocation may detect reactions with different underlying mechanisms, not detectable by the usual investigations.

CAUSES

In the perioperative setting, many simultaneous exposures occur to drugs and substances administered via different routes. Reactions occurring during or shortly after IV administration of a drug will often lead to that drug being suspected by the attending personnel. Latex and disinfectants (e.g. chlorhexidine or iodine) are not administered IV, and as absorption usually takes place through broken skin or a mucous membrane, the onset of symptoms may be delayed. Reactions to these substances can occur at any time during surgery and anesthesia and may coincide with intravenous administration of another drug, which may then be wrongly suspected to be the allergen. In addition, there may be a tendency to suspect particular drug groups such as antibiotics or NMBAs because of a perceived greater likelihood of these to be the cause. However, in the clinical situation, it is rarely possible to make a safe risk assessment, and the patient should be warned against *all* substances administered before the reaction.[41,42] Referral for allergy investigations, preferably in a highly specialized setting, should result in carefully planned testing of all suspected culprits. As some patients may react to more than one substance, investigations for all planned drugs should ideally be carried out even if a culprit is identified.

The causes of perioperative anaphylaxis have proved to show geographic variation, and although commonly implicated in the literature, NMBAs are not the most common cause of perioperative allergy in all countries.[3,4] It is important to emphasize that anaphylaxis from all causes in the perioperative setting is rare, and there is no evidence to support avoiding specific drugs or drug groups unless a specific allergy is proved/suspected.

Anesthetic Agents

Considering the wide use of both intravenous and inhalational anesthetic agents, allergic reactions are very rare. Reactions to the most commonly used barbiturate thiopental have been described but seem to be decreasing most likely due to the decreasing use.[22,70]

Propofol is probably the most widely used anesthetic agent in the Western World, and the rate of reported reactions are very rare.[68] Concerns about an increased risk of allergic reactions to propofol in patients allergic to soy, egg, or peanut have emerged in recent years because of a small content of soybean oil and egg lecithin in the propofol emulsion.[71] However, recent studies have addressed this, and these concerns are now thought to be overstated. One study failed to identify allergy to egg, soy, or peanut in patients with propofol allergy confirmed on IV challenge and also showed that patients with IgE sensitization to egg, soy, or peanut, with or without clinical allergy, had all tolerated anesthetics using propofol, if exposed.[68] Another study showed that propofol administration was safe in children with eosinophilic esophagitis and sensitization to egg, soy, or peanut.[72]

Reactions to other anesthetic agents such as ketamine and benzodiazepines have been reported rarely.[22,73]

For many years it was thought that inhalational anesthetic agents did not have allergenic potential, but a few case reports of immediate-type allergic reactions attributed to inhalational agents can be found in the literature.[74,75]

Local Anesthetics

Perioperative allergic reactions to local anesthetics (LA) are exceedingly rare.[76] When using an investigation protocol including subcutaneous provocation with culprit LA in the national reference center for perioperative allergy in Denmark, no cases of immediate-type allergy to LAs were identified over a 10-year period.[77]

Because of a small risk of false-positive testing, especially on intradermal skin testing, subcutaneous provocation has recently been recommended as the best diagnostic test in suspected allergic reactions to LA.[76] Most procedures carried out in local anesthesia lead to exposures to other substances such as latex, disinfectants, sedatives, and radiocontrast media, and these should be considered potential culprits if an allergic reaction occurs in this setting. One Norwegian study showed that other exposures were more likely to cause allergic reactions than the LA itself.[78]

Opioids and Other Analgesics

Opioids and especially the fentanyl derivatives are used during most anesthetics, but allergic reactions are only rarely described.[22,79] Morphine and other drugs such as codeine and meperidine are more likely to cause nonspecific histamine release than IgE-mediated reactions.[17]

Nonsteroidal antiinflammatory drugs (NSAIDs) and acetaminophen/paracetamol are used frequently both as premedication, at the end of surgery, and in the postoperative phase. IgE-mediated reactions to NSAIDs are very rare, and the implicated drugs usually reflect local preferences, dipyrone in Spain[6] and metamizol in Germany.[80] Reactions to acetaminophen/paracetamol are exceedingly rarely reported.

Neuromuscular Blocking Agents

For many years the NMBAs have been reported to be the most common causes of perioperative allergy in large multicenter studies from France[22,81] and studies from Australia[82,83] and Norway.[84] Centers in countries such as Denmark,[85] Sweden,[86] and the United States[87–89] have not reported the same high incidence of reactions to NMBA. The mechanism behind the majority of NMBA reactions is thought to be IgE mediated, but reactions seem to occur on first exposure to an NMBA. For years it was hypothesized that exposure to an agent outside the operating room could cause a clinically relevant cross-sensitization to NMBAs,[90] and this led to a search for this cross-sensitizing agent by a team from Norway and Sweden.[91] After a search in households in Norway and Sweden, they identified a compound called pholcodine, which was present in cough mixtures used in Norway, but not in Sweden. This compound was highly sensitizing, and it is now believed that cross-sensitization with pholcodine led to an increased risk of reactions to NMBAs in Norway, where the product was taken of the market. A decrease in the incidence of reactions to NMBAs has subsequently been reported in Norway.[92] The pholcodine story[93] has provided part of the explanation for the geographic variations in the incidence of reactions to NMBAs,[94] but differences in anesthetic practice and the performance and interpretation of skin tests are likely to also play a role. As NMBAs are all structurally similar, there is a risk of cross-sensitization to other NMBAs in patients with a confirmed reaction to one NMBA. The rate of cross-reactivity has been reported to be as high as 60%–70% in France,[95] and it is recommended to test with all NMBAs when one has tested positive. However, while the negative predictive value of skin testing with NMBAs has been reported to be very good[96] there is still a risk of false-positive testing even when using the recommended concentrations in Europe.[3,37,63,97] It is not recommended to test for all NMBAs in patients not exposed to these drugs[43] because this could lead to false-positive testing being misinterpreted as true positives, leading to the wrong conclusions being made. In every case it is thus important to ensure that testing is performed for all possible culprit drugs and not just for NMBAs because of a perceived higher risk for this group of drugs.

Reversal Agents

Reversal of neuromuscular blockade has traditionally taken place by the use of neostigmine in combination with either atropine or glycopyrrolate, and reactions to any of these drugs have been described rarely in the literature.[98,99] Recently a new reversal agent, sugammadex, has entered the market, first in Asia and Europe in 2007, and more recently it was approved for use in the United States by the FDA in 2015. Sugammadex binds specifically to the aminosteroid type of NMBAs, primarily to rocuronium, and to a lesser degree to vecuronium, and rapidly reverses the neuromuscular blockade. Reports of allergic reactions to sugammadex have been emerging especially from Japan and Australia where it has gained widespread use.[100–102] Because of the strong binding between rocuronium and sugammadex, it has been suggested that sugammadex might be useful in reducing the effects of anaphylaxis to rocuronium[103]; however, others dispute this suggestion.[104] Recently, it has been suggested that the complex formed by rocuronium and sugammadex may itself have allergenic potential.[105]

Antibiotics

Antibiotic prophylaxis is widely used in most surgical specialties, and the preferred type of antibiotic varies with specialty and between countries. The frequency of perioperative allergic reactions attributed to antibiotics have been reported to be increasing,[22] and in some centers antibiotics have been reported to be the leading cause.[89,106,107] The β-lactam antibiotics are most frequently used, and also most frequently incriminated with variations reported in the specific causative drugs, e.g. cefazolin in the United States, Belgium, and Germany[37,89,106]; cefuroxime in Denmark[41]; and penicillins and teicoplanin in the UK.[38,108] All antibiotics have the potential to cause allergic reactions and should always be included in the investigations of suspected perioperative allergic reactions. If skin testing is negative, a graded challenge should be considered because not all reactions to antibiotics will be skin test positive.[41]

Plasma Expanders

Reactions to the different types of plasma expanders, e.g. gelatins, hydroxyethyl starches, and dextrans, have been reported with varying frequency. Gelatins have been reported to cause perioperative allergic reactions in countries where these products are used.[22,109] It has been suggested that reactions to gelatins may be linked to meat allergy and perhaps to sensitization to the α-gal carbohydrate epitope.[110,111] Hydroxyethyl starches have been commonly used, and allergic reactions were only rarely reported.[112] However, recently use of these products has decreased because of suggestions of increased mortality when used in critically ill patients.[113]

When dextrans were first introduced, a relatively large number of reactions occurred. When pretreatment with dextran 1 was introduced, a marked reduction in the frequency of reactions to higher molecular weight dextrans resulted. Reactions to dextrans are still reported, attributed to either prophylaxis not being applied[114] or failing to have the desired effect.[115]

Blood and Blood Products

Blood and blood products administered in the perioperative setting may cause allergic reactions, but the diagnosis is often a diagnosis of exclusion, when investigations for all other drugs test negative. Except for patients reacting to blood products due to IgA deficiency, there are no tests that can positively identify reactions to blood or blood products at the present time.[116]

"Hidden Allergens"—Substances Not Administered IV and Not Always Documented on Charts

All exposures in the perioperative setting may cause allergic reactions, and recently focus has increased on "hidden" exposures of substances not administered IV.[3] Latex has been a well-known perioperative allergen since the late 1980s, but other substances such as disinfectants, sterilizing agents, blue dyes, hemostatic agents, bone cements, gels, and sprays have not been considered systematically in most centers. Other more well-known substances such as heparins, radiocontrast media, and antibiotics may also have been used in the perioperative setting, and documentation may not be obvious.

The identification of these exposures requires knowledge of the perioperative setting and access to all available documentation from the procedure, including anesthetic documentation and surgical notes and charts. In many cases direct contact to anesthetic and surgical personnel may be necessary to identify all exposures, as some exposures to, e.g. disinfectants, gels, and sprays may not have been documented.[3]

Latex

In the 1990s large surveys from France reported latex as the second most common allergen identified in perioperative allergic reactions.[79,117] This was thought to be caused by increased glove use in the health services all over the world due to the HIV epidemic in the late 1980s. Since then a focus on reducing the protein content and avoiding powder in latex gloves, together with implementing latex-free regimes for high-risk patients, has led to a marked decrease in perioperative allergic reactions to latex in many different countries.[4,38,106] The diagnostics of latex allergy have been improved by the introduction of recombinant allergen components. These have made it possible to distinguish between major or primary allergen components associated with clinical latex allergy, and other minor allergen components, mainly related to cross-reactivity with plants and fruit and considered of no, or doubtful, clinical relevance.[118,119]

Disinfectants

In most countries surgical disinfection is performed using either povidone iodine or chlorhexidine. Reactions to povidone iodine are only infrequently reported in the literature.[120]

Chlorhexidine is very widely used as an antiseptic, not only for skin disinfection before surgical incision, but also as an antimicrobial coating on some central venous catheters. It is also an ingredient in lubricant gels used for urinary catheterization and procedures such as colonoscopies and gynecologic and urologic procedures.[121] While it is an extremely effective disinfectant, it has also been shown to have allergenic potential. In the 1980s in Japan a number of cases of allergic reactions to chlorhexidine related to exposure on mucous membranes led to official recommendations to use only low concentrations on contact with broken skin and to avoid exposure on mucous membranes if at all possible.[122,123]

The use of chlorhexidine is increasing because of the emergence of multiresistant bacteria, and in some countries products with high concentrations of chlorhexidine are emerging for general use.[124,125] In some countries exposure to chlorhexidine is inevitable in the perioperative setting, and some centers now test with chlorhexidine in all patients with suspected perioperative allergic reactions. This practice has led to chlorhexidine being identified as the culprit allergen in 9.6% of investigated patients in Denmark[39] and 5%–8.7% in the UK[38,126] and to recommendations that perioperative allergy investigations should always include testing with chlorhexidine. There is generally low awareness of the widespread use and allergenic potential of chlorhexidine among healthcare personnel, and a recent follow-up study of chlorhexidine allergic patients showed that one-third had been accidentally reexposed to chlorhexidine in the health sector.[55] Increased vigilance about the use of chlorhexidine and its allergenic potential is needed in future, and standardized testing with chlorhexidine should be performed in all cases of potential exposure to chlorhexidine such as in the perioperative setting.[39,55]

Sterilizing Agents

Ethylene oxide is a widely used sterilizing agent for medical products used during surgery and anesthesia. Sensitization to ethylene oxide was first described in dialysis patients in the 1980s,[127] and later it was reported that patients with spina bifida may be at increased risk of allergic sensitization to ethylene oxide.[128] More recently it has been suggested that the risk of sensitization is increased in neurosurgical patients with ethylene oxide–sterilized ventriculoperitoneal shunts.[129,130] The incidence has been shown to be low in a general surgical population.[53]

Blue Dyes

Blue dyes have gained increasing use for sentinel node procedures used for identifying metastatic lymph nodes in breast cancer and malignant melanoma. There are several different blue dyes in use, but in the perioperative setting mainly patent blue, and in some centers isosulfan blue, is used.[131] Allergic reactions to patent blue have been reported to occur as often as 1:300 procedures.[132]

Oxytocin

Oxytocin can produce dose-related side effects that mimic allergic reactions with symptoms such as tachycardia, flushing, hypotension, and chest tightness.[133] It has been suggested that suspected allergic reactions may have been attributed to dose-related side effects rather than an allergic mechanism, as traditionally used doses of 10 IU intravenously have been too high.[133,134] Recent studies have shown that lower doses are equally as effective with a lower risk of inducing unwanted side effects.[134,135]

Other Hidden Exposures in the Perioperative Setting

During surgery and anesthesia exposure to a large number of substances takes place, some of which are rarely documented on anesthetic charts, and thus not considered in the case of an allergic reaction. As all of these substances have allergenic potential, a detailed account of all exposures including ultrasound gels,

disinfectant solutions/sprays/gels, local anesthetic sprays/gels, catheter gels, lubricants, bone cements, tissue sealants, artificial tears, hemostatic agents, dural sealants, bandages, dressings, etc. should be made in cases of suspected perioperative allergic reactions, and testing should be considered.[3] Information about such exposures is most reliably obtained by contact to anesthetic and/or surgical personnel present during the specific procedure.

Many of these substances contain excipients such as polyethylene glycol (PEG) or related polymers, methylcelluloses, or mannitol. PEGs are a very widely used group of polymers of varying lengths, and while they have been regarded as biologically inert, case reports of severe reactions to these compounds have emerged, including from the perioperative setting.[136–138] Reactions to PEG can occur following exposure via many different routes of administration, e.g. oral, intravenous, subcutaneous, application in wounds during surgery or on broken skin, and cross-reactivity between PEG and related polymers have been described.[136]

Methylcelluloses are excipients in a multitude of different products used in the perioperative setting including local anesthetic-, lubricant-, or ultrasound gels and artificial tears.[3] In the perioperative setting, reactions have been reported during cataract surgery,[36] but the most commonly reported administration route causing reactions to methylcelluloses has been via injection of depot steroid formulations.[139] Oral exposure seems not to induce reactions to methylcelluloses except on exposure to very large amounts, e.g. during a barium swallow.[140]

Mannitol is an excipient in intravenous formulations of several drugs, and reactions to mannitol in an intravenous formulation of paracetamol have been described.[141] Other drugs such as antibiotics may be used during surgery hidden in various products. Recently, gentamicin in bone cement used during a knee replacement is thought to have sensitized a patient to gentamicin, leading to a severe perioperative allergic reaction with cardiac arrest on subsequent intravenous exposure.[142]

ABBREVIATIONS

BAT   Basophil activation test
DAAC   Danish Anaesthesia Allergy Centre
EO   Ethylene oxide
GERAP   Groupe d'Etude des Reactions Anaphylactoides Peranesthesiques

ICON   International consensus
IDT   Intradermal test
LA   Local anesthetics
NMBAs   Neuromuscular blocking drugs
SPT   Skin prick test
UK   United Kingdom
WAO   World Allergy Organization

REFERENCES

1. Alshaeri T, Gupta D, Nagabhushana A. Peri-anaesthesia anaphylaxis (PAA): we still have not started post PAA testing to inciting anesthesia-related allergens. *Middle East J Anesthesiol.* 2016;23:465–469.

2. Garvey LH. Perioperative hypersensitivity reactions. Diagnosis, treatment and evaluation. *Curr Treat Options Allergy.* 2016;3:113–128. http://dx.doi.org/10.1007/s40521-016-0078-0.

3. Garvey LH. Old, new and hidden causes of perioperative hypersensitivity. *Curr Pharm Des.* 2016;22(45):6814–6824.

4. Mertes PM, Volcheck GW, Garvey LH, et al. Epidemiology of perioperative anaphylaxis. *Presse Med.* 2016;45:758–767.

5. Malinovsky JM, Decagny S, Wessel F, et al. Systematic follow-up increases incidence of anaphylaxis during adverse reactions in anesthetized patients. *Acta Anaesthesiol Scand.* 2008;52:175–181.

6. Lobera T, Audicana MT, Pozo MD, et al. Study of hypersensitivity reactions and anaphylaxis during anaesthesia in Spain. *J Investig Allergol Clin Immunol.* 2008;18:350–356.

7. Savic LC, Kaura V, Yusaf M, et al. Anaesthetic audit and research matrix of Yorkshire. Incidence of suspected perioperative anaphylaxis: a multicenter snapshot study. *J Allergy Clin Immunol Pract.* 2015;3:454–455.

8. Reitter M, Petitpain N, Latarche C, et al. Fatal anaphylaxis with neuromuscular blocking agents: a risk factor and management analysis. *Allergy.* 2014;69:954–959.

9. Gibbs NM, Sadleir PH, Clarke RC, et al. Survival from perioperative anaphylaxis in Western Australia 2000-2009. *Br J Anaesth.* 2013;111:589–593.

10. Johansson SG, Bieber T, Dahl R, et al. Revised nomenclature for allergy for global use: report of the nomenclature review committee of the world allergy organization. *J Allergy Clin Immunol.* October 2003;2004(113):832–836.

11. Demoly P, Adkinson NF, Brockow K, et al. International consensus on drug allergy. *Allergy.* 2014;69:420–437.

12. Ring J, Messmer K. Incidence and severity of anaphylactoid reactions to colloid volume substitutes. *Lancet.* 1977;1:466–469.

13. Krøigaard M, Garvey LH, Gilberg L, et al. Scandinavian clinical practice guidelines on the diagnosis, management and follow-up of anaphylaxis during anaesthesia. *Acta Anaesthesiol Scand.* 2007;51:655–670.

14. Mertes PM, Malinovsky JM, Jouffroy L, et al. Reducing the risk of anaphylaxis during anesthesia: 2011 updated guidelines for clinical practice. *J Investig Allergol Clin Immunol.* 2011;21:442–453.

15. Ljungstrom KG. Safety of dextran in relation to other colloids—ten years' experience with hapten inhibition. *Infusionsther Transfusionsmed.* 1993;20:206–210.

16. Lieberman P, Garvey LH. Mast cells and anaphylaxis. *Curr Allergy Asthma Rep.* 2016;16:20.

17. Baldo BA, Pham NH. Histamine-releasing and allergenic properties of opioid analgesic drugs: resolving the two. *Anaesth Intensive Care.* 2012;40:216–235.

18. McNeil BD, Pundir P, Meeker S, et al. Identification of a mast-cell-specific receptor crucial for pseudoallergic drug reactions. *Nature.* 2015;519:237–241.

19. Renauld V, Goudet V, Mouton-Faivre C, et al. Case report: perioperative immediate hypersensitivity involves not only allergy but also mastocytosis. *Can J Anaesth.* 2011;58:456–459.

20. Broesby-Olsen S, Oropeza AR, Bindslev-Jensen C, et al. Recognizing mastocytosis in patients with anaphylaxis: value of KIT D816V mutation analysis of peripheral blood. *J Allergy Clin Immunol.* 2015;135:262–264.

21. Bonadonna P, Pagani M, Aberer W, et al. Drug hypersensitivity in clonal mast cell disorders: ENDA/EAACI position paper. *Allergy.* 2015;70:755–763.

22. Dong SW, Mertes PM, Petitpain N, et al. Hypersensitivity reactions during anesthesia. Results from the ninth French survey (2005-2007). *Minerva Anesthesiol.* 2012;78:868–878.

23. Dewachter P, Mouton-Faivre C, Hepner DL. Perioperative anaphylaxis: what should be known? *Curr Allergy Asthma Rep.* 2015;15:21.

24. Nakonechna A, Dore P, Dixon T, et al. Immediate hypersensitivity to chlorhexidine is increasingly recognised in the United Kingdom. *Allergol Immunopathol (Madr).* 2014;42:44–49.

25. Garvey LH, Roed-Petersen J, Husum B. Anaphylactic reactions in anaesthetised patients—four cases of chlorhexidine allergy. *Acta Anaesthesiol Scand.* 2001;45:1204–1209.

26. Garvey LH. Practical aspects of perioperative anaphylaxis. *Trends Anaesth Crit Care.* 2013;3:320–326.

27. Melchiors BLB, Krøigaard M, Mosbech H, et al. Is isolated angioedema in the perioperative setting a symptom of allergy?—A retrospective single-centre study. Submitted.

28. Marques A, Retroz-Marques C, Mota S, et al. Postanesthetic severe oral angioedema in patients taking angiotensin converting enzyme inhibitor. *Case rep Anesthesiol.* 2014:693191.

29. Ogbureke KU, Cruz C, Johnson JV, et al. Perioperative angioedema in a patient on long-term angiotensin-converting enzyme (ACE)-inhibitor therapy. *J Oral Maxillofac Surg.* 1996;54:917–920.

30. Rasmussen ER, Mey K, Bygum A. Angiotensin converting enzyme inhibitor-induced angioedema—a dangerous new epidemic. *Acta Derm Venereol.* 2014;94:260–264.

31. Barbara DW, Ronan KP, Maddox DE, et al. Perioperative angioedema: background, diagnosis, and management. *J Clin Anesth.* 2013;25:335–343.

32. Fisher MM, Ramakrishnan N, Doig G, Rose M, Baldo B. The investigation of bronchospasm during induction of anaesthesia. *Acta Anaesthesiol Scand.* 2009;53:1006–1011.

33. Garvey LH, Belhage B, Krøigaard M, et al. Treatment with epinephrine (adrenaline) in suspected anaphylaxis during anesthesia in Denmark. *Anesthesiology.* 2011;115:111–116.

34. Ewan PW, Dugué P, Mirakian R, et al. BSACI guidelines for the investigation of suspected anaphylaxis during general anaesthesia. *Clin Exp Allergy.* 2010;40:15–31.

35. Wenande E, Mosbech H, Krøigaard M, et al. Polyethylene glycols (PEGs) and related structures—overlooked allergens in the perioperative setting? *A A Case Rep.* 2015;4:61–64.

36. Munk SJ, Heegaard S, Mosbech H, et al. Two episodes of anaphylaxis following exposure to hydroxypropyl methylcellulose during cataract surgery. *J Cataract Refract Surg.* 2013;39:948–951.

37. Antunes J, Kochuyt AM, Ceuppens JL. Perioperative allergic reactions: experience in a Flemish referral centre. *Allergol Immunopathol (Madr).* 2014;42:348–354.

38. Low AE, McEwan JC, Karanam S, et al. Anaesthesia-associated hypersensitivity reactions: seven years' data from a British bi-specialty clinic. *Anaesthesia.* 2016;71:76–84.

39. Opstrup MS, Malling HJ, Krøigaard M, et al. Standardized testing with chlorhexidine in perioperative allergy – a large single centre evaluation. *Allergy.* 2014;69:1390–1396.

40. Pumphrey RS. Lessons for management of anaphylaxis from a study of fatal reactions. *Clin Exp Allergy.* 2000;30:1144–1150.

41. Christiansen IS, Krøigaard M, Mosbech H, et al. Clinical and diagnostic features of perioperative hypersensitivity to cefuroxime. *Clin Exp Allergy.* 2015;45:807–814.

42. Krøigaard M, Garvey LH, Menné T, et al. Allergic reactions in anaesthesia: are suspected causes confirmed on subsequent testing? *Br J Anaesth.* 2005;95:468–471.

43. Brockow K, Garvey LH, Aberer W, et al. Skin test concentrations for systemically administered drugs – an ENDA/EAACI Drug Allergy Interest Group position paper. *Allergy.* 2013;68:702–712.

44. Leysen J, Bridts CH, De Clerck LS, et al. Allergy to rocuronium: from clinical suspicion to correct diagnosis. *Allergy.* 2011;66:1014–1019.

45. Caughey GH. Tryptase genetics and anaphylaxis. *J Allergy Clin Immunol.* 2006;117:1411–1414.

46. Borer-Reinhold M, Haeberli G, Bitzenhofer M, et al. An increase in serum tryptase even below 11.4 ng/mL may indicate a mast cell-mediated hypersensitivity reaction: a prospective study in Hymenoptera venom allergic patients. *Clin Exp Allergy.* 2011;41:1777–1783.

47. Garvey LH, Bech B, Mosbech H, et al. Effect of general anesthesia and orthopedic surgery on serum tryptase. *Anesthesiology.* 2010;112:1184–1189.

48. Sprung J, Weingarten TN, Schwartz LB. Presence or absence of elevated acute total serum tryptase by itself is not a definitive marker for an allergic reaction. *Anesthesiology.* 2015;122:713–714.

49. Savic L, Garside M, Savic S, et al. Anaphylaxis follow-up: making it simple—making it better. *R Coll Anaesth Bull.* 2014;87:33–37.

50. Arock M, Sotlar K, Akin C, et al. KIT mutation analysis in mast cell neoplasms: recommendations of the European Competence Network on mastocytosis. *Leukemia.* 2015;29:1223–1232.

51. Garvey LH, Krøigaard M, Poulsen LK, et al. IgE-mediated allergy to chlorhexidine. *J Allergy Clin Immunol.* 2007;120: 409–415.

52. Guttormsen AB, Johansson SG, Oman H, et al. No consumption of IgE antibody in serum during allergic drug anaphylaxis. *Allergy.* 2007;62:1326–1333.

53. Opstrup MS, Mosbech H, Garvey LH. Allergic sensitization to ethylene oxide in patients with suspected allergic reactions during surgery and anesthesia. *J Investig Allergol Clin Immunol.* 2010;20:269–270.

54. Hjortlund J, Mortz CG, Stage TB, et al. Positive serum specific IgE has a short half-life in patients with penicillin allergy and reversal does not always indicate tolerance. *Clin Transl Allergy.* 2014;4:34.

55. Opstrup MS, Poulsen LK, Malling HJ, et al. Dynamics of specific IgE in chlorhexidine allergic patients with and without accidental re-exposure. *Clin Exp Allergy.* 2016;46:1090–1098.

56. Bridts CH, Sabato V, Mertens C, et al. Flow cytometric allergy diagnosis: basophil activation techniques. *Methods Mol Biol.* 2014;1192:147–159.

57. Ebo DG, Bridts CH, Hagendorens MM, et al. Flow-assisted diagnostic management of anaphylaxis from rocuronium bromide. *Allergy.* 2006;61:935–939.

58. Uyttebroek AP, Sabato V, Leysen J, et al. Flowcytometric diagnosis of atracurium-induced anaphylaxis. *Allergy.* 2014;69:1324–1332.

59. Joint Task Force on Practice Parameters, American Academy of Allergy, Asthma and Immunology, American College of Allergy, Asthma and Immunology, et al. Drug allergy: an updated practice parameter. *Ann Allergy Asthma Immunol.* 2010;105:259–273.

60. Fatteh S, Rekkerth DJ, Hadley JA. Skin prick/puncture testing in North America: a call for standards and consistency. *Allergy Asthma Clin Immunol.* 2014;10:44–52.

61. Brockow K, Romano A, Blanca M, et al. General considerations for skin test procedures in the diagnosis of drug hypersensitivity. *Allergy.* 2002;57:45–51.

62. Bernstein IL, Li JT, Bernstein DI, et al. Allergy diagnostic testing: an updated practice parameter. *Ann Allergy Asthma Immunol.* 2008;100:S1–S148.

63. Mertes PM, Moneret-Vautrin DA, Leynadier F, et al. Skin reactions to intradermal neuromuscular blocking agent injections: a randomized multicenter trial in healthy volunteers. *Anesthesiology.* 2007;107:245–252.

64. Soetens F, Rose M, Fisher M. Timing of skin testing after a suspected anaphylactic reaction during anaesthesia. *Acta Anaesthesiol Scand.* 2012;56:1042–1046.

65. Barbaud A. Skin testing and patch testing in non-IgE-mediated drug allergy. *Curr Allergy Asthma Rep.* 2014;14:442.

66. Societe Francaises d'Anesthesie et de Reanimation. Reducing the risk of anaphylaxis during anaesthesia. Abbreviated text. *Ann Fr Anesth Reanim.* 2002;21(Suppl. 1):7–23.

67. Fisher MM, Bowey CJ. Intradermal compared with prick testing in the diagnosis of anaesthetic drugs. *Br J Anaesth.* 1997;79:59–63.

68. Asserhøj LL, Mosbech H, Krøigaard M, et al. No evidence for contraindications to the use of propofol in adults allergic to egg, soy or peanut. *Br J Anaesth.* 2016;116: 77–82.

69. Schulberg EM, Webb AR, Kolawole H. Early skin and challenge testing after rocuronium anaphylaxis. *Anaesth Intensive Care.* 2016;44:425–427.

70. Laxenaire MC, Moneret-Vautrin DA, Widmer S, et al. Anesthetics responsible for anaphylactic shock. A French multicenter study. *Ann Fr Anesth Reanim.* 1990;9: 501–506.

71. Richard C, Beaudouin E, Moneret-Vautrin DA, et al. Severe anaphylaxis to Propofol: first case of evidence of sensitization to soy oil. *Eur Ann Allergy Clin Immunol.* 2016;48:103–106.

72. Molina-Infante J, Arias A, Vara-Brenes D, et al. Propofol administration is safe in adult eosinophilic esophagitis patients sensitized to egg, soy or peanut. *Allergy.* 2014;69:388–394.

73. Ozcan J, Nicholls K, Jones K. Immunoglobulin E-mediated hypersensitivity reaction to ketamine. *Pain Pract.* June 23, 2016. http://dx.doi.org/10.1111/papr.12466.

74. Slegers-Karsmakers S, Stricker BH. Anaphylactic reaction to isoflurane. *Anaesthesia.* 1988;43:506–507.

75. Dahlem C, Cadinha S, Delgado I, et al. A rare case of sevoflurane hypersensitivity. *Eur J Anaesthesiol.* 2016;33:379–380.

76. Malinovsky JM, Chiriac AM, Tacquard C, et al. Allergy to local anesthetics: reality or myth? *Presse Med.* July 1, 2016. http://dx.doi.org/10.1016/j.lpm.2016.05.011. pii :S0755-4982(16)30129-4.

77. Kvisselgaard A, Krøigaard M, Mosbech H, et al. No cases of perioperative allergy to local anaesthetics in the Danish Anaesthesia Allergy Centre. *Acta Anaesthesiol Scand.* 2017;61:149–155.

78. Harboe T, Guttormsen AB, Aarebrot S, et al. Suspected allergy to local anaesthetics: follow-up in 135 cases. *Acta Anaesthesiol Scand.* 2010;54:536–542.

79. Laxenaire MC, Mertes PM. Anaphylaxis during anaesthesia. results of a two-year survey in France. *Br J Anaesth.* 2001;87:549–558.

80. Eckle T, Ghanayim N, Trick M, et al. Intraoperative metamizol as cause for acute anaphylactic collapse. *Eur J Anaesthesiol.* 2005;22:810–812.

81. Laxenaire MC. Substances responsible for peranesthetic anaphylactic shock. A third French multicenter study (1992-94). *Ann Fr Anesth Reanim.* 1996;15:1211–1218.

82. Fisher MM, Baldo BA. The incidence and clinical features of anaphylactic reactions during anesthesia in Australia. *Ann Fr Anesth Reanim.* 1993;12:97–104.

83. Sadleir PH, Clarke RC, Bunning DL, et al. Anaphylaxis to neuromuscular blocking drugs: incidence and cross-reactivity in Western Australia from 2002 to 2011. *Br J Anaesth.* 2013;110:981–987.

84. Harboe T, Guttormsen AB, Irgens A, et al. Anaphylaxis during anesthesia in Norway: a 6-year single-center follow-up study. *Anesthesiology.* 2005;102:897–903.

85. Garvey LH, Husum B, Roed-Petersen J, et al. Danish Anaesthesia Allergy Centre – preliminary results. *Acta Anaesthesiol Scand.* 2001;45:1290–1294.

86. Florvaag E, Johansson SG, Oman H, et al. Prevalence of IgE antibodies to morphine. Relation to the high and low incidences of NMBA anaphylaxis in Norway and Sweden, respectively. *Acta Anaesthesiol Scand.* 2005;49:437–444.

87. Gurrieri C, Weingarten TN, Martin DP, et al. Allergic reactions during anesthesia at a large United States referral center. *Anesth Analg.* 2011;113:1202–1212.

88. Guyer AC, Saff RR, Conroy M, et al. Comprehensive allergy evaluation is useful in the subsequent care of patients with drug hypersensitivity reactions during anesthesia. *J Allergy Clin Immunol Pract.* 2015;3:94–100.

89. Kuhlen Jr JL, Camargo Jr CA, Balekian DS, et al. Antibiotics are the most commonly identified cause of perioperative hypersensitivity reactions. *J Allergy Clin Immunol Pract.* 2016;4:697–704.

90. Harle DG, Baldo BA, Fisher MM. Detection of IgE antibodies to suxamethonium after anaphylactoid reactions during anaesthesia. *Lancet.* 1984;1:930–932.

91. Johansson SG, Nopp A, Florvaag E, et al. High prevalence of IgE antibodies among blood donors in Sweden and Norway. *Allergy.* 2005;60:1312–1315.

92. Florvaag E, Johansson SG, Irgens Å, et al. IgE-sensitization to the cough suppressant pholcodine and the effects of its withdrawal from the Norwegian market. *Allergy.* 2011;66:955–960.

93. Florvaag E, Johansson SG. The pholcodine story. *Immunol Allergy Clin North Am.* 2009;29:419–427.

94. Johansson SG, Florvaag E, Oman H, et al. National pholcodine consumption and prevalence of IgE-sensitization: a multicentre study. *Allergy.* 2010;65:498–502.

95. Mertes PM, Aimone-Gastin I, Guéant-Rodriguez RM, et al. Hypersensitivity reactions to neuromuscular blocking agents. *Curr Pharm Des.* 2008;14:2809–2825.

96. Ramirez LF, Pereira A, Chiriac AM, et al. Negative predictive value of skin tests to neuromuscular blocking agents. *Allergy.* 2012;67:439–441.

97. Karila C, Brunet-Langot D, Labbez F, et al. Anaphylaxis during anesthesia: results of a 12-year survey at a French pediatric center. *Allergy.* 2005;60:828–834.

98. Seed MJ, Ewan PW. Anaphylaxis caused by neostigmine. *Anaesthesia.* 2000;55:574–575.

99. Coelho D, Fernandes T, Branga P, et al. Intraoperative anaphylaxis after intravenous atropine. *Eur J Anaesthesiol.* 2007;24:289–290.

100. Tsur A, Kalansky A. Hypersensitivity associated with sugammadex administration: a systematic review. *Anaesthesia.* 2014;69:1251–1257.

101. Takazawa T, Tomita Y, Yoshida N, et al. Three suspected cases of sugammadex-induced anaphylactic shock. *BMC Anesthesiol.* 2014;14:92.

102. Sadleir PH, Russell T, Clarke RC, Maycock E, Platt PR. Intraoperative anaphylaxis to sugammadex and a protocol for intradermal skin testing. *Anaesth Intensive Care.* 2014;42:93–96.

103. Conte B, Zoric L, Bonada G, et al. Reversal of a rocuronium-induced grade IV anaphylaxis via early injection of a large dose of sugammadex. *Can J Anaesth.* 2014;61:558–562.

104. Platt PR, Clarke RC, Johnson GH, et al. Efficacy of sugammadex in rocuronium-induced or antibiotic-induced anaphylaxis. A case-control study. *Anaesthesia.* 2015;70:1264–1267.

105. Ho G, Clarke RC, Sadleir PH, Platt PR. The first case report of anaphylaxis caused by the inclusion complex of rocuronium and sugammadex. *A A Case Rep.* 2016;7(9):190–192.

106. Trautmann A, Seidl C, Stoevesandt J, et al. General anaesthesia-induced anaphylaxis: impact of allergy testing on subsequent anaesthesia. *Clin Exp Allergy.* 2016;46:125–132.

107. Gonzalez-Estrada A, Pien LC, Zell K, et al. Antibiotics are an important identifiable cause of perioperative anaphylaxis in the United States. *J Allergy Clin Immunol Pract.* 2015;3:101–105.

108. Savic LC, Garcez T, Hopkins PM, et al. Teicoplanin allergy – an emerging problem in the anaesthetic allergy clinic. *Br J Anaesth.* 2015;115:595–600.

109. Rauschenberg R, Beissert S, Bauer A, et al. Intraoperative anaphylactic reaction IV° to gelatin. *J Dtsch Dermatol Ges.* 2014;12:617–618.

110. Agarwal NS, Spalding C, Nassef M. Life-threatening intraoperative anaphylaxis to gelatin in Floseal during pediatric spinal surgery. *J Allergy Clin Immunol Pract.* 2015;3:110–111.

111. Uyttebroek A, Sabato V, Bridts CH, et al. Anaphylaxis to succinylated gelatin in a patient with a meat allergy: galactose-α(1,3)-galactose (α-gal)as antigenic determinant. *J Clin Anesth.* 2014;26:574–576.

112. Ebo DG, Hagendorens MM, Bridts CH, et al. Allergic reactions occurring during anaesthesia: diagnostic approach. *Acta Clin Belg.* 2004;59:34–43.

113. Bion J, Bellomo R, Myburgh J, et al. Hydroxyethyl starch: putting patient safety first. *Intensive Care Med.* 2014;40:256–259.

114. Zinderman CE, Landow L, Wise RP. Anaphylactoid reactions to Dextran 40 and 70: reports to the United States Food and Drug Administration, 1969 to 2004. *J Vasc Surg.* 2006;43:1004–1009.

115. Bircher AJ, Hédin H, Berglund A. Probable grade IV dextran-induced anaphylactic reaction despite hapten inhibition. *J Allergy Clin Immunol.* 1995;95:633–634.

116. Lindsted G, Larsen R, Krøigaard M, et al. Transfusion-associated anaphylaxis during anaesthesia and surgery—a retrospective study. *Vox Sang.* 2014;107:158–165.

117. Laxenaire MC. Epidemiology of anesthetic anaphylactoid reactions. Fourth multicenter survey (July 1994-December 1996). *Ann Fr Anesth Reanim.* 1999;18:796–809.

118. Kahn SL, Podjasek JO, Dimitropoulos VA, et al. Natural rubber latex allergy. *Dis Mon.* 2016;62:5–17.

119. Rolland JM, O'Hehir RE. Latex allergy: a model for therapy. *Clin Exp Allergy.* 2008;38:898–912.

120. Caballero MR, Lukawska J, Dugué P. A hidden cause of perioperative anaphylaxis. *J Investig Allergol Clin Immunol.* 2010;20:353–354.

121. Opstrup MS, Johansen JD, Garvey LH. Chlorhexidine allergy: sources of exposure in the health-care setting. *Br J Anaesth.* 2015;114:704–705.

122. Cheung J, O'Leary JJ. Allergic reaction to chlorhexidine in an anaesthetised patient. *Anaesth Intensive Care.* 1985;13:429–430.

123. Okano M, Nomura M, Hata S, et al. Anaphylactic symptoms due to chlorhexidine gluconate. *Arch Dermatol.* 1989;125:50–52.

124. Al-Niaimi A, Rice LW, Shitanshu U, et al. Safety and tolerability of chlorhexidine gluconate (2%) as a vaginal operative preparation in patients undergoing gynecologic surgery. *Am J Infect Control.* May 24, 2016. http://dx.doi.org/10.1016/j.ajic.2016.02.036. pii:S0196-6553(16)30007-4 (Epub ahead of print).

125. Pages J, Hazera P, Mégarbane B, et al. Comparison of alcoholic chlorhexidine and povidone-iodine cutaneous antiseptics for the prevention of central venous catheter-related infection: a cohort and quasi-experimental multicenter study. *Intensive Care Med.* 2016;42(9):1418–1426.

126. Krishna MT, York M, Chin T, et al. Multi-centre retrospective analysis of anaphylaxis during general anaesthesia in the United Kingdom: aetiology and diagnostic performance of acute serum tryptase. *Clin Exp Immunol.* 2014;178:399–404.

127. Poothullil J, Shimizu A, Day RP, et al. Anaphylaxis from the product(s) of ethylene oxide gas. *Ann Intern Med.* 1975;82:58–60.

128. Pittman T, Kiburz J, Steinhardt G, et al. Ethylene oxide allergy in children with spina bifida. *J Allergy Clin Immunol.* 1995;96:486–488.

129. Bache S, Petersen JT, Garvey LH. Anaphylaxis to ethylene oxide—a rare and overlooked phenomenon? *Acta Anaesthesiol Scand.* 2011;55:1279–1282.

130. Listyo A, Hofmeier KS, Bandschapp O, et al. Severe anaphylactic shock due to ethylene oxide in a patient with myelomeningocele: successful exposure prevention and pretreatment with omalizumab. *A A Case Rep.* 2014;2:3–6.

131. Scherer K, Bircher AJ, Figueiredo V. Blue dyes in medicine–a confusing terminology. *Contact Dermatitis.* 2006;54:231–232.

132. Brenet O, Lalourcey L, Queinnec M, et al. Hypersensitivity reactions to Patent Blue V in breast cancer surgery: a prospective multicentre study. *Acta Anaesthesiol Scand.* 2013;57:106–111.

133. Kjær B, Krøigaard M, Garvey LH. Oxytocin use during caesarean sections in Denmark – are we getting the dose right? *Acta Anaesthesiol Scand.* 2016;60: 18–25.

134. Kovacheva VP, Soens MA, Tsen LC. A randomized, double-blinded trial of a "rule of threes" algorithm *versus* continuous infusion of oxytocin during elective cesarean delivery. *Anesthesiology.* 2015;123:92–100.

135. Butwick AJ, Coleman L, Cohen SE, et al. Minimum effective bolus dose of oxytocin during elective caesarean delivery. *Br J Anaesth.* 2010;104:338–343.

136. Wenande E, Garvey LH. Hypersensitivity to PEG – a review. *Clin Exp Allergy.* 2016;46:907–922.

137. Yamasuji Y, Higashi Y, Sakanoue M, et al. A case of anaphylaxis caused by polyethylene glycol analogues. *Contact Dermatitis.* 2013;69:183–185.

138. Jakubovic BD, Saperia C, Sussman GL. Anaphylaxis following a transvaginal ultrasound. *Allergy Asthma Clin Immunol.* 2016;12:3.

139. Meyer MV, Zachariae C, Garvey LH. Anaphylactic shock after intradermal injection of corticosteroid. *Ugeskr Laeger.* 2015;177(4).

140. Muroi N, Nishibori M, Fujii T, et al. Anaphylaxis from the carboxymethylcellulose component of barium sulfate suspension. *N Engl J Med.* 1997;337:1275–1277.

141. Jain SS, Green S, Rose M. Anaphylaxis following intravenous paracetamol: the problem is the solution. *Anaesth Intensive Care.* 2015;43:779–781.

142. Christiansen IS, Pedersen P, Krøigaard M, et al. Anaphylaxis to intravenous gentamicin with suspected sensitization through gentamicin-loaded bone cement. *J Allergy Clin Immunol Pract.* 2016;4(6):1258–1259.

CHAPTER 22

Adverse Reactions to Contrast Media

MELANIE C. DISPENZA, MD, PHD • ANNE M. DITTO, MD

KEY POINTS

- Immediate hypersensitivity reactions to contrast media are largely nonimmunologic and can be severe and/or life-threatening.
- Low-osmolality radiocontrast media have a lower rate of adverse reactions compared with high-osmolality media.
- Skin testing and graded dose challenge are ineffective at predicting the risk of having an immediate hypersensitivity reaction to contrast media and are not recommended for routine use.
- Pretreatment with systemic steroids and antihistamines can prevent immediate hypersensitivity reactions to contrast media.
- Patients with a history of prior immediate hypersensitivity reaction to contrast media should receive pretreatment before any subsequent imaging.

INTRODUCTION

Contrast agents have proved to be powerful diagnostic tools that have allowed for great advances in medical imaging techniques. They are also some of the most frequently used drugs in the world. Contrast media is a broad term for numerous chemicals that are used for visual enhancement of intravenous, intraarterial, intrathecal, or intraluminal spaces. While they are valuable for enhancing imaging studies, they can also cause adverse reactions that can be severe and life-threatening. This chapter focuses mainly on adverse reactions to iodinated radiocontrast media (RCM), which are used in CT and radiography (Table 22.1). Gadolinium-based contrast media (GBCM), which are used during magnetic resonance imaging (MRI), are briefly discussed at the end of this chapter (Table 22.2).

IODINATED CONTRAST MEDIA
Types of Iodinated Contrast Media
Contrast agents are clear, colorless solutions that are radiopaque in radiographic imaging; thus the term "contrast dye" is a misnomer. The first organic, relatively nontoxic iodinated contrast material was developed in 1929 by Moses Swick, an intern from Mount Sinai Hospital in New York, and derivatives of this compound created the first generation of RCM, which entered routine use in medical imaging as early as the 1950s.[1] Subsequent modifications

to the original core structure allowed for decreased toxicity, with preservation of the radiopacity of the material. There are now numerous types of iodinated RCM, whose chemical structures can be broadly divided into ionic and nonionic RCM (Table 22.1). All of them share a common triiodinated benzene ring, either as a monomer or as a dimer, which has iodine atoms covalently bound to three of the six positions in the ring (Fig. 22.1). Variable side chains occupy the other three positions. Ionic media are water soluble because of the presence of a carboxyl group on the ring, whereas nonionic media are made water soluble by attachment of long hydroxylated side chains to the ring structure. Agents also differ in osmolality and are generally classified as "high" or "low" osmolality. Dimeric agents have a higher number of iodine residues per molecule; therefore, these structures can generally achieve the desired radiopacity with lower-osmolality solutions compared with monomeric agents.

Many studies have clearly shown higher rates of adverse reactions of all types with high-osmolality media compared with low-osmolality media (see Types of Adverse Reactions section).[2-11] In general, nonionic media have lower osmolality (closer to serum osmolality) than the ionic compounds, and dimers have lower osmolality than monomers. For this reason, the older ionic agents, some of which have five times the osmolality of blood, have largely been phased out in the United States. Nonionic dimers

TABLE 22.1

Types and Chemical Properties of Intravascular Iodinated Radiocontrast Media Commonly Used in the United States

Type	Generic Name	Brand Name	Iodine Content (mg/mL)	Viscosity at 37°C (mPa.s)	Osmolality (mOsm/kg H_2O)
Ionic	Iothalamate (600)	Conray (Covidien)	282	4	1400
	Iothalamate (300)	Conray 30 (Covidien)	141	1.5	600
	Iothalamate (430)	Conray 43 (Covidien)	202	2	413
	Ioxaglate meglumine/ sodium (589)	Hexabrix (Guerbet)	320	7.5	600
	Diatrizoate meglumine/ sodium (760)	MD-76 (Mallinckrodt)	370	10.5	1551
	Iodipamide (520)	Cholografin (Bracco)	257	5.6	664
Nonionic	Iohexol (302)	Omnipaque 140 (GE Healthcare)	140	1.5	322
	Iohexol (388)	Omnipaque 180 (GE Healthcare)	180	2	408
	Iohexol (518)	Omnipaque 240 (GE Healthcare)	240	3.4	520
	Iohexol (647)	Omnipaque 300 (GE Healthcare)	300	6.3	672
	Iohexol (755)	Omnipaque 350 (GE Healthcare)	350	10.4	844
	Iopromide	Ultravist 150 (Bayer HealthCare)	150	1.5	328
	Iopromide	Ultravist 240 (Bayer Healthcare)	240	2.8	483
	Iopromide	Ultravist 300 (Bayer Healthcare)	300	4.9	607
	Iopromide	Ultravist 370 (Bayer Healthcare)	370	10	774
	Iopamidol (408)	Isovue 200 (Bracco)	200	2	413
	Iopamidol (510)	Isovue 250 (Bracco)	250	3	524
	Iopamidol (612)	Isovue 300 (Bracco)	300	4.7	616
	Iopamidol (755)	Isovue 370 (Bracco)	370	9.4	796
	Ioversol (509)	Optiray 240 (Mallinckrodt)	240	3	502
	Ioversol (640)	Optiray 300 (Mallinckrodt)	300	5.5	651
	Ioversol (680)	Optiray 320 (Mallinckrodt)	320	5.8	702
	Ioversol (740)	Optiray 350 (Mallinckrodt)	350	9.0	792
	Iodixanol (550)	Visipaque 270 (GE Healthcare)	270	6.3	290
	Iodixanol (652)	Visipaque 320 (GE Healthcare)	320	11.8	290
	Ioxilan (623)	Oxilan 300 (Guerbet)	300	5.1	610
	Ioxilan (727)	Oxilan 350 (Guerbet)	350	8.1	721

Adapted ACR manual on contrast media. In: Ellis JH, ed. American College of Radiology; 2016: http://www.acr.org/quality-safety/resources/contrast-manual.

have the most favorable profile and the lowest rate of hypersensitivity reactions, but their high viscosity may limit their utility in some applications. Additionally, high costs may prohibit their use in some medical centers.

Types of Adverse Reactions

RCM can cause a range of types of adverse reactions, which can largely be divided into physiologic side effects and hypersensitivity reactions. Physiologic reactions are related to the chemical properties of

TABLE 22.2
Types and Chemical Properties of Intravascular Gadolinium-Based Contrast Agents Commonly Used in the United States

Anion	Cation	Brand Name	Chemical Structure	Relaxivity 1.5T (3T)	Viscosity at 37°C (mPa.s)	Osmolality (mOsm/kg H$_2$O)
Gadopen-tetate	Dimeglumine	Magnevist (Bayer Healthcare)	Gd-DTPA Linear Ionic	4.1 (3.7)	2.9	1960
Gadoteridol	None	Prohance (Bracco)	Gd-HP-D03A Macrocyclic Nonionic	4.1 (3.7)	1.3	630
Gadobenate	Dimeglumine	Multihance (Bracco)	Gd-BOPTA Linear Ionic	6.3 (5.5)	5.3	1970
Gadodiamide	None	Omniscan (GE Healthcare)	Gd-DTPA-BMA Linear Nonionic	4.3 (4)	1.4	789
Gadoverset-amide	None	Optimark (Mallinckrodt)	Gd-DTPA-BMEA Linear Nonionic	4.7 (4.5)	2.0	1110
Gadoxetate	Disodium	EOVIST/Primovist (Bayer Healthcare)	Gd-EOB-DTPA Linear Ionic	6.9 (6.2)	1.2	688
Gadobutrol	None	Gadavist/Gadovost (Bayer Healthcare)	Gd-BT-D03A Macrocyclic Nonionic	5.2 (5)	5.0	1603
Gadoterate	Meglumine	Dotarem (Guerbet)	Gd-DOTA Macrocyclic Ionic	3.6 (3.5)	2.4	1350
Gadofosveset	Trisodium	Ablavar/Vasovist (Lantheus)	MS-325 Linear Ionic	19 (10)	2.1	825

Adapted ACR manual on contrast media. In: Ellis JH, ed. American College of Radiology; 2016: http://www.acr.org/quality-safety/resources/contrast-manual.

RCM and are dose-dependent and infusion rate-dependent. This includes chemotoxic and vasovagal reactions. Chemotoxic reactions are often related to the osmolality of the RCM and include pain around the infusion site, warmth, flushing, and nausea. Vasovagal reactions are considered to be more severe reactions on the same spectrum, with symptoms of dizziness, hypotension, and bradycardia. These reactions are often transient and self-resolving and do not necessitate pretreatment for subsequent imaging studies. More severe chemotoxic reactions can cause nephropathy, thyroid dysfunction, and other organ toxicity, which are not further discussed in this chapter.[12-15]

RCM can cause many types of hypersensitivity reactions, including immediate hypersensitivity reactions (IHRs) and delayed hypersensitivity reactions. Systemic IHRs to RCM have historically been termed "anaphylactoid" reactions; however, this term is no longer used over concerns that it is misinterpreted to be less severe than true anaphylaxis. Thus, these reactions are now termed "nonimmunologic anaphylaxis." IHRs typically occur within 1 h of RCM administration, but some studies have shown that the majority occur during or within 5 min of RCM injection.[2] IHRs include symptoms of pruritus, urticaria, angioedema, bronchospasm, and rarely hypotension and shock. Several different classification systems have been used

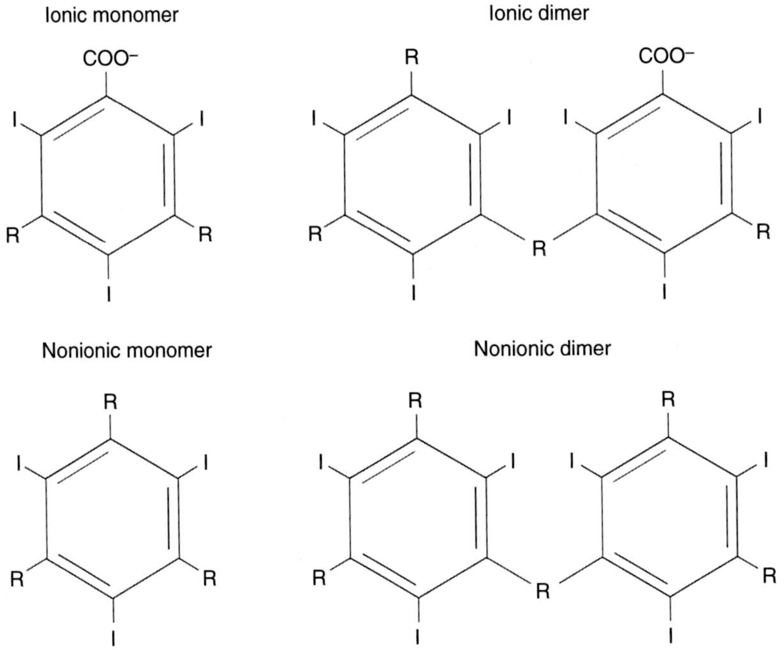

FIG. 22.1 Chemical Structure of Iodinated Contrast Agents. The central benzene ring has six positions for covalent binding. Iodine is bound to positions 2, 4, and 6, and carboxyl groups or other side chains (labeled as "R" groups) are bound to positions 1, 3, and 5.

to categorize the severity of IHRs, but the Ring and Messmer grading system may be the most commonly used in the literature.[16] Grade 1 includes generalized cutaneous or mucocutaneous symptoms, such as erythema, pruritus, urticaria, and angioedema; grade 2 encompasses mild systemic reactions, which include cutaneous symptoms plus abdominal symptoms (nausea, cramping), respiratory symptoms (shortness of breath), and/or mild tachycardia (change of over 20 beats per minute); grade 3 describes severe systemic reactions, including laryngeal edema, bronchospasm, hypoxemia, hypotension, arrhythmia, and shock; and grade 4 consists of cardiac and/or respiratory arrest. Although IHRs occur more commonly after intravenous or intraarterial administration, it should be noted that IHRs (even severe reactions including death) can also occur after administration through nonvascular routes because of absorption of RCM through mucosal barriers, for example, during urograms, arthrograms, myelograms, and hysterosalpingograms.[2,17–28]

The mechanisms of IHRs to RCM are not completely understood, but there is general consensus that they involve nonspecific mast cell and basophil activation, causing release of mediators such as histamine and tryptase.[29–32] RCM can activate mast cells and basophils

from subjects without any prior reaction to RCM in a dose-dependent fashion.[32,33] High-osmolality and ionic media may directly activate mast cells and basophils to a higher degree than low-osmolality media, which may account for the higher rates of IHR to the former compared with the latter.[33–36] Therefore, although the term "hypersensitivity" implies an immunologic mechanism, IHRs are largely nonimmunologic responses and not true IgE-mediated anaphylactic reactions. Paradoxically, IHRs to RCM display traits of both IgE-mediated and nonimmunologic mechanisms. In line with a nonimmunologic mechanism, RCM hypersensitivity reactions can be rate-dependent and dose-dependent and can also occur on first exposure, unlike IgE-mediated IHRs to other medications.[37,38] However, like IgE-mediated IHRs, severe and fatal reactions have also been reported using a fraction of a normal RCM dose.[39,40] Several other pathophysiologic mechanisms for IHR to RCM have been proposed, including complement activation and consumption, serotonin release, and activation of the bradykinin cascade.[41–46] However, the precise role of each of these mechanisms *in vivo* is unclear because *in vitro* assays demonstrate these effects in both RCM-hypersensitive patients as well as those who have never had an adverse reaction to RCM.[47,48]

A small percentage of IHR reactions to RCM may be IgE-mediated. Evidence supporting this mechanism includes the fact that serum specific IgE for RCM can be found in patients with a history of prior adverse reaction; however, the predictive value of these antibodies is unknown, because they can also be detected in patients without RCM hypersensitivity.[48,49] Additionally, there may be a higher incidence of cross-reactivity to RCM types that share similar side chains as shown by skin testing.[50] It is unclear if the presence of similar side chains allows for cross-reactivity of specific IgE binding, or if it simply imparts chemical properties that allow for nonspecific mast cell stimulation.

Numerous types of delayed hypersensitivity reactions to RCM have been documented. A variety of vague symptoms have been reported to occur more than 6 h after RCM administration in up to 14% of patients, including nausea/vomiting, abdominal cramping, fatigue, headache, dizziness, fever, and chest pain. The mechanisms for these adverse reactions are unclear, and most resolve within hours without treatment.[51] The most common delayed reaction is a maculopapular rash occurring hours to days after RCM administration.[37,52] Consistent with delayed rashes caused by other agents, these reactions are likely T cell mediated.[51,53–56] Fixed drug eruptions, drug reaction with eosinophilia and systemic symptoms (DRESS), Stevens-Johnson syndrome (SJS)/toxic epidermal necrolysis (TEN), acute generalized exanthematous pustulosis, acute respiratory distress syndrome, cutaneous vasculitis, and noncardiogenic pulmonary edema have been reported but are rare occurrences.[57–67]

Epidemiology

IHR occurrence has been reported anywhere between 2% and 60% of patients who receive ionic high-osmolality media and in 0.05% and 5.5% of those who receive nonionic low-osmolality media.[2,4,5,9,68–71] Most reactions are mild (often involving urticaria only), but severe or life-threatening reactions can occur in up to 0.4% of patients receiving ionic media versus less than 0.04% in those receiving nonionic media.[2,4,7,10,70–72] Despite the greater number of reactions with higher-osmolality RCM, some studies have suggested that the risk for fatal reaction to RCM may be the same with RCM of any osmolality, while others support a higher risk of death from ionic RCM.[4,8,27,72] It is estimated that about one-third to one-half of all IHRs occur on first exposure to RCM,[73] and up to 34.6% of patients with RCM-induced anaphylaxis develop these reactions on their first exposure to RCM.[74] The incidence of IHR appears to be lower in the pediatric population

compared with adults, presumably because of fewer prior exposures to RCM.[75,76] Children under 1 year of age are extremely unlikely to have any hypersensitivity reaction to RCM, and preadolescent children typically only have mild reactions, if any.[2,75]

By far, the most significant risk factor for having an IHR to RCM is a history of prior reaction. One study found that the incidence of hypersensitivity reactions to RCM increases cumulatively with the number of prior RCM exposures.[77] Patients with prior IHR to RCM have a 21%–60% risk of recurrent reaction on reexposure to ionic RCM.[53,55,70,71,78,79] Recurrent reactions are often similar to prior reactions, although there are some data to suggest that severe IHRs do not tend to recur as often as mild IHRs.[80] Atopic individuals with a history of asthma, allergic rhinitis, and/or food allergy are two to three times more likely to have IHR to RCM compared with nonatopic individuals, especially with high-osmolality agents.[2,71,72,81] Several studies and one meta-analysis concluded that the use of low-osmolality RCM instead of high-osmolality agents can significantly reduce (but not eliminate) the risk of IHR in atopic patients.[68,69,72,82–86] Other risk factors for IHR to RCM include female sex, advanced age, renal impairment, and possibly concurrent use of other medications such as taxanes.[74,75,77,87,88] Additionally, advanced age and history of frequent RCM exposure (more than five times) have been implicated in increasing the risk for having severe IHR and/or shock, although according to one study, age and RCM administration frequency appear to play a role in only a minority of cases involving fatal IHR to RCM.[74,89] Coronary artery disease may impart a higher risk for RCM reaction, as well as increase the likelihood of those reactions being severe and involving hemodynamic compromise.[90] The use of β-adrenergic antagonist medications was historically thought to increase the risk of having an IHR to RCM[90,91]; however, prospective studies have shown that their use may simply increase the risk of a severe reaction resistant to treatment with epinephrine but not necessarily increase the risk of any reaction.[92,93]

It is a medical myth that shellfish allergy imparts a higher risk for RCM hypersensitivity.[94] This idea may have become popular because early studies cited a slightly higher risk for reaction to high-osmolality RCM among patients with food allergy, specifically shellfish.[95] It is unclear how the link between shellfish allergy and iodine hypersensitivity came about, but this became popularly associated with iodinated RCM among both medical professionals and lay persons. Individuals with shellfish allergy have IgE specific for proteins in shellfish (namely tropomyosin), which have no relation to iodine.[96-98] Patients who have shellfish allergy have the same risk for adverse reaction to RCM as patients with asthma or other food allergies.[71,99,100] In medical centers that use low-osmolality media as standard practice, there is no need for pretreatment of shellfish-allergic patients.[100,101] Although it has been more than a decade since published guidelines including the American College of Radiology Manual on Contrast Media have recommended against routine screening for shellfish allergy, several studies have shown that many physicians still believe in this relationship, and thus, patients receive incorrect medical advice.[8,100-102] This misconception has also contributed to confusion in allergy labels in medical records. Patients may be labeled allergic to "iodine," which is ambiguous and could refer to iodinated contrast media, antiseptic solutions such as topical povidone-iodine, or shellfish (based on the patient's own perceived reaction to iodine). Allergists and other physicians should document these allergies carefully and thoroughly to avoid unnecessary pretreatment of patients with allergy to shellfish or topical iodine solution before RCM imaging studies.

Delayed reactions to RCM may be underdiagnosed, given the timing of the onset of symptoms, which typically begin days after RCM exposure. The frequency of delayed reactions to RCM has been highly variable between studies, cited as being anywhere between 0.5% and 45%, although consensus guidelines approximate the actual occurrence as being close to 2% of all patients.[53,103-111] RCM has been implicated as the third most common causative class of drugs for delayed hypersensitivity reactions, with only NSAIDs and antibiotics being more common.[112,113] The majority of these delayed reactions involve skin eruptions alone, but many can have systemic involvement as previously listed.[51,52,78,79,105,108] History of atopy or renal impairment may increase the risk of having a delayed reaction.[107] Patients with prior delayed reactions to RCM likely have a higher risk of repeat delayed reaction, which may occur in as many as 25% of patients.[52,53] Paradoxically, patients with no prior exposure to RCM also seem to have a higher incidence of delayed reaction compared with those who have received RCM without adverse reaction.[52] In contrast to IHRs, it has been suggested that delayed cutaneous reactions occur more frequently with dimeric agents.[106]

Diagnostic Testing

Diagnosis of IHR to RCM is based entirely on clinical symptoms and their chronological relation to RCM administration. Diagnostic testing is not routinely performed after a reaction, although obtaining a tryptase level within 6 h of (or, ideally 1–2 h after) the onset

of symptoms may help to distinguish an IHR from a vasovagal reaction.[114] It should be noted, however, that tryptase levels are more likely to be elevated following severe IHR reactions and may be normal following mild or moderate IHR reactions to RCM.[48,115-118]

There is no diagnostic test that can accurately predict hypersensitivity reactions to RCM. Skin prick and intradermal testing have been touted as a way to identify patients with higher risk for IHR, as suggested by several studies.[37,38,74,118-129] These studies often use undiluted RCM for skin prick testing and dilutions of 1:10 to 1:1000 for intradermal testing.[55] Generally, studies have shown that skin testing to RCM is itself safe with a very low rate of adverse reaction.[130] However, these studies are limited by small numbers of subjects and the lack of controls; therefore, it is difficult to assess the true utility of skin testing. There is general consensus that the sensitivity and specificity of skin testing for RCM are poor. In a recent meta-analysis, Yoon and colleagues showed that in patients with prior IHR to RCM, the positive skin test rate was only 3% for prick testing and 17% for intradermal testing (Table 22.3), with a very low false-positive rate among control subjects.[130] They did find better sensitivity as the severity of the IHR increased: the rate of positive intradermal skin tests was 12% in patients with prior mild IHR, 16% in those with moderate IHR, and 52% in those with severe IHR. Interestingly, several studies included in the analysis showed low cross-reactivity of skin testing between iodinated RCM types, with higher rates of positive skin testing to the culprit RCM that had caused the patient's prior IHR (23%) versus another type of RCM (3%). Skin testing may have better sensitivity when performed within 6 months of a reaction to RCM as opposed to 1 year or more.[131] However, skin testing cannot reliably identify patients who may have breakthrough reactions to RCM despite pretreatment.[129] Overall, given the low negative predictive value, skin testing is not recommended for routine use to predict hypersensitivity reactions to RCM, although the EAACI advocates use of skin testing in certain cases, such as severe IHRs or IHRs refractory to premedication.[48,55,121,127,132] A few other *in vitro* tests have been proposed to aid in predicting IHR, including basophil activation testing, leukocyte migration assays, and kallikrein conversion[45,124,127,133]; however, no large studies have been done to confirm the utility of these alternative assays, and many of these tests are experimental and not validated in most clinical laboratories.

Several small studies have suggested using graded dose challenge (either with diluted doses or with small volumes of undiluted media) as a method for predicting IHR to RCM. However, this method is not any more reliable in prediction of IHR compared with skin testing. In a large prospective study of 337,647 patients, the predictive value of using a test dose was 1.2% for ionic media and 0.0% for nonionic media, giving sensitivity values of 3.7% and 0.0%, respectively, which was consistent across all patients including those with significant atopy and/or a history of prior reaction to RCM.[132] Reactions to test doses neither correlate with reactions to a full dose of RCM, nor do they predict risk of severe reaction or death from RCM.[40,95] Additionally, test doses themselves (as small as 1 mL or less of undiluted RCM) have been reported to cause severe reactions, including death.[8,39,40,80,132,134] Therefore,

pretreatment is necessary before safely administering any dose of RCM to patients at high risk for reaction, including small test doses.

Patch testing and delayed intradermal testing (read anywhere from 24 to 96 h post placement) have been investigated as possible diagnostic methodologies for predicting delayed reactions to RCM. These methods have no utility in predicting any type of adverse reaction to RCM. For delayed hypersensitivity reactions to RCM, these studies report a very poor negative predictive value and a positive predictive value between 14% and 38%.[37,50,128,129]

TABLE 22.3
Per-Patient Positive Rates of Skin Tests in Patients With Hypersensitivity Reactions to Radiocontrast Media (RCM)

| Study | POSITIVE RATE OF SKIN TESTS | | POSITIVE RATE OF IDT ACCORDING TO... | | | | |
| | | | TESTED RCM | | SEVERITY OF IHR | | |
	SPT	IDT	Culprit RCM[a]	Alternative RCM[b]	Mild	Moderate	Severe
Dewachter et al.[120]	50% (2/4)	100% (4/4)	100% (4/4)	0% (0/4)	NS	NS	100% (4/4)
Trcka et al.[121]	Not done	4% (4/96)	NS	NS	0% (0/40)	7% (3/44)	8% (1/12)
Brockow et al.[37]	3% (4/122)	26% (32/121)	38% (24/63)	7% (8/121)	26% (24/92)	NS	28% (8/29)
Caimmi et al.[122]	0% (0/101)	15% (15/101)	NS	NS	NS	NS	NS
Dewachter et al.[118]	4% (1/24)	46% (12/26)	46% (12/26)	0% (0/26)	33% (3/9)	40% (4/10)	71% (5/7)
Goksel et al.[123]	0% (0/14)	14% (2/14)	20% (2/10)	0% (0/4)	14% (1/7)	14% (1/7)	NS
Pinnobphun et al.[124]	0% (0/63)	24% (15/63)	24% (15/63)	0% (0/63)	23% (12/53)	0% (0/5)	60% (3/5)
Kim et al.[38]	3% (1/32)	26% (12/46)	22% (10/46)	4% (2/46)	13% (4/31)	25% (2/8)	57% (4/7)
Kim et al.[74]	2% (1/51)	65% (33/51)	48% (22/46)	22% (11/51)	NS	18% (2/11)	78% (31/40)
Renaudin et al.[125]	14% (1/7)	57% (4/7)	NS	NS	NS	NS	57% (4/7)
Prieto-Garcia et al.[126]	0% (0/106)	10% (11/106)	14% (11/78)	0% (0/106)	9% (6/66)	14% (4/29)	9% (1/11)
Salas et al.[127]	3% (3/90)	6% (5/90)	6% (4/65)	2% (1/90)	0% (0/69)	11% (2/18)	100% (3/3)

The listed studies were included in a recent meta-analysis by Yoon and colleagues. Numbers in parentheses indicate the number of patients. Skin tests only included SPT and IDT, or which readings were taken within 20 min or less after testing. Positive rates of IDT were extracted using only studies that used 10⁻¹ diluted RCM for IDT.

IDT, intradermal test; *IHR*, immediate hypersensitivity reaction; *NS*, not specified; *RCM*, radiocontrast media; *SPT*, skin prick test.
[a]Positive rate of IDT tested including culprit RCM.
[b]Positive rate of IDT tested not including culprit RCM.
Adapted from Yoon SH, Lee SY, Kang HR, et al. Skin tests in patients with hypersensitivity reaction to iodinated contrast media: a meta-analysis. *Allergy*. June 2015;70(6):625–637.

Prevention of Immediate Hypersensitivity Reactions

A number of different premedication regimens have been used to prevent adverse reactions to RCM. Pretreatment is indicated for the prevention of recurrent IHR to RCM, but not for physiologic responses.[135,136] The efficacy of pretreatment in preventing delayed hypersensitivity or idiosyncratic reactions is unknown, but given the likely mechanisms underlying these reactions, pretreatment is unlikely to be of much benefit and is not currently recommended for these indications. The standard pretreatment regimen for prevention of IHR includes prednisone 50 mg orally at 13, 7, and 1 h before imaging plus diphenhydramine 50 mg orally 1 h before imaging

(Table 22.4). This regimen, which is often referred to as the "Greenberger protocol," has been standard of care for decades in preventing potentially dangerous reactions to contrast media.

The literature on premedication efficacy is complicated by the wide variety of medication regimens used each study, as well as the lack of placebo groups in most studies (as many authors argue that withholding pretreatment in patients could be fatal and therefore would be unethical) (Table 22.5). Overall, several studies have suggested that pretreatment reduces the incidence of recurrent reaction among patients with prior IHR to RCM.[5,73,86,136–141,144,146] Among patients with prior severe IHR, premedication with the above regimen of prednisone

TABLE 22.4
Pretreatment Regimens for Prevention of Immediate Hypersensitivity Reaction to Iodinated Contrast Media

	Recommended Medications	Optional Medications
Standard regimen	Prednisone 50 mg orally 13 h, 7 h, and 1 h before imaging *plus*	H2 receptor antagonist orally 1 h before imaging *and/or*
	Diphenhydramine 50 mg orally 1 h before imaging	Ephedrine 25 mg orally 1 h before imaging (withhold for severe or unstable cardiac disease) *and/or* Albuterol 4 mg orally 1 h before imaging (withhold for severe or unstable cardiac disease)
Extended regimen (for refractory IHR despite standard pretreatment)	Prednisone 50 mg orally every 6 h starting 31 h before imaging *plus*	H2 receptor antagonist orally 1 h before imaging *and/or* Ephedrine 25 mg orally 1 h before imaging (withhold for severe or unstable cardiac disease)
	Diphenhydramine 50 mg orally 1 h before imaging	*and/or* Albuterol 4 mg orally 1 h before imaging (withhold for severe or unstable cardiac disease)
Emergency protocol	Hydrocortisone 200 mg intravenously immediately and then every 4 h until imaging is complete *plus* Diphenhydramine 50 mg intramuscularly immediately before (preferably 1 h before) imaging	Albuterol 4 mg orally immediately before (preferably 1 h before) imaging (withhold for severe or unstable cardiac disease)

The standard regimen including prednisone and diphenhydramine should be used when time permits. In cases of IHRs despite receiving the standard pretreatment, anecdotal evidence has shown that an extended pretreatment regimen may be used for future imaging studies. For emergent imaging, the abbreviated emergency protocol may be used. Although ephedrine was used in early studies, it is not currently recommended for use in routine premedication, given its relative contraindication in cardiac disease.

TABLE 22.5
Studies on Breakthrough Reactions After Pretreatment

Study	Study Design; Patient Population Receiving Premedication	Imaging Modality	RCM Used	Premedication Regimen	BREAKTHROUGH REACTION RATE	
					Any Reaction	Severe Reaction
Kelly et al.[137]	Prospective cohort; included patients with prior IHR to any RCM	NS	NS	Greenberger prep	5.0% (5/101)	0% (0/101)
Zweiman et al.[138]	Prospective cohort	Intravenous urography, angiography, cholangiography	Sodium diatrizoate, methyl-glucamine diatrizoate, methyl-glucamine iodipamide	Prednisone PO in divided doses (150 mg total or an equivalent dose of another steroid) starting 18 h prior the procedure and lasting for 12 h after the procedure	9% (4/46)	0 (0/46)
Greenberger et al.[139]	Prospective cohort; included patients with prior IHR to any RCM	Intravenous, intraarterial, arthrography, myelography, pyelography	NS	Greenberger prep	6.5% (11/168)	0% (0/168)
Greenberger et al.[140]	Prospective cohort; included patients with prior IHR to any RCM	Intravenous or intraarterial infusion	NS	Greenberger prep	7.5% (24/318)	0.3% (1/318)
Greenberger et al.[141]	Prospective cohort; included patients with prior IHR to any RCM	Intravenous or intraarterial infusion	Sodium and/or methyl-glucamine iothalamate or diatrizoate	Greenberger prep Greenberger prep plus ephedrine 25 mg PO 1 h prior[a]	9.0% (42/465) 3.1% (6/192)	0.6% (3/465) 0% (0/192)
Greenberger et al.[73]	Prospective cohort; included patients with prior IHR to any RCM	Intravenous or intraarterial infusion	NS	Greenberger prep Greenberger prep plus ephedrine 25 mg PO 1 h prior[a] Greenberger prep Plus ephedrine 25 mg PO 1 h prior[a] plus cimetidine 300 mg PO 1 h prior	10.8% (45/415) 5% (9/180) 14% (14/100)	0.7% (3/415) 0% (0/180) 0% (0/100)
Ring et al.[142]	Prospective randomized cohort; included all patients receiving RCM (excluded patients with history of prior reaction to RCM)	Intravenous urography	Meglumine, amidotrizoate	Prednisolone IV divided into multiple doses (total 250mg, timing not specified) Placebo	1.5% (3/198) 4.1% (8/194)	NS NS

Continued

TABLE 22.5
Studies on Breakthrough Reactions After Pretreatment—cont'd

Study	Study Design; Patient Population Receiving Premedication	Imaging Modality	RCM Used	Premedication Regimen	BREAKTHROUGH REACTION RATE	
					Any Reaction	Severe Reaction
Lasser et al.[143]	Prospective randomized cohort; included all patients receiving RCM (excluded patients with prior reaction to any RCM)	Intravenous	Any ionic	Group 1: Methylprednisolone 32 mg PO 16 and 2 h prior	6.5% (163/2513)	0.2% (5/2513)
				Placebo PO as for group 1	9.0% (145/1603)	6.9% (11/1603)
				Group 2: Methylprednisolone 32 mg PO 2 h prior	9.4% (166/1759)	0.5% (9/1759)
				Placebo PO as for group 2	9.9% (88/888)	0.2% (2/888)
Greenberger et al.[5]	Prospective cohort; included patients with prior IHR to any RCM	NS	Iopamidol, iohexol	Greenberger prep	0.8% (1/120)	0% (0/100)
				Greenberger prep plus ephedrine 25 mg PO 1 h prior[a]	0% (0/54)	0% (0/41)
Marshall et al.[144]	Retrospective cohort; included patients with prior IHR to any RCM	NS	NS	Greenberger prep	7.7% (4/52)	0% (0/52)
				Greenberger prep plus cimetidine 300 mg PO 1 h prior	6.3% (3/48)	0% (0/48)
				Greenberger prep plus cimetidine 300 mg PO 1 h prior plus ephedrine 25 mg PO 1 h prior[a]	6.1% (3/49)	0% (0/49)
Wolf et al.[9]	Prospective cohort; included all patients receiving RCM	Intravenous urography	Diatrizoate, iohexol Iohexol	Methylprednisolone 32 mg PO 12 and 2 h prior	4.0% (32/805)	0.25% (2/805)
				Placebo	12.5% (25/200)	0% (0/200)
Lasser et al.[145]	Prospective, randomized, placebo controlled; included all patients receiving RCM	Intravenous urography; intravenous	Iohexol, ioversol	Methylprednisolone 32 mg PO 6–24 and 2 h prior placebo PO	1.7% (10/580)	0.3% (2/580)
				Placebo doses PO 6–24 and 2 h prior	4.9% (28/575)	1.6% (9/575)
Davenport et al.[146]	Retrospective; included patients with prior IHR to any RCM, multiple food or medication allergies, or moderate to severe asthma	Intravenous	Iohexol, iopromide, iopamidol	Greenberger prep	0.7% (1044/140,753) for all patients; 190 BTRs (out of unknown number of prior IHRs)	0.01% (17/140,753)
Kim et al.[147]	Retrospective; included patients with prior IHR to any RCM	Intravenous or intraarterial infusion	Iopromide, iomeprol, iopamidol, and iodixanol	Various regimens of prednisone (30–180 mg total dose) or methylprednisolone (50–187.5 mg total dose) plus H1 antihistamines and/or H2 blockers	16.7% (5/30)	3.3% (1/30)

TABLE 22.5
Studies on Breakthrough Reactions After Pretreatment—cont'd

Study	Study Design; Patient Population Receiving Premedication	Imaging Modality	RCM Used	Premedication Regimen	BREAKTHROUGH REACTION RATE	
					Any Reaction	Severe Reaction
Jingu et al.[148]	Retrospective; included patients with prior mild IHR to any RCM, asthma, or allergies (patients with prior moderate to severe IHR to RCM were excluded)	NS	NS	Methylprednisolone 32 mg PO 12 and 2 h prior plus diphenhydramine 50 mg PO 1 h prior	6.8% (8/117)	0% (0/117)
Kolbe et al.[149]	Prospective cohort; included patients with prior mild IHR (urticaria only) to any RCM	NS	NS	Diphehydramine 25–50 mg PO or IV 1 h prior	8.0% (2/25)	0% (0/25)
				Methylprednisolone 32 mg PO 12 and 2 h prior	46% (12/26)	0% (0/26)
				Methylprednisolone 32 mg PO 12 and 2 h prior plus diphehydramine 25–50 mg PO or IV 1 h prior	44% (7/16)	0% (0/16)
				No premedication	7.6% (5/66)	0% (0/66)
Mervak et al.[150]	Retrospective; included patients with prior IHR to any RCM[b]	Intravenous	Various low-osmolality RCM	Greenberger prep	2.1% (13/626)	0% (0/626)
Abe et al.[86]	Retrospective; included patients with prior IHR to any RCM, including chemotoxic reactions	Intravenous	Iopamidol, iohexol	100–500 mg hydrocortisone IV plus 10 mg chlorpheniramine 30–60 min prior Or 30 mg prednisone PO 16 and 3 h prior plus fexofenadine 30 mg PO 1 h prior	17.3% (47/271) Control group: 27.7% 61/220	0.4% (1/271) Control group: 0.5% 1/220
Jung et al.[151]	Retrospective; included patients with prior IHR to any RCM	NS	NS	Systemic steroids 13, 7, and 1 h prior (mean total prednisolone dose 95 mg)	3.2% (1/30)	NS

The literature on premedication efficacy is complicated by the wide variety of medication regimens used in each study, as well as the lack of placebo groups in many studies. The Greenberger Prep is the standard pretreatment regimen of prednisone 50 mg orally 13, 7, and 1 h before imaging, plus diphenhydramine 50 mg orally 1 h before imaging. Only studies using this pretreatment regimen or others that included systemic steroids were included in this table.

IHR, immediate hypersensitivity reaction; *NS*, not specified; *RCM*, radiocontrast media.
[a]Ephedrine was withheld for patients with unstable hypertensions or unstable angina.
[b]This study included also patients who had received pretreatment for other indications, but these are not included in the table above.

and diphenhydramine can reduce the severe recurrent reaction rate to 0.6%–0.7%.[73] The addition of ephedrine can further reduce the rate to 0%, although ephedrine is no longer recommended in routine premedication and should be avoided in patients with cardiac disease.[73] Several studies claim that premedication is not effective in preventing IHRs; however, these studies use suboptimal doses of steroids in their premedication regimens.[147] The "Lasser protocol," which includes methylprednisolone 32 mg orally 12 and 2 h before imaging plus the option of adding diphenhydramine, may not be as effective as the Greenberger protocol, although both regimens are listed as effective options in the American College of Radiology Manual on Contrast Media.[8,143,149] Antihistamines alone can prevent mild urticarial reactions in some patients but cannot prevent moderate or severe IHRs.[134,152–154]

The term "breakthrough reaction" refers to repeat IHR to RCM despite adequate pretreatment with glucocorticoids and antihistamines. Although pretreatment does reduce the overall incidence of subsequent reactions to RCM, breakthrough reactions can still occur. Some studies have suggested that pretreatment is more effective at preventing mild or moderate breakthrough reactions but is less effective at preventing severe breakthrough reactions or RCM-related deaths.[145] Breakthrough reactions are most often similar to a patient's initial reaction to RCM, although infrequently subsequent reactions can be more severe than prior ones.[155] Risk factors for having a breakthrough reaction despite adequate pretreatment include significant atopy (allergy to four or more substances), any drug allergy, and chronic corticosteroid use.[146,150] Among patients who have breakthrough reactions after receiving the Greenberger regimen, anecdotal evidence has shown that starting the protocol earlier (at 31 h before RCM administration instead of 13 h) can be efficacious in preventing further IHRs in subsequent studies (Table 22.4).

The exact mechanism of pretreatment in preventing RCM reactions is unknown, but it likely acts to stabilize mast cells and basophils. Because corticosteroids require several hours to take effect, the most effective way to reduce IHR is to use the standard pretreatment, which begins 13 h before RCM exposure. However, the need for urgent or emergent imaging often arises in the inpatient setting. In these cases, an abbreviated regimen should be started as soon as the need for imaging is known (Table 22.4). In all cases of pretreatment, the necessity for RCM use must be clearly documented in the medical record, and the patient should be made aware of the risks and benefits of the pretreatment regimen.

As with any medical treatment, the risks of giving corticosteroids must be weighed against the benefits for each patient individually. The use of systemic steroids should be used with caution in patients with diabetes, active or latent infection, peptic ulcer disease, and other comorbidities.[156] However, given the need for only a few doses before each RCM exposure, the side effects of the steroids in the standard pretreatment regimen are generally low.[145] Very few studies have performed a cost–benefit analysis of using premedication for prevention of recurrent IHRs to RCM. One study by Davenport investigated the indirect cost and potential harm in using pretreatment regimens.[150] Among 1424 inpatients who received the standard pretreatment regimen before receiving RCM, they found that pretreatment was associated with a significantly longer hospital stay and a higher nosocomial infection rate (proportional to and presumably caused by the longer length of stay).[157] However, this analysis did not compare the costs of premedication with the potential costs of having a severe or fatal reaction to RCM. Additionally, this study cannot extrapolate its findings to outpatients who receive pretreatment for scheduled outpatient imaging studies. These patients may self-administer their medications at home, which essentially negates the risk of nosocomial infection and does not impart increased usage of inpatient beds.

Approach to High-Risk Patients

Fig. 22.2 shows a general algorithm to guide the approach to patients before imaging studies that may require RCM. For all patients, the necessity of using RCM should be documented in the medical record, and the patient should be made aware of the risks and benefits of using contrast. Skin testing to RCM is not recommended given its poor positive and negative predictive values, which are not improved even in patients who have had a prior severe IHR despite pretreatment.[129] Because even low-risk patients can have severe reactions on first exposure to RCM, low-osmolality RCM should be used whenever possible in all patients, especially in those with a history of asthma or cardiovascular disease, and in those who are taking β-adrenergic blocking medications. This practice is already standard of care in many medical centers in the United States. For patients who have a history of prior reaction to any type of RCM, low-osmolality media should be used for any subsequent imaging, and pretreatment with steroids and antihistamines is recommended to prevent a severe recurrent reaction. For those with breakthrough IHR despite standard pretreatment, anecdotally there has been success with doubling the premedication period, thereby giving prednisone 50 mg orally every 6 h, starting 31 h before imaging. Currently, there are no recommendations to support or oppose premedication of atopic patients with no history of previous reaction if low-osmolality RCM is used. Significantly atopic patients who have a history of multiple food or

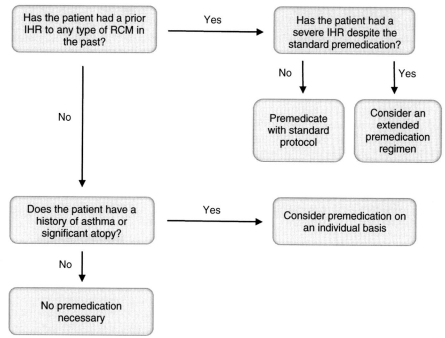

FIG. 22.2 Algorithm for Approach to Using Iodinated Radiocontrast Media (RCM) in High-Risk Patients. Low-osmolality RCM should be used for all patients whenever possible, but especially for those who have had a prior immediate hypersensitivity reaction (IHR) or who have pulmonary disease, cardiac disease, or significant atopy. For patients with a history of prior IHR, premedication with corticosteroids and antihistamines is warranted before subsequent imaging. A modified premedication regimen may be considered for patients who have IHR despite standard premedication as described in Table 22.4.

medication allergies, asthma, and/or allergic rhinitis should be considered for pretreatment on an individual basis. The risks of pretreatment need to be considered in each case, including costs, extension of hospital stay, and potential exacerbation of existing comorbidities.

The efficacy of premedication for delayed reactions to RCM is unknown.[53] For patients whose prior delayed reaction was limited to mild cutaneous symptoms, prophylaxis with corticosteroids is likely not necessary but may be considered.[8] For patients with severe delayed or idiosyncratic reactions to RCM (including DRESS, SJS/TEN, vasculitis, and others), RCM should be strictly avoided in the future.

Management of Acute Reactions

Because IHR can occur on first exposure to RCM, and timely intervention is crucial to prevent death from severe IHRs, radiologists and other staff should be prepared to treat adverse reactions for every patient (Table 22.6). For mild IHRs including urticaria, antihistamines such as diphenhydramine orally may be sufficient in most patients. The mainstay of treatment for any systemic IHR is intramuscular epinephrine (0.3–0.5 mg).

There is no absolute contraindication for epinephrine in the setting of a severe IHR to RCM. In the event of severe systemic reaction or shock, several doses of epinephrine may be required to achieve hemodynamic stability. Inhaled albuterol should be administered for bronchospasm. Further treatment should follow advanced cardiac life support guidelines, including supportive measures such as oxygen, intravenous fluids, and close monitoring. For other specific reactions such as bradycardia, pulmonary edema, and others, pharmacologic therapy should be directed at treating the specific condition. Delayed reactions may not require treatment if they involve mild rash, although antihistamines and steroids may be considered. Severe delayed reactions including DRESS, SJS/TEN, and vasculitis should be treated as they would from any other etiology.

GADOLINIUM-BASED CONTRAST MEDIA

Types of Gadolinium-Based Contrast Media

GBCM was first FDA approved for use in 1988 (see Table 22.2 for available agents in the United States).

TABLE 22.6
Management of Immediate Hypersensitivity Reactions to Radiocontrast Media

Reaction Severity	Symptoms	Therapies	Optional Therapies
Grade 1 (limited cutaneous reactions)	Generalized cutaneous or mucocutaneous symptoms such as pruritus, urticaria, and angioedema	Diphenhydramine 25–50 mg orally	Consider additional H1-receptor antagonists
Grade 2 (mild systemic reactions)	Cutaneous symptoms plus abdominal symptoms (nausea, cramping), respiratory symptoms (shortness of breath), and/or mild tachycardia (change of over 20 beats per minute)	Epinephrine 0.3 mg intramuscularly immediately (repeat every 5–15 min as needed) *plus* Supportive measures (place patient in recumbent position, treat hypotension with IVF, give O₂ via face mask, monitor vital signs)	Consider diphenhydramine 25–50 mg intravenously *and/or* Consider methylprednisolone 125 mg intravenously *and/or* For patients on β-adrenergic blockers, give glucagon 1–5 mg intravenously over 5 min, followed by infusion of 5–15 mcg/min *and/or* For bronchospasm, give albuterol 90 mcg two puffs (repeat as needed) *and/or* For hypotension refractory to epinephrine, consider giving additional vasopressors
Grade 3 (severe systemic reactions)	Laryngeal edema, bronchospasm, hypoxemia, hypotension, arrhythmia, and shock		
Grade 4 (death)	Cardiac and/or respiratory arrest	Epinephrine 0.3 mg intramuscularly (repeat every 5–15 min as needed) *plus* Resuscitation per ACLS guidelines	As for Grades 2–3

Antihistamines may be used for mild cutaneous IHRs. The mainstay of treatment for systemic reactions is intramuscular epinephrine.
ACLS, advanced cardiac life support; *IHR*, immediate hypersensitivity reaction; *IVF*, intravenous fluids.

Unlike iodinated RCM, which is radiopaque, GBCM provides contrast and enhancement of tissues during MRI by reducing the speed at which hydrogen ions revert back to their ground state after excitation. All GBCM have a core paramagnetic gadolinium (Gd^{3+}), a heavy metal ion which by itself can be directly toxic to tissues. Chelation of Gd^{3+} ions with a ligand prevents toxicity and increases the solubility and stability of the overall complex. The half-life of these agents in serum is about 2 h, and in most cases they are completely cleared within 24 h of administration.[158] The two main categories of GBCM are linear and macrocyclic, both of which can be ionic or nonionic. Macrocyclic GBCM tend to have lower dissociation constants for the Gd^{3+} ion; therefore, they are less likely than linear structures to release toxic free Gd^{3+} into circulation.[159,160] Gd^{3+} is able to compete with calcium ions (Ca^{2+}) for various cellular enzymes, which may cause tissue injury by interfering with regulatory processes, as well as by release of inflammatory mediators.[161]

Types of Adverse Reactions, Frequency, and Management

GBCM is well tolerated by the vast majority of patients, and as compared with RCM, adverse reactions are uncommon. As with RCM, physiologic reactions to GBCM can involve vague or nonspecific symptoms such as nausea, vomiting, headache, dizziness, and transient paresthesias. One physiologic reaction that is unique to GBCM is termed "transient dyspnea."[8] This feeling of subjective shortness of breath may occur in 4%–14% of patients, is self-limited, and tends to be associated with one particular type of GBCM, gadoxetate disodium.[162,163] Risk factors for having transient dyspnea are a history of having this reaction to GBCM before, history of pulmonary disease (especially COPD), and utilizing larger volumes of GBCM.[164,165] The mechanism of transient dyspnea is unclear, but it does not appear to be related to bronchospasm.[162,163] Premedication is unlikely to be of benefit for transient dyspnea and is not recommended. For future imaging, smaller volumes of GBCM can be used to help minimize the risk of recurrent reaction.[8]

IHRs to GBCM are similar to those induced by RCM; however, they occur less frequently than with RCM. Several large studies, which together include over a million patients, have estimated the IHR rate to be between 0.004% and 0.7%.[166–168] Severe or life-threatening reactions have been reported but are considered to be extremely rare, with an estimated risk between 0.001% and 0.01% of all patients. The biggest risk factor for IHR to GBCM is a history of a prior reaction, which increases the risk about eightfold compared with the rest of the population.[8] Patients with atopy and asthma may also be at higher risk for IHR. Because all types of GBCM are small molecules, it is thought that the majority of IHRs are due to nonspecific mast cell activation and not due to IgE-mediated hypersensitivity. Approach to pretreatment and management of IHR from GBCM is similar to RCM (see Fig. 22.2). Skin testing to GBCM is not currently recommended because there are no large studies to support its use.

The most serious adverse reaction to GBCM is nephrogenic systemic fibrosis (NSF), which occurs exclusively in patients who have reduced glomerular filtration rate from either acute or chronic kidney disease.[15,169–173] NSF begins days to months after GBCM administration and results in irreversible diffuse fibrosis of the skin and subcutaneous tissue. It also often affects other organs including the lungs, heart, esophagus, and skeletal muscle, and patients often develop muscle contractures or joint immobility as a result. In more severe cases, organ involvement can lead to death. The mechanisms of NSF are poorly understood, but one proposed mechanism is that free Gd^{3+} causes direct tissue damage, which results in inflammatory and profibrotic cytokine release by macrophages.[174–176] A few particular GBCMs including gadodiamide, gadoversetamide, and gadopentetate dimeglumine are associated with the greatest number of NSF cases, whereas others have been reported to cause NSF exceedingly rarely or not at all.[8] There is no effective treatment for NSF; therefore, prevention is paramount. The American College of Radiology has detailed recommendations on the approach to using GBCM in patients with renal impairment.[8]

REFERENCES

1. Swick M. The discovery of intravenous urography: historical and developmental aspects of the urographic media and their role in other diagnostic and therapeutic areas. *Bull N Y Acad Med*. 1966;42(2):128–151.
2. Katayama H, Yamaguchi K, Kozuka T, Takashima T, Seez P, Matsuura K. Adverse reactions to ionic and nonionic contrast media. A report from the Japanese Committee on the Safety of Contrast Media. *Radiology*. 1990;175(3):621–628.
3. Lieberman PL, Seigle RL. Reactions to radiocontrast material. Anaphylactoid events in radiology. *Clin Rev Allergy Immunol*. 1999;17(4):469–496.
4. Lasser EC, Lyon SG, Berry CC. Reports on contrast media reactions: analysis of data from reports to the U.S. Food and Drug Administration. *Radiology*. 1997;203(3):605–610.
5. Greenberger PA, Patterson R. The prevention of immediate generalized reactions to radiocontrast media in high-risk patients. *J Allergy Clin Immunol*. 1991;87(4):867–872.
6. Neugut AI, Ghatak AT, Miller RL. Anaphylaxis in the United States: an investigation into its epidemiology. *Arch Intern Med*. 2001;161(1):15–21.
7. Palmer FJ. The RACR survey of intravenous contrast media reactions. Final report. *Australas Radiol*. 1988;32(4):426–428.
8. ACR manual on contrast media. In: Ellis JH, ed. American College of Radiology; 2016. http://www.acr.org/quality-safety/resources/contrast-manual.
9. Wolf GL, Mishkin MM, Roux SG, et al. Comparison of the rates of adverse drug reactions. Ionic contrast agents, ionic agents combined with steroids, and nonionic agents. *Invest Radiol*. 1991;26(5):404–410.
10. Wolf GL, Arenson RL, Cross AP. A prospective trial of ionic vs nonionic contrast agents in routine clinical practice: comparison of adverse effects. *AJR Am J Roentgenol*. 1989;152(5):939–944.
11. Federle MP, Willis LL, Swanson DP. Ionic versus nonionic contrast media: a prospective study of the effect of rapid bolus injection on nausea and anaphylactoid reactions. *J Comput Assist Tomogr*. 1998;22(3):341–345.

12. Lee SY, Rhee CM, Leung AM, Braverman LE, Brent GA, Pearce EN. A review: radiographic iodinated contrast media-induced thyroid dysfunction. *J Clin Endocrinol Metab.* 2015;100(2):376–383.

13. Andreucci M, Faga T, Pisani A, Sabbatini M, Michael A. Acute kidney injury by radiographic contrast media: pathogenesis and prevention. *BioMed Res Int.* 2014;2014:362725.

14. Sandow BA, Donnal JF. Myelography complications and current practice patterns. *AJR Am J Roentgenol.* 2005;185(3):768–771.

15. Hasebroock KM, Serkova NJ. Toxicity of MRI and CT contrast agents. *Expert Opin Drug Metab Toxicol.* 2009;5(4):403–416.

16. Ring J, Messmer K. Incidence and severity of anaphylactoid reactions to colloid volume substitutes. *Lancet.* 1977;1(8009):466–469.

17. Marshall Jr WH, Castellino RA. The urinary mucosal barrier in retrograde pyelography. The role of the ureteric mucosa. *Radiology.* 1970;97(1):5–7.

18. Johenning PW. Reactions to contrast material during retrograde pyelography. *Urology.* 1980;16(4):442–444.

19. Currarino G, Weinberg A, Putnam R. Resorption of contrast material from the bladder during cystourethrography causing an excretory urogram. *Radiology.* 1977;123(1):149–150.

20. Weese DL, Greenberg HM, Zimmern PE. Contrast media reactions during voiding cystourethrography or retrograde pyelography. *Urology.* 1993;41(1):81–84.

21. Cartwright R, Cardozo L, Durling R. A retrospective review of a series of videourodynamic procedures, with respect to the risk of anaphylactoid reactions. *Neurourol Urodyn.* 2008;27(6):559.

22. Hugo 3rd PC, Newberg AH, Newman JS, Wetzner SM. Complications of arthrography. *Semin Musculoskeletal Radiol.* 1998;2(4):345–348.

23. Newberg AH, Munn CS, Robbins AH. Complications of arthrography. *Radiology.* 1985;155(3):605–606.

24. Capdeville R, Remy J. A major complication of hysterosalpingography. *J Radiol.* 1983;64(10):561–562.

25. Sanfilippo JS, Yussman MA, Smith O. Hysterosalpingography in the evaluation of infertility: a six-year review. *Fertil Steril.* 1978;30(6):636–643.

26. Grammer LC, Patterson R. Adverse reactions to radiographic contrast material. *Clin Dermatol.* 1986;4(1):149–154.

27. Spring DB, Bettmann MA, Barkan HE. Deaths related to iodinated contrast media reported spontaneously to the U.S. Food and Drug Administration, 1978-1994: effect of the availability of low-osmolality contrast media. *Radiology.* 1997;204(2):333–337.

28. Shehadi WH, Toniolo G. Adverse reactions to contrast media: a report from the Committee on Safety of Contrast Media of the International Society of Radiology. *Radiology.* 1980;137(2):299–302.

29. Simon RA, Schatz M, Stevenson DD, et al. Radiographic contrast media infusions. Measurement of histamine, complement, and fibrin split products and correlation with clinical parameters. *J Allergy Clin Immunol.* 1979;63(4):281–288.

30. Ring J, Endrich B, Intaglietta M. Histamine release, complement consumption, and microvascular changes after radiographic contrast media infusion in rabbits. *J Lab Clin Med.* 1978;92(4):584–594.

31. Ring J, Simon RA, Arroyave CM. Increased in vitro histamine release by radiographic contrast media in patients with history of incompatibility. *Clin Exp Immunol.* 1978;34(2):302–309.

32. Stellato C, de Crescenzo G, Patella V, Mastronardi P, Mazzarella B, Marone G. Human basophil/mast cell releasability. XI. Heterogeneity of the effects of contrast media on mediator release. *J Allergy Clin Immunol.* 1996;97(3):838–850.

33. Salem DN, Findlay SR, Isner JM, Konstam MA, Cohen PF. Comparison of histamine release effects of ionic and non-ionic radiographic contrast media. *Am J Med.* 1986;80(3):382–384.

34. Amon EU, Ennis M, Lorenz W, Schnabel M, Schneider C. Histamine release induced by radiographic contrast media. Comparison between pulmonary and peritoneal mast cells derived from normotensive and spontaneously hypertensive rats. *Int Arch Allergy Appl Immunol.* 1990;92(2):203–208.

35. Genovese A, Stellato C, Marsella CV, Adt M, Marone G. Role of mast cells, basophils and their mediators in adverse reactions to general anesthetics and radiocontrast media. *Int Arch Allergy Immunol.* 1996;110(1):13–22.

36. Assem ES, Bray K, Dawson P. The release of histamine from human basophils by radiological contrast agents. *Br J Radiol.* 1983;56(669):647–652.

37. Brockow K, Romano A, Aberer W, et al. Skin testing in patients with hypersensitivity reactions to iodinated contrast media – a European multicenter study. *Allergy.* 2009;64(2):234–241.

38. Kim SH, Jo EJ, Kim MY, et al. Clinical value of radiocontrast media skin tests as a prescreening and diagnostic tool in hypersensitivity reactions. *Ann Allergy Asthma Immunol.* 2013;110(4):258–262.

39. Finby N, Evans JA, Steinberg I. Reactions from intravenous organic iodide compounds: pretesting and prophylaxis. *Radiology.* 1958;71(1):15–18.

40. Fischer HW, Doust VL. An evaluation of pretesting in the problem of serious and fatal reactions to excretory urography. *Radiology.* 1972;103(3):497–501.

41. Arroyave CM, Schatz M, Simon RA. Activation of the complement system by radiographic contrast media: studies in vivo and in vitro. *J Allergy Clin Immunol.* 1979;63(4):276–280.

42. Zir LM, Carvalho AC, Hawthorne JW, Colman RW, Lees RS. Effect of contrast agents on platelet aggregation and 14C-serotonin release. *N Engl J Med.* 1974;291(3):134–135.

43. Siegle RL, Lieberman P, Rice MC. In vitro complement consumption by contrast materials and analogues: reactors vs. nonreactors. *Invest Radiol.* 1983;18(4):387–389.

44. Szebeni J. Hypersensitivity reactions to radiocontrast media: the role of complement activation. *Curr Allergy Asthma Rep.* 2004;4(1):25–30.

45. Lasser EC, Lang JH, Lyon SG, Hamblin AE, Howard MM. Prekallikrein-Kallikrein conversion rate as a predictor of contrast material catastrophies. *Radiology.* 1981;140(1):11–15.

46. Ring J, Arroyave CM, Frizler MJ, Tan EM. In vitro histamine and serotonin release by radiographic contrast media (RCM). Complement-dependent and -independent release reaction and changes in ultrastructure of human blood cells. *Clin Exp Immunol.* 1978;32(1):105–118.

47. Eloy R, Corot C, Belleville J. Contrast media for angiography: physicochemical properties, pharmacokinetics and biocompatibility. *Clin Mater.* 1991;7(2):89–197.

48. Laroche D, Aimone-Gastin I, Dubois F, et al. Mechanisms of severe, immediate reactions to iodinated contrast material. *Radiology.* 1998;209(1):183–190.

49. Mita H, Tadokoro K, Akiyama K. Detection of IgE antibody to a radiocontrast medium. *Allergy.* 1998;53(12):1133–1140.

50. Lerondeau B, Trechot P, Waton J, et al. Analysis of cross-reactivity among radiocontrast media in 97 hypersensitivity reactions. *J Allergy Clin Immunol.* 2016;137(2):633–635 e634.

51. Loh S, Bagheri S, Katzberg RW, Fung MA, Li CS. Delayed adverse reaction to contrast-enhanced CT: a prospective single-center study comparison to control group without enhancement. *Radiology.* 2010;255(3):764–771.

52. Hosoya T, Yamaguchi K, Akutsu T, et al. Delayed adverse reactions to iodinated contrast media and their risk factors. *Radiat Med.* 2000;18(1):39–45.

53. Webb JA, Stacul F, Thomsen HS, Morcos SK. Members of the Contrast Media Safety Committee of the European Society of Urogenital R. Late adverse reactions to intravascular iodinated contrast media. *Eur Radiol.* 2003;13(1):181–184.

54. Christiansen C, Pichler WJ, Skotland T. Delayed allergy-like reactions to X-ray contrast media: mechanistic considerations. *Eur Radiol.* 2000;10(12):1965–1975.

55. Brockow K, Christiansen C, Kanny G, et al. Management of hypersensitivity reactions to iodinated contrast media. *Allergy.* 2005;60(2):150–158.

56. Vernassiere C, Trechot P, Commun N, Schmutz JL, Barbaud A. Low negative predictive value of skin tests in investigating delayed reactions to radio-contrast media. *Contact Dermatitis.* 2004;50(6):359–366.

57. Miranda-Romero A, Sanchez-Sambucety P, Esquivias Gomez JI, et al. Vegetating iododerma with fatal outcome. *Dermatology.* 1999;198(3):295–297.

58. Rosado A, Canto G, Veleiro B, Rodriguez J. Toxic epidermal necrolysis after repeated injections of iohexol. *AJR Am J Roentgenol.* 2001;176(1):262–263.

59. Vaillant L, Pengloan J, Blanchier D, De Muret A, Lorette G. Iododerma and acute respiratory distress with leucocytoclastic vasculitis following the intravenous injection of contrast medium. *Clin Exp Dermatol.* 1990;15(3):232–233.

60. Goodfellow T, Holdstock GE, Brunton FJ, Bamforth J. Fatal acute vasculitis after high-dose urography with iohexol. *Br J Radiol.* 1986;59(702):620–621.

61. Savill JS, Barrie R, Ghosh S, Muhlemann M, Dawson P, Pusey CD. Fatal Stevens-Johnson syndrome following urography with iopamidol in systemic lupus erythematosus. *Postgrad Med J.* 1988;64(751):392–394.

62. Laffitte E, Nenadov Beck M, Hofer M, Hohl D, Panizzon RG. Severe Stevens-Johnson syndrome induced by contrast medium iopentol (Imagopaque). *Br J Dermatol.* 2004;150(2):376–378.

63. Belhadjali H, Bouzgarrou L, Youssef M, Njim L, Zili J. DRESS syndrome induced by sodium meglumine ioxitalamate. *Allergy.* 2008;63(6):786–787.

64. Hasdenteufel F, Waton J, Cordebar V, et al. Delayed hypersensitivity reactions caused by iodixanol: an assessment of cross-reactivity in 22 patients. *J Allergy Clin Immunol.* 2011;128(6):1356–1357.

65. Gonzalez-Estrada A, Gutta RC, Radojicic C. Prophylactic IVIG and corticosteroids for severe skin reactions post radio-contrast. *QJM.* 2015;108(10):827–828.

66. Hebert AA, Bogle MA. Intravenous immunoglobulin prophylaxis for recurrent Stevens-Johnson syndrome. *J Am Acad Dermatol.* 2004;50(2):286–288.

67. Peterson A, Katzberg RW, Fung MA, Wootton-Gorges SL, Dager W. Acute generalized exanthematous pustulosis as a delayed dermatotoxic reaction to IV-administered nonionic contrast media. *AJR Am J Roentgenol.* 2006;187(2):W198–W201.

68. Siegle RL, Halvorsen RA, Dillon J, Gavant ML, Halpern E. The use of iohexol in patients with previous reactions to ionic contrast material. A multicenter clinical trial. *Invest Radiol.* 1991;26(5):411–416.

69. Schrott KM, Behrends B, Clauss W, Kaufmann J, Lehnert J. Iohexol in excretory urography. Results of drug monitoring. *Fortschr Med.* 1986;104(7):153–156.

70. Katayama H. Survey of safety of clinical contrast media. *Invest Radiol.* 1990;25(Suppl. 1):S7–S10.

71. Shehadi WH. Adverse reactions to intravascularly administered contrast media. A comprehensive study based on a prospective survey. *Am J Roentgenol Radium Ther Nucl Med.* 1975;124(1):145–152.

72. Caro JJ, Trindade E, McGregor M. The risks of death and of severe nonfatal reactions with high- vs low-osmolality contrast media: a meta-analysis. *AJR Am J Roentgenol.* 1991;156(4):825–832.

73. Greenberger PA, Patterson R, Tapio CM. Prophylaxis against repeated radiocontrast media reactions in 857 cases. Adverse experience with cimetidine and safety of beta-adrenergic antagonists. *Arch Intern Med.* 1985;145(12):2197–2200.

74. Kim MH, Lee SY, Lee SE, et al. Anaphylaxis to iodinated contrast media: clinical characteristics related with development of anaphylactic shock. *PLoS One.* 2014;9(6):e100154.

75. Callahan MJ, Poznauskis L, Zurakowski D, Taylor GA. Nonionic iodinated intravenous contrast material-related reactions: incidence in large urban children's hospital–retrospective analysis of data in 12,494 patients. *Radiology.* 2009;250(3):674–681.

76. Dillman JR, Strouse PJ, Ellis JH, Cohan RH, Jan SC. Incidence and severity of acute allergic-like reactions to i.v. nonionic iodinated contrast material in children. *AJR Am J Roentgenol*. 2007;188(6):1643–1647.

77. Fujiwara N, Tateishi R, Akahane M, et al. Changes in risk of immediate adverse reactions to iodinated contrast media by repeated administrations in patients with hepatocellular carcinoma. *PLoS One*. 2013;8(10):e76018.

78. Munechika H, Yasuda R, Michihiro K. Delayed adverse reaction of monomeric contrast media: comparison of plain CT and enhanced CT. *Acad Radiol*. 1998;5(Suppl. 1):S157–S158.

79. Yasuda R, Munechika H. Delayed adverse reactions to nonionic monomeric contrast-enhanced media. *Invest Radiol*. 1998;33(1):1–5.

80. Shehadi WH. Contrast media adverse reactions: occurrence, recurrence, and distribution patterns. *Radiology*. 1982;143(1):11–17.

81. Bertrand P, Rouleau P, Alison D, Chastin I. Use of peak expiratory flow rate to identify patients with increased risk of contrast medium reaction. Results of preliminary study. *Invest Radiol*. 1988;23(Suppl. 1):S203–S205.

82. Barrett BJ, Parfrey PS, McDonald JR, Hefferton DM, Reddy ER, McManamon PJ. Nonionic low-osmolality versus ionic high-osmolality contrast material for intravenous use in patients perceived to be at high risk: randomized trial. *Radiology*. 1992;183(1):105–110.

83. Rapoport S, Bookstein JJ, Higgins CB, Carey PH, Sovak M, Lasser EC. Experience with metrizamide in patients with previous severe anaphylactoid reactions to ionic contrast agents. *Radiology*. 1982;143(2):321–325.

84. Holtas S. Iohexol in patients with previous adverse reactions to contrast media. *Invest Radiol*. 1984;19(6):563–565.

85. Fischer HW, Spataro RF. Use of low-osmolality contrast media in patients with previous reactions. *Invest Radiol*. 1988;23(Suppl. 1):S186–S188.

86. Abe S, Fukuda H, Tobe K, Ibukuro K. Protective effect against repeat adverse reactions to iodinated contrast medium: Premedication vs. changing the contrast medium. *Eur Radiol*. 2016;26(7):2148–2154.

87. Lang DM, Alpern MB, Visintainer PF, Smith ST. Gender risk for anaphylactoid reaction to radiographic contrast media. *J Allergy Clin Immunol*. 1995;95(4):813–817.

88. Farolfi A, Della Luna C, Ragazzini A, et al. Taxanes as a risk factor for acute adverse reactions to iodinated contrast media in cancer patients. *Oncologist*. 2014;19(8):823–828.

89. Palmiere C, Reggiani Bonetti L. Risk factors in fatal cases of anaphylaxis due to contrast media: a forensic evaluation. *Int Arch Allergy Immunol*. 2014;164(4):280–288.

90. Lang DM, Alpern MB, Visintainer PF, Smith ST. Elevated risk of anaphylactoid reaction from radiographic contrast media is associated with both beta-blocker exposure and cardiovascular disorders. *Arch Intern Med*. 1993;153(17):2033–2040.

91. Lang DM, Alpern MB, Visintainer PF, Smith ST. Increased risk for anaphylactoid reaction from contrast media in patients on beta-adrenergic blockers or with asthma. *Ann Intern Med*. 1991;115(4):270–276.

92. Aggarwal A, Smith JL, Chinnaiyan KM, et al. Beta-blocker premedication does not increase the frequency of allergic reactions from coronary CT angiography: Results from the Advanced Cardiovascular Imaging Consortium. *J Cardiovasc Computed Tomogr*. 2015;9(4):270–277.

93. Greenberger PA, Meyers SN, Kramer BL, Kramer BL. Effects of beta-adrenergic and calcium antagonists on the development of anaphylactoid reactions from radiographic contrast media during cardiac angiography. *J Allergy Clin Immunol*. 1987;80(5):698–702.

94. Drug allergy: an updated practice parameter. *Ann Allergy Asthma Immunol*. 2010;105(4):259–273.

95. Witten DM, Hirsch FD, Hartman GW. Acute reactions to urographic contrast medium: incidence, clinical characteristics and relationship to history of hypersensitivity states. *Am J Roentgenol Radium Ther Nucl Med*. 1973;119(4):832–840.

96. Reese G, Ayuso R, Carle T, Lehrer SB. IgE-binding epitopes of shrimp tropomyosin, the major allergen Pen a 1. *Int Arch Allergy Immunol*. 1999;118(2–4):300–301.

97. Reese G, Ayuso R, Lehrer SB. Tropomyosin: an invertebrate pan-allergen. *Int Arch Allergy Immunol*. 1999;119(4):247–258.

98. Coakley FV, Panicek DM. Iodine allergy: an oyster without a pearl? *AJR Am J Roentgenol*. 1997;169(4):951–952.

99. Schabelman E, Witting M. The relationship of radiocontrast, iodine, and seafood allergies: a medical myth exposed. *J Emerg Med*. 2010;39(5):701–707.

100. Beaty AD, Lieberman PL, Slavin RG. Seafood allergy and radiocontrast media: are physicians propagating a myth?. *Am J Med*. 2008;121(2). 158 e151–154.

101. Huang SW. Seafood and iodine: an analysis of a medical myth. *Allergy Asthma Proc*. 2005;26(6):468–469.

102. Baig M, Farag A, Sajid J, Potluri R, Irwin RB, Khalid HM. Shellfish allergy and relation to iodinated contrast media: United Kingdom survey. *World J Cardiol*. 2014;6(3):107–111.

103. Egbert RE, De Cecco CN, Schoepf UJ, McQuiston AD, Meinel FG, Katzberg RW. Delayed adverse reactions to the parenteral administration of iodinated contrast media. *AJR Am J Roentgenol*. 2014;203(6):1163–1170.

104. Pedersen SH, Svaland MG, Reiss AL, Andrew E. Late allergy-like reactions following vascular administration of radiography contrast media. *Acta Radiol*. 1998;39(4):344–348.

105. Panto PN, Davies P. Delayed reactions to urographic contrast media. *Br J Radiol*. 1986;59(697):41–44.

106. Schild HH, Kuhl CK, Hubner-Steiner U, Bohm I, Speck U. Adverse events after unenhanced and monomeric and dimeric contrast-enhanced CT: a prospective randomized controlled trial. *Radiology*. 2006;240(1):56–64.

107. Munechika H, Hiramatsu Y, Kudo S, et al. A prospective survey of delayed adverse reactions to iohexol in urography and computed tomography. *Eur Radiol.* 2003;13(1):185–194.

108. Sutton AG, Finn P, Campbell PG, et al. Early and late reactions following the use of iopamidol 340, iomeprol 350 and iodixanol 320 in cardiac catheterization. *J Invasive Cardiol.* 2003;15(3):133–138.

109. Sutton AG, Finn P, Grech ED, et al. Early and late reactions after the use of iopamidol 340, ioxaglate 320, and iodixanol 320 in cardiac catheterization. *Am Heart J.* 2001;141(4):677–683.

110. Vijayalakshmi K, Williams D, Wright RA, et al. A prospective, randomized trial to determine the early and late reactions after the use of iopamidol 340 (Niopam) and iobitridol 350 (Xenetix) in cardiac catheterization. *J Invasive Cardiol.* 2004;16(12):707–711.

111. Vijayalakshmi K, Kunadian B, Wright RA, et al. A prospective randomised controlled trial to determine the early and late reactions after the use of iopamidol 340 (Niopam) and iomeprol 350 (Iomeron) in cardiac catheterisation. *Eur J Radiol.* 2007;61(2):342–350.

112. Heinzerling LM, Tomsitz D, Anliker MD. Is drug allergy less prevalent than previously assumed? A 5-year analysis. *Br J Dermatol.* 2012;166(1):107–114.

113. Dona I, Blanca-Lopez N, Torres MJ, et al. Drug hypersensitivity reactions: response patterns, drug involved, and temporal variations in a large series of patients. *J Investig Allergol Clin Immunol.* 2012;22(5):363–371.

114. Schwartz LB, Yunginger JW, Miller J, Bokhari R, Dull D. Time course of appearance and disappearance of human mast cell tryptase in the circulation after anaphylaxis. *J Clin Invest.* 1989;83(5):1551–1555.

115. Brockow K, Vieluf D, Puschel K, Grosch J, Ring J. Increased postmortem serum mast cell tryptase in a fatal anaphylactoid reaction to nonionic radiocontrast medium. *J Allergy Clin Immunol.* 1999;104(1):237–238.

116. Pumphrey RS, Roberts IS. Postmortem findings after fatal anaphylactic reactions. *J Clin Pathol.* 2000;53(4):273–276.

117. Laroche D. Immediate reactions to contrast media: mediator release and value of diagnostic testing. *Toxicology.* 2005;209(2):193–194.

118. Dewachter P, Laroche D, Mouton-Faivre C, et al. Immediate reactions following iodinated contrast media injection: a study of 38 cases. *Eur J Radiol.* 2011;77(3):495–501.

119. Kvedariene V, Martins P, Rouanet L, Demoly P. Diagnosis of iodinated contrast media hypersensitivity: results of a 6-year period. *Clin Exp Allergy.* 2006;36(8):1072–1077.

120. Dewachter P, Mouton-Faivre C, Felden F. Allergy and contrast media. *Allergy.* 2001;56(3):250–251.

121. Trcka J, Schmidt C, Seitz CS, Brocker EB, Gross GE, Trautmann A. Anaphylaxis to iodinated contrast material: nonallergic hypersensitivity or IgE-mediated allergy? *AJR Am J Roentgenol.* 2008;190(3):666–670.

122. Caimmi S, Benyahia B, Suau D, et al. Clinical value of negative skin tests to iodinated contrast media. *Clin Exp Allergy.* 2010;40(5):805–810.

123. Goksel O, Aydin O, Atasoy C, et al. Hypersensitivity reactions to contrast media: prevalence, risk factors and the role of skin tests in diagnosis–a cross-sectional survey. *Int Arch Allergy Immunol.* 2011;155(3):297–305.

124. Pinnobphun P, Buranapraditkun S, Kampitak T, Hirankarn N, Klaewsongkram J. The diagnostic value of basophil activation test in patients with an immediate hypersensitivity reaction to radiocontrast media. *Ann Allergy Asthma Immunol.* 2011;106(5):387–393.

125. Renaudin JM, Beaudouin E, Ponvert C, Demoly P, Moneret-Vautrin DA. Severe drug-induced anaphylaxis: analysis of 333 cases recorded by the Allergy Vigilance Network from 2002 to 2010. *Allergy.* 2013;68(7):929–937.

126. Prieto-Garcia A, Tomas M, Pineda R, et al. Skin test-positive immediate hypersensitivity reaction to iodinated contrast media: the role of controlled challenge testing. *J Investig Allergol Clin Immunol.* 2013;23(3):183–189.

127. Salas M, Gomez F, Fernandez TD, et al. Diagnosis of immediate hypersensitivity reactions to radiocontrast media. *Allergy.* 2013;68(9):1203–1206.

128. Della-Torre E, Berti A, Yacoub MR, et al. Proposal of a skin tests based approach for the prevention of recurrent hypersensitivity reactions to iodinated contrast media. *Eur Ann Allergy Clin Immunol.* 2015;47(3):77–85.

129. Berti A, Della-Torre E, Yacoub M, et al. Patients with breakthrough reactions to iodinated contrast media have low incidence of positive skin tests. *Eur Ann Allergy Clin Immunol.* 2016;48(4):137–144.

130. Yoon SH, Lee SY, Kang HR, et al. Skin tests in patients with hypersensitivity reaction to iodinated contrast media: a meta-analysis. *Allergy.* 2015;70(6):625–637.

131. Sese L, Gaouar H, Autegarden JE, et al. Immediate hypersensitivity to iodinated contrast media: diagnostic accuracy of skin tests and intravenous provocation test with low dose. *Clin Exp Allergy.* 2016;46(3):472–478.

132. Yamaguchi K, Katayama H, Takashima T, Kozuka T, Seez P, Matsuura K. Prediction of severe adverse reactions to ionic and nonionic contrast media in Japan: evaluation of pretesting. A report from the Japanese Committee on the Safety of Contrast Media. *Radiology.* 1991;178(2):363–367.

133. Saito M, Abe M, Furukawa T, et al. Examination of patients suspected as having hypersensitivity to iodinated contrast media with leukocyte migration test. *Biol Pharm Bull.* 2014;37(11):1750–1757.

134. Schatz M, Patterson R, O'Rourke J, Nickelsen J, Northup C. The administration of radiographic contrast media to patients with a history of a previous reaction. *J Allergy Clin Immunol.* 1975;55(5):358–366.

135. Smith DC, Taylor FC, McKinney JM. Dimenhydrinate pretreatment in patients receiving intra-arterial ioxaglate: effect on nausea and vomiting. *Can Assoc Radiol J.* 1995;46(6):449–453.

136. Delaney A, Carter A, Fisher M. The prevention of anaphylactoid reactions to iodinated radiological contrast media: a systematic review. *BMC Med Imaging.* 2006;6:2.

137. Kelly JF, Patterson R, Lieberman P, Mathison DA, Stevenson DD. Radiographic contrast media studies in high-risk patients. *J Allergy Clin Immunol.* 1978;62(3):181–184.

138. Zweiman B, Mishkin MM, Hildreth EA. An approach to the performance of contrast studies in contrast material-reactive persons. *Ann Intern Med.* 1975;83(2):159–162.

139. Greenberger P, Patterson R, Kelly J, Stevenson DD, Simon D, Lieberman P. Administration of radiographic contrast media in high-risk patients. *Invest Radiol.* 1980;15(6 Suppl.):S40–S43.

140. Greenberger PA, Patterson R, Simon R, Lieberman P, Wallace W. Pretreatment of high-risk patients requiring radiographic contrast media studies. *J Allergy Clin Immunol.* 1981;67(3):185–187.

141. Greenberger PA, Patterson R, Radin RC. Two pretreatment regimens for high-risk patients receiving radiographic contrast media. *J Allergy Clin Immunol.* 1984;74(4 Pt 1):540–543.

142. Ring J, Rothenberger KH, Clauss W. Prevention of anaphylactoid reactions after radiographic contrast media infusion by combined histamine H1- and H2-receptor antagonists: results of a prospective controlled trial. *Int Arch Allergy Appl Immunol.* 1985;78(1):9–14.

143. Lasser EC, Berry CC, Talner LB, et al. Pretreatment with corticosteroids to alleviate reactions to intravenous contrast material. *N Engl J Med.* 1987;317(14):845–849.

144. Marshall Jr GD, Lieberman PL. Comparison of three pretreatment protocols to prevent anaphylactoid reactions to radiocontrast media. *Ann Allergy.* 1991;67(1):70–74.

145. Lasser EC, Berry CC, Mishkin MM, Williamson B, Zheutlin N, Silverman JM. Pretreatment with corticosteroids to prevent adverse reactions to nonionic contrast media. *AJR Am J Roentgenol.* 1994;162(3):523–526.

146. Davenport MS, Cohan RH, Caoili EM, Ellis JH. Repeat contrast medium reactions in premedicated patients: frequency and severity. *Radiology.* 2009;253(2):372–379.

147. Kim SH, Lee SH, Lee SM, et al. Outcomes of premedication for non-ionic radio-contrast media hypersensitivity reactions in Korea. *Eur J Radiol.* 2011;80(2):363–367.

148. Jingu A, Fukuda J, Taketomi-Takahashi A, Tsushima Y. Breakthrough reactions of iodinated and gadolinium contrast media after oral steroid premedication protocol. *BMC Med Imaging.* 2014;14:34.

149. Kolbe AB, Hartman RP, Hoskin TL, et al. Premedication of patients for prior urticarial reaction to iodinated contrast medium. *Abdom Imaging.* 2014;39(2):432–437.

150. Mervak BM, Davenport MS, Ellis JH, Cohan RH. Rates of breakthrough reactions in inpatients at high risk receiving premedication before contrast-enhanced CT. *AJR Am J Roentgenol.* 2015;205(1):77–84.

151. Jung JW, Choi YH, Park CM, Park HW, Cho SH, Kang HR. Outcomes of corticosteroid prophylaxis for hypersensitivity reactions to low osmolar contrast media in high-risk patients. *Ann Allergy Asthma Immunol.* 2016;117(3):304–309 e301.

152. Lee SH, Park HW, Cho SH, Kim SS. The efficacy of single premedication with antihistamines for radiocontrast media hypersensitivity. *Asia Pac Allergy.* 2016;6(3):164–167.

153. Small P, Satin R, Palayew MJ, Hyams B. Prophylactic antihistamines in the management of radiographic contrast reactions. *Clin Allergy.* 1982;12(3):289–294.

154. Bertrand PR, Soyer PM, Rouleau PJ, Alison DP, Billardon MJ. Comparative randomized double-blind study of hydroxyzine versus placebo as premedication before injection of iodinated contrast media. *Radiology.* 1992;184(2):383–384.

155. Freed KS, Leder RA, Alexander C, DeLong DM, Kliewer MA. Breakthrough adverse reactions to low-osmolar contrast media after steroid premedication. *AJR Am J Roentgenol.* 2001;176(6):1389–1392.

156. Lasser EC. Pretreatment with corticosteroids to prevent reactions to i.v. contrast material: overview and implications. *AJR Am J Roentgenol.* 1988;150(2):257–259.

157. Davenport MS, Mervak BM, Ellis JH, Dillman JR, Dunnick NR, Cohan RH. Indirect cost and harm attributable to oral 13-hour inpatient corticosteroid prophylaxis before contrast-enhanced CT. *Radiology.* 2016;279(2):492–501.

158. Bourin M, Jolliet P, Ballereau F. An overview of the clinical pharmacokinetics of x-ray contrast media. *Clin Pharmacokinet.* 1997;32(3):180–193.

159. Port M, Idee JM, Medina C, Robic C, Sabatou M, Corot C. Efficiency, thermodynamic and kinetic stability of marketed gadolinium chelates and their possible clinical consequences: a critical review. *Biometals.* 2008;21(4):469–490.

160. Fretellier N, Maazouz M, Luseau A, et al. Safety profiles of gadolinium chelates in juvenile rats differ according to the risk of dissociation. *Reprod Toxicol.* 2014;50:171–179.

161. Sherry AD, Caravan P, Lenkinski RE. Primer on gadolinium chemistry. *J Magn Reson Imaging.* 2009;30(6):1240–1248.

162. Davenport MS, Caoili EM, Kaza RK, Hussain HK. Matched within-patient cohort study of transient arterial phase respiratory motion-related artifact in MR imaging of the liver: gadoxetate disodium versus gadobenate dimeglumine. *Radiology.* 2014;272(1):123–131.

163. Davenport MS, Bashir MR, Pietryga JA, Weber JT, Khalatbari S, Hussain HK. Dose-toxicity relationship of gadoxetate disodium and transient severe respiratory motion artifact. *AJR Am J Roentgenol.* 2014;203(4):796–802.

164. Bashir MR, Castelli P, Davenport MS, et al. Respiratory motion artifact affecting hepatic arterial phase MR imaging with gadoxetate disodium is more common in patients with a prior episode of arterial phase motion associated with gadoxetate disodium. *Radiology.* 2015;274(1):141–148.

165. Davenport MS, Viglianti BL, Al-Hawary MM, et al. Comparison of acute transient dyspnea after intravenous administration of gadoxetate disodium and gadobenate dimeglumine: effect on arterial phase image quality. *Radiology.* 2013;266(2):452–461.

166. Runge VM. Safety of magnetic resonance contrast media. *Top Magn Reson Imaging.* 2001;12(4):309–314.

167. Runge VM. Safety of approved MR contrast media for intravenous injection. *J Magn Reson Imaging*. 2000;12(2):205–213.

168. Murphy KJ, Brunberg JA, Cohan RH. Adverse reactions to gadolinium contrast media: a review of 36 cases. *AJR Am J Roentgenol*. 1996;167(4):847–849.

169. Marckmann P, Skov L, Rossen K, et al. Nephrogenic systemic fibrosis: suspected causative role of gadodiamide used for contrast-enhanced magnetic resonance imaging. *J Am Soc Nephrol*. 2006;17(9):2359–2362.

170. Grobner T. Gadolinium–a specific trigger for the development of nephrogenic fibrosing dermopathy and nephrogenic systemic fibrosis? *Nephrol Dial Transplant*. 2006;21(4):1104–1108.

171. Sadowski EA, Bennett LK, Chan MR, et al. Nephrogenic systemic fibrosis: risk factors and incidence estimation. *Radiology*. 2007;243(1):148–157.

172. Wertman R, Altun E, Martin DR, et al. Risk of nephrogenic systemic fibrosis: evaluation of gadolinium chelate contrast agents at four American universities. *Radiology*. 2008;248(3):799–806.

173. Kuo PH, Kanal E, Abu-Alfa AK, Cowper SE. Gadolinium-based MR contrast agents and nephrogenic systemic fibrosis. *Radiology*. 2007;242(3):647–649.

174. Del Galdo F, Wermuth PJ, Addya S, Fortina P, Jimenez SA. NFκB activation and stimulation of chemokine production in normal human macrophages by the gadolinium-based magnetic resonance contrast agent Omniscan: possible role in the pathogenesis of nephrogenic systemic fibrosis. *Ann Rheum Dis*. 2010;69(11):2024–2033.

175. Idee JM, Fretellier N, Robic C, Corot C. The role of gadolinium chelates in the mechanism of nephrogenic systemic fibrosis: a critical update. *Crit Rev Toxicol*. 2014;44(10):895–913.

176. Newton BB, Jimenez SA. Mechanism of NSF: new evidence challenging the prevailing theory. *J Magn Reson Imaging*. 2009;30(6):1277–1283.

CHAPTER 23

Corticosteroids

IRIS M. OTANI, MD

INTRODUCTION

Corticosteroids are widely used to suppress allergic inflammation and can be easily overlooked as the causative agents of hypersensitivity reactions.[1] However, corticosteroids, and the additives and vehicles in corticosteroid preparations, have been documented to cause immediate and delayed hypersensitivity reactions. Immediate hypersensitivity reactions to corticosteroids have been reported with an estimated prevalence of 0.1% to 0.3%.[2] Delayed reactions to topical corticosteroids have been reported with a higher frequency of 0.5% to 5%.[3] Skin testing and oral graded challenges can be useful in evaluating suspected immediate hypersensitivity reactions to corticosteroids. Patch testing can be of benefit in evaluating suspected contact dermatitis caused by corticosteroids. This chapter reviews our current understanding of diagnostic allergy evaluation for immediate and delayed hypersensitivity reactions to corticosteroids.

IMMEDIATE HYPERSENSITIVITY REACTIONS

Anaphylaxis is the most commonly reported clinical presentation of immediate hypersensitivity reactions to corticosteroids, followed by isolated urticaria and isolated bronchospasm.[4] Most immediate hypersensitivity reactions occur within an hour of administration.[4,5] Methylprednisolone (41% of cases) is the most commonly implicated corticosteroid, followed by prednisolone (20%), triamcinolone (14%), and hydrocortisone (10%).[4] Reactions have been reported most frequently after administration of corticosteroids via the intravenous route (44% of cases) and oral route (26%). No clear age or gender predilection has been identified.[4,5]

As pruritus, urticaria, angioedema, and bronchospasm are prominent features of immediate hypersensitivity reactions to corticosteroids, mast cells likely play some role in the development of these reactions. However, the measurement of serum-specific IgE against corticosteroids is an unreliable measure of sensitization. This is possibly because haptenization may be necessary for corticosteroids to become allergenic.[5-7]

Skin Testing for Corticosteroids

Skin testing can be useful in the evaluation of a patient with a suspected history of immediate hypersensitivity reactions to corticosteroids. Currently, the utility of skin testing lies primarily in identifying a corticosteroid that may be tolerated by an individual with immediate hypersensitivity to a specific corticosteroid. Retrospective review of the literature suggests that the negative predictive value and specificity are high (around 88% and 97%, respectively).[5,7-18,71] Conversely, skin testing appears to have low sensitivity.[7,8,12,13,16,18-20]

Skin testing should be performed by both epicutaneous prick and intradermal steps using reported nonirritating concentrations (Table 23.1). Inclusion of intradermal skin testing likely improves sensitivity to some degree, as 25 of 80 cases reported by Patel et al. had negative epicutaneous prick testing followed by positive intradermal testing.[4] Negative skin testing must be followed by a graded challenge in a monitored setting, as five cases of positive drug challenges after negative skin testing have been reported to date in the literature.[7,12,13,16,20] Interpretation of the diagnostic value of skin testing is limited by the fact that testing protocols were not standardized between various case reports. Large systematic studies are still needed to validate predictive values of corticosteroid skin testing.

Cross-reactivity patterns have not been established for immediate hypersensitivity reactions in the way that they have been for corticosteroid-induced contact dermatitis (see Contact Dermatitis section).[9,11,16] Initial reports of corticosteroid hypersensitivity reactions suggested possible cross-reactivity between group A corticosteroids (methylprednisolone, prednisolone, hydrocortisone). However, the observed "cross-reactivity" between these corticosteroids is now thought to occur largely because of hypersensitivity to the succinate ester moiety used to solubilize these corticosteroids for intravenous administration (discussed later).[9,21] Therefore, based on our current understanding, there are no restrictions regarding which

TABLE 23.1
Non-irritating Concentrations for Skin Testing With Corticosteroids and Excipients

Corticosteroid	Skin Prick Test Dilutions (mg/mL)	Intradermal Test (IDT) Dilutions (mg/mL)
Betamethasone sodium phosphate	4	4
Betamethasone acetate	6	6
Budesonide	0.25	0.0025 0.025
Dexamethasone sodium phosphate	4	0.04 0.4 4
Hydrocortisone sodium succinate	100	1 10 25
Methylprednisolone acetate	40	0.4 4
Methylprednisolone sodium succinate	40	0.4 4
Prednisone	30	No IDT
Prednisolone	10	No IDT
Triamcinolone acetonide	40	0.4 4 40
Polyethylene glycol	10 (1:100) 100 (1:10)	0.1 (1:10,000) 1 (1:1000) 10 (1:100)
Carboxymethylcellulose	5	0.005 0.05

Data from Pryse-Phillips WE, Chandra RK, Rose B. Anaphylactoid reaction to methylprednisolone pulsed therapy for multiple sclerosis. *Neurology*. 1984;34(8):1119–1121; Nowak-Wegrzyn A, Shapiro G, Beyer K, Bardina L, Sampson H. Contamination of dry powder inhalers for asthma with milk proteins containing lactose. *J Allergy Clin Immunol*. 2004;113(3):558–560. http://dx.doi.org/10.1016/j.jaci.2003.11.015; Savvatianos S, Giavi S, Stefanaki E, Siragakis G, Manousakis E, Papadopoulos NG. Cow's milk allergy as a cause of anaphylaxis to systemic corticosteroids. *Allergy*. 2011;66(7):983–985. http://dx.doi.org/10.1111/j.1398-9995.2011.02566.x; Warshaw EM, Belsito DV, Taylor JS, et al. North American Contact Dermatitis Group patch test results: 2009 to 2010. *Dermatitis*. 2013;24(2):50–59; Isaksson M, Gruvberger B, Persson L, Bruze M. Stability of corticosteroid patch test preparations. *Contact Dermatitis*. 2000;42(3):144–148. http://dx.doi.org/10.1034/j.1600-0536.2000.042003144.x; Yim E, Baquerizo Nole KL, Tosti A. Contact dermatitis caused by preservatives. *Dermatitis*. 2014;25(5):215–231. http://dx.doi.org/10.1097/DER.0000000000000061; Wolf R, Orion E, Ruocco E, Baroni A, Ruocco V. Contact dermatitis: facts and controversies. *Clin Dermatol*. 2013;31(4):467–478. http://dx.doi.org/10.1016/j.clindermatol.2013.01.014 and Hogan DJ. Allergic contact dermatitis to ethylenediamine. A continuing problem. *Dermatol Clin*. 1990;8(1):133–136.

corticosteroids can be considered for evaluation as a possible alternative agent with skin testing and graded challenge.

Structures added during chemical modification, additives, and ingredients in corticosteroid preparations can be responsible for over one-fifth of immediate hypersensitivity reactions after corticosteroid administration.[4,9,15,20–25] This is discussed in the following sections.

Succinate ester

Hypersensitivity reactions to succinate, the most common ester added at the C21 position to increase solubility for intravenous corticosteroid preparations,[5] accounts for roughly one-tenth of reported reactions to intravenous corticosteroids.[4,9,15,20–25] Hypersensitivity reactions have not been reported to the sodium phosphate and acetate esters used to solubilize corticosteroids for intraarticular or soft tissue administration.[5]

Therefore, evaluation with both the succinate form and the unconjugated form (for example, methylprednisolone succinate and methylprednisolone) is recommended for patients who present with a history of immediate hypersensitivity reactions after succinated corticosteroid administration.

Lactose

Lactose in corticosteroids can cause immediate hypersensitivity reactions in children with IgE-mediated sensitization to cow's milk. Ten cases of milk-allergic patients who developed anaphylaxis (8/10) or urticaria (2/10) after receiving fluticasone inhaled (1/10) and methylprednisolone succinate (9/10) have been reported.[26-29] Caution is needed when choosing corticosteroid therapy for milk-allergic patients.[30]

Carboxymethylcellulose

Immediate hypersensitivity reactions to carboxymethylcellulose have been reported following intralesional and intraarticular injection of triamcinolone.[9,31-35] Carboxymethylcellulose is an osmotically active agent that could possibly cause direct mast cell activation in a manner similar to hyperosmolar radiocontrast media. Patients who experience immediate reactions after carboxymethylcellulose injections have been reported to tolerate oral administration.[36] However, anaphylaxis after oral administration of carboxymethylcellulose has also been reported.[37] This suggests that sensitized patients should not receive carboxymethylcellulose regardless of the route of administration.

Polyethylene glycol

Sensitization to polyethylene glycol is extremely rare compared with sensitization to lactose and carboxymethylcellulose. However, if evaluation with corticosteroids, milk, and carboxymethylcellulose remains unrevealing, skin testing with polyethylene glycol can be considered.[38-41]

Summary and Recommendations for Immediate Hypersensitivity Reactions

- The reported incidence of immediate hypersensitivity reactions is 0.3% to 0.5%.[2]
- Anaphylaxis, pruritus, urticaria, angioedema, and bronchospasm within 1 h of corticosteroid administration raise suspicion for corticosteroid hypersensitivity.
- Skin testing can be useful, primarily to identify alternative corticosteroids for therapeutic use. Skin testing should be performed with both epicutaneous prick and intradermal steps using nonirritating concentrations of corticosteroids. Published nonirritating concentrations are listed in Table 23.1.
- If an immediate reaction occurs after administration of an esterified corticosteroid, the reaction could be caused by either the corticosteroid itself or the ester moiety. Therefore, evaluation should include skin testing (and graded challenge if appropriate) of both the unconjugated and esterified forms (for example, methylprednisolone succinate and methylprednisolone).
- When appropriate, evaluation should include skin testing to milk, carboxymethylcellulose, and polyethylene glycol.
- A graded challenge is needed to confirm the results of negative skin testing.

CONTACT DERMATITIS

Contact dermatitis to corticosteroids occurs with a reported frequency of 0.5% to 5%,[3,42,43] more frequently in women (3:1 female:male), and most commonly among housewives (18%) followed by office workers (17%).[43] It generally presents as worsening of a preexisting dermatitis or an acute flare of eczematous dermatitis.[3] Localized edema[44,45] and erythema multiforme—like reactions[46-48] have also been reported.

Corticosteroid contact dermatitis develops via a type IV cell-mediated delayed hypersensitivity mechanism. Sensitization is generally thought to occur through the skin, with haptenization of corticosteroids occurring after skin penetration, although some patients may be sensitized via exposure to inhaled corticosteroids.[43]

Structure and Cross-Reactivity

Corticosteroids have been categorized into four reactivity groups, A to D (Coopman classification), based on clinical and structural characteristics.[49] Further subdivision of group D into D1 (less labile, halogenated) and D2 (labile, lipophilic prodrugs that penetrate the skin easily) has been established by Matura and Goossens,[3] and subdivision of group C into C1 (nonesterified) and C2 (stable esters) has been proposed by Baeck et al.[43] Cross-reactivity has been observed within corticosteroids of the same group (most commonly A, B, D2) and between corticosteroids of different groups (Table 23.2). Studies suggest that individuals are most frequently sensitized to group A corticosteroids, followed by group B corticosteroids, followed by group D2 corticosteroids.[3,43]

TABLE 23.2
Corticosteroid Groups and Observed Cross-Reactivity Patterns

Corticosteroids in Each Group • Commonly used brand	Structure	Cross-Reactivity Within Group	Cross-Reactivity With Other Groups
A: HYDROCORTISONE TYPE			
Tixocortol-21-pivalate[a] Hydrocortisone • Aveeno Anti-Itch • Cortizone • Cortaid Methylprednisolone Prednisolone	C_{21}—short-chain ester or thioester	Yes	Budesonide-(S)-isomer with group A and group D2
B: TRIAMCINOLONE ACETONIDE TYPE			
Budesonide[a] Desonide • Desonate • Desowen Fluocinolone • Capex • Synalar Triamcinolone acetonide • Kenalog	C_{16}, C_{17}—cis-ketal or -diol	Yes	Budesonide-(S)-isomer with group A and group D2
C: BETAMETHASONE TYPE			
C1 Subgroup			
Betamethasone Dexamethasone Desoximetasone • Topicort	C_{16}—methyl substitution Halogen substitution Nonesterified		Betamethasone and/or dexamethasone with group B
C2 Subgroup			
Diflucortolone valerate Fluocortolone pivalate Clocortolone pivalate • Cloderm	C_{16}—methyl substitution Halogen substitution Stable esters (-valerate, -pivalate)		No significant cross-reactivity pattern observed
D: HYDROCORTISONE-17-BUTYRATE TYPE			
D1 Subgroup			
Clobetasol-17-propionate[a] • Clobex Betamethasone dipropionate • Diprolene Mometasone furoate • Elocon Alclometasone dipropionate	C_{16}—methyl substitution Halogen substitution C_{17}—long-chain ester C_{21}—possible side chain		Rare cross-reactivity between alclometasone dipropionate and group A, budesonide, group D2
D2 Subgroup			
Hydrocortisone-17-butyrate[a] • Locoid • Locoid Lipocream Hydrocortisone valerate • Westcort	C_{16}—no methyl substitution No halogen substitution C_{17}—long-chain ester C_{21}—possible side chain	Yes	Budesonide-(S)-isomer with group A and group D2

Data from Matura M, Goossens A. Contact allergy to corticosteroids. *Allergy*. 2000;55(8):698–704. http://dx.doi.org/10.1034/j.1398-9995.2000.00121.x. Baeck M, Chemelle J-AA, Terreux R, Drieghe J, Goossens A. Delayed hypersensitivity to corticosteroids in a series of 315 patients: clinical data and patch test results. Contact Derm. 2009;61:163–75. Schalock P, Dunnick C, Nedorost S, Brod B, Warshaw E, Mowad C. American Contact Dermatitis Society Core Allergen Series. Dermatitis. 2013;24:7.
[a]Representative corticosteroid for patch test.

Patch Testing

Patch testing is the standard for identifying a causative corticosteroid in contact dermatitis.[50] The T.R.U.E. Test (Thin-layer Rapid Use Epicutaneous Test) includes a group A corticosteroid, tixocortol-21-pivalate (0.1% petrolatum), and a group B corticosteroid, budesonide (0.01% petrolatum).[50] These two corticosteroids were among the top 50 allergens identified as causative agents of contact dermatitis over a 6-year period,[51] and a combination of these two corticosteroids can identify 91% of patients with corticosteroid contact dermatitis.[52]

For some patients, patch testing with additional corticosteroids is necessary to identify the causative corticosteroid agent.[53] The North American Contact Dermatitis Group has shown that the T.R.U.E. Test alone can miss 27% of culprit allergens.[54] In their recommended core group of allergens for allergic contact dermatitis screening, they include triamcinolone acetonide (group B), clobetasol-17-propionate (group D1), and hydrocortisone-17-butyrate (group D2) in addition to tixocortol-21-pivalate and budesonide.[55] In Europe, the standard corticosteroid series includes amcinonide (0.1% ethanol), betamethasone-17-valerate (0.12% ethanol), clobetasol-17-propionate (0.25% ethanol), hydrocortisone (0.1% ethanol), hydrocortisone-17-butyrate (1% ethanol), triamcinolone acetonide (0.1% ethanol), and prednisone (1% ethanol), in addition to tixocortol-21-pivalate and budesonide.[56]

Corticosteroids must be prepared with the appropriate vehicles to ensure adequate skin penetration for patch testing. Petrolatum has been shown to be an appropriate vehicle for tixocortol-21-pivalate and budesonide, with good sensitivity and specificity.[57,58] Ethanol is an appropriate vehicle of choice for most other corticosteroids, except tixocortol-21-pivalate and budesonide as described earlier and cortisone acetate and hydrocortisone as described later.[43] A 50:50 ethanol and dimethyl sulfoxide mix is recommended for cortisone acetate and hydrocortisone to improve transepidermal penetration.[43] Including a negative control with the vehicle alone is important, especially for ethanol, as positive reactions to ethanol are not uncommon.[59] Baeck et al. provide comprehensive recommendations regarding vehicles and concentrations for corticosteroid patch testing in Table 23.2.[43]

Chromatographic purity of corticosteroids in ethanol solutions can decrease 95% to 97% by 1 month of storage at 6 to 8°C.[60] However, stability has been demonstrated for up to 1 year at −18°C.[61] Institutions that perform patch testing frequently may find

it reasonable to store corticosteroid mixtures at −18°C for 6 to 12 months. Otherwise, fresh mixtures should be prepared regularly.

As with immediate hypersensitivity reactions, ingredients in corticosteroid preparations can be responsible for irritant or allergic contact dermatitis after corticosteroid application. Suspicion is raised for sensitization to ingredients rather than the corticosteroid itself in patients who tolerate only specific formulations of corticosteroids or who have negative patch testing for corticosteroids despite a convincing history. Ingredients in topical corticosteroid preparations that have been implicated as contact allergens include parabens, formaldehyde-releasing preservatives (quaternium-15), isothiazolinones, lanolin, ethylenediamine, sorbitan sesquioleate, fragrance, and propylene glycol.[62-68] The T.R.U.E. Test includes all of these contact allergens except propylene glycol, which can be patch tested separately using a 30% aqueous solution,[69] and sorbitan sesquioleate, which can be patch tested using a 20% petrolatum preparation.[70]

Summary and Recommendations for Contact Dermatitis

- Contact dermatitis is a delayed hypersensitivity reaction to corticosteroids with a reported incidence of 0.5% to 5%.[3] Affected patients may present with worsening of preexisting dermatitis, acute flare of eczematous dermatitis, localized edema, or erythema multiforme—like reactions after topical corticosteroid treatment.
- The standard for evaluation is patch testing. A combination of tixocortol-21-pivalate (0.1% petrolatum) and budesonide (0.01% petrolatum) included in the T.R.U.E. Test identifies the majority of patients with delayed hypersensitivity to corticosteroids. For some individuals, patch testing with additional corticosteroids may be necessary to identify a causative corticosteroid.
- Observed cross-reactivity patterns are described in Table 23.2. These cross-reactivity patterns in combination with supplemental patch testing can be helpful in finding an alternative corticosteroid for therapeutic use.

REFERENCES

1. Zoorob RJ, Cender D. A different look at corticosteroids. *Am Fam Physician.* 1998;58(2):443–450.
2. Baeck M, Marot L, Nicolas J-F, Pilette C, Tennstedt D, Goossens A. Allergic hypersensitivity to topical and systemic corticosteroids: a review. *Allergy.* 2009;64(7):978–994. http://dx.doi.org/10.1111/j.1398-9995.2009.02038.x.

3. Matura M, Goossens A. Contact allergy to corticosteroids. *Allergy*. 2000;55(8):698–704. http://dx.doi.org/10.1034/j.1398-9995.2000.00121.x.

4. Patel A, Bahna S. Immediate hypersensitivity reactions to corticosteroids. *Ann Allergy Asthma Immunol*. 2015;115(3):178–182.e3. http://dx.doi.org/10.1016/j.anai.2015.06.022.

5. Kamm GL, Hagmeyer KO. Allergic-type reactions to corticosteroids. *Ann Pharmacother*. 1999;33(4):451–460.

6. Pryse-Phillips WE, Chandra RK, Rose B. Anaphylactoid reaction to methylprednisolone pulsed therapy for multiple sclerosis. *Neurology*. 1984;34(8):1119–1121.

7. Baker A, Empson M, The R, Fitzharris P. Skin testing for immediate hypersensitivity to corticosteroids: a case series and literature review. *Clin Exp Allergy*. 2015;45(3):669–676. http://dx.doi.org/10.1111/cea.12441.

8. Calogiuri GF, Muratore L, Nettis E, Ventura MT, Ferrannini A, Tursi A. Anaphylaxis to hydrocortisone hemisuccinate with cross-sensitivity to related compounds in a paediatric patient. *Br J Dermatol*. 2004;151(3):707–708. http://dx.doi.org/10.1111/j.1365-2133.2004.06102.x.

9. Venturini M, Lobera T, del Pozo MD, González I, Blasco A. Immediate hypersensitivity to corticosteroids. *J Investig Allergol Clin Immunol*. 2006;16(1):51–56.

10. Deruaz CA, Spertini F, Souza Lima F, Du Pasquier RA, Schluep M. Anaphylactic reaction to methylprednisolone in multiple sclerosis: a practical approach to alternative corticosteroids. *Mult Scler*. 2007. http://dx.doi.org/10.1177/1352458506070655.

11. Rodrigues-Alves R, Spínola-Santos A, Pedro E, Branco-Ferreira M, Pereira-Barbosa M. Immediate hypersensitivity to corticosteroids: finding an alternative. *J Investig Allergol Clin Immunol*. 2007;17(4):284–285.

12. Escobosa M, Granados C, Quesada M, López A. Anaphylaxis due to methylprednisolone. *J Investig Allergol Clin Immunol*. 2008;18(5):407–408.

13. Aranda A, Mayorga C, Ariza A, et al. IgE-mediated hypersensitivity reactions to methylprednisolone. *Allergy*. 2010;65(11):1376–1380. http://dx.doi.org/10.1111/j.1398-9995.2010.02386.x.

14. De Sousa NG, Santa-Marta C, Morais-Almeida M. Systemic corticosteroid hypersensitivity in children. *J Investig Allergol Clin Immunol*. 2010;20(6):529–532.

15. Nucera E, Lombardo C, Aruanno A, et al. "Empty sella syndrome": a case of a patient with sodium succinate hydrocortisone allergy. *Eur J Endocrinol*. 2011;164(1):139–140. http://dx.doi.org/10.1530/EJE-10-0863.

16. Rachid R, Leslie D, Schneider L, Twarog F. Hypersensitivity to systemic corticosteroids: an infrequent but potentially life-threatening condition. *J Allergy Clin Immunol*. 2011;127(2):524–528. http://dx.doi.org/10.1016/j.jaci.2010.09.030.

17. Calogiuri GF, Nettis E, Di Leo E, Muratore L, Ferrannini A, Vacca A. Long-term selective IgE-mediated hypersensitivity to hydrocortisone sodium succinate. *Allergol Immunopathol (Madr)*. 2013;41(3):206–208. http://dx.doi.org/10.1016/j.aller.2012.02.003.

18. Kim S, Kim H. Anaphylaxis induced by oral methylprednisolone in a 10-year-old boy. *Pediatr Int*. 2014;56(5):783–784. http://dx.doi.org/10.1111/ped.12341.

19. Ehret GB, Deluze C, Dayer P, Desmeules JA. Systemic allergic reaction and diffuse bone pain after exposure to a preparation of betamethasone. *Eur J Intern Med*. 2005;16(8):612–614. http://dx.doi.org/10.1016/j.ejim.2005.04.004.

20. Angel-Pereira D, Berges-Gimeno M, Madrigal-Burgaleta R, Ureña-Tavera M, Zamora-Verduga M, Alvarez-Cuesta E. Successful rapid desensitization to methylprednisolone sodium hemisuccinate: a case report. *J Allergy Clin Immunol Pract*. 2014;2(3):346–348. http://dx.doi.org/10.1016/j.jaip.2013.12.011.

21. Walker AI, Räwer H-C, Sieber W, Przybilla B. Immediate-type hypersensitivity to succinylated corticosteroids. *Int Arch Allergy Immunol*. 2010;155(1):86–92. http://dx.doi.org/10.1159/000318678.

22. Currie G, Paterson E, Keenan F, Nath S, Watt S. An unexpected response to intravenous hydrocortisone succinate in an asthmatic patient. *Br J Clin Pharmacol*. 2005;60(3):342. http://dx.doi.org/10.1111/j.1365-2125.2005.02442.x.

23. Caimmi S, Caimmi D, Bousquet P-J, Demoly P. Succinate as opposed to glucocorticoid itself allergy. *Allergy*. 2008;63(12):1641–1643. http://dx.doi.org/10.1111/j.1398-9995.2008.01894.x.

24. Gelincik A, Yazici H, Emre T, Yakar F, Buyukozturk S. An alternative approach to a renal transplant patient who experienced an immediate type systemic reaction due to methylprednisolone sodium succinate. *J Investig Allergol Clin Immunol*. 2009;19(2):162–163.

25. Koutsostathis N, Vovolis V. Severe immunoglobulin E-mediated anaphylaxis to intravenous methylprednisolone succinate in a patient who tolerated oral methylprednisolone. *J Investig Allergol Clin Immunol*. 2009;19(4):330–332.

26. Nowak-Wegrzyn A, Shapiro G, Beyer K, Bardina L, Sampson H. Contamination of dry powder inhalers for asthma with milk proteins containing lactose. *J Allergy Clin Immunol*. 2004;113(3):558–560. http://dx.doi.org/10.1016/j.jaci.2003.11.015.

27. Eda A, Sugai K, Shioya H, et al. Acute allergic reaction due to milk proteins contaminating lactose added to corticosteroid for injection. *Allergol Int*. 2009;58(1):137–139. http://dx.doi.org/10.2332/allergolint.C-07-59.

28. Savvatianos S, Giavi S, Stefanaki E, Siragakis G, Manousakis E, Papadopoulos NG. Cow's milk allergy as a cause of anaphylaxis to systemic corticosteroids. *Allergy*. 2011;66(7):983–985. http://dx.doi.org/10.1111/j.1398-9995.2011.02566.x.

29. Levy Y, Segal N, Nahum A, Marcus N, Garty B-Z. Hypersensitivity to methylprednisolone sodium succinate in children with milk allergy. *J Allergy Clin Immunol Pract*. 2014;2(4):471–474. http://dx.doi.org/10.1016/j.jaip.2014.03.002.

30. Drug allergy: an updated practice parameter. *Ann Allergy Asthma Immunol*. 2010;105(4):259–273. http://dx.doi.org/10.1016/j.anai.2010.08.002.

31. Laing ME, Fallis B, Murphy GM. Anaphylactic reaction to intralesional corticosteroid injection. *Contact Dermatitis.* 2007;57(2):132–133. http://dx.doi.org/10.1111/j.1600-0536.2007.01092.x.

32. Field S, Falvey E, Barry J, Bourke J. Type 1 hypersensitivity reaction to carboxymethylcellulose following intra-articular triamcinolone injection. *Contact Dermatitis.* 2009;61(5):302–303. http://dx.doi.org/10.1111/j.1600-0536.2009.01636.x.

33. Steiner U, Gentinetta T, Hausmann O, Pichler W. IgE-mediated anaphylaxis to intraarticular glucocorticoid preparations. *AJR Am J Roentgenol.* 2009;193(2):W156–W157. http://dx.doi.org/10.2214/ajr.09.2495.

34. Hadithy A, van Maaren M, Vermes A. Anaphylactic reactions following Kenacort-A® injection: carboxymethylcellulose is involved once again. *Contact Dermatitis.* 2011;64(3):179–180. http://dx.doi.org/10.1111/j.1600-0536.2010.01850.x.

35. Patterson DL, Yunginger JW, Dunn WF, Jones RT, Hunt LW. Anaphylaxis induced by the carboxymethylcellulose component of injectable triamcinolone acetonide suspension (Kenalog). *Ann Allergy Asthma Immunol.* 1995;74(2):163–166.

36. Bigliardi PL, Izakovic J, Weber JM, Bircher A. Anaphylaxis to the carbohydrate carboxymethylcellulose in parenteral corticosteroid preparations. *Dermatology.* 2003;207(1):100–103. http://dx.doi.org/10.1159/000070958.

37. Muroi N, Nishibori M, Fujii T, et al. Anaphylaxis from the carboxymethylcellulose component of barium sulfate suspension. *N Engl J Med.* 1997;337(18):1275–1277. http://dx.doi.org/10.1056/NEJM199710303371804.

38. Dewachter P, Mouton-Faivre C. Anaphylaxis to macrogol 4000 after a parenteral corticoid injection. *Allergy.* 2005;60(5):705–706. http://dx.doi.org/10.1111/j.1398-9995.2005.00783.x.

39. Sohy C, Vandenplas O, Sibille Y. Usefulness of oral macrogol challenge in anaphylaxis after intra-articular injection of corticosteroid preparation. *Allergy.* 2008;63(4):478–479. http://dx.doi.org/10.1111/j.1398-9995.2007.01610.x.

40. Moran D, Moynagh M, Alzanki M, Chan V, Eustace S. Anaphylaxis at image-guided epidural pain block secondary to corticosteroid compound. *Skelet Radiol.* 2012;41(10):1317–1318. http://dx.doi.org/10.1007/s00256-012-1440-3.

41. Borderé A, Stockman A, Boone B, et al. A case of anaphylaxis caused by macrogol 3350 after injection of a corticosteroid. *Contact Dermatitis.* 2012;67(6):376–378. http://dx.doi.org/10.1111/j.1600-0536.2012.02104.x.

42. Vatti R, Ali F, Teuber S, Chang C, Gershwin E. Hypersensitivity reactions to corticosteroids. *Clin Rev Allergy Immunol.* 2013;47(1):26–37. http://dx.doi.org/10.1007/s12016-013-8365-z.

43. Baeck M, Chemelle J-AA, Terreux R, Drieghe J, Goossens A. Delayed hypersensitivity to corticosteroids in a series of 315 patients: clinical data and patch test results. *Contact Dermatitis.* 2009;61(3):163–175. http://dx.doi.org/10.1111/j.1600-0536.2009.01602.x.

44. Rodríguez-Serna M, Silvestre JF, Quecedo E, Martínez A, Miguel FJ, Gauchía R. Corticosteroid allergy: report of 3 unusually acute cases. *Contact Dermatitis.* 1996;35(6):361–362.

45. Miranda-Romero A, Sánchez-Sambucety P, Bajo C, Martinez M, Garcia-Munoz M. Genital oedema from contact allergy to prednicarbate. *Contact Dermatitis.* 1998;38(4):228. http://dx.doi.org/10.1111/j.1600-0536.1998.tb05725.x.

46. Valsecchi R, Reseghetti A, Leghissa P, Cologni L, Cortinovis R. Erythema-multiforme-like lesions from triamcinolone acetonide. *Contact Dermatitis.* 1998;38(6):362–363.

47. Stingeni L, Caraffini S, Assalve D, Lapomarda V, Lisi P. Erythema-multiforme-like contact dermatitis from budesonide. *Contact Dermatitis.* 1996;34(2):154–155.

48. Calista D, Schianchi S. Erythema multiforme-like eruption induced by contact dermatitis caused by topical corticosteroids. *G Ital Dermatol Venereol.* 2008;143(3):227–228.

49. Coopman S, Degreef H, Dooms-Goossens A. Identification of cross-reaction patterns in allergic contact dermatitis from topical corticosteroids. *Br J Dermatol.* 1989;121(1):27–34.

50. Fonacier L, Sher J. Allergic contact dermatitis. *Ann Allergy Asthma Immunol.* 2014;113(1):9–12. http://dx.doi.org/10.1016/j.anai.2014.03.018.

51. Saripalli Y, Achen F, Belsito D. The detection of clinically relevant contact allergens using a standard screening tray of twenty-three allergens. *J Am Acad Dermatol.* 2003;49(1):65–69. http://dx.doi.org/10.1067/mjd.2003.489.

52. Boffa MJ, Wilkinson SM, Beck MH. Screening for corticosteroid contact hypersensitivity. *Contact Dermatitis.* 1995;33(3):149–151.

53. Camacho-Halili M, Axelrod S, Michelis M, et al. A multicenter, retrospective review of patch testing for contact dermatitis in allergy practices. *Ann Allergy Asthma Immunol.* 2011;107(6):487–492. http://dx.doi.org/10.1016/j.anai.2011.09.004.

54. Warshaw EM, Belsito DV, Taylor JS, et al. North American Contact Dermatitis Group patch test results: 2009 to 2010. *Dermatitis.* 2013;24(2):50–59. http://dx.doi.org/10.1097/DER.0b013e3182819c51.

55. Schalock P, Dunnick C, Nedorost S, Brod B, Warshaw E, Mowad C. American Contact Dermatitis Society core allergen series. *Dermatitis.* 2013;24(1):7. http://dx.doi.org/10.1097/DER.0b013e318281d87b.

56. Ljubojevic S, Lipozencic J, Basta-Juzbasic A. Contact allergy to corticosteroids and *Malassezia furfur* in seborrhoeic dermatitis patients. *J Eur Acad Dermatol Venereol.* 2010;25(6):647–651. http://dx.doi.org/10.1111/j.1468-3083.2010.03843.x.

57. Wilkinson SM, English JS. Hydrocortisone sensitivity: a prospective study of the value of tixocortol pivalate and hydrocortisone acetate as patch test markers. *Contact Dermatitis.* 1991;25(2):132–133.

58. Wilkinson SM, Beck MH. Corticosteroid contact hypersensitivity: what vehicle and concentration? *Contact Dermatitis.* 1996;34(5):305–308.

59. Matura M, Lepoittevin J-P, Arbez-Gindre C, Goossens A. Testing with corticosteroid aldehydes in corticosteroid-sensitive patients (preliminary results). *Contact Dermatitis*. 1998;38(2):106–108. http://dx.doi.org/10.1111/j.1600-0536.1998.tb05663.x.

60. Förström L, Lassus A, Salde L, Niemi KM. Allergic contact eczema from topical corticosteroids. *Contact Dermatitis*. 1982;8(2):128–133.

61. Isaksson M, Gruvberger B, Persson L, Bruze M. Stability of corticosteroid patch test preparations. *Contact Dermatitis*. 2000;42(3):144–148. http://dx.doi.org/10.1034/j.1600-0536.2000.042003144.x.

62. Yim E, Baquerizo Nole KL, Tosti A. Contact dermatitis caused by preservatives. *Dermatitis*. 2014;25(5):215–231. http://dx.doi.org/10.1097/DER.0000000000000061.

63. Wolf R, Orion E, Ruocco E, Baroni A, Ruocco V. Contact dermatitis: facts and controversies. *Clin Dermatol*. 2013;31(4):467–478. http://dx.doi.org/10.1016/j.clindermatol.2013.01.014.

64. Hogan DJ. Allergic contact dermatitis to ethylenediamine. A continuing problem. *Dermatol Clin*. 1990;8(1):133–136.

65. Asarch A, Scheinman PL. Sorbitan sesquioleate, a common emulsifier in topical corticosteroids, is an important contact allergen. *Dermatitis*. 2008;19(6):323–327.

66. Funk JO, Maibach HI. Propylene glycol dermatitis: re-evaluation of an old problem. *Contact Dermatitis*. 1994;31(4):236–241.

67. Warshaw EM, Botto NC, Maibach HI, et al. Positive patch-test reactions to propylene glycol: a retrospective cross-sectional analysis from the North American Contact Dermatitis Group, 1996 to 2006. *Dermatitis*. 2009;20(1):14–20.

68. Coloe J, Zirwas MJ. Allergens in corticosteroid vehicles. *Dermatitis*. 2008;19(1):38–42.

69. Nelson J, Mowad C. Allergic contact dermatitis: patch testing beyond the TRUE test. *J Clin Aesthet Dermatol*. 2010;3(10):36–41.

70. Pereira F, Cunha H, Dias M. Contact dermatitis due to emulsifiers. *Contact Dermatitis*. 1997;36(2):114.

71. Otani IM, Banerji A. Immediate and delayed hypersensitivity reactions to corticosteroids: evaluation and management. *Curr Allergy Asthma Rep*. 2016;16(3):18.

Index

Note: 'Page numbers followed by "f" indicate figures, "t" indicate tables, and "b" indicate boxes.'

Printed in the United States
By Bookmasters